Guidebook to the
Calcium-binding Proteins

Other books by Sambrook & Tooze Publications

Guidebook to the Cytoskeletal and Motor Proteins
Edited by Thomas Kreis and Ronald Vale

Guidebook to the Extracellular Matrix and Adhesion Proteins
Edited by Thomas Kreis and Ronald Vale

Guidebook to the Homeobox Genes
Edited by Denis Duboule

Guidebook to Cytokines and Their Receptors
Edited by Nicos A. Nicola

Guidebook to the Secretory Pathway
Edited by Jonathan Rothblatt, Peter Novick, and Tom H. Stevens

Guidebook to the Small GTPases
Edited by Marino Zerial and Lukas A. Huber

Guidebook to the
Calcium-binding Proteins

Edited by

Marco R. Celio

Co-edited by

Thomas L. Pauls and Beat Schwaller

Institute of Histology and General Embryology,
University of Fribourg,
Fribourg, Switzerland

A SAMBROOK & TOOZE PUBLICATION
AT OXFORD UNIVERSITY PRESS
1996

Oxford University Press, Walton Street, Oxford OX2 6DP

Oxford   New York
Athens   Auckland   Bangkok   Bombay
Calcutta   Cape Town   Dar es Salaam   Delhi
Florence   Hong Kong   Istanbul   Karachi
Kuala Lumpur   Madras   Madrid   Melbourne
Mexico City   Nairobi   Paris   Singapore
Taipei   Tokyo   Toronto

and associated companies in
Berlin   Ibadan

Oxford is a trade mark of Oxford University Press

Published in the United States
by Oxford University Press Inc., New York

A catalogue record for this book is available from the British Library

Library of Congress Cataloging in Publication Data
(Data available)

ISBN   0   19   859951   X   (Hbk)
ISBN   0   19   859950   1   (Pbk)

Typeset by EXPO Holdings, Malaysia
Printed in Great Britain by
The Bath Press

Preface

I originally undertook the task of editing a handbook on calcium-binding proteins with a view to becoming better acquainted with this field. Little did I realize at the time what I was letting myself in for, but it soon became apparent that it was going to be an awesome venture. The explosive growth in the number of calcium-binding proteins which has taken place in recent years was disconcerting, to say the least, and it became increasingly difficult to keep pace with the sheer body of data.

It is by no means easy to edit a book composed of 84 chapters, contributed by 121 authors from 11 countries around the world. It requires tenacity, patience, and an eye for detail. Such virtues are seldom found in one individual, and I do not count myself amongst that number. It was therefore a great relief to me to have the assistance of my collaborators Beat Schwaller and Thomas Pauls, who already have a considerable reputation in this field; together, we were able to pool our various resources and achieve the desired end. My Swiss colleagues, in addition to contributing chapters themselves, helped to trace potential authors. The response of most people contacted was very positive; indeed, only a few did not accept the invitation to write a chapter.

This is not the first book to be devoted to calcium-binding proteins, but it is perhaps the most comprehensive and useful one to date. It furnishes the reader with up-to-date information regarding most of the known calcium-binding proteins, but without drawing too extensively on the wealth of data available in many cases. Each chapter, is thus very brief and encompasses within its scope current knowledge in respect of gene sequence, protein structure, localization, and possible function; individual reference lists are limited to twenty-one pertinent citations. The key articles are indicated by an asterisk (*).

One always feels at the end of such an undertaking that one could have done better, and perhaps we could have given more weight to those proteins which are known to play important physiological roles, particularly calcium channel subtypes and c2-domain proteins (e.g. protein kinase c). But the constraints of time and space inevitably curb one's energies, and a righting of this situation must await a second edition.

It now remains for me to thank all authors who have contributed to this book under the imposed time pressures and the publishers for their support.

M.R.C.

Fribourg, Switzerland
November 1995

Dedication

This book is dedicated to Claus W. Heizmann, Zürich, who introduced many of us to the field of calcium-binding proteins.

A computer system will be available from September 1996 to accompany *Guidebook to the Calcium-binding proteins*

Due to the rapid pace of biological research, the editors and publishers of this book believe it is important that its readers are kept informed of recent developments on these proteins. For this purpose, we have established a computer database that can be accessed through the worldwide web. This database will not include the full entries shown in this book; instead the authors have been asked to add, periodically, any new information on their protein that has been published since they wrote their original entry. Authors will be asked to deposit their updates from September 1996.

The update system can be accessed using any of the standard tools for browsing the worldwide web, such as Netscape or Mosaic. The URL for information relating to this book is *http://www.oup.co.uk/guidebooks/cbp*. For information on other Sambrook & Tooze Guidebooks, start from the Oxford University Press home page at *http://www.oup.co.uk/* and follow the links to the Guidebooks series.

Contents

Part 1. EF-Hand Calcium-binding Proteins and Analogs

Part 2. Annexins

Part 3. Other Proteins

Contributors

S. Atkinson Department of Microbiology and Immunology, PO Box 138, University of Leicester, Leicester LE1 9HN, UK. Tel. +44 116 252 5094, Fax +44 116 252 5030, E-mail: vjn@leicester.ac.uk

Dorairajan Balasubramanian Centre for Cellular and Molecular Biology (CCMB), Uppal Road, Hyderabad-500 007, India. Tel. +91 40 673487, Fax +91 40 671195, E-mail: dbala@ccmb.uunet.in

Roger Barraclough Department of Biochemistry, University of Liverpool, PO Box 147, Liverpool L69 3BX, UK. Tel. +51 794 4327, Fax +51 794 4349, E-mail: brb@liv.ac.uk

Igor Bendik Molecular Oncology, Department of Research, University Hospital, Ch-4031 Basel, Switzerland. Tel. +41 61 265 2387 E-mail: bendik@ubaclu.unibas.ch

Martin W. Berchtold Institute of Veterinary Biochemistry, University of Zürich-Irchel, Winterthurerstr. 190, CH-8057 Zürich, Switzerland. Tel. +41 1 257 54 73, Fax +41 1 362 05 01, E-mail: berchtol@vetbio.unizh.ch

Claudine Blin INSERM U.120, Hôpital Robert Debré, 48 Bd Sérurier, 75019 Paris, France. Tel. +33 1400 31915, Fax +33 1400 31903, E-mail: perret@citi2.fr

Angela Boyhan Glaxo Wellcome Res. and Dev. Medicines Research Center, Gunnels Wood Road, Stevenage, Hertfordshire SG1 ZNY, UK. Tel. +44 1438 764106, Fax +44 1438 764488, E-mail: ab11372@ggR.co.uk

Karl-Heinz Braunewell Department of Neurochemistry and Molecular Biology, Federal Institute for Neurobiology, PO Box 1860, D-39008 Magdeburg, Germany. Tel. +49 391 6263 228, Fax +49 391 6263 229, E-mail: braunew@jupiter.ifn-magdeburg.de

Kristen K. Briggs Department of Zoology and Genetics, Iowa State University, Ames, IA 50011, USA. Tel. +1515 294 2358, Fax +1515 294 0345, E-mail: jorgen@iastate.edu

Alexander Burger MediGene GmbH, Lochhamerstr 11, D-82152 Martinsried, Germany. Tel. +49 8956 320, Fax +49 8956 3220, E-mail: watzmann@mips.embnet.org

Robert D. Burgoyne The Physiological Laboratory, University of Liverpool, Crown Street, Liverpool L69 3BX, UK. Tel. +44 151 794 5305, Fax +44 151 794-5337, E-mail: burgoyne@liverpool.ac.uk

H. Caohuy LCBG, NIDDK, National Institutes of Health, Bethesda, MD 20892, USA. Tel. +1301 496 3435, Fax +1301 402 3298, E-mail: hpollard@helix.nih.gov

Ernesto Carafoli Laboratory of Biochemistry III, Federal Institute of Technology (ETH), CH-8092 Zürich, Switzerland. Tel. +41 1 632 3142, Fax +41 1 632 1213.

Marco R. Celio Institute of Histology and General Embryology, University of Fribourg, CH-1705 Fribourg, Switzerland. Tel. +41 26300 8491, Fax +41 26300 9732, E-mail: marco.celio@unifr.ch

Julio E. Celis Department of Medical Biochemistry and Danish Centre for Human Genome Research, University of Aarhus, Ole Worms Allé build. 170, DK-8000 Aarhus C, Denmark. Tel. +45 89 422880, Fax +45 86 131160.

Ching-Kang Chen Department of Biochemistry, SJ-70 and Howard Hughes Medical Institute, SL-15, University of Washington, Seattle, WA98195, USA. Tel. +1 206 543 4222, Fax +1 206 543 0858, E-mail: jbhhh@u.washington.edu

Sabine Colnot INSERM U.120, Hôpital Robert Debré, 48 Bd Sérurier, 75019 Paris, France. Tel. +33 1 400 31915, Fax +33 1 400 319 03, E-mail: perret@citi2.fr

J.A. Cox Department of Biochemistry, University of Geneva, 1211, Geneva 4, Switzerland. Tel. +4122 702 6491, Fax +4122 702 6483, E-mail: cox@sc2a.unige.ch

Carl E. Creutz Department of Pharmacology, University of Virginia, Charlottesville, VA 22908, USA. Tel. +1804 924 5029, Fax +1804 982 3878, E-mail: cec3n@virginia.edu

Pierre A. de Viragh Depts of Dermatology and Cell Biology, Baylor College of Medicine, Houston, TX 77030, USA. Tel. +1713 798 6350, Fax +1713 790 0545.

John E. Donelson Department of Biochemistry, Howard Hughes Medical Institute, University of Iowa, Iowa City, IA 52242, USA.

Helena Edwards Department of Physiology, University College London, Gower Street, London WC1E 6BT, UK. Tel. +44 171 380 7744, Fax +44 171 413 8395, E-mail: ucgbsem@ucl.ac.uk

David M. Engman Departments of Pathology and Microbiology-Immunology, Northwestern University Medical School, Chicago, IL 60611, USA. Tel. +1 312 503 1267, Fax +1 312 503 1265, E-mail: dengman@casbah.acns.nwu.edu

Volker Gerke Clinical Research Group for Endothelial Cell Biology, University of Münster, Von-Esmarch Str. 56, D-48149 Münster, Germany. Tel. +49 251 83 6722, Fax +49 251 83 6748, E-mail: gerke@wwupop.uni-muenster.de

Lisa M. Godsel Departments of Pathology and Microbiology-Immunology, Northwestern University Medical School, Chicago, IL 60611, USA. Tel. +1 312 503 1267, Fax +1 312 503 1265, E-mail: dengman@casbah.acns.nwu.edu

Danilo Guerini Laboratory of Biochemistry III, Federal Institute of Technology (ETH), CH-8092 Zürich, Switzerland. Tel. +41 1 632 3142, Fax +41 1 632 1213.

Eckart D. Gundelfinger Department of Neurochemistry and Molecular Biology, Federal Institute for Neurobiology, PO Box 1860, D-39008 Magdeburg, Germany. Tel. +49 391 6263 228, Fax +49 391 6263 229, E-mail: gundelfinger@ifn-magdeburg.de

Kazuko Hanyu Institute of Biological Sciences, The University of Tsukuba, Tsukuba, Ibaraki 305, Japan. Tel. +81 298 53 6648, Fax +81 298 53 6614.

A. Harmor Department of Horticulture, 15750 Linden Dr., University of Wisconsin-Madison, WI 53706. Tel. +1 608 262 3519, Fax +1 608 262 4743, E-mail: mrs@plantpath.wisc.edu

J. Harper Department of Horticulture, 15750 Linden Dr., University of Wisconsin-Madison, WI 53706. Tel. +1 608 262 3519, Fax +1 608 262 4743, E-mail: mrs@plantpath.wisc.edu

Alexander Hauenschild Zentrum für Molekulare Neurobiologie, Institut für Neural Signalverarbeitung, Martinistr. 52, D-20246 Hamburg, Germany. Tel. +49 040 4717 4811, Fax +49 040 4717 5102, E-mail: lindemeier@zmnh.zmnh.uni-hamburg.de

James F. Head Structural Biology Group, Department of Physiology, Boston University School of Medicine, 80 E. Concord St., Boston, MA 02118, USA. Tel. +1 617 638 4396, Fax +1 617 638 4273, E-mail: jfh@medxtal.bu.edu

Claus Heilmann Department of Gastroenterology, University of Freiburg, School of Medicine, Hugstetter Str. 55, D-79106 Freiburg, Germany. Tel. +49 761 270 3402, Fax +49 761 270 3259.

Hiroyoshi Hidaka Department of Pharmacology, Nagaya University School of Medicine, 65 Tsurumai Cho, Showa-ku, Nagoya 466, Aichi, Japan. Tel. +81 52 741 211, Fax +81 52 744 2083, E-mail address: hhidaka@tsuru.med.nagoya-u.ac.jp.

Nelson D. Horseman Department of Molecular and Cellular Physiology, University of Cincinnati, College of Medicine, PO Box 670576, Cincinnati, OH 45267-0576, USA. Tel. +1 513 558-3019, Fax +1 513 558-5738, E-mail: nevidns@ucbeh.san.vc.edu

Jingru Hu Dept of Cell and Molecular Biology, Northwestern University Medical School, Chicago, IL 60611-3008, USA. Tel. +1 312 503 0697, Fax +1 312 503 7912, E-mail: vaneldik@nwo.edu

Willi Hunziker Department of Exploratory Research, Division of Vitamins and Fine Chemicals, F. Hoffmann-La Roche Ltd, CH-4002 Basel, Switzerland. Tel. +41 61 688 6226, Fax +41 61 688 5057, E-mail: hunzikew@am@rocbi

James B. Hurley Department of Biochemistry, SJ-70 and Howard Hughes Medical Institute, SL-15, University of Washington, Seattle, WA98195, USA. Tel. +1 206 543 2871, Fax +1 206 685 2320, E-mail: jbhhh@u.washington.edu

Jørgen Johansen Department of Zoology and Genetics, Iowa State University, Ames, IA 50011, USA. Tel. +1 515 294 2358, Fax +1 515 294 0345, E-mail: jorgen@iastate.edu

Kristen M. Johansen Department of Zoology and Genetics, Iowa State University, Ames, IA 50011, USA.

Tel. +1 515 294 2358, Fax +1 515 294 0345, E-mail: jorden@iastate.edu

Matthias Jost Clinical Research Group for Endothelial Cell Biology, University of Münster, Von-Esmarch Str. 56, D-48149 Münster, Germany. Tel. +49 251 83 6722, Fax +49 251 83 6748, E-mail: jost@uni-muenster.de

Masahiro Kai Department of Biochemistry, Sapporo Medical University School of Medicine, West-17, South-1, Sapporo 060, Japan. Tel. +81 11 611 2111, Fax +81 11 612 5861.

Benjamin Kaminer Department of Physiology, Boston University School of Medicine, 80 E, Concord St., Boston, MA 02118, USA. Tel. +1 617 638 4392, Fax +1 617 638 4273, E-mail: bkaminer@acs.bu.edu

Hideo Kanoh Department of Biochemistry, Sapporo Medical University School of Medicine, West-17, South-1, Sapporo 060, Japan. Tel. +81 11 611 2111, Fax +81 11 612 5861.

Barbara Kappes Department of Structural Biology, Biozentrum, University of Basel, Klingelbergstrasse 70, CH-4056 Basel, Switzerland. Tel. +41 61 267 20101, Fax +41 61 267 2109, E-mail: kappes@ubaclu.unibas.ch

Satoru Kawamura Department of Biology, Faculty of Science, Osaka University, Machikane-yama 1-1, Toyonaka, Osaka 560, Japan. Tel. +81 6 850 5436, Fax +81 6 850 5444, E-mail: kawamura@bio.sci.osaka-u.ac.jp.

William H. Klein Department of Biochemistry and Molecular Biology, University of Texas M.D. Anderson Cancer Center, 1515 Holcombe Blvd., Houston, Texas 77030, USA. Tel. +1 713 792 3646, Fax +1 713 790 0329, E-mail: wklein@utmdacc.mda.uth.tmc.edu

Masaaki Kobayashi Department of Physiology, Toho University School of Medicine, Ohta-ku, Tokyo 143, Japan. Tel. +81 3 3762 4151, Fax +81 3 3762 8225, E-mail: physiken@med.toho-u.ac.jp

Tomoyoshi Kobayashi International Institute for Advanced Research, Matsushita Electric Industrial Co., 3-4 Hikaridai, Seika, Kyoto 619-02, Japan. Tel. +81 774 98 2543, Fax +81 774 98 2575, E-mail: tomo@crl.mei.co.jp

Daniel Koch Institute of Pharmacology, University of Zürich, Winterthurerstrasse 190, CH-8057 Zürich, Switzerland. Tel. +41 1 257 59 19, Fax +41 1 257 57 08, E-mail: schaub@pharma.unizh.ch

Jacek Kuznicki Nencki Institute of Experimental Biology, 3 Pasteur str., 02-093 Warsaw, Poland. Tel. +48 2 659 3123, Fax +48 22 22 5342, E-mail: jacek@nencki.gov.pl

Mireille Lambert INSERM U.120, Hôpital Robert Debré, 48 Bd Sérurier, 75019 Paris, France. Tel. +33 1 400 31915, Fax +33 1 400 31903, E-mail: perret@citi2.fr

Angus I. Lamond Department of Biochemistry, University of Dundee, Dundee, DD1 4HN, Scotland, UK. Tel. +44 1382-345 473, Fax +44 1382-200 894, E-mail: ailamond@bad.dundee.ac.uk.

Françoise Lamy Interdisciplinary Research Institute (IRIBHN), Campus Erasme, Bldg, C, 808 route de Lennik, 1070 Brussels, Belgium. Tel. +32 2 555 4150, Fax +32 2 555 4655.

Richard D. Lane Departments of Anatomy and Neurobiology, Medical College of Ohio, PO Box 10008, Toledo, OH 43699, USA. Tel. +1 419 381 4126, Fax +1 419 381 3008, E-mail: lane@vortex.mco.edu

Djemel Lebeche Department of Physiology, Boston University School of Medicine, 80 E, Concord St., Boston, MA 02118, USA. Tel. +1 617 638 4392, Fax +1 617 638 4273, E-mail: bkaminer@acs.bu.edu

Raymond Lecocq Interdisciplinary Research Institute (IRIBHN), Campus Erasme, Bldg, C, 808 route de Lennik, 1070 Brussels, Belgium. Tel. +32 2 555 4150, Fax +32 2 555 4655.

Stefan E. Lenz Department of Neurochemistry and Molecular Biology, Federal Institute for Neurobiology, PO Box 1860, D-39008 Magdeburg, Germany. Tel. +49 391 6263 228, Fax +49 391 6263 229, E-mail: gundelfinger@inf-magdeburg.de

Anita Lewit-Bentley LURE-Centre Universitaire Paris Sud, F-91405 Orsay Cedex, France. Tel. +33 1 644 68050, Fax +33 1 644 64148, E-mail: anita@lure.u-psud.fr

Fabienne L'Horset INSERM U.120, Hôpital Robert Debré, 48 Bd Sérurier, 75019 Paris, France. Tel. +33 1 400 31915, Fax +33 1 400 31903, E-mail: perret@citi2.fr

Jürgen Lindemeier Zentrum für Molekulare Neurobiologie, Institut für Neural Signalverarbeitung, Martinistr. 52, D-20246 Hamburg, Germany. Tel. +49 040 4717 4811, Fax +49 040 4717 5102, E-mail: lindemeier@zmnh.zmnh.uni-hamburg.de

Hector Lucero Department of Physiology, Boston University School of Medicine, 80 E, Concord St., Boston, MA 02118, USA. Tel. +1 617 638 4392, Fax +1 617 638 4273, E-mail: bkaminer@acr.bu.edu

Peder Madsen Department of Medical Biochemistry and Danish Centre for Human Genome Research, University of Aarhus, Ole Worms Allé build. 170, DK-8000 Aarhus C, Denmark. Tel. +45 89 42 28 80, Fax +45 86 13 11 60.

Patrick Maurer Medical Faculty of the University of Köln, Institute for Biochemistry, Joseph-Stelzmann-Str. 52, D-50931 Köln, Germany. Tel. +49 251 478 6997, Fax +49 251 478 6977.

Michael Melkonian Universität zu Köln, Botanisches Institut I, Gyrhofstraβe 15, 50931 Köln, Germany. Tel. +49 221 470 2475, Fax +49 221 470 5181, E-mail: mmelkon@biolan.uni-koeln.de

Ronald L. Mellgren Departments of Pharmacology and Therapeutics, Medical College of Ohio, PO Box 10008, Toledo, OH 43699, USA. Tel. +1 419 381 4126, Fax +1 419 381 3008, E-mail: lane@vortex.mco.edu

Marian Meyers Albert Einstein College of Medicine, Department of Medicine/Division of Cardiology, 1300 Morris Park Avenue, Bronx, New York 10461, USA. Tel. +1 718 430 2619, Fax +1 718 430 8989.

Marek Michalak MRC Group in Molecular Biology of Membranes, Department of Biochemistry, University of Alberta, 424 Heritage Medical Research Center, Edmonton, Canada T6G 2S2. Tel. +403 492 2256, Fax +403 492 9753, E-mail: marek.michalak@ualberta.ca

Naomasa Miki Department of Pharmacology I, Osaka University School of Medicine, 2-2 Yamadoaka, Suita 565, Japan. Tel. +81 6 879 3521, Fax +81 6 879 3529, E-mail: kayamagat@pharma1.med.osaka-u.ac.jp

Stephen E. Moss Department of Physiology, University College London, Gower Street, London WC1E 6BT, UK. Tel. +0171 380 7744, Fax +0171 413 8395, E-mail: ucgbsem@ucl.ac.uk

Michiko Naka Department of Molecular and Cellular Pharmacology, Mie University School of Medicine, 2-174 Edobashi, Tsu, Mie 514, Japan. Tel. +81 592 31 5006, Fax +81 592 32 1765, E-mail: tanaka@doc.medic.mie-v.ac.jp

Patrick Nef Biochemistry Department, Sciences II, University of Geneva, 30 quai Ernest Ansermet, CH-1211, Geneva 4, Switzerland. Tel. +41 22 702 6481, Fax +41 22 702 6483, E-mail: patrick.nef@biochem.unige.ch

Yoshitake Nishimune Research Institute for Microbial Diseases, Osaka University, Yamadaoka Suita, Osaka 565, Japan. Tel. +81 6 879 8338, Fax +81 6 879 8339, E-mail: nishimun@biken.osaka-u.ac.jp

Angelika A. Noegel Max-Planck-Institute for Biochemistry, D-82152 Martinsried, Germany. Tel. +49 89 8578 2315, Fax +49 89 8578 3777, E-mail: noegel@vms.biochem.mpg.de

V. Norris Department of Microbiology and Immunology, PO Box 138, University of Leicester, Leicester LE1 9HN, UK. Tel. +44 116 252 5094, Fax +44 116 252 5030, E-mail: vjn@leicester.ac.uk

Osamu Numata Institute of Biological Sciences, The University of Tsukuba, Tsukuba, Ibaraki 305, Japan. Tel. +81 298 53 6648, Fax +81 298 53 6614, E-mail: numata@sakura.cc.tsukuba.ac.jp

Katsuo Okazaki Department of Pharmacology, Nagaya University School of Medicine, 65 Tsurumai Cho, Showa-ku, Nagoya 466, Aichi, Japan. Tel. +81 52 741 211, Fax +81 52 733 4774.

Joseph E. O'Tousa Dept. of Biological Sciences, University of Notre Dame, Notre Dame, IN 46556-0369. Tel. +1 219 631 6093, Fax +1 219 631 7413, E-mail: o'tousa.1@nd.edu

Masayuki Ozawa Department of Biochemistry, Faculty of Medicine, Kagoshima University, Kagoshima 890, Japan. Tel. +81 992 75 5246, Fax +81 992 64 5618.

Thomas L. Pauls Institute of Histology and General Embryology, University of Fribourg, CH-1705 Fribourg, Switzerland. Tel. +41 26300 8490, Fax +41 26300 9732, E-mail: thomas.pauls@unifr.ch

Christine Perret INSERM U.120, Hôpital Robert Debré, 48 Bd Sérurier, 75019 Paris, France. Tel. +33 1 400 31915, Fax +33 1 400 31903, E-mail: perret@citi2.fr

Beatrice Perron LURE-Centre Universitaire Paris Sud, F-91405 Orsay Cedex, and INSERM U332 et ICGM, 22 rue Méchain 75014-Paris, France. Tel. +31 1 4051 6442, Fax +33 1 4051 7749, E-mail: favier@lure.u-psud.fr

Tanya V. Petrova Department of Biochemistry, University of Geneva, 1211, Geneva 4, Switzerland.

Tel. +22 702 6491, Fax +22 702 6483, E-mail: tanya@sc2a.unige.ch

Harvey B. Pollard LCBG, NIDDK, National Institutes of Health, Bethesda, MD 20892, USA. Tel. +1 301 496 3435, Fax +1 301 402 3298, E-mail: hpollard@helix.nih.gov

Olaf Pongs Zentrum für Molekulare Neurobiologie, Institut für Neural Signalverarbeitung, Martinistr. 52, D-20246 Hamburg, Germany. Tel. +49 040 4717 4811, Fax +49 040 4717 5102, E-mail: lindemeier@zmnh.zmnh.vni-hamburg.de

Scott L. Pratt Department of Molecular and Cellular Physiology, University of Cincinnati, College of Medicine, PO Box 670576, Cincinnati, OH 45267-0576, USA. Tel. +1 513 558 3019, Fax +1 513 558 5738, E-mail: nevidns@vcbeh.sam.vc.edu

John A. Putkey Department of Biochemistry and Molecular Biology, University of Texas Medical School, Houston, Texas 77030, USA. Tel. +1 713 792 5600, Fax +1 713 794 4150, E-mail: jputkey@utmmg.med.uth.tmc.edu

D.J. Raine Department of Physics and Astronomy, University of Leicester, Leicester LE1 7RH, UK. Tel. +44 116 252 5094, Fax +44 116 252 5030, E-mail: vjn@leicester.ac.uk

Beat M. Riederer Institute of Anatomy, University of Lausanne, Rue du Bugnon 9, 1005 Lausanne, Switzerland. Tel. +41 21 692 5100, Fax +41 21 692 5105, E-mail: briedere@eliot.unil.ch

Michael S. Rogers Department of Biochemistry and Molecular Biology, Mayo Graduate School, Mayo Clinic and Foundation, Rochester, MN 55905, USA. Tel. +1 507 284 9372, Fax +1 507 284 2384, E-mail strehler@rcf.mayo.edu

E. Rojas LCBG, NIDDK, National Institutes of Health, Bethesda, MD 20892, USA. Tel. +1 301 496 3435, Fax +1 301 402 3298, E-mail: hpollard@helix. nih.gov

Jochen Röper Zentrum für Molekulare Neurobiologie, Institut für Neural Signalverarbeitung, Martinistr. 52, D-20246 Hamburg, Germany. Tel. +49 040 4717 4811, Fax +49 040 4717 5102, E-mail: lindemeier@zmnh.zmnh.uni-hamburg.de

Johannes Roth Institute of Experimental Dermatology, University of Münster, Von Esmarch Str. 56, D-48149 Münster, Germany. Tel. +49 251 89 77, Fax +49 251 89 536.

Françoise Russo-Marie INSERM U332 et ICGM, 22 rue Méchain 75014-Paris, France. Tel. +33 1 405 16442, Fax +33 1 405 17749, E-mail: russo@citi2.fr

Shigeharu Saitoh Department of Physiology, Toho University School of Medicine, Ohta-ku, Tokyo 143, Japan. Tel. +81 3 3762 4151, Fax +81 3 3762 8225, E-mail: physiken@med.toho-u.ac.jp

Fumio Sakane Department of Biochemistry, Sapporo Medical University School of Medicine, West-17, South-1, Sapporo 060, Japan. Tel. +81 11 611 2111, Fax +81 11 612 5861.

Beat W. Schäfer University of Zürich, Department of Pediatrics, Division of Clinical Chemistry, Steinweisstrasse 75, CH-8032, Zürich, Switzerland. Tel. +41 1 266 7553, Fax +41 1 266 7169, E-mail: schafer@wawona.vmsmail.ethz.ch

Marcus C. Schaub Institute of Pharmacology, University of Zürich, Winterthurerstrasse 190, CH-8057 Zürich, Switzerland. Tel. +41 1 257 5919, Fax +41 1 257 5708, E-mail: schaub@pharma.unizh.ch

Beat Schwaller Institute of Histology and General Embryology, University of Fribourg, CH-1705 Fribourg, Switzerland. Tel. +41 26300 8490, Fax +41 26300 9732, E-mail: beat.schwaller@unifr.ch

Anthony W. Segal Glaxo-Wellcome Research Laboratories, Langley Court, Beckenham, Kent BR3 3BS, UK. Tel. +44 181 658 2211, Fax +44 181 663 3645.

Yogendra Sharma Centre for Cellular and Molecular Biology (CCMB), Uppal Road, Hyderabad-500 007, India. Tel. +91 40 673487, Fax +91 40 671195, E-mail: dbala@ccmb.uunet.in

Clemens Sorg Institute of Experimental Dermatology, University of Münster, Von Esmarch Str. 56, D-48149 Münster, Germany, Tel. +49 251 83 65 77, Fax +49 251 89 536.

Cornelia Spamer Department of Gastroenterology, University of Freiburg, School of Medicine, Hugstetter Str. 55, D-79106 Freiburg, Germany. Tel. +49 761 270 3402, Fax +49 761 270 3259.

M. Srivastava LCBG, NIDDK, National Institutes of Health, Bethesda, MD 20892, USA. Tel. +1 301 496 3435, Fax +1 301 402 3298, E-mail: hpollard@helix.nih.gov

Jutta Steinkötter Universität zu Köln, Botanisches Institut I, Gyrhofstraße 15, 50931 Köln, Germany. Tel. +49 221 470 2475, Fax +49 221 470 5181, E-mail: jsteinko@biolan.uni-koeln.de

Emanuel E. Strehler Department of Biochemistry and Molecular Biology, Mayo Graduate School, Mayo Clinic and Foundation, Rochester, MN 55905, USA. Tel. +1 507 284 9372, Fax +1 507 284 2384, E-mail: strehler@rcf.mayo.edu

Michael R. Sussman Horticulture Department and Program in Cell and Molecular Biology, University of Wisconsin-Madison, Madison, WI 53706, USA. Tel. +1 608 262 3519, Fax +1 608 262 4743, E-mail: mrs@plantpath.wisc.edu

Ken Takamatsu Department of Physiology, Toho University School of Medicine, Ohta-ku, Tokyo 143, Japan. Tel. +81 3 3762 4151, Fax +81 3 3762 8225, E-mail: physiken@med.toho-u.ac.jp

Tohru Takemasa Department of Anatomy I, Nippon Medical School, Bunkyo-ku, Tokyo 113, Japan. Tel. +81 3 3822 2131, ext. 285, Fax +81 3 5685 3052, E-mail: takemasa@nms.ac.jp

Toshio Tanaka Department of Molecular and Cellular Pharmacology, Mie University School of Medicine, 2-174 Edobashi, Tsu, Mie 514, Japan. Tel. +81 592 31 5006, Fax +81 592 32 1765, E-mail: tanaka@doc.medic. mie-u.ac.jp

Monique Thomasset INSERM U.120, Hôpital Robert Debré, 48 Bd Sérurier, 75019 Paris, France. Tel. +33 1 400 31915, Fax +33 1 400 31903, E-mail: perret@citi2.fr

Christine A. Towle Orthopedic Research Laboratories, Massachusetts General Hospital and Harvard Medical

School, Boston, MA 02114, USA. Tel. +1 617 724 3744, Fax +1 617 724 7396.

M. Trinei Department of Microbiology and Immunology, PO Box 138, University of Leicester, Leicester LE1 9HN, UK. Tel. +44 116 252 5094, Fax +44 116 252 5030, E-mail: vjn@leicester.ac.uk

Linda J. van Eldik Dept Cell and Molecular Biology, Northwestern University Medical School, Chicago, IL 60611-3008, USA. Tel. +1 312 503 0697, Fax +1 312 503 0007, E-mail: vaneldik@nwu.ed

Ikuo Wada Department of Biochemistry, Sapporo Medical University School of Medicine, West-17, South-1, Sapporo 060, Japan. Tel. +81 11 611 2111, ex. 2294, Fax +81 11 612 5861, E-mail: wada@cc. sapmed.ac.jp

Yoshio Watanabe University of Joubu, Toyatsuka 634, Isesaki, Gumma 372, Japan. Tel. +81 270 32 1011, Fax. +81 270 32 1021.

Karsten Weis EMBL, Meyerhofstrasse 1, Postfach 102209, D-69017 Heidelberg, Germany. Tel. +49 6221 387 328, Fax +49 6221 387 518, E-mail: weis@embl-heidelber.de

Athula H. Wikramanayake Department of Biochemistry and Molecular Biology, University of Texas M.D. Anderson Cancer Center, 1515 Holcombe Blvd., Houston, Texas 77030, USA. Tel. +1 713 792 3646, Fax +1 713 790 0329.

Kanato Yamagata Department of Pharmacology I, Osaka University School of Medicine, 2-2 Yamadoaka, Suita 565, Japan. Tel. +81 6 879 3521, Fax +81 6 879 3529, E-mail: kyamagat@pharma1.med.osaka-u.ac.jp

Danna B. Zimmer Department of Pharmacology, University of South Alabama, Mobile, AL 36688, USA. Tel. +1 334 460 7056, Fax +1 334 460 6798, E-mail: dzimmer@jaguar1.usouthal.edu

Abbreviations

AA	amino acid
AAS	atomic absorption spectrometry
ADR	arrested development of righting response
AP1	activator protein 1
ASL	arginosuccinate lyase
ATH	avian thymic hormone
ATPase	adenosine triphosphatase
Baa	basic amphiphilic alpha-helix
BAPTA	1,2-bis (2-aminophenoxy) ethane-N,N,N',N'-tetraacetic acid
Bb	basal body
BiP	immunoglobulin binding protein
bp	base pair
BSA	bovine serum albumin
CaBPs	calcium-binding proteins
CACY	calcyclin
CaM	calmodulin
cAMP	cyclic adenosine monophosphate
CAP	calcyclin-associated annexin
CAR	cancer-associated retinopathy
CaVP	calcium vector protein
CaVPT	calcium vector target protein
cDNA	complementary DNA
CDPKs	calmodulin-domain protein kinases
cGMP	cyclic guanosine monophosphate
CHO	Chinese hamster ovary
CKII	casein kinase II
CLP	calmodulin-like protein
Cn	calcineurin
CNS	central nervous system
CR	calretinin
CS	calsequestrin
CSc	calsequestrin, cardiac muscle isoform
CSs	calsequestrin, skeletal muscle isoform
CTER	calmodulin, troponin C, ELC, RLC
CV	clathrin-coated vesicles
d-frq	*Drosophila* frequenin
DGK	diacylglycerol kinase
DMSO	dimethylsulfoxide
DNaseI	deoxyribonuclease I
DTNB	5,5'-dithiobis(2-nitrobenzoic acid)
EcaSt/PDI ER	calcistorin/protein disulfide isomerase
EDTA	ethylenediaminetetraacetic acid
EGF	epidermal growth factor
EGTA	ethylene glycol-bis(βaminoethyl ether) N,N,N',N'-tetraacetic acid
EJP	excitatory junctional potential
ELC	(myosin) essential light chain
EM	electron microscopy
ER	endoplasmic reticulum
ERE	estrogen-responsive element
FcaBP	flagellar calcium-binding protein

flup	frequenin-like ubiquitous protein
FPLC	fast protein liquid chromatography
frq	frequenin
GABA	gamma-aminobutyric acid
GC	guanylyl cyclase
GDB	Genome Database
GFAP	Glial fibrillary acidic protein
GRE	glucocorticoid response elements
GRK	G-protein-coupled receptor kinase
GST	glutathione-S-transferase
GTP	guanosine 5'-triphosphate
GTPase	guanosine triphosphatase
HDEL	His-Asp-Glu-Leu
HEK	human embryonic kidney
ICAM-1	intercellular adhesion molecule-1
IEP	isoelectric point
IFN-γ	interferon-γ
Ig	immunoglobulin
IHS	*in situ* hybridization
INF-α	interferon-α
ir	immunoreactivity
IRBP	interphotoreceptor retinoid binding protein
ISA	intestine-specific annexin
LBP	luciferin-binding protein
LC	(myosin) light chains
LTD	long-term depression
LTP	long-term potentiation
LTR	long terminal repeat
mAB	monoclonal antibody
MAP	microtubule associated protein
MHC	myosin heavy chain
MIF	migration inhibitory factor
MLCK	myosin light chain kinase
MLCP	myosin light chain phosphatase
NAD	nicotinamide adenine dinucleotide
NADP(H)	nicotinamide adenine dinucleotide phosphate (reduced)
NBBCs	nucleus–basal body connectors
N-CAM	neural cell adhesion molecule
NCAP	neuron-specific CaBPs
NCS	neuronal calcium sensors
NF1	nuclear factor 1
NF-AT	nuclear factor for activation of T cells
NGF	nerve growth factor
NLS	nuclear localization signal
NMR	nuclear magnetic resonance
NRK	normal rat kidney
nt	nucleotide
OM	oncomodulin
PARV	parvalbumin
PCR	polymerase chain reaction
PDE	phosphodiesterase

PDGF	platelet-derived growth factor	SDS-PAGE	sodium dodecyl sulfate polyacrylamide gel electrophoresis
PDI	protein disulfide isomerase		
PF	profilaggrin	SPB	spindle pole body
PfCPK	*Plasmodium faciparum* calcium-dependent protein kinase	SR	sarcoplasmic reticulum
		STAT	signaling transducers and activators of transcription
PKC	protein kinase C		
PMA	phorbol myristate	TCA	trichloroacetic acid
PMCA	plasma membrane Ca^{2+} ATPase	TGF-β	transforming growth factor-β
PMNs	polymorphonuclear neutrophils	TH	trichohyalin
PS	phosphatidylserine	TIP	tonoplast integral protein
PV	parvalbumin	Tn	troponin
RACE	rapid amplification of cDNA ends	TnC	troponin C
RCN	reticulocalbin	TNF-α	tumor necrosis factor-α
RK	rhodopsin kinase	TPA	12-*O*-tetradecanoyl-phorbol-13-acetate
RLC	(myosin) regulatory light chain		
RNase	ribonuclease	TSH	thyroid stimulating hormone
ROS	rod outer segment	UV	ultraviolet
RT-PCR	reverse transcriptase polymerase chain reaction	VAC	vascular anticoagulant
		VDR	vitamin D receptor
Rv	recoverin	VDRE	vitamin D-responsive element
SCP	sarcoplasmic CaBPs	VSV	vesicular stomatitis virus

Techniques for measuring the binding of Ca^{2+} and Mg^{2+} to calcium-binding proteins

All the Ca^{2+}-binding proteins (CaBPs) have affinities for Ca^{2+} which are fine tuned to handle the intracellular Ca^{2+} signal, i.e. an oscillating and transient increase of free Ca^{2+} from 10^{-7} M at rest to 0.5 to 2×10^{-6} M during stimulation. Unless their metal-free form shows some physiological activity, as was in fact demonstrated in one case for yeast calmodulin (Geiser et al. 1991), binding of Ca^{2+} is the most important way CaBPs can be useful to the cell. The affinities of CaBPs for Ca^{2+} vary considerably; moreover for a given protein the affinity for Ca^{2+} can be strongly affected by Mg^{2+}; e.g. in the absence of Mg^{2+} parvalbumins display affinity constants for Ca^{2+} (K_{Ca}) of 10^9 to 10^7 M^{-1} which are decreased to 10^7 to 10^6 M^{-1} in the presence of millimolar concentrations of Mg^{2+} (Wnuk et al. 1982). On the other hand calmodulin shows affinity constants of the order of 10^5 M^{-1} and these values are nearly not affected by Mg^{2+} (Milos et al. 1986). Some CaBPs show much lower affinities: for instance calmodulin-like protein (Durussel et al. 1993) displays K_{Ca} values of around 10^4 M^{-1} and S100 proteins of 3 to 6×10^3 M^{-1} (Pedrocchi et al. 1994). The reasons for these important differences in affinities for proteins, which by default are all supposed to be active in the cytosol, is not clear, but it must be kept in mind that factors such as the interaction of the CaBPs with target proteins may dramatically alter their affinity for Ca^{2+} (Keller et al. 1982). Moreover in the case of calmodulin it has been shown that the rather low affinity for Ca^{2+} is compensated by its high cellular concentration and huge excess over the target enzymes (Cox 1988).

For a better understanding of the mode of action of these proteins at the molecular level, it is necessary to identify all the equilibria constants and to quantify their thermodynamic parameters. In essence, one has to know as precisely as possible the binding constants of a given CaBP for Ca^{2+} and for Mg^{2+} and, when an activator protein is involved, the binding constants of the complex for Ca^{2+} and the affinity of the metal-free and metal-bound CaBP for the target protein. This chapter deals with the currently used methods for quantifying the binding of Ca^{2+} and Mg^{2+} to CaBPs and summarizes the highlights concerning the best characterized proteins in this respect. Since most of the methods require initial removal of the metal ions from the protein, a short first section is devoted to this topic.

▪ Metal ion removal from CaBPs

All the methods for metal binding described below require a strict control of the Ca^{2+} and Mg^{2+} levels and hence of the contamination of the buffers and protein solutions by these ions. Whereas the natural contamination of solutions by Mg^{2+} is negligible (below 0.05 µM), Ca^{2+} contamination is several µM. Therefore all solutions used must be rendered "calcium-free" (i.e. below 0.2 µM) by treatment with Chelex 100 resin (Bio-Rad Laboratories) or with the EDTA resin, first described by Haner et al. (1984). To avoid or reduce Ca^{2+} contamination all solutions must be kept in plastic containers, which have been soaked in 1 N HCl and rinsed with bidistilled water. In the second step Ca^{2+} must be removed from the CaBPs by methods which do not alter the binding properties and which eventually remove also any foreign Ca^{2+} chelator from the protein solution. The softest protein decalcifications are done at neutral pH under non-denaturing conditions, but one can take advantage of the fact that many of the CaBPs are surprisingly stable and easily accommodate reversible denaturation. A panoply of fast (taking 1 hour or less) methods is listed below, together with references to recent applications. It may be useful to distinguish between the mild and harsher methods.

A. Mild methods:

1) After addition of 1 to 10 mM EDTA the protein solution is chromatographed on Sephadex G-25 equilibrated in the "Ca^{2+}-free" working buffer (Starovasnik et al. 1993; Petrova et al. 1995). There is a risk that complexes of weak affinity are formed between the protein and EDTA and that these are not completely dissociated by the gel filtration. To increase the efficiency of metal removal with even lower chelator concentrations, one can first remove most of the Ca^{2+} by dialysis against 1 mM EDTA, then perform the gel filtration chromatography.

2) After addition of 1 mM EDTA the protein is precipitated by ultra pure ammonium sulfate to over 90% saturation (Milos et al. 1986). The precipitate is washed several times with a solution of saturated ammonium sulfate, then dissolved in the working buffer and passed over a Sephadex G-25 column in the same buffer. The decalcification can be monitored by Ca^{2+} measurements with atomic absorption on the washings. A last washing step can be done with saturated ammonium sulfate which is acidified to pH 4 in order to decrease the affinity of CaBP for EDTA and as a result the risk of contaminating the sample with EDTA.

3) Passage of the protein solution over a column of Chelex 100 (Beckingham 1991) or of EDTA-agarose (Eberhard and Erne 1991) equilibrated in the working buffer. It must be noted that the Ca^{2+} exchange leads to proton exchange, thus necessitating strong pH buffers. In

this method the protein is in fact not perfectly equilibrated in the working buffer.

B. Somewhat harsher methods:

1) Acidification of the protein solution to pH 2 followed by Sephadex G-25 chromatography at pH 2 and acid neutralization (Maune et al. 1992a).

2) Denaturation of the protein in 6 M guanidine HCl at pH 8.0 followed by Sephadex G-25 chromatography in the working buffer (Starovasnik et al. 1992).

3) Protein precipitation by addition of 3% trichloroacetic acid (TCA), resolubilization, and repeated precipitation. At the end the dissolved protein is put on a Sephadex G-25 column equilibrated in the working buffer (Haiech et al. 1981). As in 2) the process can be followed by atomic absorption spectrometry (AAS).

The last method has been applied successfully in my laboratory for calmodulin, calmodulin-like protein, oncomodulin, parvalbumin, troponin C, Nereis SCP and its N- and C-terminal domains, CaVP, CACY and CAPL, calreticulin and calsequestrin, and the neuronal proteins NCS-1 and vilip. In some cases we compared the Ca^{2+}-binding data from samples obtained by either the TCA method or methods 1) or 2): no significant differences were detected. In contrast the Ca^{2+}-binding properties of amphioxus SCPs and the complex CaVP.CaVPT, as well as certain mutant forms of parvalbumin are damaged by the TCA method, and can better be treated with method 1).

■ Protein concentration

In quantitative investigations a precise estimation of the protein concentration is of utmost importance. Since nearly always pure proteins are involved in ion binding studies, spectrophotometry using the molar extinction coefficient at 280 nm is the most convenient method. This coefficient can be determined on a sample of which the protein content has been determined by dry weight or by quantitative amino acid analysis including norleucine as an internal standard.

■ Ca^{2+} binding

The first question to be solved after one realizes that a given new protein contains one or more EF-hand motifs is, if it really binds Ca^{2+}. For this purpose easily accessible qualitative methods exist such as the Ca^{2+}-dependent mobility shift in PAGE in the presence or absence of SDS (Cox and Stein 1981; Garrigos et al. 1991), detection using the $^{45}Ca^{2+}$-overlay method (Maruyama et al. 1984) or interaction with the Ca^{2+} homologs Eu^{3+} and Tb^{3+} (Henzle et al., 1991). Different optical methods, especially circular dichroism, fluorimetry and difference UV spectrophotometry, can be performed in most laboratories and lead to a valid diagnosis provided ion-binding leads to signal changes. Filtration (Nakamura et al., 1991) and precipitation (Sakane et al., 1991) methods implying $^{45}Ca^{2+}$ as well as a $^{45}Ca^{2+}$/Chelex 100 competition assay (Benzonana et al., 1972) yield semi-quantitative information. But quantitative information, leading to the evaluation of the physiological significance of Ca^{2+}-binding to a protein, can not be gathered by these methods. Special methods have been developed since 1970 for the determination of binding curves. The next sections deal with the three most common methods to determine Ca^{2+}-binding isotherms.

1. Equilibrium dialysis

For measuring the affinity between a small ligand and a protein the equilibrium dialysis method is in principle the most simple one (Potter and Gergely 1975; Wnuk et al., 1979). In this method an equilibrium is established on both sides of a solute-permeable, but protein-impermeable membrane. In practice, aliquots of a protein solution (approximately 20 to 100 μM of binding sites) are simultaneously equilibrated against a series of buffers of increasing ion concentrations. After 24 hours the concentrations of the protein and of total ligand in both compartments are measured. The difference in ligand concentration between both compartments corresponds to bound ligand, which can be directly related to the protein concentration. Ion measurements can be done by AAS or by liquid scintillation counting, provided $^{45}Ca^{2+}$ was added from the beginning of the experiments. A major complication is that it is impossible to decontaminate buffers of physiological ionic strength to free Ca^{2+} values lower than 0.2 μM. In order to attain free Ca^{2+} levels of 10^{-9} to 10^{-5} M, it is thus necessary to "clamp" the free Ca^{2+} by including EGTA in the dialysis experiments. The free Ca^{2+} concentration in the protein-free compartment is then calculated using a computer program such as COMICS (Perrin and Sayce 1967) taking into account the constants of EGTA + Ca^{2+} and EGTA + H^+ and the total concentrations of EGTA and Ca^{2+}. Mg^{2+}-binding can be measured in a similar manner, providing EDTA is used to clamp the concentration of the ion. Even with this complication the method is quite simple and needs minimal equipment. Moreover, a non-negligible advantage is that Ca^{2+} does not have to be removed beforehand from the protein (provided AAS is used to measure the Ca^{2+} concentration). But some negative points must be mentioned: 1) The length of the equilibration precludes determination on labile, sticky or hydrolysis-susceptible proteins; 2) In the EGTA buffering system the free Ca^{2+} v. total Ca^{2+} relationship is not linear and lacks precision in the 10^{-7} to 2×10^{-5} M range, i.e. in the zone one usually wants to cover; 3) Some CaBPs themselves interact with the chelator, leading to modified or supplementary binding (Chiancone et al., 1986); 4) The workload is quite heavy and the number of manipulations requires maximal attention of the experimenter, especially when $^{45}Ca^{2+}$ is present.

2. Fluorescent or light absorbing ion indicators

The principle in this method is competition for Ca^{2+} of the CaBP with an indicator whose binding parameters are well known and whose degree of saturation can be quantified exactly by optical means (Linse et al., 1987, 1993; Eberhard and Erne 1991a,b). To the mixture of protein and indicator-increasing Ca^{2+} concentrations are added until the indicator is saturated. If the physical and optical properties of the indicator are the same in the presence and absence of protein, one can determine the free Ca^{2+} concentration as indicated by the following equation:

Eq. 1 $\quad [Ca^{2+}] = \Delta S_i / (\Delta S_{max} - \Delta S_i) \, K_{indicator}$

where $[Ca^{2+}]$ is the concentration of free Ca^{2+}, ΔS_i and ΔS_{max} are the optical signal change at titration point i and at the end (maximal saturation of chelator), respectively, and $K_{indicator}$ the affinity constant of the indicator (one assumes a 1 to 1 stoichiometry with Ca^{2+}). The value of $K_{indicator}$ under the experimental conditions can be determined by a separate titration of the indicator alone. Protein-bound Ca^{2+} (Ca_{bound}) is then calculated as follows:

Eq.2 $\quad Ca_{bound} = Ca_{Tot} - [Ca^{2+}] - \{K_{indicator} \, C_{indicator} \, [Ca^{2+}]/(1 + K_{indicator} \, [Ca^{2+}])\}$

where Ca_{Tot} and $C_{indicator}$ are the concentrations of added Ca^{2+} and of the indicator, respectively. If the protein concentration is in large excess over that of the indicator the last factor of Eq. 2 can be neglected.

Many Ca^{2+} indicators are available which show either fluorescence or absorbance signal changes. In the latter case the amplitude of the signal change is smaller, thus requiring higher $C_{indicator}$ values; i.e. usually comparable to the protein concentration (around 20 µM). Fluorescent probes are used at submicromolar concentrations while the protein concentration is 2 to 3 µM. Therefore, spectrophotometric more than the fluorimetric titrations suffer from the risk that the protein may interact with the indicator. It is then safe to demonstrate, e.g. by fluorescence anisotropy, that no such interaction occurs (Eberhard and Erne 1991a). A second advantage of the fluorimetric over absorbance titration is that the spectra of the indicator often show an isosbestic point, a wavelength where no ligand-induced changes occur during the titration. Indeed, the precision is much higher when the signal at the wavelength of maximal fluorescence change is rationed to the signal at the isosbestic wavelength. An important consideration is the choice of the indicator with respect to its affinity for Ca^{2+}. Ideally the affinity of the indicator for Ca^{2+}, K_{Ca}, should be slightly lower than that of the lowest affinity sites of the protein. Fortunately, many indicators have been developed with different affinities for Ca^{2+}, ranging from 10^7 M^{-1} (Quin 2) to 5×10^5 M^{-1} (5,5'-Br$_2$BAPTA). If a CaBP shows pronounced negative cooperativity or displays more than one site with markedly different affinities, the indicator method is not recommended. A last caveat is the selectivity of the indicator, especially if one wants to determine the Ca^{2+}-binding properties in the presence of physiological concentrations of Mg^{2+}. Ideally, the Ca^{2+}/Mg^{2+}-selectivity ratio should be higher than 10 000. Indicators with a low selectivity ratio can in fact be used to determine the Mg^{2+}-binding parameters of a CaBP by similar Mg^{2+}-titration experiments in the absence of Ca^{2+} (i.e. in the presence of EGTA).

3. Flow dialysis

Technically this method is inspired by the flow reactor where an immobile solution (upper compartment) is separated from the lower compartment by a semi-permeable membrane which retains the protein but not the small ligands; the lower chamber is continuously flushed with the working buffer (Colowick and Womack 1969). Flow dialysis is based on the principle that the amount of Ca^{2+} diffusing per unit of time from the upper compartment through the dialysis membrane is proportional to the concentration of free Ca^{2+} in that compartment. If the Ca^{2+} pool in the upper compartment is tagged with $^{45}Ca^{2+}$, this rate can be measured by determining the concentration of the isotope in the effluent of the lower chamber (for commodity called here cpm$_i$), which is collected in a fraction collector. After perfusion with 4 times the volume of the lower chamber a steady state is reached for which the rates for isotope entering and leaving the lower chamber are practically equal, as indicated by the next equation:

Eq.3 $\quad dcpm_i/dt = D \, [Ca^{2+}] - cpm_i \, (f/V) = 0$
$\quad\quad$ hence: $[Ca^{2+}]_i = cpm_i \, f/(V.D)$

where D is a constant depending on both the diffusion properties of Ca^{2+} and the geometry of the dialysis apparatus, f is the flow rate of buffer through the lower chamber, and V is the volume of this chamber. In essence Eq. 3 indicates that after a steady state is reached, the concentration of isotope (cpm$_i$) in the effluent becomes a true measure of free $[Ca^{2+}]$ in the upper compartment. After each addition of unlabeled Ca^{2+} to the upper chamber, a new equilibrium is established and a new steady state of cpm$_i$ is reached. The parameters $f/(V.D)$ are not directly determined; instead a large excess (with respect to the binding capacity of the protein) of cold Ca^{2+} is added at the end of the titration, so that all Ca^{2+} and $^{45}Ca^{2+}$ in the upper compartment can be considered as free. The corresponding cpm$_{end}$ value is an index standing for 100% free $[Ca^{2+}]$ and the ratio of cpm$_i$/cpm$_{end}$ represents thus the fraction of *free* Ca^{2+} in the upper compartment. From the known total Ca^{2+} concentration at each increment the concentration of free and bound Ca^{2+} in the upper chamber are calculated. This data treatment would be sufficient if three factors were negligible: 1) the dilution (Fdil$_i$, or dilution factor) in the upper chamber by the increments; 2) the losses (Floss$_i$, or loss factor) of $^{45}Ca^{2+}$ and total Ca^{2+}; 3) the Ca^{2+} (and of tracer $^{45}Ca^{2+}$) contamination in upper chamber at the start of the experiment. For these reasons the following additional parameters must be measured:

• The initial Ca^{2+} contamination, $[Ca^{2+}]_{contam.}$: After the cell is mounted, the upper chamber is filled with the protein solution and tracer $^{45}Ca^{2+}$ is added; then 250 µl is withdrawn to measure the Ca^{2+} concentration by AAS. In order to decrease the contamination, it is indicated to wash the upper compartment with the working buffer before introducing the protein solution.

• The initial (CPM$_{init}$) and final $^{45}Ca^{2+}$ counts (CPM$_{end}$) in the upper compartment: The ΔCPM factor, defined as

(CPM$_{init}$ − CPM$_{end}$)/CPM$_{init}$, determines the total loss of Ca^{2+} in the upper chamber, which can vary substantially (from 10 to 20%) depending on the profile of free Ca^{2+} change in this chamber during the experiment. The fraction of free Ca^{2+}, $f_{[Ca^{2+}]i}$, after increment i is as follows:

Eq.4 $f_{[Ca^{2+}]i}$ = (cpm$_i$ Fdil$_i$ Floss$_i$) / (cpm$_{end}$ Fdil$_{end}$ Floss$_{end}$)

with Fdil$_i$ = Vol$_i$ / Vol$_{init.}$ and Fdil$_{end}$ = Vol$_{end}$ / Vol$_{init.}$
and Flossi = 1 + ΔCPM {$\Sigma_{(i = 1\ to\ n)}$cpm$_i$ / $\Sigma_{(i = 1\ to\ end)}cpm_i$}
The total Ca^{2+} concentration, Catot$_i$, after increment i is:

Eq.5   Catot$_i$ = ([Ca^{2+}]$_{contam.}$ + Σ[Ca^{2+}]$_{increm.i}$) / Fdil$_i$

The free Ca^{2+} concentration corresponds to $f_{[Ca^{2+}]i}$ Catot$_i$ and the protein-bound Ca^{2+} is then calculated by Ca^{2+}$_{bound}$ = Ca$_{Tot}$ − [Ca^{2+}].

In practice the following experimental conditions are used for most of the CaBPs. The flow device, with either a stirred lower chamber (Womack and Colowick 1973) or a spiral groove (Feldmann 1978) was mounted using Spectrapor membranes, which were boiled twice: once in EDTA alkalinized water and once in bidistilled water. The upper chamber contains 750 µl of a protein solution of 60 µM Ca^{2+}-binding sites. From this chamber 250 µl is withdrawn just after the addition of tracer ^{45}Ca^{2+}. The lower chamber with a volume of 50 µl is perfused at a flow rate of 1 ml/min and the effluent is collected in fractions of 0.4 ml. Every 2 minutes increments of Ca^{2+} are added so that the total Ca^{2+} concentrations in the upper compartment vary according to an exponential scale until a value of 2 to 3 mM is attained. The samples of the fraction collector are supplemented with scintillation liquid and counted to over 98% precision. A flow dialysis profile is shown in Fig. 1. Occasionally the determination of the maximal plateau can lead to an underestimation (Krause et al., 1991), especially with proteins of low affinity for Ca^{2+}. In this case one can increase the chase Ca^{2+} concentration to over 10 mM in order to assure that virtually all Ca^{2+} is free. However, it is advised not to add Ca^{2+} to levels such that ionic strength and Donnan effects change too much, because the method is based on the assumption that the diffusion parameters remain strictly constant during the whole flow dialysis experiment. If such problems arise it is advised to find the real maximal plateau by acidifying the protein solution in the upper chamber to pH 4 to 5 so that Ca^{2+} dissociates from the protein and all Ca^{2+} is free. Alternatively, or if the protein precipitates upon acidification, one can measure with a Ca^{2+}-selective electrode the free Ca^{2+} concentration (Krause et al., 1991) in the upper chamber after the flow experiment. The real plateau value is then equal to cpm$_{end}$ (Ca$_{Tot}$ / [Ca^{2+}]$_{end}$). An example of treatment of the raw data of Fig. 1 is given in Table 1. This method has

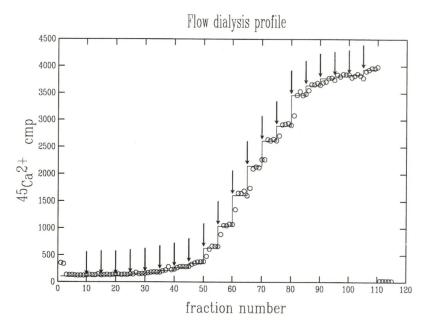

Figure 1. Time course of a flow dialysis experiment with 21 increments of Ca^{2+}. The experiment was carried out at 25 °C in 50 mM Tris–HCl, pH 7.5, 130 mM KCl, 10 mM MgCl$_2$ with 32 µM of a chimaeric protein (parvalbumin with the CD site of oncomodulin). The volumes of the upper and lower compartments were 500 µl and 50 µl, respectively; the flow rate was 1 ml/min, the volume of a fraction 0.4 ml. Ca^{2+}$_{contam.}$ was 10 µM; ΔCPM was 0.066. The titration (done by the MicroLab 2200) consisted of additions at each arrow of 1 to 4 µl of the following stock solutions of Ca^{2+}: 0.625, 3.05, 9.58, 82.5 mM and the final chase was done with 1 µl of 1 M Ca^{2+}. The treatment of these raw data to yield free and protein-bound Ca^{2+} is demonstrated in Table 1.

Table 1. Treatment of the raw data of flow dialysis

No.	cpm raw	cpm corr.	$[Ca^{2+}]_{tot}$ (μM)	$[Ca^{2+}]_{free}$ (%)	$[Ca^{2+}]_{free}$ (μM)	$[Ca^{2+}]_{bound}$ (μM)	Ca^{2+}/Prot.
1	102	102	10.00	2.28	0.228	9.77	0.305
2	103	103	11.23	2.30	0.259	10.97	0.343
3	115	116	12.45	2.60	0.324	12.13	0.379
4	116	117	14.88	2.62	0.389	14.49	0.453
5	140	142	17.29	3.17	0.549	16.74	0.523
6	163	166	23.27	3.71	0.863	22.41	0.700
7	213	217	29.23	4.84	1.420	27.82	0.869
8	264	269	35.17	6.01	2.110	33.05	1.033
9	345	353	41.08	7.88	3.240	37.84	1.182
10	625	643	52.83	14.35	7.580	45.25	1.414
11	1035	1071	64.49	23.91	15.400	49.07	1.534
12	1604	1668	82.97	37.23	30.900	52.08	1.627
13	2146	2246	101.38	50.12	50.800	50.57	1.580
14	2610	2756	137.97	61.50	84.900	53.12	1.660
15	2887	3079	174.29	68.70	120.000	54.56	1.705
16	3455	3716	332.30	82.92	276.000	56.74	1.773
17	3637	3948	489.71	88.08	431.000	58.36	1.823
18	3769	4136	802.73	92.30	741.000	61.82	1.932
19	3807	4233	1267.80	94.45	1200.000	70.36	2.199
20	3838	4332	1879.72	96.65	1820.000	62.91	1.966
21	3934	4482	3755.88	100.00	3756.000	–	–

cpm_{init}: 50 480; cpm_{end}: 47 150.
Protein concentration: 32 μM.
Concentration of contaminant Ca^{2+}: 10 μM.

allowed us to determine quite easily and precisely the Ca^{2+} affinities of various proteins with K_{Ca} values varying from 3×10^7 to 2×10^3 M^{-1}. It is our experience that the precision is greatly improved by automation of the pipetting of the increments.

■ Mg²⁺ binding

Under physiological ionic conditions at low Ca^{2+} concentrations many EF-hand containing CaBPs interact with Mg^{2+} with affinities ranging from 10^2 to 10^5 M^{-1}. The binding of Mg^{2+} to CaBPs can be measured by equilibrium dialysis or by the fluorescent indicator method, but unfortunately not by flow dialysis since there is no stable radioactive isotope of Mg^{2+} with a long enough half-life time. In the equilibrium dialysis method the concentration of the ion can be "clamped" with EDTA (Wnuk et al., 1979; Cox and Stein 1981). The indicator method is hampered by the fact that the commercially available indicators, such as Magnesium Orange, Mag-Fura Red or Mag-quin-2, have affinity constants of 300 to 700 M^{-1}, implying that they are useful for proteins with a K_{Mg} of 3×10^3 M^{-1} at the utmost. A method well suited for Mg^{2+}-binding studies is equilibrium gel filtration, first proposed by Hummel and Dryer (1962).

Hummel–Dryer method
The equilibrium gel filtration method (Hummel and Dryer 1962) takes advantage of the fact that on a gel filtration column a protein is rapidly and efficiently brought to equilibrium with the buffer in which the gel matrix is equilibrated. In practice 0.5 to 1 ml of a protein solution is applied to a 0.8×40 cm column of Sephadex G-25 equilibrated in the working buffer plus a given concentration of free Mg^{2+}, and eluted at 0.4 ml/min. In the eluent fractions the protein concentration is monitored by its UV absorbance and Mg^{2+} by AAS. Analysis of three protein-containing fractions across the protein peak allows us to verify if equilibrium is reached, which is the case when the bound Mg^{2+} to protein ratio is the same in the three fractions. In the method originally proposed the protein sample was loaded without any addition of ligand, thus creating a positive peak at the elution position of the protein and a negative one where small molecules are eluted. The surfaces of the positive and negative peak are identical. However, in Mg^{2+}-binding experiments it is preferable for kinetic reasons that the loaded protein already contains Mg^{2+}. A practical and rapid way of generating a Mg^{2+}-binding isotherm is to chromatograph first the CaBP in buffer containing 1 mM Mg^{2+} and, after analysis, rechromatograph each of the protein-containing fractions on columns equilibrated in lower Mg^{2+} concentrations (from 50 to 500 μM). Excess Mg^{2+} dissociates and a new equilibrium is rapidly reached. When performing Hummel–Dryer experiments in buffer containing less than 50 μM Mg^{2+}, the flow rate must be reduced to 0.1 ml/min and care must be taken to pre-equilibrate the protein load with Mg^{2+}. Since generating a correct isotherm takes 3 to 5 days, the determination of the Mg^{2+}-binding isotherms now constitutes the rate-limiting step in the unraveling of the ion-binding parameters of a given CaBP.

■ Analysis of the binding data

1. Stoichiometric, microscopic and intrinsic constants

The above methods yield model-independent isotherms which describe the global binding of the ion to the protein. They provide macroscopic, also named stoichiometric binding constants, K_n, which refer to the binding of the first, second, etc. Ca^{2+} ion to the protein (Cornish-Bowden and Koshland 1975; for an excellent review, see Linse and Forsén 1995). The most general description of equilibria in terms of stoichiometric binding is provided by the Adair–Klotz model (Klotz and Hunston 1979), which analyses the binding data in terms of a set of constants that describe the binding of the first, second, ..., nth Ca^{2+} ion to the protein. The binding data then obey the following equation:

Eq.6
$$r = \frac{(K_1[Ca^{2+}] + 2K_1K_2[Ca^{2+}]^2 + \ldots nK_1K_2\ldots K_n[Ca^{2+}]^n)}{(1 + K_1[Ca^{2+}] + K_1K_2[Ca^{2+}]^2 + \ldots + K_1K_2\ldots K_n[Ca^{2+}]^n)}$$

where r is the ratio of bound Ca^{2+} per protein and n is the number of Ca^{2+}-binding sites. These stoichiometric (or macroscopic) binding constants yield information on the pace of the successive binding steps, but *not* on the affinity constants (= association constants) of any particular site. In a CaBP with four functional Ca^{2+}-binding sites I, II, III, and IV and the affinity constants k_I, k_{II}, k_{III}, and k_{IV} (called microscopic or site binding constants) related to each site, the relationship between K_n and these constants is as follows (Cornish-Bowden and Koshland 1975; Saroff 1992):

Eq.7
$$K_1 = k_I + k_{II} + k_{III} + k_{IV}$$
$$K_1K_2 = k_Ik_{II} + k_Ik_{III} + k_Ik_{IV} + k_{II}k_{III} + k_{II}k_{IV} + k_{III}k_{IV}$$
$$K_1K_2K_3 = k_Ik_{II}k_{III} + k_Ik_{II}k_{IV} + k_Ik_{III}k_{IV} + k_{II}k_{III}k_{IV}$$
$$K_1K_2K_3K_4 = k_Ik_{II}k_{III}k_{IV}$$

Only ion titrations using optical probes which monitor Ca^{2+} binding to a given site (Kilhoffer et al., 1992; Trigo-Gonzales et al., 1992), will yield information on the microscopic constants. It should be noticed that the microscopic k values may change during the binding process, e.g. the affinity of site II for Ca^{2+} may be different depending upon the presence or not of Ca^{2+} in site I. Cornish-Bowden and Koshland (1975) analysed the binding isotherm in terms of the intrinsic affinity constants, K'_n, whose meaning is intuitively the easiest understood since it represents the mean affinity constant of site n in a protein. If all the microscopic constants are identical there is only *one* intrinsic constant and the relation between stoichiometric and intrinsic constant is as follows: $K1 = 4 K'$; $K_2 = 3/2 K'$, $K_3 = 2/3 K'$ and $K_4 = 1/4 K'$. If the k values do *not* change during the titration (i.e. in a non-cooperative system) , but are different, the four different intrinsic constants, K'_1, K'_2, K'_3, and K'_4, describe the binding isotherm. In many instances, as in this book, the metal binding parameters are expressed as dissociation constants K_D, since these are closest to the notion of

the Ca^{2+} concentration which induces half maximal binding or response: in most (simplified) cases $K_D = 1/K'$.

In the case of positive cooperativity in a two-site system the relationship between the intrinsic constants is as follows: $K'_1 < K'_2$ and the degree of allostery is given either by the ratio $k_{I,II}/k_I$ or by $\Delta G = \Delta G_{I,II} - \Delta G_I$, i.e. by the difference between the change in free energy when Ca^{2+} binds to a given site (here site I) in the presence ($\Delta G_{I,II}$) or absence (ΔG_I) of bound Ca^{2+} to the second site (Linse et al., 1991a,b). However, a much more popular cooperativity index is given by the empirical Hill model, with:

Eq.8 $r = n K^{nH} [Ca^{2+}]/(1 + K^{nH} [Ca^{2+}])$

were n is the number of sites, n_H the Hill coefficient and K an apparent binding constant, not related to the stoichiometric, intrinsic, or macroscopic constants (Cornish-Bowden and Koshland 1975). Linearization of Eq. 8 yields the widely used Hill function:

Eq.9 $\log \{r/(n - r)\} = \log K + n_H \log [Ca^{2+}]$

2. The Ca^{2+}/ Mg^{2+} antagonism

In most cases the affinities of CaBPs for Ca^{2+} are modulated by millimolar concentrations of Mg^{2+}, either by direct competition at so-called Ca^{2+}/ Mg^{2+} mixed sites, or by indirect antagonism in proteins with Ca^{2+}-specific sites. A primordial task after the Ca^{2+}-binding isotherms have been collected at different Mg^{2+} concentrations is to determine which model of antagonism is functioning.

1) In the model of *direct competition* the EF-hand site binds either Ca^{2+} or Mg^{2+} and the shift of the isotherms to higher $[Ca^{2+}]$ upon increasing the Mg^{2+} concentrations is unlimited. The competition model obeys the following equation:

Eq.10 $K_{Ca}/K_{Ca}.app = 1 + K_{Mg} [Mg^{2+}]$

where K_{Ca} and $K_{Ca}.app$ are the Ca^{2+}-binding constants in the absence and presence of Mg^{2+}, respectively, and K_{Mg} is the Mg^{2+}-binding constant in the absence of Ca^{2+}. Examples of the analysis of simple competition models have been presented for troponin C (Potter and Gergely 1975) and parvalbumin (Moeschler et al., 1980); complex, but still direct competition models have been described for sarcoplasmic Ca^{2+}-binding proteins (Wnuk et al., 1982), especially for NSCP, the sarcoplasmic Ca^{2+}-binding protein of *Nereis* (Engelborghs et al., 1990; Luan-Rilliet et al., 1992).

2) *Indirect Mg^{2+}- Ca^{2+} antagonism* is exemplified by calmodulin (Milos et al., 1986). In this protein Mg^{2+} does not bind to the same sites as Ca^{2+}, but to auxiliary sites, physically different from the EF-hand sites (Milos et al., 1989). Calmodulin can bind 4 Ca^{2+} and 4 Mg^{2+} simultaneously. The Ca^{2+} and Mg^{2+}-binding sites influence each other's affinity due to negative free energy coupling between the sites. The scheme that accounts for the whole phenomenon is as follows (for each individual site, S):

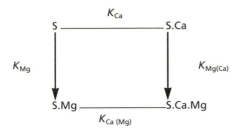

where K_{Ca} and K_{Mg} are the association constants for Ca^{2+} and Mg^{2+}, respectively, in the absence of the other ligand, and $K_{Ca(Mg)}$ and $K_{Mg(Ca)}$ the corresponding constants in the presence of infinite concentrations of the second ligand. The amount of bound ligand per mole of site is given by (see Cox et al., 1982; Milos et al., 1986):

Eq.11

$$\text{bound } Ca^{2+}/\text{site} = \frac{1 + (K_{Mg(Ca)}\,[Mg^{2+}])^{-1}}{1 + (K_{Ca\,(Mg)}\,[Ca^{2+}])^{-1} + (1 + K_{Ca}[Ca^{2+}])^{-1}\,(K_{Mg(Ca)}\,[Mg^{2+}])^{-1}}$$

Similarly:

$$\text{bound } Mg^{2+}/\text{site} = \frac{1 + (K_{Ca(Mg)}\,[Ca^{2+}])^{-1}}{1 + (K_{Mg(Ca)}\,[Mg^{2+}])^{-1} + (1 + K_{Mg}[Mg^{2+}])^{-1}\,(K_{Ca(Mg)}\,[Ca^{2+}])^{-1}}$$

It should be noted that, as in the model of straight competition, upon increasing the Mg^{2+} concentrations the Ca^{2+}-binding isotherms shift to higher free Ca^{2+} concentrations, but in this model the shift is not unlimited and levels off at the isotherm dictated by $K_{Ca(Mg)}$.

■ Conformational studies confirm and complement direct binding data

The binding of ions to EF-hand CaBPs usually leads to conformational changes. Recent studies indicate that the secondary structure is nearly unaltered, but that angles and distances between structural motifs change (Declerq et al., 1991; Skelton et al., 1994). If Tyr and Trp residues are involved in this change, fluorimetry and difference spectrophotometry constitute very adequate methods to follow the binding of Ca^{2+} or Mg^{2+}. Independent of the information they yield on the quality of the conformational change (more or less hydrophobic exposure, accessibility to quenchers, charge effects, etc.), the two methods may help to determine stoichiometries, to provide good estimates of the values of the affinity constants, etc. Of the two methods, fluorimetry is the more sensitive one: correct measurements are done on 1 μM solutions of Trp-containing proteins and on 15 μM solutions if the protein contains Tyr but not Trp residues. The method is well suited to evaluate the affinity of a CaBP for Mg^{2+} (most often in the 5×10^4 to 10^3 M^{-1} range). Ca^{2+}-titrations can only be envisioned providing the free $[Ca^{2+}]$ is controlled with EGTA. Difference spectrophotometry is optimal on protein solutions with an optical density at 280 nm of 1 to 1.5 unit, corresponding to a

protein solution of 70 to 500 μM, depending on the size of the protein and the presence or absence of Trp. This method is thus indicated for the determination of Ca^{2+} stoichiometries and for estimates of the affinity for Mg^{2+}.

It must be noticed that quite often conformational changes do not follow the mean saturation of the protein, but are linked to the saturation of a given site or pair of sites. For example in calmodulin the Tyr fluorescence (Burger et al., 1984) or spectrophotometric (Klee 1977) changes are strictly concomitant with the binding of Ca^{2+} to the paired domain in the C-terminal half. In other cases the conformational changes are sequential, i.e. they closely follow the appearance of a well-defined $CaBP.Ca_n$ species and n can even be different for different types of conformational probes. An example of this behavior is crayfish SCP $\alpha 2$, where the α-helical content changes with binding of the second, the Trp fluorescence with binding of the third, and thiol reactivity with binding of the fourth Ca^{2+} ion (Wnuk et al., 1981).

■ Anthology of Ca^{2+}-binding to CaBPs

Although there exist 32 distinct subfamilies of EF-hand proteins (Kawasaki and Kretsinger 1994), detailed ion-binding studies have been carried out on seven to eight members only. Below are summarized the most characteristic features of the best studied CaBPs, with emphasis on what they have added recently to our knowledge on ion interaction to EF-hand motifs.

Calmodulin and its complexes with targets

The Ca^{2+}-binding properties of calmodulin, its different natural and mutant forms, have been intensively studied by different groups. Whereas very similar binding isotherms have been reported under comparable ionic conditions, much debate has centered on the binding model, i.e. on the relation between the microscopic affinity and the stoichiometric binding constants (Cox 1988; Kilhoffer et al., 1992). The now prevailing model is based on diversified studies on calmodulins from yeast, plants, and higher animals, as well as on mutant forms and calmodulin fragments. The N- and C-terminal globular domains appear to bind Ca^{2+} independently of each other (Linse et al., 1991a; Maune et al., 1992a,b) and the fragmented, isolated domains show the same ion-binding properties as in the whole protein (Minowa and Yagi 1984). Within the paired domain positive cooperativity exists, at least in the C-terminal domain, and this cooperativity can be modulated by mutations of Asp to Asn in the Y coordinating position of sites II and III (Waltersson et al., 1993). The two sites in the N-terminal domain display a lower affinity than those in the C-terminus, which is more accentuated in calmodulins from plants (Yoshida et al., 1983) and in calmodulin-like protein (Durussel et al., 1993b) than in the animal protein. All these calmodulins possess exclusively Ca^{2+}-specific sites, except calmodulin-like protein, which possesses both Ca^{2+}-specific and Ca^{2+}-Mg^{2+} mixed sites.

Upon complex formation of calmodulin with its target(s) the Ca^{2+}-binding properties are dramatically changed (Keller *et al.*, 1982; Mamar-Bachi and Cox 1987). In the case of the complex with smooth muscle myosin light chain kinase the binding curve becomes strongly cooperative. A quantitative model of energy linkage is as follows (Mamar-Bachi and Cox 1987):

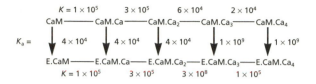

where the K values are the stoichiometric (macroscopic) Ca^{2+}-binding constants and K_a the enzyme association constants. The unusual strong affinity increase upon binding of the third Ca^{2+} indicates that only $CaM.Ca_3$ and $CaM.Ca_4$ are the competent forms for enzyme-activation. The finding that upon binding of the third Ca^{2+} calmodulin acquires its activating potential, has been observed for different enzymes (Cox 1988). Recently the strong increase in affinity has also been documented for the case of calmodulin interaction with synthetic peptides representing the calmodulin-binding domain of the plasma membrane calcium pump (Yazawa *et al.*, 1992) and myosin light chain kinase (Porumb *et al.*, 1994).

Troponin C
The publication in 1975 of the detailed Ca^{2+} and Mg^{2+}-binding properties of skeletal muscle troponin C was a landmark in the field of divalent ion interactions with CaBPs (Potter and Gergely 1975). Troponin C contains a pair of high affinity, Ca^{2+}–Mg^{2+} mixed sites in the C-terminal half and a pair of low affinity Ca^{2+}-specific sites in the N-terminal half. As in calmodulin, there is little ion-induced interaction between the two globular domains (Li *et al.*, 1994). Ca^{2+}-binding to the low affinity site(s) is the triggering event of muscular contraction, whereas ion-binding to the high-affinity sites is necessary for anchoring the protein to the troponin complex (Cox *et al.*, 1981). When skeletal or cardiac troponin C is incorporated in the respective troponins, the affinity for Ca^{2+} is increased by a factor of 10 to 50, and this for all the sites (for summary, see Ebashi and Ogawa 1988). An interesting strategy of modulating *in vitro* the Ca^{2+}-affinity of troponin C is the manipulation of the energetically unfavorable solvent-exposed hydrophobic patches by genetic engineering: replacement of these hydrophobic residues that make up the N-terminal patch by hydrophilic ones increases the affinity up to five fold (Pearlstone *et al.*, 1992; da Silva *et al.*, 1993). Thus, modifications far away from the Ca^{2+}-binding sites can profoundly affect the affinity.

Myosin light chains
Type II myosins contain two different light chains, the regulatory and essential light chains, which both are derived from a 4 EF-hand containing ancestor protein,

but have been subjected to a strong evolutionary drift. All myosins display one Ca^{2+}-Mg^{2+} mixed site, which is located on the regulatory light chain; the latter can be dissociated by treatment with EDTA while retaining its Ca^{2+}–Mg^{2+}-binding capacity (Bagshaw and Kendrick-Jones 1979). Only site I is functional in the regulatory light chain. Molluscan myosins are unique by the fact that they possess a direct Ca^{2+} regulatory mechanism (Kendrick-Jones *et al.*, 1976). These myosins contain in addition to the Ca^{2+}–Mg^{2+}-mixed site a Ca^{2+}-specific site, located in the essential light chain (Kwon *et al.*, 1990). This latter site disappears upon dissociation of the regulatory light chain from myosin, because the regulatory light chain is necessary to maintain the native structure of whole myosin and in particular of the Ca^{2+}-specific site of the essential light chain. The recently resolved crystal structure has confirmed the binding model for both types of light chains (Xie *et al.*, 1994) and identified the Ca^{2+}-specific site as site I in the essential light chain. Interestingly, this is a new type of EF-hand site, rich in liganding α-carbonyl groups.

Calbindin D-9k
Calbindin D-9k is ideally suited as a model for a better understanding of the chemical rules that govern the affinity of an EF-hand, especially since this is a small protein consisting of only two paired EF-hand sites. Moreover, it most likely constitutes the prototype of a cooperative system within a "2-site domain". The two sites are of the high-affinity, Ca^{2+}-specific type and contain one canonical (site II) and one particular (site I) EF-hand sequence pattern. Deactivating mutations in site I lead to affinity decrease in this site, but do not significantly alter the affinity of site II for Ca^{2+} (Johansson *et al.*, 1990). Fragmentation of the protein in the middle leads to formation of a heterodimer with strongly decreased affinity constants for Ca^{2+} (Finn *et al.*, 1992). These results suggest that, as far as the configuration of the two-sites domain remains preserved, the affinity of the canonical site is not influenced by the particular EF-hand site. Recently important progress was achieved regarding the pronounced positive cooperativity in Ca^{2+}-binding, which can be manipulated either by neutralization of negative charges (Linse *et al.*, 1988) or, more specifically, by a E60D mutation (Linse *et al.*, 1994). The molecular basis of this type of cooperativity seems to reside in the direct contact between site I and II by a bridging Glu60 (Linse *et al.*, 1991b; Skelton *et al.*, 1994).

Parvalbumin and oncomodulin
The protein pair parvalbumin–oncomodulin constitutes an ideal platform to pin down the rules that govern the Ca^{2+}–Mg^{2+} selectivity and the affinity of the EF-hand motif since they behave like twins with a single different birthmark. The two proteins show 50% sequence identity, bind non-cooperatively 2 Ca^{2+} ions and display very similar crystal structures in their Ca^{2+}-saturated form (Ahmed *et al.*, 1990; McPhalen *et al.*, 1994). But, parvalbumin possesses two high-affinity Ca^{2+}–Mg^{2+} mixed sites (Wnuk *et al.*, 1982), whereas oncomodulin contains one

high-affinity, Ca^{2+}–Mg^{2+} mixed site (the EF site at the C-terminal end) *and* one low-affinity, Ca^{2+}-specific site (the CD site) (Hapak *et al.*, 1989; Cox *et al.*, 1990). Interestingly, parvalbumin is the only CaBP of which the three-dimensional structure of the Mg^{2+}-binding form could be resolved (Declerq *et al.*, 1991). Site-directed mutagenesis is now used to change the selectivity of the CD site in either parvalbumin or oncomodulin. Residues in the CD loop of oncomodulin do not seem to be major determinants of the selectivity (MacManus *et al.*, 1989; Palmisano *et al.*, 1990). The structural integrity of the mutant proteins is checked by monitoring the conformational properties of a Trp inserted in the hydrophobic core (MacManus *et al.*, 1989; Pauls *et al.*, 1993). Recently a new aspect was highlighted by studying parvalbumin with inactivated sites: despite the fact that the affinities for Ca^{2+} and Mg^{2+} for the symmetrical paired two-site domain are the same, one of the sites is structurally dominant (Pauls *et al.*, 1994).

Sarcoplasmic Ca^{2+}-binding proteins

Although SCPs (sarcoplasmic Ca^{2+}-binding protein) are considered to be the functional counterparts of parvalbumins in invertebrates, their ion-binding properties are among the most complex encountered in simple proteins (Wnuk *et al.*, 1982; Cox 1990). Crustacean SCPs display three functional ion-binding sites with pronounced positive and negative cooperativity. Moreover the Ca^{2+}-binding is antagonized in a complex way by Mg^{2+}, leading to a reinforcement of the positive cooperativity of Ca^{2+}-binding, concomitant with a decrease in affinity for Ca^{2+}. Annelid SCP possesses one high-affinity and two low-affinity (dormant) sites. It binds the first Ca^{2+} to a well-defined site (probably site I), which leads to a strong increase in affinity of the two remaining dormant sites. This sequential model is also valid for the binding of Mg^{2+}: the increase in affinity as a consequence of the first binding step leads to pronounced positive cooperativity. Research on *Nereis* SCP also allowed a problem of the structure–function relationship to be solved: which structural elements determine whether a CaBP is an activator rather than a buffer and *vice versa*? Activators are elongated and possess important solvent-exposed hydrophobic surfaces, which are metastable and seek stabilization by interaction with their target. SCPs display a very compact structure with the N- and C-terminal paired domains strongly "glued" together and are thus very stable by themselves (Durrussel *et al.*, 1993a). Understanding of the complexity of ion-binding to SCPs is greatly improved by the recent elucidation of the three-dimensional structure of the annelid (Cook *et al.*, 1991) and amphioxus SCP (Cook *et al.*, 1993).

Neuron-specific Ca^{2+}-binding proteins

Recently the existence of a new subfamily of neuron-specific Ca^{2+}-binding proteins (NCaP) of 22 to 26 kDa was reported (for the most recent report, see Palczewski *et al.*, 1994). NCaPs can be subdivided in two groups: the A-type NCaPs, e.g. recoverin and visinin, are exclusively present in light-sensitive organs, and possess two canonical EF-hands in sites II and III. B-type NCaPs, e.g. vilip and NCS-1, are expressed in various neuronal tissues including the retina and the brain, and possess three canonical EF-hands in sites II, III and IV. Recoverin was reported to bind two Ca^{2+} ions, but in the crystal Ca^{2+} was found only in site III, likely because the region of site II is too highly mobile (Flaherty *et al.*, 1993). No detailed Ca^{2+}-binding studies have been reported on the A-type NCaPs, but detailed metal-binding studies on two B-type NCaPs, namely vilip and NCS-1, revealed some surprising features (Cox *et al.*, 1994). These proteins possess two active Ca^{2+}/Mg^{2+}-binding sites although three canonical EF-hand motifs are present in their sequence. Moreover, they markedly differ in their Ca^{2+}- and Mg^{2+}-binding characteristics. Vilip shows quite simple metal-binding properties with two Ca^{2+}-binding sites of equal, rather low affinity for Ca^{2+}. In this protein Ca^{2+}-binding is weakly antagonized by Mg^{2+}. NCS-1 binds two Ca^{2+} with a tenfold higher affinity than vilip and with a high degree of positive cooperativity. Although for both proteins the Ca^{2+}/Mg^{2+}-binding is mutually exclusive, the high K'_{Mg} values determined by direct binding studies are 30- to 100-fold higher than those obtained by applying the competition equation, indicating that the antagonism is indirect. The problems of stoichiometry, cooperativity, and of Mg^{2+}-antagonism in the NCaP subfamily deserve further investigation.

■ The take-home message from 20 years of Ca^{2+}-binding studies

The *first* message is that the majority of CaBPs have multiple Ca^{2+}-binding sites, which allows a lot of sophistication in the binding isotherms. In the case of activating CaBPs the "multi-site" property also provides a mechanism of strong energy linkage (better on-off behavior) without having to adopt extremely high, and therefore nearly irreversible, Ca^{2+} affinities. The *second* message is that for different CaBPs, especially the buffering ones, Mg^{2+} is nearly as important as Ca^{2+}; it not only lowers the Ca^{2+} affinity to the physiological range, but, by acting differently in different Ca^{2+}-binding sites, can strongly alter the isotherms. Moreover, the abundant CaBPs such as parvalbumin and SCPs can be instrumental in transforming changes in the Ca^{2+} concentration to changes in the Mg^{2+} concentration. The *third* message is that there is a very complex relation between the amino acid sequence and the Ca^{2+} affinity or Ca^{2+}–Mg^{2+} selectivity. The rules have not yet been laid down, and the many studies towards this goal indicate that the Rosetta stone is not yet found. The *fourth* message is that CaBPs can provide excellent models for better understanding of positive cooperativity; from the direct, short distance cooperativity in calbindin D-9k to the long distance cooperativity in *Nereis* SCP, implying an allosteric pathway through the molecule.

The few examples mentioned above show a bewildering diversity of thermodynamic behavior of different

CaBPs. Moreover, the kinetics of Ca^{2+}- and Mg^{2+}-binding, deliberately not treated in this methodological review, adds a new dimension to the action of CaBPs in the cell. As paraphrased from a recent review (Williams 1994) "the kinetics rather than thermodynamics will ultimately explain how the Ca^{2+} signal can control events of very different time scales such as muscle contraction (10^{-3} s), metabolic control (10^{-1} s), and protein synthesis (up to hours)". Since at present time, the ion-binding properties of only a minority of the known CaBPs are explored, and even fewer kinetic studies have been performed, a lot of excitement is still ahead.

■ References

Ahmed, F.R., Przybyska, M., Rose, D.R., Birnbaum, G.I., Pippy, M.E., and MacManus, J. (1990) Structure of oncomodulin refined at 1.85 Å resolution. J. Mol. Biol. **216**, 127–140.

Bagshaw, C.R. and Kendrick-Jones, J. (1979) Characterisation of homologous divalent metal ion binding sites of vertebrate and molluscan myosin using electron paramagnetic resonance spectroscopy. J. Mol. Biol. **130**, 317–336.

Beckingham, K. (1991) Use of site-directed mutations in the individual Ca^{2+}-binding sites of calmodulin to examine Ca^{2+}-induced conformational changes. J. Biol. Chem. **226**, 6027–6030.

Benzonana, G., Capony, J.-P., and Pechère, J.-F. (1972) The binding of calcium to muscular parvalbumin. Biochim. Biophys. Acta **278**, 110–116.

Burger, D., Cox, J.A., Comte, M., and Stein, E.A. (1984) Sequential conformational changes in calmodulin upon binding of calcium. Biochemistry **23**, 1966–1971.

Chiancone, E., Thulin, E., Boffi, A., Forsén, S., and Brunori, M. (1986) Evidence for the interaction between the calcium indicator 1,2-bis(o-aminophenoxy)ethan-N,N,N',N'-tetraacetic acid and calcium-binding proteins. J. Biol. Chem. **261**, 16306–16308.

Colowick, S.P. and Womack, F.C. (1969) Binding of diffusible molecules by macromolecules: rapid measurement by rate of dialysis. J. Biol. Chem. **244**, 774–777.

Cook, W.J., Ealick, Y.S., Babu, Y.S., Cox, J.A., and Vijay-Kumar, S. (1991) Three-dimensional structure of a sarcoplasmic calcium binding protein. J. Biol. Chem. **266**, 652–656.

Cook, W.J., Jeffrey, L.C., Cox, J.A., and Vijay-Kumar, S. (1993) Structure of a sarcoplasmic calcium-binding protein from amphioxus refined at 2.4 A resolution. J. Mol. Biol. **229**, 461–471.

Cornish-Bowden, A. and Koshland, D.E. (1975) Diagnostic uses of the Hill (Logit and Nernst) plots. J. Mol. Biol. **95**, 201–212.

Cox, J.A. (1988) Interactive properties of calmodulin. Biochem. J. **249**, 621–629.

Cox, J.A. (1990) Calcium vector protein and sarcoplasmic calcium-binding proteins from invertebrate muscle. In *Stimulus-response coupling: the role of intracellular calcium* (eds J.R. Dedman and V.L. Smith) pp. 83–107 CRC Press, Boca Raton, FL.

Cox, J.A. and Stein, E.A. (1981) Characterization of a new sarcoplasmic calcium-binding protein with magnesium-induced cooperativity in the binding of calcium. Biochemistry **20**, 5430–5436.

Cox, J.A., Comte, M., and Stein, E.A. (1981) Calmodulin-free skeletal muscle troponin C prepared in the absence of urea. Biochem. J. **195**, 205–211.

Cox, J.A., Comte, M., and Stein, E.A. (1982) Activation of human erythrocyte Ca^{2+}-dependent Mg^{2+}-activated ATPase by calmod-

ulin and calcium: quantitative analysis. Proc. Natl. Acad. Sci. USA **79**, 4265–4269.

Cox, J.A., Comte, M., Malnoë, A., Burger, D., and Stein, E.A. (1984) Mode of action of the regulatory protein calmodulin. In *Metal ions in biological systems* (ed. H. Sigel), Vol. 17, pp. 215–275, New York, Basel.

Cox, J.A., Milos, M., and MacManus, J.P. (1990) Calcium and magnesium-binding properties of oncomodulin. Direct binding studies and microcalorimetry. J. Biol. Chem. **265**, 6633–6637.

Cox, J.A., Durussel, I., Comte, M., Nef, S., Nef, P., Lenz, S.E., and Gundelfinger, E.D. (1994) Cation binding and conformational changes in vilip and NCS-1, two neuron-specific calcium-binding proteins. J. Biol. Chem. **269**, 32807–32813.

da Silva, A.C.R., de Araujo, A.H.B., Herzberg, O., Moult, J., Sorenson, M., and Reinach, F.C. (1993) Troponin-C mutants with increased calcium affinity. Eur. J. Biochem. **213**, 599–604.

Declerq, J.P., Tinant, B., Parello, J., and Rambaud, J. (1991) Ionic interactions with parvalbumins. Crystal structure determination of pike 4.10 parvalbumin in four different ionic environments. J. Mol. Biol. **220**, 1017–1039.

Durussel, I., Luan-Rilliet, Y., Petrova, T., Takagi. T., and Cox, J.A. (1993*a*) Cation binding and conformation of tryptic fragments of *Nereis* sarcoplasmic calcium-binding protein: Calcium-induced homo- and heterodimerization. Biochemistry **32**, 2394–2400.

Durussel, I., Rhyner, J.A., Strehler, E.E., and Cox, J.A. (1993*b*) Cation binding and conformation of human calmodulin-like protein. Biochemistry **32**, 6089–6094.

Ebashi, S. and Ogawa, Y. (1988) Troponin C and calmodulin as calcium receptors: mode of action and sensitivity to drugs. In Handbook of experimental pharmacology (ed. P.F. Baker), pp. 31–56. Springer-Verlag, Berlin.

Eberhard, M. and Erne, P. (1991*a*) Analysis of calcium binding to α-lactalbumin using a fluorescent calcium indicator. Eur. J. Biochem. **202**, 1333–1338.

Eberhard, M. and Erne, P. (1991*b*) Calcium binding to fluorescent calcium indicators: calcium green, calcium orange and calcium crimson. Biochem. Biophys. Res. Commun. **180**, 209–215.

Engelborghs, Y., Mertens, K., Willaert, K., Luan-Rilliet, Y., and Cox, J.A. (1990) Kinetics of conformational changes in *Nereis* sarcoplasmic calcium-binding protein upon calcium- and magnesium binding. J. Biol. Chem. **265**, 18801–18815.

Feldmann, K. (1978) New devices for flow dialysis and ultrafiltration for the study of protein-ligand interactions. Anal. Biochem. **88**, 225–235.

Finn, B.E., Kördel, J., Thullin, E., Sellers, P., and Forsén, S. (1992) Dissection of calbindin D9k into two Ca^{2+}-binding subdomains by a combination of mutagenesis and chemical cleavage. FEBS Lett. **298**, 211–214.

Flaherty, K.M., Zozulya, S., Stryer, L., and McKay, D.B. (1993) Three-dimensional structure of recoverin, a calcium sensor in vision. Cell **75**, 709–716.

Garrigos, M., Dechamps, S., Viel, A., Lund, S., Champeil, P., Moller, J.V., and le Maire, M. (1991) Detection of Ca^{2+}-binding proteins by electrophoretic migration in the presence of Ca^{2+} combined with ^{45}Ca^{2+} overlay of protein blots. Anal. Biochem. **194**, 82–88.

Geiser, J.R., van Tuinen, D., Brockerheff, S.E., Neff, M.M., and Davis, T.N. (1991) Can calmodulin function without binding calcium? Cell **65**, 949–959.

Haiech, J., Klee, C.B., and Demaille, J.G. (1981) Effects of cations on affinity of calmodulin for calcium: ordered binding of calcium ions allows the specific activation of calmodulin-stimulates enzymes. Biochemistry **20**, 3890–3897.

Haner, M., Henzl, M.T., Raissouni, B., and Birnbaum, E.R. (1984) Synthesis of a new chelating gel: removal of Ca^{2+} ions from parvalbumin. Anal. Biochem. **138**, 229–234.

Hapak, R.C., Lammers, P.J., Palmisano, W.A., Birnbaum, E.R., and Henzl, M.T. (1989) Site-specific substitution of glutamate for aspartate at position 59 of rat oncomodulin. J. Biol. Chem. **264**, 18751–18760.

Henzl, M.T., Serda, R.E., and Boschi, J.M. (1991) Identification of a novel parvalbumin in avian thymic tissue. Biochem. Biophys. Res. Commun. **177**, 881–887.

Hummel, J.P., and Dryer, W.J. (1962) Measurement of protein-binding phenomena by gel filtration. Biochim. Biophys. Acta **63**, 530–532.

Johansson, C., Brodin, P., Grundström, T., Thulin, E., Forsén, S., and Drakenberg, T. (1990) Biophysical studies of engineered mutant proteins based on calbindin D_{9k} modified in the pseudo EF-hand. Eur. J. Biochem. **187**, 455–460.

Kawasaki, H. and Kretsinger, R. (1994) Calcium-binding proteins 1: EF-hands. Protein Profile **1**, 343–517.

Keller, C.H., Olwin, B.B., LaPorte, D.C., and Storm, D.R. (1982) Determination of the free-energy coupling for binding of calcium ions and troponin I to calmodulin. Biochemistry **21**, 156–162.

Kendrick-Jones, J., Szentkiralyi, E.M., and Szent-Györgyi, A.G (1976) Regulatory light chains in myosins. J. Mol. Biol. **104**, 747–775.

Kilhoffer, M.-C., Kubina, M., Travers, F., and Haiech, J. (1992) Use of engineered proteins with internal tryptophan reporter groups and perturbation techniques to probe the mechanism of ligand-protein interactions: investigation of the mechanissm of calcium binding to calmodulin. Biochemistry **31**, 8098–8106.

Klee, C.B. (1977) Conformational transition accompanying the binding of Ca^{2+} to the protein activator of 3',5'-cyclic adenosine monophosphate phosphodiesterase. Biochemistry **16**, 1017–1024.

Klotz, I.M. and Hunston, D.L. Protein affinities for small molecules: conceptions and misconceptions. Arch. Biochem. Biophys. **193**, 314–428.

Krause, K.H., Milos, M., Luan-Rilliet, Y., Lew, D.P., and Cox, J.A. (1991) Thermodynamics of cation-binding to rabbit skeletal muscle calsequestrin. Evidence for distinct Ca^{2+}- and Mg^{2+}-binding sites. J. Biol. Chem. **266**, 9453–9459.

Kwon, H., Goodwin, E.B., Nyitray, L., Berliner, E., O'Neall-Hennessey, E., Melandri, F.D., and Szent-Györgyi, A.G. (1990) Isolation of the regulatory domain of scallop myosin: role of the essential light chain in calcium binding. Proc. Natl. Acad. Sci. USA **87**, 4771–4775.

Li, M.X., Chandra, M., Pearlstone, J.R., Racher, K.I., Trigo-Gonzales, G., Borgford, T., Kay, C.M., and Smillie, L.B. (1994) Properties of isolated recombinant N and C domains of chicken troponin C. Biochemistry **33**, 917–925.

*Linse, S. and Forsén, S. (1995) Determinants that govern high-affinity calcium binding. Adv. Second Mess. Phosphoprot. Res. **30**, 89–151.

Linse, S., Brodin, P., Drakenberg, T., Thulin, E., Sellers, P., Elmdén, K., Grundström, T., and Forsén, S. (1987) Structure-function relationship in EF-hand proteins. Protein engineering and biophysical studies on calbindin D9k. Biochemistry **26**, 6723–6735.

Linse, S., Brodin, P., Johansson, C., Grundström, T., and Forsén, S.(1988) The role of protein surface charges in ion binding. Nature **335**, 651–652.

Linse, S., Helmerson, A., and Forsén, S. (1991a) Calcium binding to calmodulin and its globular domains. J. Biol. Chem. **266**, 8050–8054.

Linse, S., Johansson, C., Brodin, P., Thulin, E., Grundström, T., Drakenberg, T., and Forsén, S.(1991b) Electrostatic contributions to the binding of Ca^{2+} in calbindin D_{9k}. Biochemistry **30**, 154–162.

Linse, S., Thulin, E., and Sellers, P. (1993) Disulfide bonds in homo- and heterodimers of EF-hand subdomains of calbindin D_{9k}: stability, calcium binding, and NMR studies. Protein Sci. **2**, 985–1000.

Linse, S., Bylsma, N.R., Drakenberg, T., Sellers, P., Forsén, S., Svensson, L.A., Tajtsev, V., and Marek, J. (1994) A calbindin D_{9k} mutant with reduced calcium affinity and enhanced cooperativity. Metal ion binding, stability, and structural chances. Biochemistry **33**, 12478–12486.

Luan-Rilliet, Y., Milos, M., and Cox, J.A. (1992) Thermodynamics of cation binding to *Nereis* sarcoplasmic calcium-binding protein. Direct binding studies, microcalorimetry and conformational changes. Eur. J. Biochem. **208**, 133–138.

MacManus, J.P., Hutnik, C.M.L., Sykes, B.D., Szabo, A.G., Williams, T.C., and Banville, D (1989) Characterisation and site-specific mutagenesis of the calcium-binding protein oncomodulin produced by recombinant bacteria. J. Biol. Chem. **264**, 3470–3477.

McPhalen, C.A., Sielecki, A.R., Santarsiero, B.D., and James, M.N.G. (1994) Refined crystal structure of rat parvalbumin, a mammalian α-lineage parvalbumin, at 2.0 Å resolution. J. Mol. Biol. **235**, 718–732.

Mamar-Bachi, A. and Cox, J.A. (1987) Quantitative analysis of the free energy coupling in the system calmodulin, calcium, smooth muscle myosin light chain kinase. Cell Calcium **8**, 473–482.

Maruyama, K., Mikawa, T., and Ebashi, S. (1984) Detection of calcium binding proteins by ^{45}Ca autoradiography on nitrocellulose membrane after sodium dodecyl sulfate gel electrophoresis. J. Biochem. (Tokyo) **95**, 511–519.

Maune, J.F., Beckingham, K., Martin, S.R., and Bayley, P.M. (1992a) Circular dichroism studies on calcium binding to two series of Ca^{2+}-binding site mutants of *Drosophila melanogaster* calmodulin. Biochemistry **31**, 7779–7786.

Maune, J.F., Klee, C.B., and Beckingham, K. (1992b) Ca^{2+} binding and conformational change in two series of point mutations to the individual Ca^{2+}-binding sites of calmodulin. J. Biol. Chem. **267**, 5286–5295.

Milos, M., Schaer, J.-J., Comte, M., and Cox, J.A. (1986) Calcium-proton and calcium-magnesium antagonisms in calmodulin. Biochemistry **25**, 6279–6287.

Milos, M., Comte, M., Schaer, J.-J., and Cox, J.A. (1989) J. Inorganic Biochem. **36**, 11–25.

Minowa, O. and Yagi, K. (1984) Calcium binding to tryptic fragments of calmodulin. J. Biochem. **96**, 1175–1182.

Moeschler, H., Schaer, J.-J., and Cox, J.A. (1980) A thermodynamic analysis of the binding of calcium and magnesium ions to parvalbumin. Eur. J. Biochem. **111**, 73–78.

Nakamura, M., Yamanobe, T., Suyemitsu, T., Komukai, M., Kan, R., Okinaga, S., and Arai, K. (1991) A new membrane-associated Ca^{2+}-binding protein of rat spermatogenic cells: its purification and characterization. Biochem. Biophys. Res. Commun. **176**, 1358–1364.

Palczewski, K., Subbaraya, I., Gorczyca, W.A., Helekar, B.S., Ruiz, C.C., Ohguro, H., Huang, J., Zhao, X., Crabb, J.W., Johnson, R.S., Walsh, K.A., Gray-Keller, M.P., Detwiler, P.B., and Baehr, W. (1994) Molecular cloning and characterization of retinal photoreceptor guanylyl cyclase-activating protein. Neuron **13**, 395–404.

Palmisano, W.A., Trevino, C.L., and Henzl, M.T. (1990) Site-specific replacement of amino acid residues within the CD binding loop of rat oncomodulin. J. Biol. Chem. **265**, 14450–14456.

Pauls, T.L., Durussel, I., Cox, J.A., Clark, I., Szabo, A.G., Gagné, S.M., Sykes, B.D., and Berchtold, M.W. (1993) Metal binding properties of recombinant rat parvalbumin wildtype and F102W mutant. J. Biol. Chem. **268**, 20897–20903.

Pauls, T.L., Durussel, I., Berchtold, M.W., and Cox, J.A. (1994) Inactivation of individual Ca^{2+}-binding sites in the paired EF-hand domain of parvalbumin reveals asymmetrical metal-binding properties. Biochemistry **33**, 10393–10400.

Pearlstone, J.R., Borgford, T., Chandra, M., Oikawa, K., Kay, C.M., Herzberg, O., Moult, J., Herklotz, A., Reinach, F.C., and Smillie, L.B. (1992) Construction and characterization of a spectral probe mutant of troponin C: application to analyses of mutants with increased Ca^{2+} affinity. Biochemistry **31**, 6545–6553.

Pedrocchi, M., Schäfer, B.W., Durussel, I., Cox, J.A., and Heizmann, C.W. (1994) Purification and characterization of the recombinant human calcium-binding S100 proteins, CAPL and CACY. Biochemistry **33**, 6732–6738.

Perrin, D.D. and Sayce, I.G. (1967) Computer calculation of equilibrium concentrations in mixtures of metal ions and complexing species. Talanta **14**, 833–842.

Petrova, T.V., Comte, M., Takagi, T., and Cox, J.A. (1995) Thermodynamic and molecular properties of the interaction between amphioxus calcium vector protein and its 26 kDa target. Biochemistry **34**, 312–318.

Porumb, T., Yau, P., Harvey, T.S., and Ikura, M. (1994) A calmodulin-target peptide hybrid molecule with unique calcium-binding properties. Prot. Engin. **7**, 109–115.

Potter, J.D. and Gergely, J. (1975) The calcium and magnesium binding sites on troponin and their role in the regulation of myofibrillar ATPase. J. Biol. Chem. **250**, 4628–4633.

Sakane, F., Yamada, K., Imai, S., and Kanoh, H. (1991) Porcine 890-kDa diacylglycerol kinase is a calcium-binding and calcium/phospholipid dependent enzyme and undergoes calcium-dependent translocations. J. Biol. Chem. **266**, 7096–7100.

Saroff, H.A. (1992) Analysis of individual-site binding data. Anal. Biochem. **205**, 143–150.

Skelton, N.J., Kördel, J., Akke, M., Forsén, S., and Chazin, W.J. (1994) Signal transduction versus buffering activity in Ca^{2+}-binding proteins. Struct. Biol. **1**, 239–245.

Starovasnik, M.A., Su, D.-R., Beckingham, K., and Klevit, R.E. (1992) A series of point mutations reveal interactions between the calcium-binding sites of calmodulin. Protein Sci. **1**, 245–253.

Starovasnik, M.A., Davis, T.N., and Klevit, R.E. (1993) Similarities and differences between yeast and vertebrate calmodulin: an examination of the calcium binding and structural properties of calmodulin from the yeast *Saccharomyces cerevisiae*. Biochemistry **32**, 3261–3270.

Trigo-Gonzales, G., Racher, K., Burtnick, L., and Borgford, T. (1992) A comparative spectroscopic study of tryptophan probes engineered into high- and low-affinity domains of recombinant chicken troponin C. Biochemistry **31**, 7009–7015

Waltersson, Y., Linse, S., Brodin, P., and Grundström, T. (1993) Mutational effects on the cooperativity of Ca^{2+}-binding in calmodulin. Biochemistry **32**, 7866–7871.

Williams, R.J.P. (1994) Calcium-binding proteins in normal and transformed cells. Cell Calcium **16**, 339–346.

Wnuk, W., Cox, J.A., Kohler, L.G., and Stein, E.A. (1979) Calcium and magnesium binding properties of a high-affinity calcium-binding protein from crayfish sarcoplasm. J. Biol. Chem: **254**, 5284–5289.

Wnuk, W., Cox, J.A., and Stein, E.A. (1981) Structural changes induced by calcium and magnesium in a high affinity protein from crayfish sarcoplasm. J. Biol. Chem. **256**, 11538–11544.

Wnuk, W., Cox, J.A., and Stein, E.A. (1982) Parvalbumin and other soluble sarcoplasmic Ca-binding proteins. In *Calcium and cell function*, (ed. W.Y. Cheung), Vol. II, Academic Press Inc. pp. 243–278.

Womack, F.C. and Colowick, S.P. (1973) Rapid measurement of binding of ligands by rate of dialysis. Methods Enzymology **27**, 464–471.

Xie, X., Harrison, D.H., Schlichting, I., Sweet, R.M., Kalabokis, V.N., Szent-Györgyi, A.G., and Cohen, C. (1994) Structure of the regulatory domain of scallop myosin at 2.8 Å resolution. Nature **368**, 306–312.

Yazawa, M.,Vorherr, T., James, P., Carafoli, E., and Yagi, K. (1992) Binding of calcium by calmodulin: influence of the calmodulin binding domain of the plasma membrane calcium pump. Biochemistry **31**, 3171–3176.

Yoshida, M., Minowa, O., and Yagi, K. (1983) Divalent cation binding to wheat calmodulin. J. Biochem. **94**, 1925–1933.

■ *J.A. Cox:*
Department of Biochemistry,
University of Geneva,
1211, Geneva 4, Switzerland,
Tel. (022) 702 64 91
Fax (022) 702 64 83
E-mail cox sc2a.unige.ch

1

EF-Hand Calcium-binding Proteins and Analogs

Introduction to EF-hand calcium-binding proteins

Introduction

The superfamily of EF-hand helix–loop–helix Ca^{2+}-binding proteins represents the largest and best characterized group embraced by this highly homologous class of molecules. At the present time, 39 subfamilies (11 of which have come to light in the last 5 years alone), embodying more than 250 proteins in all, have been described, and the number being discovered continues to escalate (reviewed by Kawasaki and Kretsinger 1994; Nakayama and Kretsinger 1994). All of these proteins share a common structural motif, which consists of a Ca^{2+}-binding loop flanked by two α-helices orientated almost perpendicularly with respect to one another. The designation "EF-hand" derives from a description of the C-terminal E-helix–loop–F-helix Ca^{2+}-binding site in parvalbumin (Fig. 1; Kretsinger and Nockolds 1973). This motif permits reversible binding of Ca^{2+}, with dissociation constants lying in the nanomolar to micromolar range (0.001–10 µM), i.e., corresponding to the cytoplasmic levels of this divalent cation in resting and stimulated cells, respectively.

History

Parvalbumin was not only the first EF-hand Ca^{2+}-binding protein to be purified (Henrotte 1955), sequenced (Pechére et al. 1971) and crystallized (Kretsinger et al. 1971), but it was also the first of this entire class of molecules to be extracted; this took place in 1934, when it was recognized as a low molecular weight, water soluble, acidic protein (Deuticke 1934). Calmodulin (reviewed by Cheung 1980) and the troponin complex (reviewed by Ebashi 1980) were both identified in 1963, but the former was recognized to be a Ca^{2+}-binding protein only in 1973 (Teo and Wang 1973); the Ca^{2+}-binding subunit of the later (troponin C) was isolated two years earlier (Greaser and Gergely 1971). S100A1 and S100b were extracted from brain tissue in 1965 (Moore 1965) and vitamin D-induced calbindin D-28k from chicken intestine in 1966 (Wassermann and Taylor 1966); the latter was subsequently found to exist in a number of other tissues (Wassermann and Fullmer 1982). The structure, encoding gene sequence, pattern of expression and physiological functions of these proteins have been extensively studied in some cases (e.g. calmodulin and troponin C), whereas in others [e.g. CAM-related gene product (CRGP)], only the cDNA sequence has been identified.

The "EF-hand" Ca^{2+}-binding site

The typical canonical EF-hand Ca^{2+}-binding site consists of an α-helix (residues 1–10), a loop around the Ca^{2+} ion

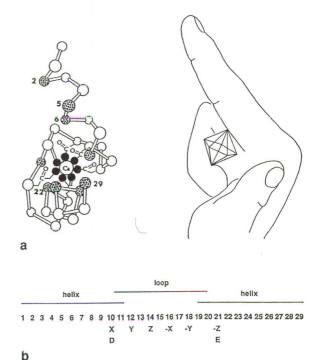

a

| helix | loop | helix |

1 2 3 4 5 6 7 8 9 10 11 12 13 14 15 16 17 18 19 20 21 22 23 24 25 26 27 28 29
              X   Y   Z   -X -Y   -Z
              D   E

b

Fig. 1 The EF-hand Ca^{2+}-binding motif. In each EF-hand motif, two α-helices, orientated at approximately 90° with respect to one another, flank a 12 amino acid-containing loop. The Ca^{2+} ion is coordinated by seven oxygen ligands (•) in a pentagonal bipyramid arrangement; five amino acid residues at positions X, Y, Z, -X and -Y provide one oxygen ligand, whereas the residue at position -Z provides two. As indicated, Asp (D) and Glu (E) are usually found at positions 10 and 21, respectively. The three-dimensional structure of the EF-hand site can be simulated by the right hand, with the extended thumb and index finger representing the α-helices and the bent middle finger indicating the Ca^{2+}-binding loop. [Modified from Moncrief et al. 1990.]

(residues 10–21), and a second α-helix (residues 19–29), which is oriented almost at right angles to the first (Fig. 1; reviewed by Kawasaki and Kretsinger 1994). The Ca^{2+} ion is coordinated by 7 oxygen ligands, which are furnished by acidic residues within the side chains, carbonyl groups of the peptide backbone and bridging water molecules; the spatial configuration thereby contrived is most aptly described as a pentagonal bipyramid (reviewed by Strynadka and James 1989; McPhalen et al. 1991). The three-dimensional structure of the EF-hand site can be simulated by the right hand, with the index finger representing the E-helix, the bent middle finger symbolizing the Ca^{2+}-binding loop, and the thumb depicting the F-helix (Fig. 1; Kretsinger and Nockolds 1973). Although most proteins within this category contain the typical EF-hand motif, a degree of divergence is nonetheless encountered in the first Ca^{2+}-binding site of the S100 proteins and in *Aquipecten* essential myosin light chain. In these proteins two additional residues occur in the first Ca^{2+}-binding loop.

The Ca^{2+}-binding loop also contains a β-pleated sheet, which is important for the pairing of two EF-hands into a tandem domain, also termed HLH domain (Strynadka and James 1989; McPhalen et al. 1991). The double EF-hand motif appears to be a basic structural feature common to all EF-hand Ca^{2+}-binding proteins, and it seems to be important for the internal organization of tandem domains during protein folding (Shaw et al. 1990) as well as for the functional properties of invidual Ca^{2+}-binding sites (Maune et al. 1992; Britto et al. 1993; Pauls et al. 1994).

■ Two types of EF-hand Ca^{2+}-binding sites

Using flow dialysis, gel filtration and diverse fluorescent techniques, the metal-binding properties of EF-hand Ca^{2+}-binding proteins have been extensively studied (Linse and Forsén 1995; see also chapter by J.A. Cox). Two distinct types of Ca^{2+}-binding sites have been distinguished on the basis of differences in selectivity and affinity for Ca^{2+} and Mg^{2+} binding, namely, a mixed Ca^{2+}/Mg^{2+} site and a Ca^{2+}-specific site (Haiech et al. 1979; Wnuk et al. 1982).

The mixed Ca^{2+}/Mg^{2+} sites bind Ca^{2+} with high affinity and Mg^{2+} with moderate affinity in a competitive manner (dissociation constants: $K_{Ca} = 10^{-7}–10^{-9}$ M; $K_{Mg} = 10^{-3}–10^{-5}$ M). Under physiological conditions, i.e., at low resting levels of Ca^{2+}, they are occupied by Mg^{2+}; when the intracellular Ca^{2+} concentration is elevated, Mg^{2+} is replaced by Ca^{2+}, a reaction which is characterized by slow kinetics. These sites are believed to play an important role in temporal buffering and transport of Ca^{2+}.

In comparison with mixed Ca^{2+}/Mg^{2+} sites, the affinity range spanned for Ca^{2+}-specific sites is two orders of magnitude lower with respect to Ca^{2+} binding and reduced still further in the case of Mg^{2+} ($K_{Ca} = 10^{-5}–10^{-7}$ M; $K_{Mg} = 10^{-1}–10^{-2}$ M). Mg^{2+} ions thus have only a minor effect on Ca^{2+} binding. In the resting cell, Ca^{2+}-specific sites are considered to be in a metal-free state, and hence in readiness to bind Ca^{2+} ions directly, with fast kinetics, when intracellular levels of this cation are raised. These sites are believed to be responsible for Ca^{2+}-dependent regulatory functions involved in protein activation.

■ Protein structure

The tertiary structure of EF-hand Ca^{2+}-binding proteins has been studied in detail by X-ray crystallography and multidimensional NMR (reviewed by Strynadka and James 1989; Kawasaki and Kretsinger 1994). Such analyses have revealed the presence of a tandem domain, composed of two helix–loop–helix Ca^{2+}-binding sites linked by peptides 5 to 10 residues in length. The invidual binding sites are integrated via antiparallel β-sheet hydrogen bonds between the two Ca^{2+}-binding loops, and by intra- and interhelical hydrophobic interactions between the amphipathic helices. The tandem domain can be visualized as a cup, the bottom of which is formed by the Ca^{2+}-binding loops and the sides by the α-helices, with the outside and rim covered by charged, hydrophilic residues and the inside lined by the relatively exposed hydrophobic ones (reviewed by Strynadka and James 1989; Linse and Forsén 1995). Each tandem domain represents a structurally conserved architectural unit. Differences between proteins involve mainly modifications to the peptide chains linking adjacent EF-hand motifs, and structural additions to the N-termini of the tandem domain itself.

Most of the EF-hand Ca^{2+}-binding proteins contain four EF-hand motifs (e.g. calmodulin, troponin C, essential light chain, regulatory light chain; see Table 1 and the review by Kawasaki and Kretsinger 1994), which are organized into two tandem domains. In the case of calmodulin, this arrangement has been likened to the form of a dumb-bell. However, proteins possessing two (e.g. S100, diacyl-glycerol kinase and α-actinin), six (calbindin D-28k and calretinin) or eight (SPEC-like protein) EF-hand motifs also exist, and it is believed that these too are organized into tandem domains.

Proteins containing an odd number of EF-hand motifs, namely, one (psoriasin), three (parvalbumin, aequorin and protein phosphatase) or five (*Plasmodium falciparum* surface membrane protein), have also been described; in these cases, one site must necessarily remain unpaired. In the case of parvalbumin, the "missing" EF-hand site is known to be lost by deletion from cDNA whereas in other proteins, it may still be present but modified beyond recognition.

■ Localization/distribution

EF-hand Ca^{2+}-binding proteins are found in all living organisms, from prokaryotes to eukaryotes, and in the latter, throughout the entire plant (fungi included) and animal kingdoms. With the exception of S100b and avian thymic hormone, which can be found in the blood stream, they are localized principally within the cell; in only a few cases are they found associated with membranes or organelles. An increasing number of EF-hand Ca^{2+}-binding proteins with different developmental and tissue-specific patterns of expression are being discovered (for review, see Heizmann and Braun 1990). Recoverin, visinin and S-modulin, for example, are found exclusively in the brain, whereas parvalbumin and calbindin D-28k are also found in other tissues. They are of great interest morphologically in that they render possible selective visualization of cells, pathways and nuclei in a manner not previously possible. Yet again, there are other members which are restricted to specific cells, such as troponin C distributed in skeletal and cardiac muscle fibres, or present ubiquitiously, such as calmodulin in all

Table 1. Subfamilies of EF-hand Ca²⁺-binding proteins

#	Name	Kingdom	Function	Structure	1	2	3	4	5	6	7	8
1	Calmodulin	APFPr	+	X	+	+	+	+/−				
2	Troponin C	A	+	X	+/−	+	+/−	+				
3	Essential light chain (myosin)	A F	+	X	&/−	+/−	+/−	+/−				
4	Regulatory light chain (myosin)	A FPr	+	X	+	−	−	−				
5	Troponin, nonvertebrate	A	+	?	−	+	+/−	+				
6*	Cal1-*C. elegans*	A	+	?	+	+	+	+				
7	Squidulin-*Loligo*	A	?	?	+	+	+	+				
8	Centrin	APFPr	?	?	+	+/−	+/−	+				
9	Ca-dependent protein kinase (*Plasmodium*)	P	+	? ::::	+	+	+	+				
10*	LAV1-*Physarum*	F	?	? ::::	+	+	+	+				
11*	EFH5	P	?	?	−	+/−	+/−	−				
12	Calcineurin	A FPr	+	?	+	+	+	+				
13	Calcyphosine-*Canis*	A	?	?	+	+	+	?				
14	Calbindin D-28k	A	?	?	+	+/−	+	+	+	−		
15	Parvalbumin	A	?	X		−	+	+				
16	S100's	A	?	X	&/−	+						
17	Diacylglycerol kinase	A	+	? ::::	+	+::::						
18	α-Actinin	A	+	? ::::	+/−	+/−						
19	rdgC protein phosphatase-*Drosophila*	A	+	? ::::	−	::−::	+	+				
20*	*Strongylocentrotus* Ca²⁺-binding protein	A	?	?	+/−	+	+	+/−				
21	SPEC-resembling protein	A	?	?	+	+	+	+	+	+	+	−
22	Aequorin and luciferin-binding protein	A	+	?	+	::−::	+	+				
23	Ca²⁺ vector protein-*Branchiostoma*	A	?	?	−	−	+	+				
24	Flagelar calcium-binding protein-*Trypanosoma*	Pr	?	?	+	+	+	+				
25	Calpain and Sorcin	A	+	? (::)	+	+	−	−				
26*	Surface protein-*Plasmodium*	Pr	?	? ::::	+	+	+	+	+::::			
27	Sarcoplasmic Ca²⁺-binding protein	A	?	X	+	+/−	+	+/−				
28	Visinin and recoverin	A	+	X	−	+	+	−				
29*	Calerythrin, *Saccharopolyspora erythrea*	Proc	?	?	+	+	+	+				
30	*Tetrahymena* Ca²⁺-binding protein (TCBP)	Pr	?	?	−	+	+	+				
31	Calmodulin-related protein-*Homo*	A	?	?	+	+						
32	Calmodulin domain protein kinase	P Pr	+	? ::::	+	+	+	+				
33*	PM 129 from *Arabidopsis thaliana*	P	?	?	+	+	+	+				
34*	Calmodulin-like protein from *Arabidopsis*	P	?	?	+	+	+	+				
35*	pCAST clone from *Solanum tuberosum*	P	?	?	+	−	+	+				
36	Trichohyalin and Profilaggrin	A	?	?	+	+::::						
37	Reticulocalbin	A	?	?	+	+	+	+	+	+		
38	Psoriasin (S100A7)	A	?	?	::−::	+						

The 39 subfamilies of EF-hand Ca²⁺-binding proteins; members indicated by an asterisk are not discussed in this book. In instances where the generic name is given, the relevant protein has been found in only one species. Under *Kingdom*, information respecting the known occurrence of the named protein in animal (A), plant (P), fungus (F), protist (Pr) or procaryote (Proc) divisions is given. The column headed *Function* reveals whether this has been elucidated (+) or not (?). Under *Structure*, the symbols "x" and "?" denote whether this has been elucidated (by crystal/solution (NMR) analysis) or not, respectively; the designation ":::::" indicates that non-EF-hand domains form part of the chimeric protein and are located either at the N- or C-terminal sides of the tandem EF-hands (see also under "Number of EF-hand sites"); "(::)" used in conjunction with calpain and sorcin denotes that the former possesses an N-terminal sulphydryl protease domain whereas the latter does not. The number of EF-hand sites characterizing a particular subfamily of proteins ranges from one to eight, indicated accordingly by the appropriate digit. For each site, the observed or inferred Ca²⁺-binding facility is represented as being present (+), present or absent according to the source from which material was derived (+/−), or absent (−); with respect to parvalbumin, site 1 is inferred to have been deleted during evolution; the symbol "&" indicates unique Ca²⁺-ion coordinations in site 1 of S100 and molluscan essential myosin light chain; "::−::", used in reference to site 2 of protein phosphatase and aequorin, denotes that the corresponding region is not recognizable as an EF-hand homologue (which does not, of course, exclude the possibility of its having diverged beyond recognition). [Table and legend modified from Kawasaki and Kretsinger 1994.]

eukaryotic cells. The tissue distribution of EF-hand Ca^{2+}-binding proteins varies considerable between species, and use of this criterion as a means of delineating function is thus not dependable. The complexity of the situation may be readily appreciated when one bears in mind that for a given organism, tissue-specific differences in the temporal regulation of Ca^{2+}-binding protein expression also exist [e.g. expression of calbindin-D28k and calretinin in developing chick pineal gland (Bastianelli and Pochet 1994) and retina (Ellis et al. 1991)].

Genomic localization, gene structure and protein expression

No general chromosomal clustering of genes encoding for different EF-hand Ca^{2+}-binding proteins has been recognized, suggesting the absence of selective pressure for maintaining such an association (reviewed by Berchtold 1993). The sole exception is represented by the S100 family, for which at least 10 genes are grouped together on human chromosome 1q12-25 (Schäfer et al. 1995; see also chapter S100 proteins). All S100 genes have an intron which separates the two exons encoding for the EF-hand sites, and this indicates that the latter may have evolved from a single ancestral gene by duplication. It is not at present clear whether clustering in this case results from recent divergence in default of chromosomal rearrangements or from the existence of a selective pressure for maintaining gene proximity. Several of the EF-hand Ca^{2+}-binding protein genes conserved in human and mouse genomes (e.g. the IDH1 – and myosin light-chain genes MLCF1F/MLC3F) map to known syntenic groups, i.e. regions comprising genes which remain together during chromosomal translocation, and it is hypothesized that this latter phenomenon took place prior to divergence of these species (reviewed by Berchtold 1993). For human calmodulin, three genes (CaM I–III) have been detected on three different chromosomes. Although they code for an identical protein, these genes have highly diverging nucleotide sequences, which exploit the redundancy of the genetic code; several pseudogenes and expressed intronless calmodulin-like genes are also known to exist (Fischer et al. 1988; Koller and Strehler 1988).

Analysis of 35 intron sites within 15 subfamilies of EF-hand protein genes has revealed that 13 of these are located between domains and 22 within them (reviewed by Kretsinger and Nakayama 1993). The positions occupied by intra- and interdomainal introns follow a random distribution, which argues strongly against the importance of exon shuffling in the evolution of EF-hand homolog proteins. Exons do not, therefore, correspond to, or define, the structural and functional EF-hand sites. On the other hand, many intron sequences have diverged in parallel with the exon and protein sequences, and intron/exon junctions are highly conserved in subfamilies. Of the 7 exons known in calbindin D-28k and calretinin genes, junctional regions are precisely maintained with respect both to phase and position (Wilson et al. 1988). Taken together, these findings suggest that EF-hands have evolved by a complex pattern of gene duplication,

gene rearrangements (transposition) and splicing (reviewed by Berchtold, 1993).

EF-hand Ca^{2+}-binding proteins, with the notable exception of calmodulin, are expressed in a tissue- and cell-specific pattern. The expression of calmodulin by multiple genes in higher organisms may fulfil a protective role against deleterious mutations in any one of these (Fischer et al. 1988). Differential patterns of expression have been observed for CaM I and CaM II genes in rat tissue (Nojima et al. 1987), and on the basis of these and other data, it has been concluded that the former represents the housekeeping gene, controlling the basal level of calmodulin, whereas the other(s) are expressed in a tissue-specific fashion. The high degree to which calmodulin is conserved in different species is believed to reflect its being the target for a large number of interacting molecules.

Several genes of EF-hand Ca^{2+}-binding proteins are known to be transcriptionally regulated, for instance S100A7 (psoriasin) by retinoic acid (Hoffmann et al. 1994) and calbindin-D9k by glucocorticoids or 1,25-dihydroxy vitamin D_3 (Christakos et al. 1992); the latter also induces the expression of intestinal calbindin-D-28k, and recent promotor analysis of the murine gene encoding this protein has revealed the presence of several vitamin D-responsive elements (Christakos et al. 1992; Takeda et al. 1994).

Functions: Ca^{2+} signal transducer, enzymes and Ca^{2+} buffers

Three important functional aspects can be assigned to EF-hand Ca^{2+}-binding proteins: the mediation of Ca^{2+} signals, a direct Ca^{2+}-dependent enzymatic activity, and the buffering of the cytosolic Ca^{2+} concentration.

Members of the first group interact with target proteins in a Ca^{2+}-dependent manner, thereby modulating protein activation. For example, the binding of Ca^{2+} to calmodulin induces marked conformational changes, which enable it to interact with, and regulate the activity of a large number of different target proteins (reviewed by Veigl et al. 1984; Cohen and Klee 1988; Crivici and Ikura 1995). In contrast, troponin C, which has a very similar overall structure to calmodulin (Herzberg and James 1985), is involved solely in the Ca^{2+}-dependent regulation of skeletal and heart muscle contraction.

Proteins within the second group manifest direct Ca^{2+}-dependent enzymatic activity. Currently, several subfamilies have been described, including aequorin, Ca^{2+}-dependent protein kinase, calcineurin, diacylglycerol-kinase, rdgC serine/threonine phosphatase, calpain and calmodulin domain protein kinase. Calcineurin, for example, is a Ca^{2+}- and calmodulin-dependent protein phosphatase with two subunits, and it is the EF-hand-containing one which is regulatory (Liu and Storm 1989; Jain et al. 1993).

Members of the third group do not interact with other proteins but themselves act as intracellular Ca^{2+}-buffers, thereby modulating the free cytosolic levels of this cation. Parvalbumin (reviewed by Pauls et al. 1996) and sarcoplasmic Ca^{2+}-binding protein (reviewed by Cox

1990) belong to this category. They are believed to exert an important influence on the Ca^{2+}/Mg^{2+}-exchange system in fast skeletal muscle fibers of vertebrates and invertebrates, respectively.

For the majority of EF-hand Ca^{2+}-binding proteins, no specific function, other than the ability to bind Ca^{2+} ions, has been elucidated. For some proteins of the 'buffer'-type (e.g. calbindin-D-28k, calretinin and parvalbumin), a possible role in protecting cells from Ca^{2+} overload has been proposed; their presence could help to efficiently buffer prolonged Ca^{2+} transients which would otherwise lead to cytotoxic effects. Several groups have shown that overexpression of Ca^{2+}-binding proteins in culture systems can modulate Ca^{2+} transients and protect cells from apoptosis due to elevated levels of this cation (Dowd et al. 1992; Lledo et al. 1992). The development of several neurodegenerative diseases has been attributed to the failure of such a protective mechanism.

■ EF-hand Ca^{2+}-binding proteins in disease and as diagnostic tools

The expression of several EF-hand Ca^{2+}-binding proteins is known to be modified in various human diseases. The level of calmodulin, an important regulator in proliferation and cell cycle progression (reviewed by Cohen and Klee 1988; Means et al. 1991), is increased several-fold in tumour cells (Watterson et al. 1976; Chafouleas et al. 1981; Van Eldik and Burgess 1983) and tissue (MacManus et al. 1981; Wei and Hickie 1981), as are the cerebrospinal fluid and blood levels of astrocytic S100b protein in patients with cerebral infarction, transient ischaemic attacks, haemorrhagy, head injury (Persson et al. 1987) or Down's syndrome (Griffin et al. 1989). Reduced profilaggrin expression or conversion to filaggrin has been observed in patients with ichthyosis, dry-skin disease (see chapter by de Viragh). Nonetheless, it still remains to be established whether modified expression of these proteins is the cause or consequence of these disease conditions. Albeit so, various Ca^{2+}-binding proteins have been implemented as diagnostic tools. Antibodies against S100b are used to diagnose and classify tumours of glial and other origin (Kahn et al. 1983; Van Eldik et al. 1986), and calretinin is known to be a marker for colon cancer cells (Gotzos et al. 1992 and unpublished observations) and mesotheliomas (Gotzos et al. 1996). In certain human neurodegenerative disorders, such as Alzheimer's, Huntington's and Parkinson's disease, calbindin D-28k, parvalbumin and S100 may have a protective capacity (reviewed by Heizmann and Braun 1992; Andressen et al. 1993) since cells containing one or other of these proteins appear to be more resistant to cell death. This proposal is, however, still controversial, and further studies are required to put it on a firm footing.

■ References

Andressen, C., Blümcke, I., & Celio, M.R. (1993) Calcium-binding proteins: selective markers of nerve cells. Cell Tissue Res. 271, 181–208.

Bastianelli, E., & Pochet, R. (1994) Calbindin-D28K, calretinin, and recoverin immunoreactivities in developing chick pineal gland. J. Pineal Res. 17, 103–111.

Berchtold, M.W. (1993) Evolution of EF-hand calcium-modulated proteins. V. The genes encoding EF-hand proteins are not clustered in mammalian genomes. J. Mol. Evol. 36, 489–496.

Brito, R.M.M., Krudy, G.A., Negele, J.C., Putkey, J.A., & Rosevear, P.R. (1993) Calcium plays distinctive structural roles in the N- and C-terminal domains of cardiac troponin C. J. Biol. Chem. 268, 20966–20973.

Chafouleas, J.G., Pardue, R.L., Brinkley, B.R., Dedman, H.R., & Means, A.R. (1981) Regulation of intracellular levels of calmodulin and tubulin in normal and transformed cells. Proc. Natl. Acad. Sci. USA 78, 996–1000.

Cheung, W.Y. (1980) Calmodulin plays a pivotal role in cellular regulation. Science 207: 19–27.

Christakos, S., Gill, R., Lee, S., & Li, H. (1992) Molecular aspects of the calbindins. J. Nutr. 122, 678–682.

Cohen, P., & Klee, C.B. (1988) Calmodulin. Elsevier, Amsterdam – New York – Oxford.

Cox, J.A. (1990) The role of intracellular calcium binding proteins. In: Stimulus Response coupling (J.-R. Dedman and Smith, V.L. ed.) pp. 266–269, CRC Press, Boca Raton, Ann Arbor, Boston.

Crivici, A., & Ikura, M. (1995) Molecular and structural basis of target recognition by calmodulin. Ann. Rev. Biophys. Biomol. Struct. 24, 85–116.

Deuticke, H.J. (1934) Ueber die Sedimentationskonstante von Muskelproteinen. Hoppe Seyler's Z. physiol. Chemie. 224: 216–228.

Dowd, D.R., MacDonald, R.N., Komm, B.S., Haussler, M.R., & Miesfeld, R.L. (1992) Stable expression of the calbindin-D28K complementary DNA interferes with the apoptotic pathway in lymphocytes. Mol. Endocrinol. 6 (11), 1843–1848.

Ebashi, S. (1980) Regulation of muscle contraction. Proc. R. Soc. London B. 207: 259–286.

Ellis, J.H., Richards, D.E., & Rogers, J.H. (1991) Calretinin and calbindin in the retina of the developing chick. Cell Tissue Res. 264, 197–208.

Fischer, R., Koller, M., Flura, M., Mathews, S., Strehler-Page, M.A., Krebs, J., Penniston, J.T. Carafoli, E., & Strehler, E.E. (1988) Multiple divergent mRNAs code for a single human calmodulin. J. Biol. Chem. 263, 17055–62.

Greaser, M.L. and Gergely, J. (1971) Reconstitution of troponin activity from three protein components. J. Biol. Chem. 246, 4226–4233.

Griffin, W.S., Stanley L.C., Ling, C., White, L., MacLeod V., Perrot L.J., White C.L., Araoz, C. (1989) Brain interleukin 1 and S-100 immunoreactivity are elevated in Down syndrome and Alzheimer disease. Proc. Natl. Acad. Sci. (USA) 86, 7611–7615.

Gotzos, V., Schwaller, B., Heztl, N., Bustos-Castillo, M., & Celio, M.R. (1992) Expression of the calcium-binding protein calretinin in WiDr cells and its correlation to their cell cycle. Exp. Cell Res. 202, 292–302.

Gotzos, V., Vogt, P. & Celio M.R. (1996) Calretinin as a marker of mesotheliomas of the epithelial type. Path. Res. Pract., 192, 1–9.

Haiech, J., Derancourt, J., Pechére, J.-F., & Demaille, J.G. (1979) Magnesium and calcium binding to parvalbumins: Evidence for differences between parvalbumins and an explanation of their relaxing function. Biochemistry 18, 2752–2758.

Heizmann, C.W., & Braun, K. (1990) Calcium binding proteins: Molecular and functional aspects. In: The role of calcium in biological systems (ed. L.J. Anghileri) 5, pp. 21–66, CRC Press.

Heizmann, C.W., & Braun, K. (1992) Changes in Ca^{2+}-binding proteins in human neurodegenerative disorders. Trends Neurosci. 15, 259–264.

Henrotte, J.G. (1955) A crystalline constituent from myogen of carp muscle. Nature 169, 968–969.

Herzberg, O., & James, M.N.G. (1985) Structure of the calcium regulatory muscle protein troponin-C at 28 Å resolution. Nature **313**, 653–659.

Hoffmann, H.J., Olsen, E., Etzerodt, M., Madsen, P., Thogersen, H.C., Kruse, T., & Celis, J.E. (1994) Psoriasin binds calcium and is upregulated by calcium to levels that resemble those observed in normal skin. J. Invest. Dermatol. **103**, 370–375.

Jain, J., McCaffrey, P.G., Miner, Z., Kerppola, T.K., Lambert, J.N., Verdine, G.L., Curran, T., & Rao, A. (1993) The T-cell transcription factor NFAT$_p$ is a substrate for calcineurin and interacts with Fos and Jun. Nature **365**, 352–355.

Kahn, H.J., Marks, A., Thom, H., & Baumal, R. (1983) Role of antibody to S100 protein in diagnostic pathology. Ann. J. Clin. Pathol. **79**, 314–347.

Kawasaki, H., & Kretsinger, R.H. (1994) Calcium-binding proteins 1: EF-hands. Protein Profile **1**, 343–517.

Koller, M., & Strehler, E.E. (1988) Characterization of an intronless human calmodulin-like pseudogene. FEBS Lett. **239**, 121–128.

Kretsinger, R.H., & Nakayama, S. (1993) Evolution of EF-hand calcium-modulated proteins. IV. Exon shuffling did not determine the domain compositions of the EF-hand proteins. J. Mol. Evol. **36**, 477–488.

Kretsinger, R.H., & Nockolds, C.E. (1973) Carp muscle calcium-binding protein. II. Structure determination and general description. J. Biol. Chem. **248**, 3313–3326.

Kretsinger, R.H., Nockolds, C.E., Coffee, C.J., & Bradshaw, R.A. (1971) The structure of a calcium binding protein from a carp muscle. Cold Spring Harbor Symp. Quant. Biol. **36**, 217–220.

Linse, S., & Forsén, S. (1995) Determinants that govern high-affinity calcium-binding. Adv. Second Mess. and Phosphoprot. Res. **30**, 89–151.

Liu, Y., & Storm, D.R. (1989) Dephosphorylation of neuromodulin by calcineurin, J. Biol. Chem. **264**, 12800–12804.

Lledo, P.-M., Somasundaram, B., Morton, A.J., Emson, P.C., & Mason, W.T. (1992) Stable transfection of calbindin-D28k into the GH3 cell line alters calcium currents and intracellular calcium homeostasis. Neuron **9**, 943–954.

MacManus, J.P., Braceland, B.M., Rixon, R.H., Whitfield, J.F., & Morris, H.P. (1981) An increase in calmodulin during growth of normal and cancerous liver in vivo. FEBS Lett. **133**, 99–102.

Manune, J.F., Klee, C.B., & Beckingham, K. (1992) Ca^{2+} binding and conformational change in two series of point mutations to the individual Ca^{2+}-binding sites of calmodulin. J. Biol. Chem. **267**, 5286–5295.

McPhalen, C.A., Strynadka, N.C., & James, M.N. (1991) Calcium-binding sites in proteins: a structural perspective. Adv. Protein Chem. **42**, 77–144.

Means, A.R., VanBerkum, M.F., Bagchi, I., Lu, K.P., & Rasmussen, C.D. (1991) Regulatory functions of calmodulin. Pharmacol. Ther. **50**, 255–70.

Moore, B. (1965) A soluble protein characteristic of the nervous system. Biochem. Biophys. Res. Commun. **19**: 739–744.

Nakayama, S., & Kretsinger, R.H. (1994) Evolution of EF-hand family of proteins. Ann. Rev. Biophys. Biomol. Struct. **23**, 473–507.

Nojima, H., Kishi, K., & Sokabe, H. (1987) Multiple calmodulin mRNA species are derived from two distinct genes. Mol. Cell. Biol. **7**, 1873–1880.

Pauls, T.L., Durussel, I., Berchtold, M.W., & Cox, J.A. (1994) Inactivation of individual Ca^{2+}-binding sites in the paired EF-hand domain of parvalbumin reveals asymmetrical metal-binding properties. Biochemistry **33**, 10393–10400.

Pauls, T.L., Cox, J.A. & Berchtold, M.W. (1996) The Ca^{2+} binding proteins parvalbumin and oncomodulin: New structural and functional findings. Biochim. Biophys. Acta, in press.

Pechère, J.-F., Capony, J.P., Ryden, L., & De Maille, J. (1971) The amino acid sequence of the major parvalbumin from hake muscle. Biochem. Biophys. Res. Commun. **43**, 1106–1111.

Persson L., Hardemark H.G., Gustafsson J. Rundstrom G. Mnedl I., Esscher T., Pahlman S. (1987) S-100 protein and neuron-specific enolase in cerebrospinal fluid and serum: markers of cell damage in human central nervous system. Stroke **18**, 911–918.

Schäfer, B.W., Wicki, R., Engelkamp, D., Mattel, M.G., & Heizmann, C.W. (1995) Isolation of a YAC clone covering a cluster of nine S100 genes on human chromosome 1q21: Rationale for a new nomenclature of the S100 calcium-binding protein family. Genomics **25**, 638–643.

Shaw, G., Hodges, R.S., & Sykes, B.D. (1990) Calcium-induced peptide association to form an intact protein domain: H NMR structural evidence. Science **249**, 280–283.

Strynadka, N.C.J., & James, M.N.G. (1989) Crystal structures of the helix-loop-helix calcium-binding proteins. Ann. Rev. Biochem. **58**, 951–998.

Takeda, T., Arakawa, M., & Kuwano, R. (1994) Organization and expression of the mouse spot35lcalbindin-D28k gene: identification of the vitamin D-responsive promoter region. Biochem. Biophys. Res. Commun. **204**, 889–897.

Teo, T.S. and Wang, J.H. (1973) Mechanism of activation of a cyclic adenosine-3'-5'-monophosphate diesterase from rat heart. J. Biol. Chem. **248**: 5950–5955

VanEldik, L.J., Jensen, R.A., Ehrenfried, B.A., & Whetsell Jr., W.O. (1986) Immunohistochemical localization of S100b in human nervous system tumours by using monoclonal antibodies with specificity for the S100b polypeptide. J. Histochem. Cytochem. **34**, 977–982.

VanEldik, L.J., & Burgess, W.H. (1983) Analytical subcellular distribution of calmodulin and calmodulin binding proteins in normal and virus-transformed fibroblasts. J. Biol. Chem. **258**, 4539–4547.

Veigl, M.L., Vanaman, T.C., & Sedwick, W.D. (1984) Calcium and calmodulin in cell growth and transformation. Biochim. Biophys. Acta **738**, 21–48.

Wassermann, R.H. & Fullmer C.S. (1982) Vitamin D- induced calcium-binding protein. In: Cheung W.Y. (Ed.) Calcium and cell function. Academic Press, New York, pp. 175–216.

Wasserman, R.H., & Taylor, A.N. (1966) Vitamin D3-induced calcium-binding protein in chick intestinal mucosa. Science **152**, 791–793.

Watterson, D.M., VanEldik, L.J., Smith, R.E., & Vanaman, T.C. (1976) Calcium-dependent regulatory protein of cyclic nucleotide metabolism in normal and transformed chicken embryo fibroblasts. Proc. Natl. Acad. Sci. USA **73**, 2711–2715.

Wei, J.-W., & Hickie, R.A. (1981) Increased content of calmodulin in Morris hepatoma 5123 t.c.(h). Biochem, Biophys. Res. Commun. **100**, 1562–1568.

Wilson, P.W., Rogers, J., Harding, M., Pohl, V., Pattyn, G., & Lawson, D.E.M. (1988) Structure of chick chromosomal genes for calbindin and calretinin. J. Mol. Biol. **200**, 615–625.

Wnuk, W., Cox, J.A., & Stein, E.A. (1982) Parvalbumins and other soluble high-affinity calcium-binding proteins from muscle. **In:** Calcium and Cell Function (W.Y. Cheung ed.) 2, pp. 243–278, Academic Press, New York.

■ *Marco R. Celio*
Thomas L. Pauls
Beat Schwaller
Institute of Histology and General Embryology,
University of Fribourg,
CH-1705 Fribourg, Switzerland.
Tel.: +41 26300 84 91
Fax: +41 26300 97 32
Emails: marco.celio@unifr.ch
thomas.pauls@unifr.ch
beat.schwaller@unifr.ch

Alpha-actinin

Alpha-actinin is a component of the actin filament system and present in muscle and non-muscle cells. In vitro it causes the gelling of an F-actin solution by its bundling and crosslinking activity. Direct binding of Ca²⁺ to typical EF-hands regulates the activity in non-muscle alpha-actinins.

Alpha-actinin was first isolated from muscle cells (Ebashi and Ebashi 1965). It is present at the Z-discs where it is proposed to crosslink ends of both parallel and antiparallel arrays of actin filaments (Endo and Masaki 1982; Meyer and Aebi 1990). In non-muscle cells it is located in cell–cell and cell–extracellular matrix junctions, and along actin filaments in fibroblasts. It belongs to a family of F-actin binding proteins that includes spectrin, dystrophin, gelation factor, filamin and fimbrin and is defined by similar and functionally homologous actin binding domains (Hemmings *et al*. 1992). Alpha-actinin is an elongated molecule consisting of two identical subunits with a molecular mass of approximately 100 kDa. In the homodimer the subunits have an antiparallel arrangement (Wallraff *et al*. 1986; Imamura *et al*. 1988). Each subunit contains an N-terminal F-actin binding site which is followed by a central rod domain formed by four spectrin-like alpha-helical repeats. Two EF-hands at the C-terminus are responsible for the Ca²⁺ regulation of non-muscle alpha-actinin. In an incomplete form they are also present in skeletal muscle alpha-actinins which exhibit a Ca²⁺-independent crosslinking activity. Mutational analyses of the two EF-hands of *Dictyostelium* alpha-actinin, a typical non-muscle alpha-actinin, indicate that they have a different impact on the activity of the molecule (Witke *et al*. 1993). The more N-terminal EF-hand is the low affinity Ca²⁺-binding site and regulates the crosslinking activity, the C-terminal EF-hand represents the high affinity binding site for Ca²⁺.

■ Identification/isolation

Alpha-actinin was isolated from striated muscle based on its activity to gel an actin solution (Ebashi and Ebashi 1965). It can also be isolated in high amounts from smooth muscle and non-muscle tissues (Endo and Masaki 1982).

■ Gene and sequence

cDNA sequences are available for alpha-actinin from *Dictyostelium discoideum* (EMBL/GenBank Y00689), chicken brain (EMBL/GenBank M74143), chicken non-muscle (EMBL D26597), chicken skeletal muscle, human non-muscle (GenBank M31300), *Drosophila* (EMBL/GenBank/DDBJ X51753). The genomic structures of *D. discoideum* alpha-actinin, *Drosophila* and human alpha-actinin are known. *Drosophila* alpha-actinin is located within subdivision 2C of the X-chromosome. A single gene gives rise to one non-muscle and two muscle isoforms by differential splicing (Roulier *et al*. 1992). The human gene is on chrommosome 14.

■ Protein

The protein is a three-domain polypeptide, the homologies among alpha-actinins extend throughout the polypeptide.

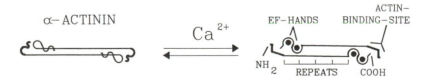

Figure 1. Proposed interaction between the Ca²⁺- and actin binding sites in *D. discoideum* alpha-actinin (Noegel *et al*. 1987). The alpha-actinin molecule is a Ca²⁺ inhibited, rod-shaped homodimer whose subunits are organized in an antiparallel fashion. The N-terminal region contains the actin binding site (bold lines), the extended structure is based on spectrin-like repeats with a high alpha-helix potential, and at the C-terminus of each subunit two EF-hands are the structural basis of the regulation by Ca²⁺. Binding of Ca²⁺ changes the conformation of the EF-hands, thus disturbing the interaction of the opposite actin binding site with the actin filament.

▪ Antibodies

Monoclonal and polyclonal antibodies recognizing the protein in muscle and non-muscle cells are available commercially from Sigma Chemicals.

▪ Anatomical localization

Alpha-actinin is a component of myofibrils and cytoskeleton. It is present in Z-bands of muscle fibres and in cell membrane-associated structures and intracellular structures corresponding to dense plaques and dense bodies. In non-muscle cells actin filaments are decorated, in amoeboid motile cells a diffuse staining of the cytosol is observed.

▪ Biological regulation

Autoregulation of its synthesis has been reported for non-muscle cells (Schulze *et al.* 1989). In *D. discoideum* the protein and RNA are present throughout development (Witke *et al.* 1986).

▪ Mutagenesis studies

Mutants lacking alpha-actinin have been described in *D. discoideum* and *Drosophila*. In *D. discoideum* the mutant cells were only marginally impaired with regard to growth. Other aspects of *D. discoideum* biology such as motility and development were not altered (Wallraff *et al.* 1986; Schleicher *et al.* 1988). Serious impairment of development was observed when double mutants lacking alpha-actinin and the gelation factor, a crosslinking protein with comparable structure and function (Noegel *et al.* 1989), were constructed (Witke *et al.* 1992). In *Drosophila* alpha-actinin mutations cause either lethal or flightless phenotypes (Fyrberg *et al.* 1990).

▪ Interactions

In focal adhesions alpha-actinin is associated with integrins, where it binds directly to the β1 subunit (Otey *et al.* 1990). An interaction with the intercellular adhesion molecule-1 (ICAM-1) was also reported (Carpén *et al.* 1992). Other interaction partners are clathrin (Merisko *et al.* 1988) and zyxin (Crawford *et al.* 1992). By binding Phosphatidyl inositol 4,5-bis-phosphate (PIP_2) it might be involved in signal transduction (Fukami *et al.* 1994).

▪ References

Carpén, O., Pallai, P., Staunton, D.E., and Springer, T.A. (1992) Association of intercellular adhesion molecule-1 (ICAM-1) with actin-containing cytoskeleton and α-actinin. J. Cell Biol. **118**, 1223–1234.

Crawford, A., Michelsen, J.W., and Beckerle, M.C. (1992) An interaction between zyxin and α-actinin. J. Cell Biol. **116**, 1381–1393.

Ebashi, S. and Ebashi F. (1965) α-Actinin, a new structural protein from striated muscle. I. preparation and action on actomyosin-ATP interaction. J. Biochem. **58**, 7–12.

Endo, T. and Masaki, T. (1982) Molecular properties and functions *in vitro* of chicken smooth muscle α-actinin in comparison with those of striated-muscle α-actinins. J. Biochem. **92**, 1457–1468.

Fukami, K., Endo, T., Imamura, M., and Takenawa, T. (1994) α-Actinin and vinculin are PIP_2-binding proteins involved in signaling by tyrosine kinase. J. Biol. Chem. **269**, 1518–1522.

Fyrberg, E., Kelly, M., Ball, E., Fyrberg, C., and Reedy, M.C. (1990) Molecular genetics of *Drosophila* alpha-actinin: mutant alleles disrupt Z disc integrity and muscle insertions. J. Cell Biol. **110**, 1999–2011.

Hemmings, L., Kuhlman, P.A., and Critchley, D.R. (1992) Analysis of the actin-binding domain of α-actinin by mutagenesis and demonstration that dystrophin contains a functionally homologous domain. J. Cell Biol. **116**, 1369–1380.

Imamura, M., Endo, M., Kuroda, T., Tanaka, T., and Masaki, T. (1988) Substructure and higher structure of chicken smooth muscle α-actinin molecule. J. Biol. Chem. **263**, 7800–7805.

Merisko, E.M., Welch, J.K., Chen, T.-Y., and Chen, M. (1988) α-Actinin and calmodulin interact with distinct sites on the arms of the clathrin trimer. J. Biol. Chem. **263**, 15705–15712.

Meyer, R.K. and Aebi, U. (1990) Bundling of actin filaments by α-actinin depends on its molecular length. J. Cell Biol. **110**, 2013–2023.

Noegel, A., Witke, W., and Schleicher M. (1987) Calcium-sensitive non-muscle α-actinin contains EF-hand structures and highly conserved regions. FEBS Lett. **221**, 391–396.

Noegel, A.A., Rapp, S., Lottspeich, F., Schleicher, M., and Stewart, M. (1989) The *Dictyostelium* gelation factor shares a putative actin binding site with α-actinins and dystrophin and also has a rod domain containing six 100-residue motifs that appear to have a cross-beta conformation. J. Cell Biol. **109**, 607–618.

Otey, C.A., Pavalko, F. M., and Burridge, K. (1990) An interaction between α-actinin and the β integrin subunit *in vitro*. J. Cell Biol. **111**, 721–729.

Roulier, E.M., Fyrberg, C., and Fyrberg, E. (1992) Perturbations of *Drosophila* α-actinin cause muscle paralysis, weakness, and atrophy but do not confer obvious nonmuscle phenotypes. J. Cell Biol. **116**, 911–922.

Schleicher, M., Noegel, A., Schwarz, T., Wallraff, E., Brink, M., Faix, J., Gerisch, G., and Isenberg, G. (1988) A *Dictyostelium* mutant with severe defects in α-actinin: its characterization using cDNA probes and monoclonal antibodies. J. Cell Sci. **90**, 59–71.

Schulze, H., Huckriede, A., Noegel, A.A., Schleicher, M., and Jockusch, B.M. (1989) α-actinin synthesis can be modulated by antisense probes and is autoregulated in non-muscle cells. EMBO J. **8**, 3587–3593.

Wallraff, E., Schleicher, M., Modersitzki, M., Rieger, D., Isenberg, G., and Gerisch. G. (1986) Selection of *Dictyostelium* mutants defective in cytoskeletal proteins: use of an antibody that binds to the ends of α-actinin rods. EMBO J. **5**, 61–67.

Witke, W., Schleicher, M., Lottspeich, F., and Noegel, A. (1986) Studies on the transcription, translation, and structure of α-actinin in *Dictyostelium discoideum*. J. Cell Biol. **103**, 969–975.

Witke, W., Schleicher, M., and Noegel A.A. (1992) Redundancy in the microfilament system: Abnormal development of *Dictyostelium* cells lacking two F-actin cross-linking proteins. Cell **68**, 53–62.

Witke, W., Hofmann, A., Köppel, B., Schleicher, M., and Noegel A.A. (1993) The Ca²⁺-binding domains in non-muscle type α-actinin: Biochemical and genetic analysis. J. Cell Biol. **121**, 599–606.

■ Angelika A. Noegel:
Max-Planck-Institute for Biochemistry,
D-82152 Martinsried
Germany
Tel.: +49 89 8578 2315
Fax: +49 89 8578 3777
E-mail: noegel@vms.biochem.mpg.de

Calbindin D-28K

Calbindin D-28k is an intracellular soluble Ca²⁺-binding protein which, together with calretinin, constitutes the six EF-hand-domain branch of the troponin C superfamily of Ca²⁺-binding proteins. Calbindin D-28k shows a tissue-specific expression pattern, in some of the tissues its expression is regulated by vitamin D.

Calbindin D-28k from various species was found to consist of 261 (mammalian) or 262 (avian) amino acids as deduced from the corresponding cDNA sequences. The molecular weight and IEP of the human protein are 30,025 and 4.54, respectively. Calbindin D-28k (similar to most other EF-hand proteins) has a rather rigid structure and readily renatures after heat- or chemical denaturaton.

■ Alternative names

Vitamin D-dependent Ca²⁺-binding protein (Wassermann and Taylor 1966), CaBP.

■ Identification/isolation

Calbindin D-28k was first observed in the chicken duodenal mucosa as a protein which is induced by vitamin D (Wassermann and Taylor 1966). Since vitamin D was also found to induce the absorption of Ca²⁺ from the intestinal lumen, the possibility of a link was obvious. Indeed, Breddermann and Wasserman (1974) found that calbindin D-28k binds with high affinity 3–4 moles of Ca²⁺ per mole of protein. The original purification procedure included a heat denaturation step. More recent procedures take advantage of the differing properties of the protein in the presence or absence of Ca²⁺, e.g. a Ca²⁺-mediated elution from cation exchange chromatography (Friedlander and Norman 1980). Calbindin D-28k can easily be produced in an active conformation in *E. coli* (Gross *et al.* 1988).

■ Gene and sequence

Calbindin cDNAs from various species, including human (Genebank accession number: X06661), rat (M31178;

M27839), mouse (M21531), chicken (Hunziker 1986) and *Drosophila* (X68566), were cloned and sequenced. Interestingly, the deduced amino acid sequences show the presence of six EF-hand domains which most likely arose by gene duplication in evolution. Domains two and six have mutated some of the amino acids required for the coordination of the Ca²⁺ ion and thus have probably lost their Ca²⁺-binding ability. A comparison of the coding sequences among the different species shows a high degree of conservation during evolution, e.g. 80% sequence identity between chicken and mammals, which is similar to that of cytochrome *c* (Hunziker and Schrickel 1988). Surprisingly, the four intact and the two degenerated EF-hand domains show a similar degree of conservation during evolution, suggesting, apart from the Ca²⁺-binding, the presence of an additional conservation pressure (Hunziker and Schrickel 1988).

Genomic calbindin D-28k clones were isolated from the chicken (Minghetti *et al.* 1988) and the human (I., Bendik, and Hunziker, W., unpublished observation). The human gene spans more than 20 kb, the coding sequence is interrupted by 10 introns and it was mapped to chromosome 8 (Parmentier *et al.* 1991). Reticulocalbin and ERC-55, two other Ca²⁺-binding proteins with six EF-hands, have a different gene structure and thus are not closely related to calbindin D-28k or calretinin.

■ Protein

The classical source of the protein has been the chicken intestinal mucosa, where it is present as 1–3% of the cytoplasmic protein. Most studies on the protein were aimed at its Ca²⁺-binding property, in the absence of any other known physiological function.

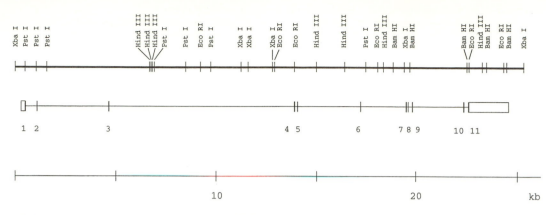

Figure 1. Restriction map of the human calbindin D-28k gene. Selected restriction sites of the human calbindin D-28 gene are shown in the top line. The exons (numbered) and introns (–) are shown below.

Antibodies

Classically, antisera were raised against the protein purified from chicken intestine. Interestingly, these antisera were found to cross-react with calbindin D-28k over a broad spectrum of animal species, including humans. Some of the antisera were later found to cross-react with calretinin, a closely related Ca²⁺-binding protein. Calbindin D-28k monoclonal antibodies that do not cross-react with calretinin are available from Swant.

Anatomical localization

Calbindin D-28k shows a tissue-specific expression pattern. In fishes calbindin D-28k is restricted to the nervous system. In amphibians and birds it also occurs in the enterocytes of the intestine, in the cells of the distal tubules of the kidney, in β-cells of the pancreas and in subpopulations of nerve cells in the nervous system (Wassermann and Fullmer 1982). In mammals calbindin D-28k persists in all these tissues with the exception of the enterocytes from which it has disappeared, being replaced by calbindin-D9k. Antibodies against calbindin D-28k are increasingly used for neuroanatomical studies of the vertebrate nervous system because they give excellent cytoarchitectural staining and visualize a Golgi-like cellular morphology (Celio 1990). They even label entire pathways and sometimes whole functional systems (for review, see Baimbridge et al. 1992 Andressen et al. 1993;). Calbindin D-28k in the brain is discussed as a buffer which may modulate cytosolic Ca²⁺ transients and thus protect nerve cells (Heizmann and Braun 1992).

Biological activities

Calbindin D-28k has one very high affinity Ca²⁺-binding site (K_d : 0.1–1 nM) located in EF-hand 1, and 2–3 sites with an affinity in the μM range (Gross et al. 1987, 1988, 1993). Aside from its Ca²⁺-binding property no physiological func-

tion is thus far established. Speculations on its function range from a pure Ca²⁺ buffer that keeps Ca²⁺ in the cytoplasm below toxic levels on the one hand, to a Ca²⁺-dependent regulatory function analogous to that of calmodulin, on the other. Calbindin D-28k has also been associated with neurodegenerative diseases such as Alzheimer's or Parkinson's disease (Heizmann and Braun 1992).

Biological regulation

Calbindin D-28k is upregulated in the kidney and the pancreas (also in the enterocytes of the intestine in amphibians and birds) by 1,25-dihydroxyvitamin D₃ (the active metabolite of vitamin D), by a mechanism similar to that of other steroid hormones. A vitamin D receptor-binding response element was described in the chicken (Boland et al. 1991) and mouse (Gill and Christakos 1993; Takeda et al. 1994) genes. In certain brain areas NGF (Iacopino et al. 1992) or glucocorticoids (Iacopino and Christakos 1990) were reported to induce the expression of calbindin D-28k.

Mutagenesis studies

Several rat calbindin D-28k mutants have been expressed in *E. coli* and their Ca²⁺-binding properties have been analysed. Mutant proteins with a deletion of EF-hand 2 or EF-hand 6, or a combined deletion of EF-hands 2+6, were found to still bind Ca²⁺ (Gross et al. 1993). Even more surprisingly, a protein containing only EF-hands 1+2 of calbindin D-28k was found to contain one Ca²⁺-binding site with a very high affinity similar to the very high affinity site of the wildtype protein (Gross et al. 1993).

References

Andressen, C., Blümcke, I., and Celio, M.R. (1993) Calcium-binding proteins–selective markers of nerve cells. Cell Tissue Res. **271**, 181–208.

Baimbridge, K.G., Celio, M.R., and Rogers, J.H. (1992) Calcium-binding proteins in the nervous system. Trends in Neuroscience **15**, 259–264.

Boland, R., Minghetti, P.P., Lowe, K.E., and Norman, A.W. (1991) Sequences near the CCAAT region and putative 1, 25-dihydroxyvitamin D3-response element and further upstream novel regulatory sequences of calbindin-D28k promoter show DNase I footprinting protection. Mol. Cell Endocrinol. **75**, 57–63.

Bredderman, P.J. and Wasserman, R.H. (1974) Chemical composition, affinity for calcium and some related properties of the vitamin D-dependent calcium-binding protein. Biochemistry **13**, 1687–1694.

Celio, M.R. (1990) Calbindin D-28k and parvalbumin in the rat nervous system. Neuroscience **35**, 375–475.

Friedlander, E.J. and Norman, A.W. (1980) Purification of chick intestinal calcium-binding protein In *Methods in enzymology*, vol. 67, 504–508. Academic Press.

Gill, R.K. and Christakos, S. (1993) Identification of sequence elements in mouse calbindin-D28k gene that confer 1, 25-dihydroxyvitamin D_3- and butyrate-inducible responses. Proc. Natl. Acad. Sci. USA. **90**, 2984–2988.

Gross, M.D., Nelssestuen, G.L. and Kumar, R. (1987) Observations on the binding of lanthanides and calcium to the vitamin D-dependent chick intestinal calcium binding protein; implications regarding calcium binding protein function. J. Biol. Chem. **262**, 6539–6545.

Gross, M.D., Kumar, R. and Hunziker, W. (1988) Expression in *Escherichia coli* of full length and mutant rat brain calbindin D28. J. Biol. Chem. **263**, 14426–14432.

Gross, M.D., Gosnell, M., Tsarbopoulos, A., and Hunziker, W. (1993) A functional and degenerate pair of EF hands contains the very high affinity calcium-binding site of calbindin-D28K. J. Biol. Chem. **268**, 20917–20922.

Heizmann, C.W. and Braun, K. (1992) Changes in calcium-binding proteins in human neurodegenerative disorders. Trends in Neuroscience **15**, 303–308.

Hunziker, W. (1986) The 28-kDa vitamin D-dependent calcium-binding protein has a six-domain structure. Proc. Natl. Acad. Sci. USA **83**, 7578–7582.

Hunziker, W. and Schrickel, S. (1988) Rat brain calbindin D28: six domain structure and extensive homology with chicken calbindin D28. Mol. Endo. **2**, 465–473.

Iacopino, A.M. and Christakos, S. (1990) Corticosterone regulates calbindin-D28k mRNA and protein levels in rat hippocampus. J. Biol. Chem. **265**, 10177–10180.

Iacopino, A.M., Christakos, S., Modi, P., and Altar, C.A. (1992) Nerve growth factor increases calcium binding protein (calbindin- D28K) in rat olfactory bulb. Brain Res. **578**, 305–310.

Minghetti, P.P., Cancela, L., Fujisawa, Y., Theofan, G., and Norman, A.W. (1988). Molecular structure of the chicken vitamin D-induced calbindin-D28k gene reveals eleven exons, six Ca^{2+}-binding domains, and numerous promoter regulatory elements. Mol. Endo. **2**, 355–367.

Parmentier, M., Passage, E., Vassart, G., and Mattei, M.G. (1991) The human calbindin D28k (CALB1) and calretinin (CALB2) genes are located at 8q21.3–>q22.1 and 16q22–>q23, respectively, suggesting a common duplication with the carbonic anhydrase isozyme loci. Cytogenet. Cell Genet. **57**, 41–43.

Takeda, T., M., Arakawa, and Kuwano, R. (1994) Organization and expression of the mouse spot 35/calbindin-D28k gene: identification of the vitamin D-responsive promoter region. Biochem. Biophys. Res. Commun. **204**, 889–897.

Wassermann, R.H. and Fullmer, C.S. (1982) Vitamin D-induced calcium-binding protein. *In Calcium and cell function*, pp. 175–216. II. Academic Press, New York.

Wassermann, R.H. and Taylor, A.N. (1966) Vitamin D_3 induced calcium-binding protein in chick intestinal mucosa. Science **152**, 791–793.

■ *Willi Hunziker:*
Dept. of Exploratory Research,
Division of Vitamins & Fine Chemicals,
F. Hoffmann-La Roche LTD,
CH-4002 Basel, Switzerland
Tel.: +4161 688 6226
Fax: +4161 688 5057
E.mail: Hunzikew@am@rocbi
Igor Bendik:
Molecular Oncology,
Dept. of Research,
University Hospital,
CH-4031 Basel, Switzerland
Tel.: +41 61 265 2387
E-mail: Bendik@ubaclu.unibas.ch

Calretinin

Calretinin (CR) is a cytosolic Ca²⁺-binding protein abundant in the nervous system and is also expressed in several adenocarcinoma cell lines. Hypothetical functions in nerve cells include Ca²⁺-buffering in resting cells and a protective role against a Ca²⁺ overload under pathological conditions.

Human calretinin (CR) has a calculated molecular mass of 31.5 kDa, migrates on SDS gels with an apparent molecular mass of 29 kDa and has an isoelectric point of 5.1. It consists of six EF-hand domains with high sequence homology to calbindin D-28k. Truncated forms of human calretinin arise by alternative splicing in cancer cell lines (Schwaller *et al.* 1995) and have calculated molecular masses of 22 and 20.5 kDa (see chapter on Calretinin-22k).

In the adult, CR is expressed mainly in distinct subpopulations of nerve cells in the central and peripheral nervous system of vertebrate and invertebrate species (Fig. 1). During rat development, CR-immunoreactivity (ir) is also transiently expressed in non-neuronal cells. CR has been detected in adenocarcinoma cell lines (Fig. 1; Gotzos *et al.* 1992). In nerve cells CR is a soluble cytosolic protein but immuno electron microscopy in cancer cells has revealed a preferential association of CR with microtubules of the mitotic spindle during mitosis (Gotzos *et al.* 1992). In nerve cells, CR is discussed as a Ca²⁺-buffer which may protect neurons against Ca²⁺ overload (Lukas and Jones 1994; Möckel and Fischer 1994).

■ Alternative names

29 kDa protein (Pochet *et al.* 1985), protein 10 (Winsky *et al.* 1989).

■ Isolation/identification

A partial chick calretinin cDNA clone was found in a library produced from chick retina mRNA (Rogers 1987). The human calretinin cDNA was isolated from a λgt11 expression library by Parmentier (1989) using an antiserum against calbindin D-28k which cross-reacted with a second protein of 29 kDa in Western blots. CR protein was identified on two-dimensional polyacrylamide gels from cytosolic extracts from guinea-pig brain and was purified by a series of chromatographic steps, including a DEAE-cellulose column loaded in the presence or absence of Ca²⁺ ions followed by gel-filtration (Winsky *et al.* 1989). Purified recombinant CR (human: Schwaller *et al.* 1993; rat: Strauss *et al.* 1994a) produced in *E.coli* were tested in ⁴⁵Ca²⁺ overlay and Western blots and were

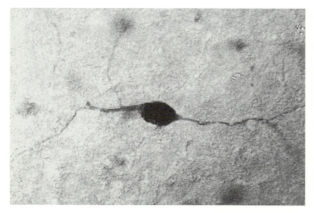

A

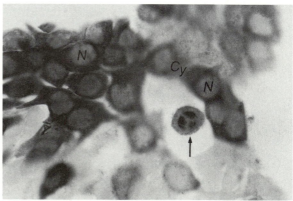

B

Figure 1. (A) CR immunoreactive neurons of rat neocortex. These cells often display bipolar or bitufted morphologies (taken from Schwaller *et al.* 1993). **(B)** In the human colon adenocarcinoma cell line WiDr, CR is expressed in the cytoplasm of interphase cells (Cy, cytoplasm; N, nucleus; taken from Gotzos *et al.* 1992). CR is associated with the tripolar spindle of a mitotic WiDr cell (arrow).

found to have similar properties as the purified native protein.

Gene and sequences

The sequence of chick (Cheung et al. 1993: GenBank accession number X62866), human (Parmentier and Lefort 1991; X56667), rat (Strauss and Jacobowitz 1993; X66974), and mouse calretinin (Rogers 1993; X73985 (partial sequence)) are highly homologous. The intron positions of the chick and human CR genes known up to date are exactly in the same positions as in the calbindin D-28k gene (Wilson et al. 1988) suggesting that the CR gene also comprises 11 exons. All introns known (2–9) are in phase 0 except intron 7 which is phase 2. The introns are not consistently placed with respect to the coding regions of the tandemly repeated EF-hand domains.

The human CR gene is located on chromosome 16 (Parmentier 1989).

Protein

CR consists of six EF-hand domains (three tandem repeats) of which four or five bind Ca^{2+} (Fig. 2). Domains VI and possibly II are aberrant and do not bind ions. The amino acid sequences of the species known are highly conserved within EF-hand domains as well as in regions connecting the domains. The deduced amino acid sequences of rat and chicken are 98% and 85% identical to human calretinin. For mouse CR, the identity is also

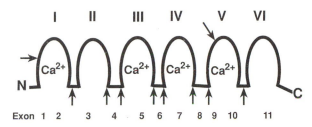

Figure 2. EF-hand structure of CR. The presumed intron/exon junctions are marked by arrows.

98% for the sequence known, not including approximately 30 amino acids at the N-terminal, which are not sequenced yet. The evolutionary rate of amino acid substitutions per 100 residues per 10^9 years was calculated to be in the order of 3.8 for CR, similar to that for another highly conserved protein, cytochrome $c_{(5)}$. The human gene is located on chromosome 16 (Parmentier et al. 1989).

Antibodies

Antibodies specific for calretinin, which do not cross-react with calbindin D-28k or other known CaBPs, are commercially available through Swant and Chemicon (see addresses at the end of the book).

Localization

Antibodies against CR have been used in a large number of studies on the peripheral and central nervous system. CR is an excellent marker for neurons in the submucous and myenteric plexi of the gastrointestinal tract and for various types of nerve cells in the brain (Résibois and Rogers 1992). The literature on the distribution of this protein in the brain is steadily increasing. Recently, the protein has also been detected in the interstitial cells of the rat ovary (Pohl et al. 1992), the avian thymus (Kiraly and Celio, 1993) and the Leydig cells of rat testis (Strauss et al. 1994b).

Biological activities

Purified chicken calretinin was used in equilibrium dialysis in vitro and Ca^{2+}-binding sites (4.5 ± 0.5 / molecule) and binding affinities (K_d: 0.3–0.5 μM) were almost identical as for calbindin D-28k (3.5 ± 0.4 / molecule; same K_d) (Cheung et al. 1993). A role for CR in the inhibition of a Ca^{2+}-dependent phosphorylation of a synaptic membrane protein (Yamaguchi et al. 1991) has been suggested, but recently it was demonstrated that the inhibition was due to small amounts of phosphate present in the preparation of CR (Winsky and Kuznicki 1995). An involvement of calretinin in the cell cycle of WiDr cells has been postulated because CR-immunoreactivity was strongest in phase G1 and mitosis (Gotzos et al. 1992). Down-regulation of CR in WiDr cells by antisense oligodeoxynucleotides led to the inhibition of the cell cycle at two specific checkpoints, thus further supporting a role for CR in the cell cycle (Gander et al. 1996). No other biochemical or biological studies have been published concerning the function of CR.

References

Cheung, W.-T., Richards, D.E., and Rogers, J.H. (1993) Calcium binding by chick calretinin and rat calbindin-D28k synthesised in bacteria. Eur. J. Biochem. **215**, 401–410.

Gander, J.-Ch., Gotzos, V., Fellay, B., and Schwaller, B. (1995) Inhibition of the proliferative cycle and apoptotic events in

WiDr cells after down-regulation of the calcium-binding protein calretinin using antisense oligodeoxynucleotides (submitted).

*Gotzos, V., Schwaller, B., Hetzel, N., Bustos-Castillo, M., and Celio, M.R. (1992) Expression of the calcium binding protein calretinin in WiDr cells and its correlation with the cell cycle. Exp. Cell Res. **202**, 292–302.

Kiraly, E. and Celio, M.R. (1993) Parvalbumin and calretinin in the avian thymus. Anat. Embryol. **188**, 339–344.

Lukas, W. and Jones K.A. (1994) Cortical neurons containing calretinin are selectively resistant to calcium overload and excitotoxicity in vitro. Neurosci. **61**, 307–316.

Möckel, V. and Fischer G. (1994) Vulnerability to excitotoxic stimuli of cultured rat hippocampal neurons containing the calcium-binding proteins calbindin D28k and calretinin. Brain Res. **648**, 109–120.

Parmentier, M. (1989) The human calbindins: cDNA and gene cloning. Adv. Exp. Med. Biol. **255**, 233–240.

*Parmentier, M. and Lefort A. (1991) Structure of the human brain calcium-binding protein and its expression in bacteria. Eur. J. Biochem. **196**, 79–85.

Parmentier, M., Szpirer,J., Levan,G., and Vassart, G. (1989) The human genes for calbindin 27 and 29 kDa proteins are located on chromosomes 8 and 16, respectively. Cytogenet. Cell Genet. **52**, 85–87.

Pochet, R.,Parmentier, M., Lawson, D.E.M., and Pasteels, J.L. (1985) Rat brain synthesizes two "vitamin D-dependent" CaBP's. Brain Res. **345**, 251–256.

Pohl, V., Van Ramplebergh, J., Mellaert, S., and Pochet, R. (1992) Calretinin in rat ovary: an *in situ* hybridization and immuno-histochemical study. Biochim. Biophys. Acta **1160**, 87–94.

Résibois, A. and Rogers, J.H. (1992) Calretinin in the rat brain: an immunohistochemical study. Neuroscience. **46**, 101–134.

*Rogers, J.H. (1987) Calretinin: a gene for a novel CaBP expressed principally in neurons. J. Cell. Biol. **105**, 1343–1353.

Rogers, J.H. (1993) unpublished.

Schwaller, B., Buchwald, P., Blümcke, I., Celio, M., and Hunziker, W. (1993) Characterization of a polyclonal antiserum against the purified human recombinant calcium binding protein calretinin. Cell Calcium **14**, 639–648.

*Schwaller, B., Celio, M.R., and Hunziker, W. (1995) Alternative splicing of calretinin mRNA leads to different forms of calretinin. Eur. J. Biochem. **230**, 424–430.

Strauss K.I. and Jacobowitz, D.M. (1993) Nucleotide sequence of rat calretinin cDNA. Neurochem. Int. **22**, 541–546.

Strauss, K.I., Kuznicki, J., Winsky, L., and Jacobowitz, D.M. (1994a) Expression and rapid purification of recombinant rat calretinin–similarity to native calretinin. Protein Expression and Purification **5**, 187–191.

Strauss, K.I., Isaacs, K.R., Ha, Q.N., and Jacobowitz, D.M. (1994b) Calretinin is expressed in the Leydig cells of rat testis. Biochim. Biophys. Acta **1219**, 435–440.

Wilson, P.W., Roger, J., Harding, M., Pohl, V., Pattyn, G., and Lawson, D.E.M. (1988) Structure of chick chromosomal genes for calbindin and calretinin. J. Mol. Biol. **200**, 615–625.

Winsky, L. and Kuznicki, J. (1995) Distribution of calretinin, calbindin D28k and parvalbumin in subcellular fractions of rat cerebellum: Effects of calcium. J. Neurochemistry **65**, 381–388.

*Winsky, L., Nakata H., Martin, B.M., and Jacobowitz, D.M. (1989) Isolation, partial amino acid sequence, and immunohistochemical localization of a brain-specific calcium-binding protein. Proc. Natl. Acad. Sci. USA **86**, 10139–10143.

Yamaguchi, T., Winsky, L., and Jacobowitz, D.M. (1991) Calretinin, a neuronal calcium binding protein, inhibits phosphorylation of a 39 kDa synaptic membrane protein from rat brain cerebral cortex. Neurosci. Lett., **131**, 79–82.

■ *Beat Schwaller:*
Institute of Histology and General Embryology, University of Fribourg, CH-1705 Fribourg, Switzerland Tel.:+41 26300 84 90 Fax:+41 26300 97 32 E-mail: beat.schwaller@unifr.ch

Calretinin-22k and -20k

Calretinin-22k and -20k (CR-22k and -20k) are isoforms of calretinin, most likely as the result of alternative splicing. The mRNA coding for CR-22k has been detected in several colon adenocarcinoma cell lines. The proteins expressed in E. coli are able to bind Ca^{2+}, but with a lower capacity than the full-length protein. While the distribution of CR-22k in WiDr cells is mainly cytosolic, specific conditions lead to an accumulation of the protein in the nucleus, suggesting a different function from full-length calretinin.

Up to now, the mRNAs could only be detected in colon carcinoma cell lines (e.g. WiDr, Co115/3, HT-29), although there is growing evidence that the mRNA coding for CR-22k, as well as the protein, is present during rat embryogenesis (D.M. Vogt Weisenhorn, unpublished).

■ Isolation/identification

In a cDNA library constructed from WiDr mRNA, besides several clones coding for calretinin, clones containing deletions of 40 and 94 nucleotides were isolated (Schwaller *et al.* 1995). These deletions coincided exactly with the presumed exon 8, or 8 and 9. In Western blots of cytosolic extracts from Co115/3 cells, a second band of 23–24 kDa indicative of CR-22k was detected using the polyclonal antiserum 7696 against calretinin (Schwaller *et al.* 1993). In WiDr cell extracts the concentrations of CR-20k and -22k were below the detection limit of the Western blot techniques used.

■ Gene and sequences

The sequences of the two mRNAs are identical to the published sequence of human CR (Parmentier and Lefort

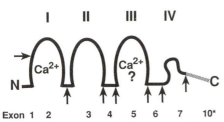

Figure 1. EF-hand structure of CR-22k. The presumed intron/exon junctions are marked by arrows. The unique C-terminal amino acids are depicted in grey.

Calretinin-20k (CR-20k) contains 179 amino acid residues (1–178 identical to CR) and an Ala residue at position 179. The calculated molecular weight is 20 660 and the isoelectric point is 4.86. As for CR-22k, EF-hand IV is very likely to be non-functional.

Sequence comparison of the C-terminal amino acids of CR-22k with the GenBank revealed several interesting homologies (Fig. 2). Secondary structure predictions for the C-terminal region of CR-22k suggest an alpha-helical conformation (Chou-Fasmann algorithms using the gcg software). The consensus residues are located on the same region of the helix as modelled.

1991; X56667) except for the deletion of 40 (CR-20k) and 94 (CR-22k) nucleotides within the coding region. The deletions coincide exactly with the presumed exon 8, or 8 and 9, according to the positions of the chick CR introns. All introns known (2–9) are in phase 0 (between codons) except intron 7, where the alternative splicing occurs, which is in phase 2 (between the second and third nucleotide of the codon).

Protein

Human calretinin-22k (CR-22k) consists of 192 amino acid residues and has a calculated molecular mass of 22 155 Da. It migrates on SDS gels with an apparent molecular mass of 23–24 kDa and has a calculated isoelectric point of 4.93. It is identical to full-length CR up to amino acid 178 followed by 14 additional amino acids as depicted in Fig. 2. The protein consists of four EF-hand domains, number IV most likely not functional, since F-helix IV is not intact and the 14 amino acid substitution (compared to full-length CR) does not confer to the EF-hand consensus sequence (Fig. 1).

Antibodies

Antibodies specific for the C-terminal 14 amino acid residues of CR-22k were produced, but are not commercially available (Gander et al. 1996, submitted).

Localization

Antibodies against CR-22k have been used in immunohistochemical stainings of colon adenocarcinoma cell lines. The distribution of the protein is cytosolic, as for the full-length protein. In WiDr cells treated with 1,25-dihydroxyvitamin D_3 for 48 h (10^{-9} M), an accumulation of CR-22k in the nucleus is evident (Fig. 3). The effect is transient and reaches a peak after 48–72 h treatment (Schwaller et al. 1996, in preparation).

Biological activities

CR-20k and -22k expressed in E. coli are able to bind Ca^{2+} ions as demonstrated in a $^{45}Ca^{2+}$ overlay blot (Schwaller

```
CR-22k human                              -IEAATLTSMSWMPF*    11
CR-22k rat (hypothetical)                 -MEAATSMRTSWTPS*     9
CB-32 Drosophila (hypothetical)           -TIAAPLKMRSSKAS*     5
Fibronectin-bovine                        -QEALSQTTISWTPF-     9
GADD153                                  #MAAESLPFSFGTLSSWELW-  3
Heat-shock protein hsp 25 (chick)        #MAERRVPFTFLTSPSWEPF-  7
Heat-shock protein hsp 27 (mouse)        #MTERRVPFSLLRSPSWEPF-  6
Kinesin-like protein (Drosophila)         -GEATTVSSISWMPL-     8
putative DNA-binding protein              -xEASSSLSTSLPPS-     8
Annexin VI (alternative spliced form)     -QVAAEILEIADTPS-     4

CONSENSUS SEQUENCE                        -EAAUJUU-SW-PX
nr. of cons. residues at that position (out of -5745655-97-77
10) U: Ser or Thr; J: Leu or Ser, X: Ser or Phe  |  ||  ||  |
```

Figure 2. Sequence comparison of the C-terminal region of human CR-22k with proteins stored in the GenBank (GenEMBL or SwissProt). The C-terminus of a protein is marked by an asterisk (*) and the N-terminus by the symbol (#). The numbers on the right side represent the number of residues confirming to the consensus sequence. The residues 3, 6, 7, 10, 11, 14, which are on the same side of the alpha-helix (helical wheel representation), are marked by a vertical line (|) and are also the most conserved residues.

et al. 1995). No other biological activities have been reported.

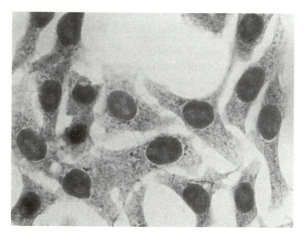

Figure 3. Nuclear localization of CR-22k in WiDr cells treated with with 1,25-dihydroxyvitamin D3.

■ References

Gander, J.-Ch., Bustos-Castillo, M., Hunziker, W., Celio, M.R., and Schwaller, B. (1995) The calcium-binding protein calretinin-22k, an alternative splicing product of the calretinin gene is present in several colon adenocarcinoma cell lines (submitted).

Parmentier, M. and Lefort, A. (1991) Structure of the human brain calcium-binding and its expression in bacteria. Eur. J. Biochem. **196**, 79–85.

Schwaller, B., Buchwald, P., Blümcke, I., Celio, M., and Hunziker, W. (1993) Characterization of a polyclonal antiserum against the purified human recombinant calcium binding protein calretinin. Cell Calcium **14**, 639–648.

*Schwaller, B., Celio, M.R., and Hunziker, W. (1995) Alternative splicing of calretinin mRNA leads to different forms of calretinin. Eur. J. Biochem. **230**, 424–430.

■ *Beat Schwaller:*
Institute of Histology and General Embryology,
University of Fribourg,
CH-1705 Fribourg,Switzerland
Tel.:+41 26300 84 90
Fax:+41 26300 97 32
E-mail: beat.schwaller@unifr.ch

Calcineurin

Calcineurin (Cn) is a Ca²⁺/calmodulin-dependent protein phosphatase, composed of a catalytic and a regulatory subunit. It has been found in the brain, where it is one of the most abundant calmodulin-binding proteins. Recently it was demonstrated that calcineurin is the target of immunosuppressant drugs (cyclosporin, FK-506). This observation indicated that calcineurin is a necessary component in the activation of T cells.

Calcineurin is a heterodimeric protein phosphatase composed of a 61 000 Da catalytic subunit (CnA) and a 15 000–17 000 Da regulatory subunit (CnB). It has been purified from bovine brain (Klee *et al.* 1988) and was shown to be a Ca²⁺/calmodulin-dependent protein phosphatase (Stewart *et al.* 1982). The two subunits could be dissociated under denaturing conditions, and after partial renaturation it was possible to demonstrate that the phosphatase activity was associated with CnA (Klee *et al.* 1988). The sequence of the bovine brain CnB has high homology with calmodulin and it was possible to show that CnB binds Ca²⁺ with high affinity (Klee *et al.* 1988). Although very similar, calmodulin and CnB could not substitute for each other, i.e. they have different binding sites on the CnA and both of them are needed for full activation of the phosphatase (Stemmer and Klee 1994). The Ca²⁺ activation mediated by the CnB is only 10% of the maximal activation obtained in the presence of calmodulin, but the lack of CnB has a dramatic influence on the basal activity of the CnA (Milan *et al.* 1994).

CnA is encoded by two genes in human, rat, yeast, and *Drosophila melanogaster* (Cyert *et al.* 1991; Guerini and Klee 1991; Guerini *et al.* 1992). On the contrary, only one gene for CnB could be found in all species tested so far (Cyert *et al.* 1991; Guerini and Klee 1991; Guerini *et al.* 1992).

Calcineurin was shown to bind the immunosuppressant drugs cyclosporin and FK-506, complexed to their cellular receptors (cyclophilin and FKB-506 binding protein), in a Ca²⁺/calmodulin-dependent manner. As a consequence this inhibits phosphatase activity toward peptide substrates (Liu *et al.* 1991). *In vivo* studies with T cells confirmed these observations (Clipstone and Crabtree 1992; O'Keefe *et al.* 1992), leading to the proposal that calcineurin represents the link between external stimuli and the activation of the interleukin-2 gene promoter. These observations stimulated the search for the amino acids involved in the interaction with immunosuppressant drugs. In two recent publications the cyclophilin–cyclosporin complex was shown to bind primarily to CnB

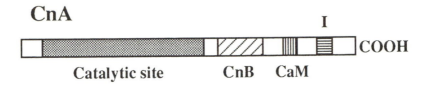

CnA

Catalytic site CnB CaM I COOH

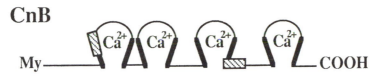

CnB

My — Ca²⁺ Ca²⁺ Ca²⁺ Ca²⁺ — COOH

Figure 1. Structural domains of calcineurin. The upper part of the scheme represents calcineurin A (CnA) functional domains. CnB, calcineurin-binding domain; CaM, calmodulin-binding domain; I, inhibitory domain. The lower part represents the calcineurin B (CnB) functional domains. My, myristoylated N-terminus of CnB. CnB contains four EF-hand Ca²⁺-binding sites. The striped boxes indicate the latch region which has been suggested to bind immuno-suppressant drugs (see also text).

(Li and Handschumacher 1993) and more precisely to amino acids in the latch region (Milan *et al.* 1994), which comes in closer contact once CnB is bound to CnA (Fig. 1).

■ Alternative names

Calcineurin, Ca²⁺-calmodulin-dependent protein phosphatase, (protein)-phosphatase 2B.

■ Isolation/identification

Calcineurin is generally purified from bovine brain tissue, where it is very abundant (Klee *et al.* 1983). The soluble fraction after homogenization can be fractionated by ionic exchange chromatography: Cn is recovered at lower salt concentration. This fraction is then further purified by affinity chromatography on a calmodulin-Sepharose column, and subsequently by gel filtration or chromato-focusing. Calcineurin is known to be present in different tissues and the basic scheme described above can be used in most cases (Klee *et al.* 1988).

■ Genes and sequences

cDNA sequences for both CnA and CnB have been obtained from rat, mouse, human, *Drosophila melanogaster* and yeast (*Saccharomyces cerevisiae*) (CnB accession numbers: M87508, D14568, M30773; CnA: M29550, M29551, D90035, D90036, M64839, M64840, J05479, J05480, M29275). The CnB subunit has a much higher level of conservation than the CnA and only one gene for it has been found. The possibility of an alternative splicing for the CnB has been indicated by recent data (Chang *et al.* 1994). At least two genes for the CnA are present in yeast, *Drosophila melanogaster*, human and rat, and alternative splicing of these has been described (Guerini and Klee 1991). The gene for the CnAa has been mapped to the human chromosome 8 (Muramatsu and Kincaid 1992). The promoter region of the CnAa has been determined (Chang *et al.* 1992), indicating that while no TATA and CCAT boxes are present, its sequence is similar to that of the housekeeping gene promoters.

■ Protein

The CnA can be divided into different functional domains (Fig. 1). The 300 amino acids in the centre of the protein, highly homologous to other protein phosphatases, contain the catalytic region of CnA (Guerini and Klee 1991). At the N-terminus of the protein, where the two CnA genes differ the most, an unusual stretch of polyprolines has been found, which was proposed to be important for the control of the activity of the enzyme (Guerini and Klee 1989). The CnB- and the CaM-binding domains are located at the C-terminus of the phosphatase (Fig. 1). In addition, an inhibitory domain was also found (Guerini and Klee 1991). As in the case of the CaM-binding proteins, in the absence of calmodulin, the inhibitory domain comes in close contact with the catalytic region, repressing the phosphatase activity. The inhibition is relieved after binding to calmodulin.

CnB belongs to the family of EF-hand proteins and it has been shown to bind Ca²⁺ with submicromolar affinity (Klee *et al.* 1988). The sequence is very similar to that of troponinC and calmodulin, and four canonical EF Ca²⁺-binding sites could be identified (Fig. 1). The CnB subunit is myristoylated at its N-terminal glycine (Klee *et al.* 1988), a property that could influence the distribution of the Cn in the cells, but a definitive function for this post-translational modification is lacking at the moment.

■ Biological function

Calcineurin is, among the protein phosphatases, the one with the narrowest substrate specificity and, due to the regulation by Ca^{2+}/calmodulin, is the candidate for second messenger regulation (Cohen and Cohen, 1989). DARP32 and phosphatase inhibitor-I are among the preferred substrate of calcineurin. Both proteins are involved in the control of the activity of protein phosphatase I, supporting the idea of a phosphatase activation cascade by second messengers. Recently, studies have indicated that the inhibitor-I/calcineurin complex may play an important role in hippocampal long-term depression (Mulkey *et al.* 1994).

The discovery that the phosphatase activity of calcineurin could be inhibited by immunosuppressant drugs (Liu *et al.* 1991) established a link between the biological action of these drugs and the activation the T cell: immunosuppression is likely to be the result of the inhibition of calcineurin. In fact, calcineurin was shown to mediate the dephosphorylation of the NF-AT (nuclear factor for activation of T cells) protein complex (McCaffrey *et al.* 1993) which is believed to be necessary for the translocation of the NF-AT to the nucleus.

■ References

Chang, C.D, Takeda T., Mukai, H., Shuntoh, H., Kuno, T., and Tanaka, C. (1992) Molecular cloning and characterization of the promoter region of the calcineurin A gene. Biochem. J. **288**, 801–805.

Chang, C.D, Mukai, H., Kuno, T., and Tanaka, C. (1994) cDNA cloning of an alternative isoform of the regulatory subunit of Ca^{2+}/calmodulin-dependent protein phosphatase (calcineurin Ba2). Biochim. Biophys. Acta **1217**, 174–180.

Clipstone N.A. and Crabtree G.R. (1992) Identification of calcineurin as a key signalling enzyme in T-lymphocyte activation. Nature **357**, 695–697.

Cohen, P. and Cohen P.T.W. (1989) Protein phosphatases come of age. J. Biol. Chem. **2645**, 21435–21438.

Cyert M.S., Kunisawa, R., Kaim. D., and Thorner J. (1991) Yeast has homologues (CNA1 and CNA2 gene products) of mammalian calcineurin, a calmodulin-regulated phospho-protein phosphatase. Proc. Natl. Acad. Sci. USA **88**, 7376–7380.

Guerini D. and Klee C.B. (1989) Cloning of human calcineurin A: evidence for two isozymes and identification of a polyproline structural domain. Proc. Natl. Acad. Sci. USA **86**, 9183–9187.

Guerini D. and Klee C.B. (1991) Structural diversity of Calcineurin, a Ca^{2+} and calmodulin-stimulated protein phosphatase. Adv. Prot. Phosphatases **6**, 391–410.

Guerini D., Montell C., and Klee C.B. (1992) Molecular cloning and characterization of the genes encoding the two subunits of *Drosophila melanogaster* calcineurin. J. Biol. Chem **267**, 22542–22549.

Klee, C.B., Krinks, M.H., Manalan, A.S., Cohen, P., and Stewart, A.A. (1983). Isolation and characterization of bovine brain calcineurin; a calmodulin-stimulated protein phosphatase. Meth. Enzymol. **102**, 227–244.

Klee, C.B., Draetta, G.L., and Hubbard, M.J. (1988) Calcineurin. Adv. Enzymol. **61**, 149–200.

Li W. and Hanschumacher R.E. (1993) Specific interaction of the cyclophilin–cyclosporin complex with the B subunit of calcineurin. J. Biol. Chem. **268**, 14040–14044.

Liu, J., Farmer, J.D.Jr., Friedman, J., Weissman, I., and Schreiber, S.L. (1991) Calcineurin is a common target of cyclophilin–cyclosporin A and FKBP–FK 506 complexes. Cell **66**, 807–815.

McCaffrey, P.G., Perrino, B.G., Soderling, T.R., and Rao, A. (1993) NF-ATp, a T lymphocyte DNA-binding protein that is a target for calcineurin and munosuppressive drugs. J. Biol. Chem. **268**, 3747–3752.

Milan D., Griffith, J., Su, M., Price, E.R., and McKeon F. (1994) The latch region of calcineurin B is involved in both immuno-suppressant-immunophilin complex docking and phosphatase activation. Cell **79**, 437–447.

Mulkey, R.M., Endo, S., Shenolikar, S., and Malenka, R.C. (1994) Involvement of a calcineurin inhibitor-phosphatase cascade in hippocampal long-term depression. Nature **369**, 486–488.

Muramatsu, T. and Kincaid, R., (1992) Molecular cloning and chromosomal mapping of the human gene for the testis-specific catalytic subunit of calmodulin-dependent protein phosphatase (calcineurin A). Biochem. Biophys. Res. Comm. **188**, 265–271.

O'Keefe, S.J., Tamura, J., Kincaid, R.L., Tocci, M.J., and O'Neill, E.A. (1992) FK506 and CsA-sensitive activation of the interleukin-2 promoter by calcineurin. Nature **357**, 692–694.

Stemmer P.M. and Klee C.B. (1994) Dual calcium ion regulation of calcineurin by calmodulin and calcineurin B. Biochemistry **33**, 6859–6866.

Stewart, A.A., Ingebritsen, T.S., Manalan, A., Klee, C.B., and Cohen P. (1982) Discovery of a Ca^{2+} and calmodulin-dependent protein phosphatase. FEBS Lett. **137**, 80–84.

■ *Danilo Guerini:*
  Laboratory of Biochemistry III,
  Federal Institute of Technology (ETH),
  CH-8092 Zürich, Switzerland
  Tel.: +41 1 632 31 42
  Fax: +41 1 632 12 13

Calcyphosine

Calcyphosine (p24) is a Ca²⁺-binding protein located in the cytosol and is present in numerous tissues. p24 was initially identified as being a major phosphorylated substrate for cyclic AMP-dependent protein kinase following stimulation of dog thyroid cells by thyrotropin (Lecocq et al. 1979). The role of p24 is as yet unknown. All cells where p24 has been found are epithelial and of the secretory type, which leads us to propose the hypothesis that calcyphosine may play a role in the regulation of ionic transport.

Dog calcyphosine (p24) has an isoelectric point of 5.4 and a calculated molecular mass of 21 104 Da, comparable to the apparent molecular mass of 24 kDa previously estimated by SDS-polyacrylamide gel electrophoresis (Lecocq *et al.* 1979; Lefort *et al.* 1989). It clearly belongs to the calmodulin superfamily of proteins binding Ca²⁺ ions through 'EF hands' (Lefort *et al.* 1989). p24 is subjected to multiple regulation in dog thyroid cells. It is rapidly phosphorylated during the full functional activation of the cell through the cyclic AMP cascade; it is not phosphorylated in response to acetylcholine which activates the Ca²⁺-phosphatidylinositol cascade and has some similar but mostly opposite effects to thyroid stimulating hormone (TSH). Its synthesis is enhanced by TSH and cyclic AMP analogues which trigger cell proliferation and maintain expression of the differentiated thyrocyte phenotype; it is decreased by epidermal growth factor (EGF) and 12-*O*-tetradecanoyl-phorbol-13-acetate (TPA), which also trigger cell proliferation but repress expression of differentiation (Lecocq *et al.* 1990). Assuming a cytosolic localization of calcyphosine in the dog thyrocyte, we calculate that its concentration is 30 μM (Lecocq *et al.* 1995).

◼ Alternative names

Protein 5 (Lecocq *et al.* 1979), protein 5' (Lamy *et al.* 1986; Lamy *et al.* 1989), p24 (Lefort *et al.* 1989).

◼ Isolation/identification

p24 is a thyroid protein which can be identified by two-dimensional gel electrophoresis on the basis that its synthesis and phosphorylation are up-regulated by thyrotropin and cyclic AMP agonists. A method for purifying p24 in its native form by a procedure involving three chromatographic steps has been published (Lecocq *et al.* 1995).

◼ Gene and sequences

p24 was cloned from a λgt11 cDNA library using a polyclonal antibody raised against the protein recovered from a Western blot spot (Lefort *et al.* 1989). The EMBL/GenBank/DDBJ Nucleotide Sequence Database accession number is X14047. An open reading frame of 189 codons would encode a polypeptide of calculated molecular mass of 21 104 Da. The primary structure of the encoded polypeptide contains a serine residue (serine 40) which could be phosphorylated by the cyclic AMP-dependent protein kinase. This primary structure reveals significant similarities with most of the Ca²⁺-binding proteins containing EF-hand domains, particularly with calmodulin (Lefort *et al.* 1989). A polypeptide expressed predominantly in olfactory receptor neurons and sharing extensive amino acid identity with calcyphosine has been described (Nemoto *et al.* 1993). A protein from the abdominal muscle of the crayfish with 44% sequence identity to calcyphosine has recently been described (Sauter *et al.* 1995).

◼ Protein

p24 consists of four EF-hand domains, two of which show deviation from the consensus 'EF hand'. The first lacks a glycine residue (position 39) which is considered essential to the shape of Ca²⁺-binding domains. The arginine replacing it belongs to the putative target site for phosphorylation by cAMP-dependent protein kinase. The fourth domain displays an insertion of 17 residues at position 160 which disrupts its structure and, most probably, makes it non-functional. The ability of p24 to bind Ca²⁺ has been demonstrated using ⁴⁵Ca²⁺ (Lefort *et al.* 1989).

◼ Antibodies

A specific rabbit polyclonal antibody was raised in a rabbit (Lecocq *et al.* 1990) and is available from the authors.

◼ Localization

Immunohistochemical studies reveal that calcyphosine is located in the cytosol and is present in numerous tissues including various endocrine glands (thyroid, pancreas, adrenal, pituitary gland) and epithelia (respiratory, digestive, urinary, genital, skin) (Halleux *et al.*, manuscript in preparation).

◼ Biological activities

The role of calcyphosine is as yet unknown. As calcyphosine is found in several tissues, it is not a protein involved in the specialized iodine metabolism of the thyrocyte. All the cells expressing calcyphosine are epithelial and of the secretory type, which leads us to propose the hypothesis that calcyphosine may play a role in the regulation of ionic transport.

■ References

Halleux *et al.* (1995), in preparation.

*Lamy, F., Roger, P.P., Lecocq, R., and Dumont, J.E. (1986) Differential protein synthesis in the induction of thyroid cell proliferation by thyrothropin, epidermal growth factor or serum. Eur. J. Biochem. **155**, 265–272.

Lamy, F., Roger, P., Lecocq, R., and Dumont, J.E. (1989) Protein synthesis during induction of DNA replication in thyroid epithelial cells: evidence for late markers of distinct mitogenic pathways. J. Cell Physiol. **138**, 568–578.

*Lecocq, R., Lamy, F., and Dumont, J.E. (1979) Pattern of protein phosphorylation in intact stimulated cells: thyrotropin and dog thyroid. Eur. J. Biochem. **102**, 147–152.

Lecocq, R., Lamy, F., and Dumont, J.E. (1990) Use of two-dimensional gel electrophoresis and autoradiography as a tool in cell biology: the example of the thyroid and the liver. Electrophoresis **11**, 200–212.

Lecocq, R., Lamy, F., Erneux, C., and Dumont, J.E. (1995) Rapid purification and identification of calcyphosine, a Ca^{2+}-binding protein phosphorylated by protein kinase A. Biochem. J. **306**, 147–151.

*Lefort, A., Lecocq, R., Libert, F., Lamy, F., Swillens, S., Vassart, G., and Dumont, J.E. (1989) Cloning and sequencing of a calcium-binding protein regulated by cyclic AMP in the thyroid. EMBO J. **8**, 111–116.

Nemoto, Y., Ikeda, J., Katoh, K., Koshimoto, H., Yoshihara, Y., and Mori, K. (1993) R2D5 Antigen: a calcium-binding phosphoprotein predominantly expressed in olfactory receptor neurons. J. Cell Biol. **123**, 963–976.

Sauter, A., Staudenmann, W., Hughes, G. and Heizmann C. (1995) A novel EF-hand Ca^{2+}-binding protein from abdominal muscle of crustaceans with similarity to calcyphosine from dog thyreoidea. Eur. J. Biochem. **227**, 97–101.

■ *Raymond Lecocq and Françoise Lamy:*
Interdisciplinary Research Institute (IRIBHN),
Campus Erasme, Bldg. C,
808 route de Lennik,
1070 Brussels, Belgium
Tel.: 32 2 5554150
Fax: 32 2 5554655

Calmodulin

Calmodulin (CaM) is a small (about 17 kDa), ubiquitously expressed, 4 EF-hand Ca^{2+}-binding protein that appears to be the primary calcium sensor in eukaryotic cells. Calmodulin acts as a calcium signal-transmitting subunit for a multitude of different proteins in mammalian cells. CaM is highly conserved throughout eukaryotic species, and no naturally occurring mutations have as yet been identified in multicellular organisms. Calmodulin appears to act primarily by binding and sequestering self-interacting (e.g. autoinhibitory) domains in its target proteins, but other modes of action may also be found in the case of individual enzymes.

Calmodulin (CaM) and similar proteins are found in all eukaryotic organisms studied so far (Cohen and Klee 1988). Several bacterial species also produce calmodulin homologues (Onek and Smith 1992). Calmodulin appears to be a primary sensor of Ca^{2+} transients in eukaryotic cells. It is a dumb-bell-shaped, heat stable, acidic protein (p*I* 3.9–4.3) with a molecular mass of approximately 17 kDa (148 amino acid residues in vertebrates). Calmodulin migrates on SDS-polyacrylamide gels with an apparent mobility of 15 kDa in the presence of Ca^{2+} and an apparent mobility of 21 kDa in its absence (Burgess *et al.* 1980).

CaM regulates multiple cellular functions including intermediary metabolism, secretion, motility, signal transduction, and cell growth and division (Means and Dedman 1980; Cohen and Klee 1988; Gnegy 1993; Hinrichsen 1993; Lu and Means 1993). Some CaM is required for viability in all cells, although its levels vary considerably between cell types. The exact nature of a cell's CaM requirement is unknown, although at least in yeast it appears to be partially independent from its Ca^{2+}-binding function (Geiser *et al.* 1991; Ohya and Botstein 1994).

■ Alternative names

Cyclic nucleotide phosphodiesterase activator protein (PAF), Modulator protein, calcium-dependent regulator protein (CDR).

■ Identification/isolation

Calmodulin was initially identified in 1970 as a protein which activates cyclic nucleotide phosphodiesterase (reviewed in Cheung *et al.* 1978). It was later shown that

CaM binds to phenothiazine drugs in the presence of Ca^{2+}, and affinity chromatography using these compounds superseded other purification methods. Finally in 1983 it was shown that CaM binds to phenyl sepharose in a Ca^{2+}-dependent manner, thus obviating the need for specialized resins in CaM purification (Vogel *et al.* 1983).

Genes and amino acid sequences

In vertebrates, a multigene family comprising at least three (e.g. humans and rodents) or four (teleost fish) different, maximally divergent genes encodes an identical 148 amino acid protein. In these organisms, as well as in many plant species (e.g. *Arabidopsis thaliana*), calmodulin represents a rare example of the "multiple genes–one protein" principle. By contrast, a single gene for calmodulin has been identified in several invertebrates, including budding and fission yeast, the slime mold *Dictyostelium discoideum*, the filamentous fungus *Aspergillus nidulans*, the mollusk *Aplysia californica*, and the insect *Drosophila melanogaster*. Calmodulin genes have now been cloned from over 50 different eukaryotic species, including plants, animals, protists, and fungi. In several species (e.g. the sea urchin *Arbacia punctulata* and the plants *Arabidopsis thaliana* and *Petunia hybrida*) two or more genes code for closely related but non-identical calmodulin isoforms.

CaM amino acid sequences among multicellular eukaryotes are nearly identical (>90% among mammals, fruit flies, and plants). An optimal alignment of known CaM sequences and a comparison with the computer-derived consensus calmodulin sequence is shown in Table 1.

The calmodulin genes of some invertebrate species are intronless (e.g. in *Saccharomyces cerevisiae*) whereas multiple intron interruptions are the rule for vertebrate and plant calmodulin genes (five in the human genes). Several intron locations are highly conserved in calmodulin genes from widely divergent species (a striking example is the intron following the ATG initiation codon; this intron is present in the *Schizosaccharomyces pombe* gene and in all mammalian calmodulin genes); however, non-conserved intron locations are also found in several (mostly plant v. vertebrate) calmodulin genes. Calmodulin genes vary in size from less than 1 kb (intronless CaM genes) to about 15 kb (mammalian and *Drosophila* intron-containing CaM genes). Mammalian CaM genes appear to be dispersed in the genome: the human CALM1, CALM2, and CALM3 genes are located on chromosomes 14q24–q31, 2p21.1–21.3, and 19q13.2–13.3, respectively.

Protein

Several post-translational modifications of CaM have been reported, including acylation of the amino terminus, (tri-) methylation of Lys115, and phosphorylation of Ser81, Ser101, Thr79, Thr117, Tyr99, and Tyr138 in vertebrate CaM (Cheung *et al.* 1978; Sacks *et al.* 1992;

Williams *et al.* 1994). A variable, but significant fraction of calmodulin in hepatocytes has been shown to be phosphorylated *in vivo* on Thr79, Ser81, and Ser101 (Quadroni *et al.* 1994). The functional significance of these post-translational modifications is not as yet entirely clear although phosphorylation does affect both solubility and Ca^{2+} affinity to some extent.

CaM consists of two pairs of 2 EF-hand domains connected by a flexible tether. Spectroscopic studies of Ca^{2+}-binding isotherms on wildtype and selectively mutated CaMs suggest that under physiological ionic strength conditions CaM contains two high-affinity ($K_d < 10^{-5}$ M) binding sites in the carboxy terminus and two lower affinity (K_d 10^{-4} to 10^{-5} M) sites in the amino terminus (reviewed in Cohen and Klee 1988; Weinstein and Mehler 1994). Positive cooperativity of Ca^{2+} binding has been demonstrated for each pair of binding sites, but appears to be particularly pronounced for the (high-affinity) C-terminal sites; by contrast, Ca^{2+} binding cooperativity between the N- and C-terminal lobe sites is less obvious (reviewed in Weinstein and Mehler 1994). When measured in the presence of target peptides, the Ca^{2+} affinity of CaM is increased, apparently as a result of a decreased Ca^{2+} off-rate constant for at least three of the binding sites (Suko *et al.* 1986). CaM also has significant affinities for other divalent cations, although only Mg^{2+} may be physiologically significant. At the free Mg^{2+} concentrations found in the cell, at least two and probably all four Ca^{2+} binding sites of Ca^{2+}-free CaM are occupied by Mg^{2+}. During Ca^{2+} signaling, exchange of Ca^{2+} for Mg^{2+} is likely to limit the rate at which Ca^{2+} binds to the amino terminal half of CaM. However, in the carboxyl half, the fast off-rate of Mg^{2+} makes Ca^{2+} binding diffusion/dehydration limited, and thus any Mg^{2+} binding will have little effect on Ca^{2+} on-rates.

Structure and target recognition

The X-ray crystal structure of CaM in its Ca^{2+}-liganded form has been solved and refined to a resolution of 1.7 Å (Chattopadhyaya *et al.* 1992; see Fig. 1A). In contrast to the crystal structure which suggests a well-defined central helix linking the two globular domains in the dumb-bell-shaped CaM molecule, NMR solution structure data indicate a considerable flexibility for the central helix, which may serve as a variable extension joint to allow dynamic changes in the relative positioning of the two globular lobes towards each other (reviewed in Weinstein and Mehler 1994).

The nature and mechanism underlying the conformational changes involved in CaM substrate recognition have been extensively studied (recently reviewed in Török and Whitaker 1994). Briefly, upon Ca^{2+} binding CaM undergoes a conformational change that exposes hydrophobic pockets on the underside of each pair of EF hands. In the presence of target peptide, a further conformational change results in the flexible linker between the two heads being dramatically bent, partially unwound and wrapped around the target peptide. As a

Table 1. Amino acid sequences of known calmodulins and alignment with a computer-generated consensus sequence (bottom line). Hyphens indicate identity with the consensus, dots denote the absence of residues at the corresponding positions. Sequence definitions and SwissProt accession numbers are listed separately. A single entry is made whenever an identical protein sequence is found in different species. A GenBank accession number is indicated if the protein sequence is not found in SwissProt. Original references for each sequence can be retrieved from the corresponding SwissProt or GenBank entry

```
Calm_Emeni     --s----- vs-y------ -------q-- ---------- -----s-s-- ---------- n--------- --m-------
Calm_Neucr     --s----- vs-------- -------q-- --------l- -----s-s-- ---------- n--------- --m-------
Call_Plafa     m--k----- -s-------- -------... ---------- ---------- -----i-t-- ---------- -------l--
Calm_Plafa     m--k----- -s-------- ---------- ---------- ---------- -----i-t-- ---------- -------l--
Calm_Style     --n------ ---------- ---------- ---------- ---------- ---------- ---------- -s--------
Calm_Tetpy     --------- ---------- ---------- ---------- ---------- ---------- ---------- -s--------
Calm_Parte     -e------ --------a- ---------- ---------- ---------- ---------- ---------- -s------e
Calm_Lyces     -e------ ---------- -------c-- ---------- ---------- ----s---- q-------- -n------
Calm_Soltu     -e------ ---------- -------c-- ---------- ---------- ---s-a--- q-------- -n------
Cal2_Pethy     -e------ ---------- -------c-- ---------- ---------- ---------- q-------- -n------
Call_Arath     ........ -----==== -------c-- ---------- ---------- ---------- ---------- -n--k---
Cal4_Arath     -----d-- -s-------- -------c-- ---------- ---------- ---------- ---------- -n--k---
Calm_Horvu     -----dd- ---------- -------c-- ---------- ---------- ---------- ---------- -n------
Calm_Zmays     -----d-- ---------- -------c-- ---------- ---------- ---------- ---------- -n------
Call_Pethy     -----dd- -s-------- -------c-- ---------- ---------- ---------- ---------- -n------
Calm_Medsa     -----d-- -s-------- -------c-- ---------- ---------- ---------- ---------- -n------
Cal2_Arath     -----dd- -s-------- -------c-- ---------- ---------- ---------- ---------- -n------
Cal6_Arath     -----d-- -s-------- -------c-- ---------- ---------- ---------- ---------- -n------
Calm_Brydi     -----dd- -s-------- -------c-- ---------- ---------- ---------- ---------- -n------
Calm_Wheat     -----d--n -s-------- -------c-- ---------- ---------- ---------- ---------- -n------
Calm_Achkl     -------- -------g-- ---------- ---------- v--------- ---------- ---------- --m-----
Calm_Phyin     -------- ---------- ---------- ---------- ---------- ---------- ---------- --m-----
Calm_Eleel     -------- ---------- ---------- ---------- ---------- ---------- ---------- --m--k---
Calm_Human     -------- ---------- ---------- ---------- ---------- ---------- ---------- --m-----
Calm_Patsp     -------- ---------- ---------- ---------- ---------- ---------- -d-------- --m-----
Calm_Pyusp     -------- ---------- ---------- ---------- ---------- ---------- -d-------- --m-----
Calm_Drome     -------- ---------- ---------- ---------- ---------- ---------- ---------- --m-----
Calm_Stija     -------- ---------- ---------- ---------- ---------- ---------- ---------- --m-----
Call_Arbpu     ........ ..-------- ---------- ---------- ---------- ---------- ---------- --m------e
Calm_Metse     -------- ---------- ---------- ---------- ---------- ---------- -d-------- --m-----
Calm_Pleco     ----s--- -s-------- ---------- ---------- ---------- ---------- ---------- --m----e
Calm_Euggr     -ea--h-- ---------- ---------- ---------- ---------- -------q- -s-------- ----s---h-
Calm_Trybb     ----sn-- -s-------- ---------- ---------- ---------- -------q- -s-------- -------q-
Calm_Chlre     aante------ ---------a- ---------- ---------- ----s----- ---------- ---------- --m------e
Calm_Dicdi     asqes----- ---------- -------s-- ---------- ---------- ---------- --n------ --m----q-
Calm_Pncar     msneqn----- -s-------- -------s-- -----i---- ---------- ---v------ ---------- -am-------
Calm_Nagru     msreaisnne----- ---------- ---------- -------s-- ---------- h--------- -------t-- --m-k----
Calm_Lytpi     ........ ---------- ---------- ---------- ---------- ---------- .......... .....k----
Calm_Schpo     mttrn---d- ----r----- --r-q--n-- sn---v---- ---s-a---- ---------- -------t-- --m-----
Calm_Canal     m-ek-s-q- ---------- ----s--k-- ---------- -----s-s-- t-------vn sd-s------ --n-----
Calm_Yeast     mssn---- --------a- ----nn-s-s ss--a----- --ls-s---v n-lm--i-v- --hq-e-s-- -a--s-ql-s
Consensus      ADQLTEEQ IAEFKEAFSL FDKDGDGTIT TKELGTVMRS LGQNPTEAEL QDMINEVDAD GNGTIDFPEF LTLMARKMKD


Calm_Emeni     ---------- -k---r-n-- ---------- --si------ d--------- -q----r-d- n---ql--q-
Calm_Neucr     ---------- -k---r-n-- ---------- --si------ d--------- -q----r-d- n---ql--q-
Call_Plafa     --t---li-- -----r-d- y---d----- ---------n ---------- ---------- -------i--
Calm_Plafa     --t---li-- -----r-d- y---d----- ---------n ---------- ---------- -------i--
Calm_Style     --t---lv-- -k---r---- l--------- ---------- ---------- -v----h--- ----r-----
Calm_Tetpy     --t---li-- -k---r---- l--------- ---------- ---------- ------h--- ----r-----
Calm_Parte     q-----li-- -k---r---- l--------- ---------- d--------- ------h--- ----r--vs-
Calm_Lyces     ------lk-- -k-----q-- ---------- ---------- ---------- ------v--- ----r-l---
Calm_Soltu     ------lk-- -k-----q-- ---------- ---------- ---------- ------v--- ----r-l---
Cal2_Pethy     ------lk-- -k-----q-- y----dv--- ---------- ---------- -m----v--- ----r-l---
Call_Arath     ------lk-- -------q-- ---------- ---------- ---e------ -v-------- ------i----
Cal4_Arath     ------lk-- -------q-- ---------- ---------- ---e------ -v-------h -----i----
Calm_Horvu     ------lk-- -------q-- ---------- ---------- ---------- -v-------- ------v---
Calm_Zmays     ------lk-- -------q-- ---------- ---------- ---------- -v-------- ------v---
Call_Pethy     ------lk-- -------q-- ---------- ---------- ---------- -v-------- ------v---
Calm_Medsa     ------lk-- -------q-- ---------- ---------- ---------- -v-------- ------v---
Cal2_Arath     ------lk-- -------q-- ---------- ---------- -------k-- -v-------- -----v----
Cal6_Arath     ------lk-- -------q-- --------- ---------s- ---------- -v-------- -----v----
Calm_Brydi     ------lk-- -------q-- ---------- ---------- ---------- -v----t-- -----v----
Calm_Wheat     ------lk-- -------qd- ---------- ---------- ---------- -v-------- ------v---
Calm_Achkl     -------l-- -qg------- ---------m ---------- ---------- ---------- ---------s-
Calm_Phyin     -------l-- -k-------- ----------i ---------- ---------- ---------- ---------s-
Calm_Eleel     ---------- ---------- y--------- ---------- ---------- ------v-- ---q--t--
Calm_Human     ---------- ---------- y--------- ---------- ---------- ------v-- ---q--t--
Calm_Patsp     ---------- -------d-- ---------- ---------- ---------- ------v-- ----t-ts-
Calm_Pyusp     ---------- ---------- ---------- ---------- ---------- ------v-- ----t-ts-
Calm_Drome     ---------- ---------- ---------- ---------- ---------- ------v-- ----t-ts-
Calm_Stija     ---------- ---------- y--------- ---------- ---------- ------v-- ----t-ts-
Call_Arbpu     ---------- ---------- ---------- ---------- ---------- ------v-- ----a-ts-
Calm_Metse     ---------- -------d- ---------- ---------- ---------- ------v-- -------ts-
```

Table 1. *Continued*

```
Calm_Pleco    -------k--  -k--------  y---------  ----------  n---------  ----------  -------ls-
Calm_Euggr    --t-----k--  -k--------  ----------  ----------  ----------  -v--------  -------s-
Calm_Trybb    s------k--  -k--------  ---------i  ----------  ----------  -v--------  -------s-
Calm_Chlre    --h-d-l---  -k--------  ----------  ------se  ----------  -v----v--  -r--tsgatddkdkk ghk
Calm_Dicdi    --t-------  -k--------  y---------  --s------n  ----------  -l-----v--  d------ivrn
Calm_Pncar    v---------  -k--------  i---------  ----------  ----------  -v----vidy  s------ls-
Calm_Nagru    --n----k--  -k--------  ----q-----  --c-------  ----------  -----n----  t------q-
Calm_Lytpi    ----------  ----------  y-rl-.....  ..........  ..........
Calm_Schpo    --n-------  -k--------  --tve--t--  l-s---r-sq  ---ad-----  -t----v---  ---srviss-
Calm_Canal    ---a--a--  -k--rn-d-  k------l  l-si----s-  ad--q--k--  -tnn--e-di  q--tllla--
Calm_Yeast    n---q-ll--  -k----n-d-  -------k--  l-si------  a---d-l--v  s.--s-e-i  qq-aallsk.
Consensus     TDSEEEIREA  FRVFDKDGNG  FISAAELRHV  MTNLGEKLTD  EEVDEMIREA  DIDGDGQINY  EEFVKMMMAK
```

Cal1_Arath P25854 arabidopsis thaliana (mouse-ear cress). calmodulin-1 (fragment). 8/92 136aa
Cal1_Pethy P27162 petunia hybrida (petunia), daucus carota (carrot), lilium longiflorum (trumpet lily), and malus domestica (apple). calmodulin. 8/92 148aa
Cal2_Arath P25069 arabidopsis thaliana (mouse-ear cress) 2/3/5, and Brassica napus Naehan. calmodulin. 10/93 148aa
Cal2_Pethy P27163 petunia hybrida (petunia). calmodulin 2/4. 8/92 148aa
Cal4_Arath Translation of GB Z12022 arabidopsis thaliana (mouse-ear cress). calmodulin 4 6/93 148aa
Cal6_Arath Translation of GB Z12024 arabidopsis thaliana (mouse-ear cress). calmodulin 6 6/93 148aa
Call_Arbpu P05932 arbacia punctulata (punctuate sea urchin). calmodulin beta (fragment). 8/92 138aa P05934 strongylocentrotus purpuratus (purple sea urchin). calmodulin (fragment). 11/88 80aa
Call_Plafa Translation of GB X56950 plasmodium falciparum. calmodulin 5/91 145aa
Calm_Achkl P15094 achlya klebsiana. calmodulin. 8/92 148aa
Calm_Brydi P34792 bryonia dioica (red bryony). calmodulin. 2/94 148aa
Calm_Canal P23286 candida albicans (yeast). calmodulin. 3/92 149aa
Calm_Chlre P04352 chlamydomonas reinhardtii. calmodulin. 4/90 162aa
Calm_Dicdi P02599 dictyostelium discoideum (slime mold). calmodulin. 2/94 151aa
Calm_Drome P07181 drosophila melanogaster (fruit fly), locusta migratoria (migratory locust), and aplysia californica (california sea hare). calmodulin. 4/88 148aa
Calm_Eleel P02594 electrophorus electricus (electric eel). calmodulin. 5/91 148aa
Calm_Emeni P19533 emericella nidulans (aspergillus nidulans), and aspergillus oryzae. calmodulin. 4/93 148aa
Calm_Euggr P11118 euglena gracilis. calmodulin. 5/92 148aa
Calm_Horvu P13565, P29612 hordeum vulgare (barley), oryza sativa (rice),soybean 2, and vigna radiata. calmodulin. 11/88 148aa
Calm_Human P02593 homo sapiens (human), oryctolagus cuniculus (rabbit), bos taurus (bovine), rattus norvegicus (rat), mus musculus (mouse), gallus gallus (chicken), xenopus laevis (african clawed frog), oncorhynchus sp. (salmon), ducks, and arbacia punctulata (punctuate sea urchin). 7/86 148aa
Calm_Lyces P27161 lycopersicon esculentum (tomato). calmodulin. 8/92 148aa
Calm_Lytpi P05935 lytechinus pictus (painted sea urchin). calmodulin (fragment). 4/90 30aa
Calm_Medsa P17928 medicago sativa (alfalfa),soybean 1/3, and vigna radiata (clone pMBCaM-1). calmodulin. 8/92 148aa
Calm_Metse P02596 metridium senile (brown sea anemone) (frilled sea anemone), and renilla reniformis (sea pansy). calmodulin. 7/86 148aa
Calm_Nagru Translation of GB U04381 naegleria gruberi. flagellar calmodulin. 3/94 ***aa
Calm_Neucr Q02052 neurospora crassa. calmodulin. 2/94 148aa
Calm_Parte P07463 paramecium tetraurelia. calmodulin. 6/94 148aa
Calm_Patsp P02595 patinopecten sp. (scallop). calmodulin. 11/88 148aa
Calm_Phyin P27165 phytophthora infestans (potato late blight fungus).calmodulin. 8/92 148aa
Calm_Plafa P24044 plasmodium falciparum. calmodulin. 5/92 149aa
Calm_Pleco P11120 pleurotus cornucopiae (cornucopia mushroom). calmodulin. 2/91 148aa
Calm_Pncar Translation of GB L05572 pneumocystis carinii. calmodulin. 8/93 ***aa
Calm_Pyusp P11121 pyuridae sp. (sea squirt). calmodulin. 7/89 148aa
Calm_Schpo P05933 schizosaccharomyces pombe (fission yeast). calmodulin. 7/89 150aa
Calm_Soltu P13868 solanum tuberosum (potato). calmodulin. 8/92 148aa
Calm_Stija P21251 stichopus japonicus (sea cucumber). calmodulin. 4/88 148aa
Calm_Style P27166 stylonychia lemnae. calmodulin. 4/93 148aa
Calm_Tetpy P02598 tetrahymena pyriformis, tetrahymena thermophila. calmodulin. 7/93 148aa
Calm_Trybb P04465, P18061 trypanosoma brucei brucei, trypanosoma brucei gambiense, and trypanosoma cruzi. calmodulin. 5/92 148aa
Calm_Wheat P04464 triticum aestivum (wheat). calmodulin. 11/88 149aa
Calm_Yeast P06787 saccharomyces cerevisiae (baker's yeast). calmodulin. 8/92 147aa
Calm_Zmays Translation of GB X74490, P04353 zea mays (maize), and spinacia oleracea (spinach). calmodulin. 6/94 148aa

result, the hydrophobic pockets in each head line up next to each other on the same side of the target helix. There the two pairs of EF-hand domains form an elongated hydrophobic patch with significant methionine content (methionine puddle) that is presumed to allow flexibility in calmodulin–target interaction and thus permit binding to a wide range of targets. The peptide-induced conformational change may be stabilized by a latch region in the loop between EF hands in both domains (see Fig. 1; O'Neil and DeGrado 1990; Török and Whitaker 1994; Weinstein and Mehler 1994).

◼ Interactions

Calmodulin has been shown to interact with well over 100 different proteins (see Table 2 for a comprehensive list). Affinities for bona-fide CaM targets are usually in the nanomolar range. By contrast, the physiological relevance of CaM regulation of proteins/peptides with micromolar CaM affinities is less obvious. In general, CaM seems to bind to targets only in the presence of Ca^{2+}, although there are exceptions, such as phosphorylase kinase, in which CaM binds to targets in the absence of

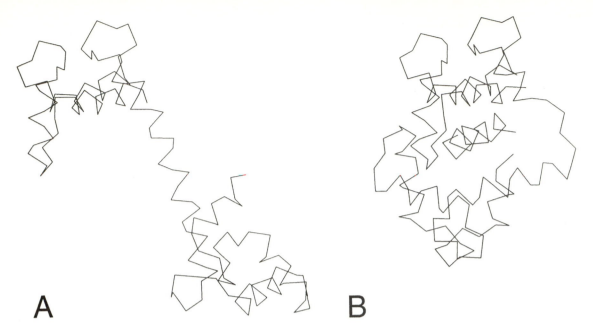

A   B

Figure 1. (A) Alpha-carbon trace of the crystal structure of vertebrate calcium-calmodulin. **(B)** Alpha-carbon trace of calcium-calmodulin bound to the cognate peptide of smooth muscle myosin light chain kinase. Note the latch region to the left of the peptide and the unwinding of the central tether (right). The amino termini (top) have been optimally aligned in this view of the structures shown in (A) and (B). Coordinates were obtained from the Brookhaven Protein Database.

Ca^{2+} and then undergoes a regulatory conformational change upon Ca^{2+} binding. There is also a class of proteins, likely involved in the regulation of CaM availability (see Table 2), which have a greater affinity for Ca^{2+}-free than for Ca^{2+}-bound CaM. In addition, see below for the evidence of entirely Ca^{2+}-independent functions of CaM in yeast.

■ Antibodies

Polyclonal and monoclonal CaM-specific antibodies are available from several commercial sources, including Calbiochem and Sigma Immunochemicals.

■ Anatomical localization

CaM is found in all cells and tissues. In mammals, it is particularly abundant in brain and testis. Total CaM concentrations have been determined in a number of vertebrate tissues and range from a few micromolar to over 30 μM. Intracellularly, CaM is found both in the cytosol as well as in membrane-bound fractions. CaM has also been detected in the nucleus but not in mitochondria or the endoplasmic reticulum. The precise subcellular localization of CaM and its dynamics are not well understood, but the regulated redistribution of CaM among different cellular compartments and between the cytosol and the nucleus appears to play an important role for the proper regulation of CaM function (Bachs *et al.* 1992; Gnegy 1993).

■ Biological activities

As is to be expected in the case of a protein with such a large number and variety of targets (Table 2), CaM has been shown to be required for a bewildering multitude of cellular processes, including, but not limited to: gene regulation, DNA synthesis, cell cycle progression, mitosis, cytokinesis, cytoskeletal organization, muscle contraction, signal transduction, ion homeostasis, exocytosis, and metabolic regulation (Means and Dedman 1980; Cohen and Klee 1988; Bachs *et al.* 1992; Gnegy 1993; Hinrichsen 1993; Lu and Means 1993).

■ Biological regulation

CaM mRNA and protein levels have been shown to be regulated in a tissue, developmental, and cell cycle specific manner (Gnegy 1993; Lu and Means 1993). Although several studies indicate the possibility of differential regulation of the multiple CaM transcripts in plants and vertebrates, most (vertebrate) cells co-express all CaM transcripts, albeit at varying levels. CaM has been shown to be up-regulated in the tumors and in tumor-derived cell lines in several types of cancer (Rasmussen and Means 1989); however, it has also been recently

Table 2. Comprehensive list of calmodulin binding proteins (last updated in March 1995).

Protein Kinases/Phosphatases
CaM kinase I/V
CaM kinase II
CaM kinase III/EF-2 kinase
CaM kinase IV/protein kinase Gr
CaM kinase kinase
Bovine heart CaM kinase
80 kDa CaM kinase
Glycogen synthase kinase 3a/Protein kinase FA/*tau* kinase/42 kDa MAP kinase
Myosin heavy chain kinase (*Acanthamoeba*)
Myosin light chain kinase
Phosphorylase kinase
Calcineurin/Protein phosphatase-2b

Signalling Proteins
Adenylyl cyclase (I, III, VIII)
Cyclic 3'-5'-nucleotide phosphodi-esterase
Dopamine β monooxygenase
EGF receptor
G-protein βγ subunits
Guanylyl cyclase (*Tetrahymena*)
Insulin receptor complex
IP3 kinase
Nitric oxide synthase (I, II, III)
Phospholipase A2

Ion Transporters
Ca^{2+}-dependent K+ channel (*Paramecium*)
Ca^{2+}-dependent Na+ channel (*Paramecium*)
Cardiac 116-picosiemen chloride channel
IP_3 receptor Ca^{2+} release channel
Na^+–Ca^{2+} exchanger (cardiac type)
Na^+-H+ exchanger 1 (NHE1)
Olfactory cyclic nucleotide gated cation channel
Phospholamban
Photoreceptor cGMP-gated cation channel (240 kDa subunit)
Plasma membrane Ca^{2+} ATPase
Ryanodine receptor Ca^{2+} release channel
trpl (*Drosophila*)

Potential Regulators of CaM Location/Availability
MARCKS
MRP/MacMARCKS/F52
Neurogranin/RC3

Neuromodulin/GAP43/GAP48/B50/F1/ P-57/pp46/IGLOO/protein 4
pp170
Proacrosin, Acrosin

Nucleic Acid Regulating Proteins
CaM-BP-68 (nuclear regulator of DNA synthesis, associated with DNA polymerase α-primase)
DNA Pol α complex proteins M_r 48, 55, 80, 120, 150–200
ECa proteins (E-box, Ca^{2+}/CaM-binding bHLH transcription factors) SEF2-1/ITF2, E2A, E12, E47, Max
hnRNP A2
hnRNP C
p62 (nuclear matrix associated, dsDNA binding)
p68 RNA helicase

Cytoskeletal Proteins
α/β-Adducin
Caldesmon h & l
Calponin
Clathrin light chains a & b
Cytosynalin
Desmocalmin
Dynein
Dystrophin
α-Dystroglycan
α-Fodrin/α-Spectrin
Keratocalmin
Kinesin light chain
Myosin I
Myosin III (nina C)
Myosin V
Myosin VI
Myosin IX
MAP-2
Nebulin
Plastin/Fimbrin
Protein 4.1
Utrophin
Synapsin I
Syntrophin/59 DAP/Syn
tau
Tubulin
Twitchin

Other Proteins with Known Functions
Calmodulin *N*-methyl transferase
C-CAM/Cell-CAM 105/Ecto-ATPase
Chromogranin A
FKBP 52

FKBP 59/HBI (heat shock protein binding immunophilin)
Glutamate decarboxylase (plant)
HSP (heat shock protein) 26, 70, 90, 100
NAD kinase
Nuf1p/SPC110p (yeast)
Phosphofructokinase
Ribosomal protein L19
Succinate dehydrogenase
Translation elongation factor EF1a (*Trypanosoma brucei*, higher plants)
VSG (*Trypanosoma brucei*)

Natural Peptides
C-type natriuretic peptide/bSVSP15
Growth hormone releasing factor
Mastoparan
Melittin
NPY-25
VIP/vasoactive intestinal peptide

Proteins of Unknown Function
BSP (bovine seminal plasma) A1, A2, A3
BSP 30 kDa
Calspermin
CaM-BP55 (electric eel)
CAP (CaM acceptor protein)/CAP-23, CAP-45, CAP-60
CBP-100/CaMBP-100
65-CMBP (65 K vesicle-associated integral membrane protein)
High molecular weight (175 KDa) CaMBP
1G5 (a vesicle-associated protein with kinase homology, but no activity)
NAP-22

Proteins with Binding of Questionable Relevance
ACTH (low μM affinity)
Bombesin (60–90 μM affinity)
β-Endorphin (low μM affinity)
Glucagon (low μM affinity)
Histone H1 (inactivated CaM binds histones)
α-MSH (60–90 μM affinity)
Smooth muscle myosin (20–30 μM affinity)
Somatostatin (60–90 μM affinity)
Substance P (low μM affinity)
Tropomyosin (μM affinity)

There are also proteins of almost any electrophoretic mobility that have been shown to bind calmodulin in overlay experiments; however, these are not included in this table unless they have been further characterized. Not all binding has been shown to be physiologically relevant. This table may contain omissions or duplications, especially such as are not obvious in the relevant literature. The authors request that additions and/or corrections be communicated to them at the address at the end of this article. Specific references for each of the entries are available from the authors upon request.

reported that mRNA levels of at least one CaM gene transcript (human CALM1) are dramatically down-regulated in some cancers. These observations have not as yet yielded a discernible general pattern in CaM regulation. CaM levels have been shown to be regulated at the transcriptional, post-transcriptional, and translational levels but the interplay between and relative importance of the diverse regulatory mechanisms are largely unknown.

Mutagenesis studies

Extensive site-directed mutagenesis studies on vertebrate and invertebrate (*Drosophila*) CaM, as well as analyses of *in vivo* generated CaM mutants in *Paramecium* and yeast have yielded considerable information on the roles of various amino acids in CaM Ca^{2+}-binding properties, structure, and function. In addition, considerable work with mutant CaMs and synthetic peptides has defined some requirements for CaM-binding sequences, resulting in the identification of the so-called Baa (basic amphiphilic alpha-helix) motif in numerous CaM-binding proteins (O'Neil and DeGrado 1990).

No natural mutants of any of the vertebrate CaM genes exist. However, in yeast and *Paramecium*, (partial) loss of CaM function mutants have been characterized that are temperature sensitive and/or result in behavioral dysfunction (Hinrichsen 1993; Ohya and Botstein 1994). These mutants have allowed the identification and dissection of several independent CaM functions such as the differential effects of the N- and C-terminal lobes on diverse ion channels (reviewed by Hinrichsen 1993; Saimi and Kung 1994). A thought-provoking study has also shown the ability of site-directed CaM mutants that fail to bind Ca^{2+} to rescue CaM-deficient haploid yeast spores, suggesting an essential role for CaM in its Ca^{2+}-free form at least in this organism (Geiser *et al.* 1991).

References

Bachs, O., Agell, N., and Carafoli, E. (1992) Calcium and calmodulin function in the cell nucleus. Biochim. Biophys. Acta **1113**, 259–268.

Burgess W.H., Jemiolo, D.K., and Kretsinger, R.H. (1980) Interaction of calcium and calmodulin in the presence of sodium dodecyl sulfate. Biochim. Biophys. Acta **623**, 257–270.

Chattopadhyaya, R., Meador, W.E., Means, A.R., and Quiocho, F.A. (1992) Calmodulin structure refined at 1.7 Å resolution. J. Mol. Biol. **228**, 1177–1192.

Cheung, W.Y., Lynch T.J., and Wallace R.W. (1978) An endogenous Ca^{2+}-dependent activator protein of brain adenylate cyclase and cyclic nucleotide phosphodiesterase. Adv. Cycl. Nucleotide Res. **9**, 233–251.

*Cohen, P. and Klee, C.B. (ed.) (1988) Calmodulin. In *Molecular aspects of cellular regulation*, Vol. 5. Elsevier, Amsterdam.

Geiser, J.R., van Tuinen, D., Brockerhoff, S.E., Neff, M.M., and Davis, T.N. (1991) Can calmodulin function without binding calcium? Cell **65**, 949–959.

Gnegy, M.E. (1993) Calmodulin in neurotransmitter and hormone action. Annu. Rev. Pharmacol. Toxicol. **32**, 45–70.

*Hinrichsen, R.D. (1993) Calcium and calmodulin in the control of cellular behavior and motility. Biochim. Biophys. Acta **1155**, 277–293.

*Lu, K.P. and Means, A.R. (1993) Regulation of the cell cycle by calcium and calmodulin. Endocrine Rev. **14**, 40–58.

Means, A.R. and Dedman, J.R. (1980) Calmodulin–an intracellular calcium receptor. Nature **285**, 73–77.

Ohya, Y. and Botstein, D. (1994) Diverse essential functions revealed by complementing yeast calmodulin mutants. Science **263**, 963–966.

O'Neil, K.T. and DeGrado, W.F. (1990) How calmodulin binds its targets: sequence independent recognition of amphiphilic a-helices. Trends Biochem. Sci. **15**, 59–64.

Onek, L.A. and Smith, R.J. (1992) Calmodulin and calcium mediated regulation in prokaryotes. J. Gen. Microbiol. **138**, 1039–1049.

Quadroni, M., James, P., and Carafoli, E. (1994) Isolation of phosphorylated calmodulin from rat liver and identification of the *in vivo* phosphorylation sites. J. Biol. Chem. **269**, 16116–16122.

Rasmussen, C.D. and Means, A.R. (1989) Calmodulin, cell growth and gene expression. Trends Neurosci. **12**, 433–438.

Sacks, D.B., Davis, H.W., Crimmins, D.L., and McDonald, J.M. (1992) Insulin-stimulated phosphorylation of calmodulin. Biochem. J. **286**, 211–216.

Saimi, Y. and Kung, C. (1994) Ion channel regulation by calmodulin binding. FEBS Lett. **350**, 155–158.

Suko J., Wyskovsky W., Pidlich J., Hauptner R., Plank B., and Hellmann G. (1986) Calcium release from calmodulin and its C-terminal or N-terminal halves in the presence of the calmodulin antagonists phenoxybenzamine and melittin measured by stopped-flow fluorescence with Quin 2 and intrinsic tyrosine. Inhibition of calmodulin-dependent protein kinase of cardiac sarcoplasmic reticulum. Eur. J. Biochem. **159**, 425–434.

Török, N. and Whitaker, M. (1994) Taking a long, hard look at calmodulin's warm embrace. BioEssays **16**, 221–224.

Vogel, H.J., Lindahl. L., and Thulin, E. (1983) Calcium-dependent hydrophobic interaction chromatography of calmodulin, troponin C and their proteolytic fragments. FEBS Lett. **157**, 241–246.

*Weinstein, H. and Mehler, E.L. (1994) Ca^{2+}-binding and structural dynamics in the functions of calmodulin. Ann. Rev. Physiol. **56**, 213–236.

Williams J.P., Jo, H., Sacks, D.B., Crimmins, D.L., Thoma, R.S., Hunnicutt, R.E., Radding, W., Sharma, R.K., and McDonald, J.M. (1994) Tyrosine phosphorylated calmodulin has reduced biological activity. Arch. Biochem. Biophys. **315**, 119–126.

■ *Michael S. Rogers and Emanuel E. Strehler: Department of Biochemistry and Molecular Biology, Mayo Graduate School, Mayo Clinic and Foundation, Rochester, MN 55905, USA.*
Tel.: +507 284 9372
Fax: +507 284 2384
E-mail: strehler@rcf.mayo.edu

Calmodulin-like proteins

Calmodulin-like proteins are a diverse group of EF-hand proteins whose amino acid sequence is most homologous to that of calmodulin (CaM) from the corresponding species, but still differs to such a degree that functional differences are to be expected (operationally differences of > 10% in amino acid sequence). These proteins are likely to be functionally distinct, but they share with calmodulin their small size and many biophysical characteristics (e.g. Ca^{2+}-induced conformational changes, target-induced conformational changes, and Ca^{2+}-affinity changes). A number of gene products which have originally been called calmodulin-related or calmodulin-like because of their (partial) sequence similarity with calmodulin are, in fact, significantly larger than CaM and contain additional domains that indicate their functional divergence from CaM. These members of the EF-hand family of calcium-binding proteins will not be considered in this entry but are separately listed where appropriate (e.g. the calmodulin-like gene and the touch-sensitive calmodulin-related gene products Tch-2 and Tch-3 from Arabidopsis, *or the "calmodulin family" proteins TCBP-23 and TCBP-25 from* Tetrahymena).

Several genes and pseudogenes have been identified with predicted amino acid sequences closely matching that of CaM, including intronless and intron-containing pseudogenes, with and without appropriate open reading frames. At present, evidence for expression has only been claimed in the case of seven such genes, one each in chicken (Stein *et al.* 1983), rat (Nojima and Sokabe 1986), *Caenorhabditis elegans* (Salvato *et al.* 1986), human (Koller and Strehler 1988), *Arabidopsis* (Ling and Zielinski 1993), *Drosophila* (Fyrberg *et al.* 1994), and *Petunia* (H. Fromm, E. Carlenor, and N.-H. Chua, unpublished).

In the first case, Northern blot hybridization suggested expression of a chicken calmodulin-like gene product, cCM1 in striated muscle (Stein *et al.* 1983). Failure to isolate the predicted protein product from these tissues led to the discovery that the probe used cross-reacts with troponin C mRNA (Putkey *et al.* 1987). It thus appears that this gene sequence is not expressed. Similar results have apparently been obtained upon careful examination of the rat intronless pseudogene (Nojima *et al.* 1987).

Of the remaining five actively transcribed genes, the expression pattern and/or the product of only one (the human CLP (NB-1) gene) has so far been further characterized.

■ Identification/isolation

The *C. elegans* calmodulin-like gene *cal-1* was isolated by screening a nematode genomic DNA library under low stringency conditions with a human CaM cDNA probe (Salvato *et al.* 1986).

Human CLP (calmodulin-like protein) was originally cloned as a putative pseudogene in screening a genomic DNA library for calmodulin genes (Koller and Strehler 1988). It was independently identified by subtractive hybridization of RNA from normal and chemically immortalized breast epithelial cells and named NB-1 (Yaswen *et al.* 1990). Bacterially expressed CLP has been purified by phenyl-Sepharose chromatography in a manner identical to that used for the purification of CaM (Rhyner *et al.* 1992; Yaswen *et al.* 1992).

cDNAs encoding the *Arabidopsis* CaBP-22 calmodulin-related protein were isolated from a leaf cDNA library (Ling and Zielinski 1993).

cDNAs corresponding to the *Drosophila* calmodulin-related gene were isolated by low stringency screening of pupal-stage cDNA libraries with a *Drosophila* CaM gene probe (Fyrberg *et al.* 1994).

■ Gene and sequence

Gene Bank (GB) and Swiss protein data base (SwissProt) accession numbers for the expressed calmodulin-like proteins are: *C. elegans cal-1* (GB X04259, SwissProt P04630), human CLP/NB-1 (GB X13461, SwissProt P27482), *Arabidopsis* CaBP-22 (GB Z12136, SwissProt P30187), *Drosophila* (GB X76045), *Petunia Cal-3* (GB M80831, SwissProt P27164). See Table 1 for a comparison of these sequences with the calmodulin consensus.

The *C. elegans cal-1* gene is about 0.8 kb in size, contains a single intron of 55 bp and is located 52 to 68% from the left end of linkage group IV (Salvato *et al.* 1986). The human CLP gene is intronless, generates a mRNA of about 1.4 kb (Yaswen *et al.* 1990) and is located on chromosome 10p13-ter (Berchtold *et al.* 1993). The *Drosophila* gene is intronless and is located on chromosome 3 division 97A (Fyrberg *et al.* 1994).

■ Protein

Human CLP shares several traits with calmodulin, including the ability to bind four Ca^{2+} (although with an average eightfold lower affinity) (Rhyner *et al.* 1992). CLP also shows an affinity for magnesium similar to that of calmodulin and it undergoes an electrophoretic mobility shift in the presence of Ca^{2+} (17 to 14.5 kDa), although this shift is less dramatic than that of CaM. Like CaM, CLP

Table 1. Amino acid sequences of expressed calmodulin-like proteins, and optimal alignment with the calmodulin consensus sequence.

```
Cal3_Pethy                          -------d    d--s------  ---------c              ----------  ----------
Call_Human                          --------    --vt------  ---------c  ---r------  --r--ms-i-
Call_Drome  mse-----                -------d--  vq---e-t-k  -a-r----l-  -t-------   --l---a-ae
Call_Caeel  maipsnlmqf  sediik---p  -e-d-r---   mm-----n--  -s-----ia-  ----------q -ile------
Cbp2_Arath              m-nkf--r    q--s--r-q-  -vy--n---h  ---e-f-a--  -----l-l-q- ---ee--ds-
 CaM Cnsns              ADQLTE      EQIAEFKEAF  SLFDKGDGT   ITTKELGTVM  RSLGQNPTEA  ELQDMINEVD

Cal3_Pethy  ----------  --n-----                -------lk  ---------q
Call_Human  r-----v---  ---gm-----  ----n-----             ---v------  -----r----  s---------
Call_Drome  nnn--qln-t  --cgi--kq-  re--t---m-  ---ki--r--  d----p--i-  f---i-----v ----i-----
Call_Caeel  i----q-e--  --cvm-k-m-  -e---.-m--              --v-t-q-f-  yf--vhm-mqf se-------k
Cbp2_Arath  l--d---n-t  ---ca--...  ---y--kdlk  kd--l--i-k  --------m-  y-r--i-rw-q ----i--i-k
 CaM Cnsns  ADGNGTIDFP  EFLTLMARKM  KDTDSEEEIR  EAFRVFDKDG  NGFISAAELR  HVMTNLGEKL  TDEEVDEMIR

Cal3_Pethy  ---v------  -------v--  -nrrrriee  skrsvnsnis  rsnngrkvrk  rdrctil
Call_Human  a--t-----v  ------rvlv  s-
Call_Drome  ---f----m-  ------w-is  q-
Call_Caeel  -v-v----e-  d--------s  nq
Cbp2_Arath  a--v------  --r--arl--  --nqghdtky dttggtlerd  laagvaknii  aapmdfikn   fealfs
 CaM Cnsns  EADIDGDGQI  NYEEFVKMMM  AK
```

The sequences are: Cal3_Pethy, *Petunia hybrida* calmodulin-related protein; Call_Human, *Homo sapiens* calmodulin-like protein (CLP/NB-1); Call_Drome, *Drosophila melanogaster* calmodulin-related gene product; Call_Caeel, *Caenorhabditis elegans* calmodulin-like protein; Cbp2_Arath, *Arabidopsis thaliana* 22 kDa calmodulin-like protein (CaBP-22). The calmodulin consensus sequence (CaM Cnsns) was derived from a compilation of all known bona fide CaM sequences (see separate entry for calmodulin in this guidebook). Hyphens indicate identity with the consensus, dots denote the absence of residues and were introduced to optimize the alignment.

can be purified on phenyl-Sepharose and other hydrophobic interaction matrices (Rhyner, *et al.* 1992; Yaswen *et al.* 1992). In addition, CLP undergoes conformational changes upon calcium binding that are reminiscent of those displayed by CaM (Durussel *et al.* 1993). CLP can also activate the 3′,5′-cyclic nucleotide phosphodiesterase to the same V_{max} as CaM, albeit with a sevenfold higher K_{act}.

Despite these similarities, CLP is functionally distinct from calmodulin as evidenced by its inability to stimulate the plasma membrane calcium pump to the same extent as calmodulin (Rhyner *et al.* 1992). It has been suggested that CaM may in fact have two binding modes, one compact as observed in the cases of CaM kinase, smooth muscle myosin light chain kinase and the plasma membrane calcium pump, and the other more elongated as may be the case with phosphodiesterase (Török and Whitaker 1994). Results with phosphodiesterase and the plasma membrane calcium pump suggest that CLP's ability to assume the compact structure observed in cocrystals of CaM with CaM kinase or smooth muscle myosin light chain kinase peptides may be impaired, while the hypothetical more elongated structure remains accessible.

■ Anatomical localization

Arabidopsis CaBP-22 mRNA appears to be specifically expressed in the leaves of the plant (Ling and Zielinski 1993).

The gene product known alternatively as CLP and NB-1 protein (normal breast 1) has been shown to be expressed in a highly tissue-restricted and cell-type specific manner in normal stratified and pseudostratified epithelial cells of breast, cervix, prostate, and skin. This protein may also be localized to the nucleus during portions of the cell cycle and to the spindle during mitosis (Yaswen *et al.* 1992).

■ Biological activities and regulation

The regulation and expression pattern of CLP suggest a role for this protein in cell cycle regulation and/or differentiation. CLP is down-regulated in immortalized cells and epithelial cancer cells both in culture and in primary isolates (Yaswen *et al.* 1990, 1992). Whether this down-regulation is required for, or merely coincident with, immortalization and transformation is uncertain. CLP's activity may include a role as a putative tumor suppressor, as evidenced by the apparent incompatibility of CLP expression and the transformed phenotype (Yaswen *et al.* 1990, 1992). This property is opposite to that of CaM, which is required for cell cycle progression and growth and which has been reported to be up-regulated in many transformed cells. CLP also differs from CaM in that it is apparently unable to rescue lethal yeast CaM mutants (unpublished observation cited in Yaswen *et al.* 1992), although human CaM (Davis and Thorner 1989) and mutant CaMs with dramatically reduced Ca^{2+} affinity are both able to do so (Geiser *et al.* 1991).

■ References

Berchtold, M.W., Koller, M., Egli, R., Rhyner, J.A., Hameister, H., and Strehler, E.E. (1993) Localization of the intronless gene coding for calmodulin-like protein CLP to human chromosome 10p13-ter. Hum. Genet. **90**, 496–500.

Davis, T.N. and Thorner, J. (1989) Vertebrate and yeast calmodulin, despite significant sequence divergence, are functionally interchangeable. Proc. Natl. Acad. Sci. USA **86**, 7909–7913.

Durussel, I., Rhyner, J.A., Strehler, E.E., and Cox, J.A. (1993) Cation binding and conformation of human calmodulin-like protein. Biochemistry **32**, 6089–6094.

Fyrberg, C., Parker, H., Hutchison, B., and Fyrberg, E. (1994) *Drosophila melanogaster* genes encoding three troponin-C isoforms and a calmodulin-related protein. Biochem. Genet. **32**, 119–135.

Geiser, J.R., van Tuinen, D., Brockerhoff, S.E., Neff, M.M., and Davis, T.N. (1991) Can calmodulin function without binding calcium? Cell **65**, 949–959.

Koller, M. and Strehler, E.E., (1988) Characterization of an intronless human calmodulin-like pseudogene. FEBS Lett. **239**, 121–128.

Ling, V. and Zielinski, R.E. (1993) Isolation of an *Arabidopsis* cDNA sequence encoding a 22 kDa calcium-binding protein (CaBP-22) related to calmodulin. Plant Mol. Biol. **22**, 207–214.

Nojima, H. and Sokabe, H. (1986) Structure of rat calmodulin processed genes with implications for a mRNA-mediated process of insertion. J. Mol. Biol. **190,** 391–400.

Nojima, H. Kishi, K., and Sokabe, H. (1987) Multiple calmodulin mRNA species are derived from two distinct genes. Mol. Cell. Biol. **7**, 1873–1880.

Putkey, J.A., Carroll, S.L., and Means, A.R. (1987) The non-transcribed chicken calmodulin pseudogene cross-hybridizes with mRNA from the slow-muscle troponin C gene. Mol. Cell. Biol. **7**, 1549–1553.

Rhyner, J.A., Koller, M., Durussel-Gerber, I., Cox, J.A., and Strehler, E.E. (1992) Characterization of the human calmodulin-like protein expressed in *Escherichia coli*. Biochemistry **31**, 12826–12832.

Salvato, M., Sulston, J., Albertson, D., and Brenner, S. (1986) A novel calmodulin-like gene from the nematode *Caenorhabditis elegans*. J. Mol. Biol. **190**, 281–290.

Stein, J.P., Munjaal, R.P., Lagace, L., Lai, E.C., O'Mally, B.W., and Means, A.R. (1983) Tissue specific expression of a chicken calmodulin pseudogene lacking intervening sequences. Proc. Natl. Acad. Sci. USA **80**, 6485–6489.

Török, K. and Whitaker, M. (1994) Taking a long, hard look at calmodulin's warm embrace. Bioessays **16**, 221–224.

Yaswen, P., Smoll, A., Peehl, D.M., Trask, D.K., Sager, R., and Stampfer, M.R. (1990) Down-regulation of a calmodulin-related gene during transformation of human mammary epithelial cells. Proc. Natl. Acad. Sci. USA **87**, 7360–7364.

Yaswen, P., Smoll, A., Hosoda, J., Parry, G., and Stampfer, M.R. (1992) Protein product of a human intronless calmodulin-like gene shows tissue-specific expression and reduced abundance in transformed cells. Cell Growth Diff. **3**, 335–345.

■ *Michael S. Rogers and Emanuel E. Strehler:*
Department of Biochemistry and Molecular Biology,
Mayo Graduate School, Mayo Clinic and Foundation,
Rochester, MN 55905, USA
Tel.: +507 284 9372
Fax: +507 284 2384
E-mail: strehler@rcf.mayo.edu

Calpains

Calpains (μ- and m-) are non-lysosomal cysteine proteinases present in most mammalian tissues in varying amounts and have been detected in all vertebrate species tested. Activation in vitro requires 1–100 μM, and 0.1–1 mM levels of Ca^{2+} for μ- and m-calpain, respectively. Suggested functions for the calpains include a role in modulating intracellular signal transduction, cell division, platelet activation, and memory formation.

Calpains are heterodimers composed of a large (80 kDa) and a small (30 kDa) subunit that associate in a non-covalent manner. The same small subunit is identical in both isozymes, μ- and m-calpain, whereas the 80 kDa large subunits have only 60% identity. The proteinase activity is located in the large subunit, as is a calmodulin-like Ca^{2+}-binding domain. The small subunit contains a second calmodulin-like Ca^{2+}-binding domain and a glycine-rich hydrophobic domain. Although the calpains appear to require non-physiological Ca^{2+} concentrations for activity for most protein substrates, there is evidence that the Ca^{2+} requirement in the intracellular environment can be several orders of magnitude lower (Mellgren 1991). Autoproteolysis of μ-calpain reduces the Ca^{2+} concentration for activation and involves cleavage of the N-terminal regions of both subunits, resulting in a 76 kDa large subunit and a 18 kDa small subunit (Saido *et al.*

1992). Autoproteolytic activation of m-calpain takes place in the presence of phosphatidylinositol which reduces the Ca^{2+} requirement to the 50 μM range (Coolican and Hathaway 1984). The activation involves autoproteolysis of the N-terminal regions of both subunits of m-calpain, resulting in a 78 kDa large subunit and a 18 kDa small subunit (Hathaway *et al.* 1982).

■ Alternative names

μ-Calpain: Mu-calpain, calpain I, μ-CANP (Ca^{2+}-activated neutral proteinase), and CDP I (Ca^{2+}-dependent proteinase I).

m-Calpain: Calpain II, m-CANP (Ca^{2+}-activated neutral proteinase), CANP-2, and CDP II (Ca^{2+}-dependent proteinase II).

■ Identification/isolation

μ-Calpain can be isolated by conventional purification techniques from human erythrocytes or from striated muscle (Mellgren 1991). The gene structure of the 80 kDa subunit was first identified for chicken μ-calpain by Suzuki and his colleagues who used oligonucleotide probes synthesized according to partial amino acid sequences. The chicken cDNA was then used as a probe to isolate the human and rabbit μ-calpain gene. The structures of the human, rabbit, and porcine 30 kDa subunits were then determined by this same research group (reviewed by Suzuki 1990).

m-Calpain can be isolated in mg amounts from mammalian skeletal muscle by conventional purification techniques (Dayton et al. 1976). The gene structure of the 80 kDa subunit of m-calpain was first identified for the chicken protein by Suzuki (1990). Recently, the enzymatically active recombinant rat m-calpain heterodimer has been expressed in E. coli (Graham-Siegenthaler et al. 1994).

■ Gene and sequence

The large and small subunits of both μ- and m-calpain can be divided into four and two domains, respectively (Fig. 1). The molecular mass of the human μ-calpain large subunit primary translation product is 81.9 kDa and that for the small subunit is 28.3 kDa. The gene for the chicken large subunit is composed of 21 exons. Sequence comparisons between the μ- and m-calpain large subunits from the same species show about 60% identity (Suzuki 1990). Many of the exon–intron borders correspond closely with the borders of the domains, suggesting that the large subunit is formed from the fusion of multiple genes. The rabbit small subunit is composed of 11 exons whose borders again correspond with domain borders. The 5′-upstream region of both large and small subunit genes has multiple translation promoter elements and regulatory regions. Strong sequence homology in the upstream region of the two subunits indicates that they are co-regulated at the transcription level. Recently four new calpain large subunit genes have been identified by Sorimachi et al. (1994), including three which are tissue specific for skeletal muscle (nCL-1) or stomach (nCL-2 and nCL-2′). GenBank accession numbers: μ-calpain large subunit from pig (U01180); calpain homolog expressed in Drosophila melanogaster (Z46891, Z46892); skeletal muscle specific calpain 3 from human (X85030, X85031, X85032); calpain small subunit from rat (U10861).

■ Protein

Domain I of the large subunit contains the N-terminal amino acids which are removed during auto-activation (Fig. 1). Domain II contains the cysteine protease active region. Domain III is suspected of possessing a calmodulin-binding domain that may play a role in controlling the proteinase activity of domain II (Suzuki et al. 1987). Domain IV of the large subunit and IV′ of the small

subunit each contain a calmodulin-like domain with four EF-hand structures for Ca^{2+} binding (Suzuki 1990). Domains IV and IV′ contain the sites of attachment between the large and small subunit as well as for interaction with membranes. Domain V of the small subunit contains a glycine-rich hydrophobic region that may also play a role in membrane attachment. This region is completely removed during autocatalytic activation. m-Calpain, having a greater net negative charge than μ-calpain at neutral pH, binds more tightly to anion exchange columns and hence can be eluted separately. Swiss-Prot accession number for calpains: μ-calpain large subunit from rabbit (P06815), human (P07384), pig (P35750), chicken (P00789); m-calpain large subunit from human (P17655), rabbit (P06814), rat (Q07009); skeletal muscle specific calpain P94 large subunit from rat (P16259), human (P20807).

■ Antibodies

The murine monoclonal antibody P-6, produced against the μ-calpain large subunit from human erythrocytes (Lane et al. 1992), is available from Swant and Chemicon. This antibody shows no cross-reactivity with either the calpain small subunit or the m-calpain large subunit.

A rabbit polyclonal antiserum, PC-1 produced against m-calpain large subunit from human placentas (Lane et al. 1992), is available from Swant and Chemicon. This antibody shows minimal cross-reactivity with either the calpain small subunit or the μ-calpain large subunit. The murine monoclonal antibody P-1, produced against m-calpain small subunit from bovine myocardium (Mellgren and Lane 1990) is available from Chemicon. This antibody recognizes the calpain small subunit from either μ– or m-calpain.

■ Localization

At the subcellular level μ- and m-calpain are localized to the I-band and Z-disks of skeletal muscle (Dayton and Schollmeyer 1981; Yoshimura et al. 1986). In the brain, μ-calpain-like immunoreactivity has been seen in the neuronal somatic cytoplasm and extends into the proximal dendritic processes, whereas m-calpain-like immunoreactivity has been seen in the neuronal cell bodies, glial cells, and myelinated-axons. (Hamakubo et al. 1986). μ-Calpain is present in the cytoplasm, spindle apparatus, and cell membrane of dividing A431 cells, and in the

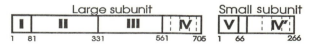

Figure 1. Domain structure of the calpain large and small subunits. Dashed vertical lines denote the location of EF-hand structures (adapted from Suzuki 1990).

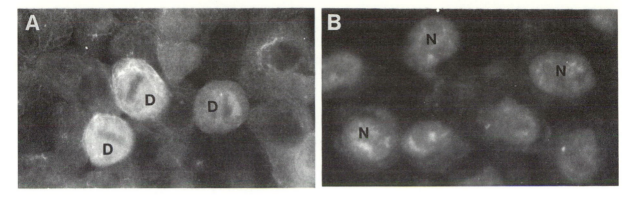

Figure 2. (A) μ-Calpain immunolocalization in the human A431 epidermal carcinoma cell line. Note the intense staining of the dividing cells, D. (B) In the human C-33A cervical carcinoma cell line, μ-Calpain is concentrated in the nuclei, N.

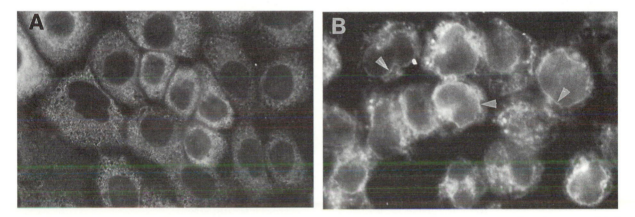

Figure 3. (A) m-Calpain immunolocalization (A) in the cytoplasm of human A431 epidermal carcinoma cell line; (B) in the cytoplasm and nuclear envelopes (arrows) of C33A cervical carcinoma cells.

nuclei of cultured C-33A cervical carcinoma cells (Lane *et al.* 1992; Fig. 2). m-Calpain is present in the cytoplasm of interphase A431 cells (Fig. 3), and the cytoplasm, spindle poles, and midbodies of mitotic A431 cells (Lane *et al.* 1992). Cell-specific localization of μ- and m-calpain has been noted in the convoluted tubules of the kidney (Murachi and Yoshimura 1985) and striated ducts of the submandibular gland (Murachi and Yoshimura 1985). β-cells of the islets of Langerhans (Kitahara *et al.* 1985), and keratinocytes (Miyachi *et al.* 1986) express μ-calpain, whereas endocrine cells in the human pituitary gland contain m-calpain (Kitahara *et al.* 1985).

■ Biological activities

A large number of endogenous proteins have been identified as substrates for calpain-mediated proteolysis *in vitro* (for a review, see Takahashi 1990). These include myofibrillar proteins, cytoskeletal proteins, hormone receptors, protein kinases, and other enzymes. Proteolysis of most substrates is limited, so that large fragments are produced, compared with the more extensive cleavages produced by most other endoproteases. μ-Calpain appears to be a substrate for the nuclear energy-dependent protein uptake system (Mellgren and Lu 1994).

■ Interactions

In the presence of Ca^{2+}, both μ- and m-calpain are bound and inactivated by calpastatin, a large protein (apparent molecular mass = 110 to 130 kDa on SDS-PAGE). The calpastatin contains multiple inhibitory domains that block the calpain proteinase activity. Calpastatin may function in protecting specific membranes and intracellular organelles from calpain-mediated proteolysis (for review, see Mellgren and Lane 1990).

■ References

Coolican, S.A. and Hathaway, D.R. (1984) Effect of L-a-phos-phatidylinositol on a vascular smooth muscle Ca²⁺-dependent protease. J. Biol. Chem. **259**, 11627–11630.

Dayton, W.R. and Schollmeyer, J.V. (1981) Immunocytochemical localization of a calcium-activated protease in skeletal muscle cells. Exp. Cell Res. **136**, 423–433.

Dayton, W.R., Goll, D.E., Zeece, M.G., Robson, R.M., and Reville, W.J. (1976) A Ca²⁺-activated protease possibly involved in myofibrillar protein trunover. Purification from porcine muscle. Biochemistry **15**, 2150–2158.

Graham-Siegenthaler, K., Gauthier, S., Davies, P.L., and Elce, J.S. (1994) Active recombinant rat calpain II. Bacterially produced large and small subunits associate both *in vivo* and *in vitro*. J. Biol. Chem. **269**, 30457–30460.

Hamakubo, T., Kannagi, R., Murachi, T., and Matus, A. (1986) Distribution of Calpains I and II in rat brain. J. Neurosci. **6**, 3103–3111.

Hathaway, D.R., Werth, D.K., and Haeberle, J.R. (1982) Limited autolysis reduces the Ca²⁺-requirement of a smooth muscle Ca²⁺-activated protease. J. Biol. Chem. **257**, 9072–9077.

Kitahara, A., Ohtsuki, H., Kirihata, Y., Yamagata, Y., Takano, E., Kannagi, R., and Murachi, T. (1985) Selective localization of calpain 1 (the low calcium requiring form of calcium-dependent cysteine proteinase) in B-cells of human pancreatic islets. FEBS Lett. **184**, 120–124.

Lane, R.D., Allan, D.M., and Mellgren, R.L. (1992) A comparison of the intracellular distribution of μ-calpain, m-calpain and calpastatin in proliferating human A431 cells. Exp. Cell Res. **203**, 5–16.

Mellgren, R.L. (1991) Proteolysis of nuclear proteins by μ-calpain and m-calpain. J. Biol. Chem. **266**, 13920–13924.

Mellgren, R.L. and Lane, R.D. (1990) The regulation of calpains by interaction with calpastatin. In *Intracellular calcium-dependent proteolysis* (ed. R. L. Mellgren and T. Murachi), pp. 55–74. CRC Press, Boca Raton, Florida.

Mellgren, R.L. and Lu, Q. (1994) Selective nuclear transport of μ-calpain. Biochem. Biophys. Res. Comm. **204**, 544–550.

Miyachi, Y., Yoshimura, N., Suzuki, S., Hamakubo, T., Kannagi, R., Imamura, S., and Murachi, T. (1986) Biochemical demonstration and immunohistochemical localization of calpain in human skin. J. Invest. Dermatol. **86**, 346–349.

Murachi, T. and Yoshimura, N. (1985) Intracellular localization of low and high calcium-requiring forms of calpains. Prog. Clin. Biol. Res. **198**, 165–174.

Saido, T.C., Nagao, S., Shiramine, M., Tsukaguchi, M., Sorimachi, H., Murofushi, H., Tsuchiya, T., Ito, H., and Suzuki, K. (1992) Autolytic transition of μ-calpain upon activation as resolved by antibodies distinguishing between pre- and post-autolysis forms. J. Biochem. (Tokyo) **111**, 81–86.

Sorimachi, H., Saido, T.C., and Suzuki, K. (1994) New era of calpain research; Discovery of tissue-specific calpains. FEBS Lett. **343**, 1–5.

Suzuki, K. (1987) Calcium activated neutral protease: domain structure and activity regulation. Trends Biochem. Sci. **12**, 103–105.

Suzuki, K. (1990) The structure of calpains and the calpain gene. In *Intracellular calcium-dependent proteolysis* (ed. R. L. Mellgren and T. Murachi), pp. 25–36. CRC Press, Boca Raton, Florida.

Takahashi, K. (1990) Calpain substrate specificity. In *Intracellular calcium-dependent proteolysis* (ed. R. L. Mellgren and T. Murachi), pp. 55–74. CRC Press, Boca Raton, Florida.

Yoshimura, N., Murachi, T., Heath, R., Kay, J., Jasani, B., and Newman, G.R. (1986) Immunogold electron-microscopic localization of calpain I in skeletal muscle of rats. Cell Tissue Res. **244**, 265–270.

■ *Richard D. Lane[1] and Ronald L. Mellgren[2]:*
Departments of [1]Anatomy and Neurobiology, and
[2]Pharmacology and Therapeutics,
Medical College of Ohio,
PO Box 10008,
Toledo, OH 43699, USA
Tel.: +1 419 381 4126
Fax: +1 419 381 3008
E-mail: Lane@vortex.mco.edu

Calmodulin-domain protein kinase

Calmodulin-domain protein kinases (CDPKs) are calcium-activated protein kinases that do not require exogenous calmodulin for activity since they contain a calmodulin-like domain as a part of their primary protein structure. CDPK activity has been found in plant genera from algae to higher plants, and also in protists, such as Plasmodium *and* Paramecium. *In plants, CDPKs are encoded by a large gene family, and both cytoplasmic and membrane-bound activities have been reported. Information on the biological function of most CDPKs has not yet emerged.*

In plant extracts, the predominant calcium-stimulated protein kinases are CDPKs, an abbreviation for cal-modulin-domain protein kinases, sometimes referred to as calcium-dependent protein kinases (for a recent review, see Roberts and Harmon 1992). As shown in Fig. 1, the enzyme consists of an amino terminal domain of variable size (from 3 to 20 kDa), a serine/threonine-type protein kinase catalytic domain (about 30 kDa), a junction domain that appears to contain a pseudosubstrate site (approximately 30 amino acids) and a carboxy terminal calmodulin-like domain (about 20 kDa) that in most cases contains four EF-hand motifs (Harper *et al.* 1991).

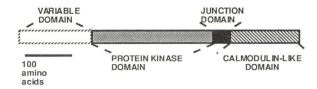

Figure 1. Modular structure of a calmodulin-domain protein kinase.

Alternative names

CDPK (Roberts and Harmon 1992) originally stood for calcium-dependent protein kinase, based on the biochemical characteristics of the isolated proteins. Now that the structure of the protein is understood from sequence analysis, CDPK may also refer to calmodulin-domain protein kinase. CPK (i.e. CPK1, CPK2) is proposed as the nomenclature for individual CDPK genes (Hrabak et al., in press).

Isolation/identification

CDPK was first purified to homogeneity from the cytosolic fraction of soybean tissue culture cells (Putnam-Evans et al. 1990). This purified protein was microsequenced and also used to generate the monoclonal antibodies described below. Enzyme activity and immunoreactive protein were subsequently found associated with plasma membrane vesicles purified from oat roots. Limited proteolysis of purified oat CDPK suggested that an approximately 10 kDa N- or C-terminal domain was responsible for attachment to the membrane (Schaller et al. 1992). CDPK-like protein kinase activity (i.e. Ca^{+2}-activated, but calmodulin-insensitive) has been identified in extracts of many plant species and has been localized to a number of different cell fractions (Roberts and Harmon 1992).

Genes and sequences

The first complete CDPK amino acid sequence was deduced from the cDNA sequence of a clone isolated from soybean cells (Harper et al. 1991, GenBank accession number: M64987). Subsequent studies in the model higher plant, *Arabidopsis thaliana*, have demonstrated that there is a large gene family containing at least 11 members encoding this enzyme (Harper et al. 1992, L14771; Urao et al.1994, D21805, D21806, D28582; Hrabak et al., in press). They all share the conserved 50 kDa kinase-junction-calmodulin tripartite structure, but vary in the length and sequence of the amino terminal variable domain. Most (but not all) of the *Arabidopsis* CDPK cDNAs sequenced thus far predict a protein with a motif that may result in post-translational addition of an N-terminal myristate moiety (Han and Martinage 1992). Myristoylation has been shown to be important for the

association of some proteins with the plasma membrane (Kamps et al. 1985). Some isoforms also contain a "PEST" motif in the variable domain. This motif is correlated with rapid protein turnover (Rogers et al. 1986). CDPK cDNA sequences have also been derived from the protists *Paramecium* (Kim 1994) and *Plasmodium* (Zhao et al. 1993; X67288), as well as higher plants including rice (Kawasaki et al. 1993; D13436), corn (Estruch et al. 1994; L27484), and carrot (Suen and Choi 1991; X56599).

Protein

Due to proteolysis during homogenization, it has been difficult to obtain large quantities of purified CDPK from plant tissues. An "affinity sandwich" technique has been utilized to produce *Arabidopsis* CDPK proteins using an *E. coli* expression system (Binder et al. 1994). The CDPK is produced as a fusion protein, with glutathione-S-transferase attached to its amino terminal end and a hexahistidine tract attached to its carboxy terminal domain. Two-step affinity purification yielded a purified CDPK fusion protein that had a maximal specific activity and an affinity for Ca^{2+} resembling the native enzyme purified from soybean cells. CDPKs are the only protein kinases cloned from higher plants which have been unequivocally shown to encode proteins that exhibit calcium-stimulated protein kinase activity.

Antibodies

Currently there are no commercially available antibodies specific for CDPK.

Anatomical localization

Indirect immunofluorescence microscopy, using a monoclonal antibody that recognizes an epitope in the protein kinase domain, labeled cytoskeletal microfilaments of onion root cells and *Tradescantia* pollen tubes (Putnam-Evans et al. 1989). This may mean that the enzyme plays a role in the cessation of cytoplasmic streaming, which occurs when there is a transient Ca^{2+} rise during action potentials in algae and plants.

Biological activities

The only well-characterized CDPK substrate is nod26, a carrier protein involved in nutrient transport across the peribacteroid membrane of nitrogen-fixing nodules in legumes (Weaver and Roberts 1992; Weaver et al. 1994). *In vitro* studies have implicated two other membrane proteins as possible substrates of CDPK in plants: the plasma membrane H^+-ATPase (Schaller and Sussman 1988) and TIP, the major tonoplast integral protein, which appears to be a water channel (Johnson and Chrispeels 1992).

Biological regulation

Some lipids activated CDPK three- to fivefold above that seen with Ca^{2+} alone, but the lipid specificity for this stimulation of protein kinase activity does not resemble that of protein kinase C, nor is there a lipid-induced change in Ca^{2+} affinity (Harper *et al.* 1992).

Genetic and biochemical studies indicate that the mechanism of Ca^{2+} activation involves a Ca^{2+}-induced alleviation of inhibition by a pseudosubstrate sequence present in the junction domain. Once Ca^{2+} is bound, the calmodulin-like carboxy-terminal domain prevents the attached pseudosubstrate domain from blocking catalytic activity (Harmon *et al.* 1994; Harper *et al.* 1994).

References

Binder, B.M., Harper, J.F., and Sussman, M.R. (1994) Characterization of an *Arabidopsis* calmodulin-like domain protein kinase purified from *Escherichia coli* using an affinity sandwich technique. Biochemistry **33**, 2033–2041.

Estruch, J.J., Kadwell, S., Merlin, E., and Crossland, L. (1994) Cloning and characterization of a maize pollen-specific calcium-dependent calmodulin-independent protein kinase. Proc. Natl. Acad. Sci. USA **91**, 8837–8841.

Gordon, J.I., Duronio, R.J., Rudnick, D.A., Adams, S.P., and Gokel, G.W. (1991) Protein N-myristoylation. J. Biol. Chem. **266**, 8647–8650.

*Harmon, A.C., Yoo, B.C., and McCafery, C. (1994) Pseudosubstrate inhibition of CDPK, a protein kinase with a calmodulin-like domain. Biochemistry **33**, 7278–7287.

*Harper, J.F., Sussman, M.R., Schaller, G.E., Putnam-Evans, C. Charbonneau, H., and Harmon, A.C. (1991) A calcium-dependent protein kinase with a regulatory domain similar to calmodulin. Science **252**, 951–954.

Harper, J.F., Binder, B.M., and Sussman, M.R. (1992) Calcium and lipid regulation of an *Arabidopsis* protein kinase expressed in *Escherichia coli*. Biochemistry **32**, 3282–3290.

*Harper, J.F., Huang, J.F., and Lloyd, S.J. (1994) Genetic identification of an autoinhibitor in CDPK, a protein kinase with a calmodulin-like domain. Biochemistry **33**, 7267–7277.

Hrabak, E. M., Dickmann, L. J., Satterlee, J. S., and Sussman, M. R. The calmodulin-domain protein kinase (CDPK) gene family of *Arabidopsis thaliana* contains at least eleven members Plant Molec. Biol. (in press).

Johnson K. D. and Chrispeels, M.J. (1992) Tonoplast-bound protein kinase phosphorylates tonoplast intrinsic protein. Plant Physiol. **100**, 1787–1795.

Kamps, M.P., Buss, J.E., and Sefton, B.M. (1985) Mutation of amino-terminal glycine of p60srс prevents myristoylation and morphological transformation. Proc. Natl. Acad. Sci. USA **82**, 4625–4628.

Kawasaki, T., Hayashida, N., Baba, T. , Shinozaki, K., and Shimada, H. (1993) The gene encoding a CDPK located near the *sbe1* gene encoding starch branching enzyme I is specifically expressed in developing rice seeds. Gene **129**, 183–189.

Kim, K. (1994) Cloning and characterization of calcium-dependent protein kinases from *Paramecium tetraurelia*. PhD thesis, University of Wisconsin-Madison.

Putnam-Evans, C., Harmon, A.C., Palevitz, B.A., Fechheimer, M., and Cormier, M.J. (1989) Calcium-dependent protein kinase is localized with F-actin in plant cells. Cell Motility and the Cytoskeleton **12**, 12–22

Putnam-Evans, C., Harmon, A.C., and Cormier, M.J. (1990) Purification and characterization of a novel calcium-dependent protein kinase from soybean. Biochemistry **29**, 2488

*Roberts, D.M. and Harmon, A.C. (1992) Calcium-modulated proteins: targets of intracellular calcium signals in higher plants. Ann. Rev. Plant Physiol. Plant Mol. Biol. **43**, 375–414.

Rogers, S., Wells, R., and Rechsteiner, M. (1986) Amino acid sequences common to rapidly degraded proteins: the PEST hypothesis. Science **234**, 364–368.

Schaller, G. E. and Sussman, M. R. (1988) Phosphorylation of the plasma membrane proton ATPase of oat roots by a calcium-stimulated protein kinase. Planta **173**, 509–518.

Schaller, G. E., Harmon, A.C., and Sussman, M.R. (1992) Characterization of a calcium and lipid dependent protein kinase associated with the plasma membrane of oat. Biochemistry **31**, 1722–1727.

Suen, K. L. and Choi, J. H. (1991) Isolation and sequence analysis of a cDNA clone for a carrot calcium-dependent protein kinase: Homology to calcium-calmodulin-dependent protein kinases and to calmodulin. Plant Molecular Biology **17**, 581–590.

Urao, T., Katagiri, T., Mizoguchi, T., Yamaguchi-Shinozaki, K., Hayashida, N., and Shinozaki, K. (1994) Two genes that encode Ca^{2+}-dependent protein kinases are induced by drought and high-salt stresses in *Arabidopsis thaliana*. Mol. Gen. Genet. **244**, 331–340.

Weaver, C.D. and Roberts, D.M. (1992) Determination of the site of phosphorylation of nodulin 26 by the calcium-dependent protein kinase from soybean nodules. Biochemistry **31**, 8954–8959.

Weaver, C.D., Shomer, N.H., Louis, C.F., and Roberts, D.M. (1994) Nodulin 26, a nodule-specific symbiosome membrane protein from soybean, is an ion channel. J. Biol. Chem. **269**, 17858.

Zhao, Y., Kappes, B., and Franklin, R.M. (1993) Gene structure and expression of an unusual protein kinase from *Plasmodium falciparum* homologous at its carboxyl terminus with the EF hand calcium-binding proteins. J. Biol. Chem. **268**, 4347–4354.

■ *Michael R. Sussman, Estelle M. Hrabak, and John S. Satterlee:*
Horticulture Department and Program in Cell and Molecular Biology,
University of Wisconsin-Madison,
Madison, WI 53706, USA
Tel.: +1 608 262 3519
Fax: +1 608 262 4743
E-mail: mrs@plantpath.wisc.edu

Centrin

Centrin is a cytoskeletal Ca²⁺-binding EF-hand protein present in animal, plant, fungal, and protist cells. Mutational analyses, as well as its association with centrosomes, spindle pole bodies, and basal bodies, suggest that it plays a fundamental role in the cell cycle dependent duplication, functional assembly, and positioning of centrosomes.

Centrin in green algae has a calculated molecular mass (M_r) of 19.3 kDa (*Scherffelia dubia*) or 19.5 kDa (*Chlamydomonas reinhardtii*) and migrates in SDS-PAGE with an apparent molecular mass of 20 kDa. It exists in two isoforms with p/s of 4.7 and 4.6, depending on the phosphorylation state of the protein. Centrin consists of four EF-hand, Ca²⁺-binding domains and an additional N-terminal domain of 23 to 31 amino acids. The Ca²⁺-binding domains are collinear to calmodulin and congruent with the CTER subfamilies (calmodulin, troponin C, ELC, and RLC) of EF-hand proteins (Nakayama and Kretsinger 1994). The N-terminal domain is highly vari-able among known sequences; however, in algae and land plants it represents a helical and amphipathic domain deduced from amino acid sequences.

■ Alternative names

Caltractin (Huang *et al.* 1988a; Lee and Huang 1993; Ogawa and Shimizu 1993). The yeast protein homologous to centrin is called cdc31p (Baum *et al.* 1986; Biggins and Rose 1994).

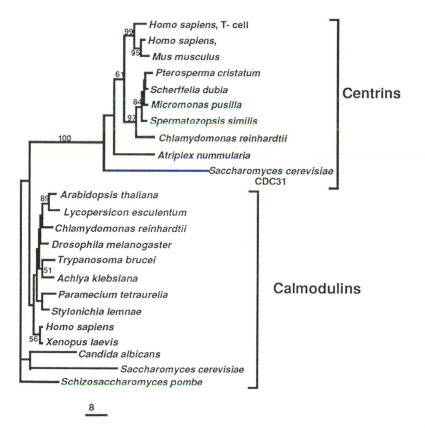

Figure 1. Phylogeny of centrin and calmodulin coding regions (1st and 2nd codon positions of the four domains and interdomains, i.e. 274 positions) constructed with the neighbor-joining method based on structural distances between the sequences. Bootstrap values ≥50 of 100 resamplings are indicated at the nodes of the branches; the scale indicates the distance that corresponds to 8% sequence divergence.

Identification/isolation

Centrin was purified from isolated rhizoplasts or basal body complexes of the green algae *Tetraselmis striata* and *Chlamydomonas reinhardtii*, by high salt extractions and hydrophobic interaction chromatography (Salisbury *et al.* 1986; Huang *et al.* 1988*a*). An alternative purification protocol based on KJ-extraction and ammonium sulfate precipitation is described by Höhfeld *et al.* (1994). Isolation of recombinant centrin expressed in *E. coli* was performed by hydrophobic interaction chromatography and ion exchange chromatography (Weber *et al.* 1994). Cdc31p, expressed in *E. coli*, was purified by anion exchange and hydroxyapatite chromatography (Spang *et al.* 1993). Biggins and Rose (1994) purified cdc31p by non-denaturing polyacrylamide gel electrophoresis and electroelution of the cdc31p band.

Gene and sequence

The sequence of the cdc31 gene product was identified from the temperature sensitive mutant of *Saccharomyces cerevisiae* (Baum *et al.* 1986; GenBank accession number: M14078). Centrin cDNAs have been isolated and sequenced from *Chlamydomonas reinhardtii* (Huang *et al.* 1988*b*; X12634), *Atriplex nummularia* (Zhu *et al.* 1992; M90970), *Scherffelia dubia* (Bhattacharya *et al.* 1993; X69220), mouse testis (Ogawa and Shimizu 1993; D16301), and two isoforms from human cells. The latter have been isolated from two different cell types, namely T-cell lymphoblastic leukemia cells (MOLT-4) (Lee and Huang 1993; X72964) and HeLa cells (Errabolu *et al.* 1994; U03270). Isolation and characterization of the centrin gene locus from *Chlamydomonas reinhardtii* (Lee *et al.* 1991; X57973) revealed that the positions of the six introns do not correlate with the domain structure of the protein or with other EF-hand protein coding regions. Further partial sequences encoding the four EF-hand domains were obtained by RT-PCR amplification from several green algae, namely *Spermatozopsis similis*, *Tetraselmis striata* (Bhattacharya *et al.* 1993; X70657, X70693, respectively), *Pterosperma cristatum* (X83766) and *Micromonas pusilla* (X83765). Green algal centrin genes have been shown to be single-copy-coding regions (Huang *et al.* 1988*b*; Bhattacharya *et al.* 1993).

All known centrin sequences are highly conserved and represent a subfamily with congruence to the CTER group of EF-hand proteins (Bhattacharya *et al.* 1993; Nakayama and Kretsinger 1994).The phylogeny of centrin- and calmodulin-coding regions (Fig. 1) verifies the distinctness of these two subfamilies. The yeast protein cdc31p is obviously a member of the centrin subfamily, although its sequence is highly derived.

Protein

All centrins consist of four EF-hand domains which are presumably all capable of Ca^{2+} coordination deduced from the canonical EF-hand model (Nakayama and Kretsinger

1994). The Ca^{2+} affinity of recombinant centrin from *Chlamydomonas reinhardtii* has been determined. It coordinates four Ca^{2+} ions, two with high ($K_d = 1.2 \times 10$–6 M) and two with low ($K_d = 1.6 \times 10$–4 M) affinity. Centrin undergoes Ca^{2+}-dependent structural changes as can be deduced from altered electrophoretic mobility in non-denaturing gel electrophoresis and ^{1}H-NMR analyses (Weber *et al.* 1994).

The two isoforms of centrin in *Tetraselmis striata* represent phosphorylated α and dephosphorylated β forms of the protein. The relative amount of the isoforms ranges from 2:1 to 1:1, perhaps related to the contraction or relaxation status of the rhizoplasts (Salisbury *et al.* 1986). A consensus sequence for cAMP-dependent protein kinase phosphorylation is present in all known complete centrin coding regions (e.g. position serine167 in *Chlamydomonas* or serine166 in *Scherffelia*).

Localization

Centrin was first characterized as a component of the striated flagellar roots (rhizoplast, system II fibers) in the basal body (Bb) complex of the green alga *Tetraselmis striata* (Salisbury *et al.* 1984). Within the green algal cytoskeleton, centrin occurs in the nucleus–basal body connector, the distal connecting fiber linking the two Bbs and the flagellar transitional region (Schulze *et al.* 1987) (Fig. 2). These structures have been shown to perform Ca^{2+}-dependent contractions (Salisbury *et al.* 1984; Sanders and Salisbury 1994). Centrin-containing structures have also been characterized in various protists (Melkonian *et al.* 1992) as well as in the multi-layered structure of the basal body complex of spermatogenous cells of bryophytes and pteridophytes (Vaughn *et al.* 1993). In *Saccharomyces cerevisiae* the centrin homologue, cdc31p, was localized to the half bridge of spindle pole bodies or the bridge interconnecting them after their duplication (Spang *et al.* 1993). In immunofluorescence analyses centrin was localized to the centrosomes of interphase and mitotic vertebrate (HeLa) cells (Lee and Huang 1993).

Mutagenesis studies

The mutant vfl2 of *Chlamydomonas reinhardtii* is defective in correct localization and segregation of basal bodies as well as flagellar autonomy (Taillon *et al.* 1992; Sanders and Salisbury, 1994). The mutant cells lack centrin-containing fibers and contain reduced quantities of centrin. It was shown that the mutation resulting in this phenotype is a single amino acid replacement (Glu to Lys) in position 101 of the centrin molecule (Taillon *et al.* 1992).

The phenotype of the yeast mutant CDC31 is characterized by defective SPB duplication, resulting in large budded cells with increased levels of ploidy, a single large SPB, and absence of satellites (Spang *et al.* 1993).

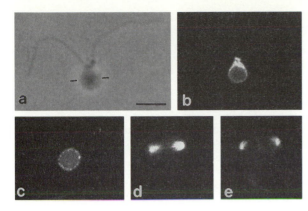

Figure 2. Analysis of isolated cytoskeletons of *Chlamydomonas reinhardtii cw 15+* with polyclonal anti-centrin (Höhfeld *et al.* 1994). (a) Phase-contrast image of an isolated cytoskeleton from *Chlamydomonas reinhardtii cw 15+*, bar: 5 μm. (b) Immunofluorescence corresponding to the region of the basal bodies and the nucleus–basal body connectors (NBBCs) partially enclosing the anterior part of the karyoskeleton labeled with anti-centrin. (c) Top view of an isolated cytoskeleton, focused on the nucleus (plane indicated in a) showing fibrous extensions of NBBCs–probably 16–on the nuclear surface. (d) and (e) Double-label indirect immunofluorescence of a mitotic *Chlamydomonas reinhardtii cw 15+* cell showing the mitotic spindle, visualized by anti-tubulin labeling (d); centrin (e) is localized to the poles of the of the miotic spindle. (Courtesy of Dr K.-F. Lechtreck.)

■ Interactions

Interactions between the two spindle pole body components cdc31p and kar1p in yeast were characterized by Biggins and Rose (1994). Both genes were identified from cell cycle (CDC31) and karyogamy (KAR1) mutants of *Saccharomyces cerevisiae*, which exhibit similar phenotypes. From binding assays and mutational analyses, it was concluded that kar1p is required for cdc31p localization to the spindle pole bodies. Other putative centrin-binding proteins are under investigation.

■ References

Baum, P., Furlong, C., and Byers, B. (1986) Yeast gene required for spindle pole body duplication: Homology of its product with Ca²⁺-binding proteins. Proc. Natl. Acad. Sci. USA **83**, 5512–5516.

*Bhattacharya, D., Steinkötter, J., and Melkonian, M. (1993) Molecular cloning and evolutionary analysis of the calcium modulated contractile protein, centrin, in green algae and land plants. Plant Mol. Biol. **23**, 1243–1254.

Biggins, S. and Rose, M.D. (1994) Direct interaction between yeast spindle pole body components: Kar1p is required for cdc31p localization to the spindle pole. J. Cell Biol. **125**, 843–852.

Errabolu, R., Sanders, M.A., and Salisbury, J.L. (1994) Cloning of a cDNA encoding human centrin, an EF-hand protein of

centrosomes and mitotic spindle poles. J. Cell Sci. **107**, 9–16.

Höhfeld, I., Beech, P.L., and Melkonian, M. (1994) Immunolocalization of centrin in *Oxyrrhis marina* (Dinophyceae). J. Phycol. **30**, 474–489.

Huang, B., Watterson, D.M., Lee, V.D., and Schibler, M.J. (1988*a*) Purification and characterization of a basal body associated protein. J. Cell Biol. **107**, 121–131.

Huang, B., Mengersen, A., and Lee, V.D. (1988*b*) Molecular cloning of cDNA for caltractin , a basal body-associated Ca²⁺ binding protein: Homology in its protein sequence with calmodulin and the CDC31 gene product. J. Cell Biol. **107**, 133–140.

*Lee, V.L. and Huang, B. (1993) Molecular cloning and centrosomal localization of human caltractin. Proc. Natl. Acad. Sci. USA **90**, 11039–11043.

Lee, V.L., Stapleton, M., and Huang, B. (1991) Genomic structure of *Chlamydomonas* caltractin. J. Mol. Biol. **221**, 175–191.

Melkonian, M., Beech, P.L., Katsaros, C., and Schulze, D. (1992) Centrin-mediated cell motility in algae. In (ed. M. Melkonian, Algal cell motility), pp. 179–221. Chapman & Hall, New York.

Nakayama, S. and Kretsinger, R.H. (1994) Evolution of the EF hand family of proteins. Ann. Rev. Biophys. Biomol. Struct. **23**, 473–507.

Ogawa, K. and Shimizu, T. (1993) cDNA sequence for mouse caltractin. Biochim. Biophys. Acta **1216**, 126–128.

Salisbury, J.L., Baron, A., Surek, B., and Melkonian, M. (1984) Striated flagellar roots Isolation and partial characterization of a calcium-modulated contractile organelle. J. Cell Biol. **99**, 962–970.

Salisbury, J.L., Aebig, K.W., and Coiling, D.E. (1986) Isolation of the calcium-modulated contractile protein of striated flagellar roots. Meth. Enzymol. **134**, 408–414.

Sanders, M.A. and Salisbury, J.L. (1994) Centrin plays an essential role in microtubule severing during flagellar excision in *Chlamydomonas reinhardtii*. J. Cell Biol. **124**, 795–805.

Schulze, D., Robenek, H., McFadden, G.I., and Melkonian, M. (1987) Immunolocalization of a Ca²⁺-modulated contractile protein in the flagellar apparatus of green algae: the nucleus-basal body connector. Eur. J. Cell Biol. **45**, 51–61.

*Spang, A., Courtney, I., Fackler, U., Matzner, M., and Schiebel, E. (1993) The calcium-binding protein cell division cycle 31 of *Saccharomyces cerevisiae* is a component of the half bridge of the spindle pole body. J. Cell Biol. **123**, 405–416.

Taillon, B.E., Adler, S.A., Suhan, J.P., and Jarvik, J.W. (1992) Mutational analysis of centrin: An EF-hand protein associated with three distinct contractile fibers in the basal body apparatus of *Chlamydomonas*. J. Cell Biol. **119**, 1613–1624.

Vaughn, K.C., Sherman, T.D., and Renzaglia, K.S. (1993) A centrin homologue is a component of the multilayered structure in bryophytes and pteridophytes. Protoplasma **175**, 58–66.

Weber, C., Lee, V.D., Chazin, W.J., and Huang, B. (1994) High level expression in *Escherichia coli* and characterization of the EF-hand calcium-binding protein caltractin. J. Biol. Chem. **269**, 15795–15802.

Zhu, J.-K., Bressan, R.A., and Hasegawa, P.M. (1992) An *Atriplex nummularia* cDNA with sequence relatedness to the algal caltractin gene. Plant Physiol. **99**, 1734–1735.

■ *Jutta Steinkötter and Michael Melkonian:*
Universität zu Köln,
Botanisches Institut I,
Gyrhofstrasse 15,
50931 Köln, Germany
Tel.: +49 221 470 2475
Fax: +49 221 470 5181
E-mail: jsteinko@biolan.uni-koeln.de
mmelkon@biolan.uni-koeln.de

Diacylglycerol kinase

Diacylglycerol kinase (DGK) reverses the normal flow of phospholipid biosynthesis by phosphorylating diacylglycerol back to phosphatidic acid. DGK consists of a number of isozymes with different enzymological properties. The three isozymes so far sequenced, however, share highly conserved regions including two sets each of EF-hand and zinc finger structures. Despite structural similarities these isozymes are expressed markedly differently, depending on the cell types.

Diacylglycerol kinase (DGK) has been detected in almost all the tissues and cells examined. Within the cells the DGK activity is associated with the nuclear matrix (Payrastre *et al.* 1992) and cytoskeletons (Payrastre *et al.* 1991) in addition to the major soluble and membrane-bound forms (Kanoh *et al.* 1990). Reflecting such variable enzyme localizations, several DGKs with distinct molecular masses have been purified from the cytosol of porcine brain and thymus (83 and 150 kDa; Kanoh *et al.* 1992), human platelet cytosol (58, 75, and 150 kDa; Yada *et al.* 1990), rat brain (110 and 150 kDa; Kato and Takenawa 1990), and recently from bovine testicular membranes (58 kDa; Walsh *et al.* 1994). The 58 kDa testicular enzyme is specific to the 2-arachidonoyl type of diacylglycerol, whereas other DGKs possess no specificity with regard to the acyl compositions of diacylglycerol. The 58 kDa isozyme may thus be involved in a transient accumulation of arachidonoyl-enriched phosphatidic acid known to occur in the early stage of cell stimulation. The 83 kDa enzyme (DGKα) was the first to be sequenced by molecular cloning (Sakane *et al.* 1990; Schaap *et al.* 1990; Goto *et al.* 1992), followed by rat brain 90 kDa (DGKβ, Goto and Kondo, 1993) and human retina 89 kDa isozymes (DGKγ, Kai *et al.* 1994). The three sequenced DGKs are tentatively designated according to their order of cDNA cloning (Kai *et al.* 1994). In the case of DGKγ, a catalytically inactive enzyme with an internal deletion of 25 amino acid residues is expressed in human cells other than the retina and brain, which express only a full-length enzyme.

■ Isolation/identification

DGK was first identified as a Ca^{2+}-binding protein by ^{45}Ca overlay assay using DGKα purified from porcine thymus cytosol (Sakane *et al.* 1991*a*). DGKα bound two mol of Ca^{2+} per mol enzyme in a cooperative manner (Hill coefficient: 1.4) with an apparent K_D value of 300 nM. The tandem repeat of EF-hand motifs was subsequently confirmed to be the Ca^{2+} binding sites using various truncation and deletion mutants of DGKα expressed in *E. coli* (Sakane *et al.* 1991*b*). The porcine and human homologues of DGKα, sharing more than 90% identical amino acid sequence, were cloned from cDNA libraries prepared from porcine thymus (Sakane *et al.* 1990; accession number: X53256) and Jurkat cell mRNAs (Schaap *et al.*

1990; X62535), respectively. The porcine DGKα cDNA was used as a probe to clone rat DGKα cDNA (Goto *et al.* 1992; S49760) from rat brain cDNA library. This work subsequently resulted in the cloning of rat DGKβ by a low-stringency screening of the same cDNA library (Goto and Kondo 1993; D16100). DGKγ was initially obtained by the reverse transcriptase/polymerase amplification of HepG2 mRNA using amplimers designed on the basis of amino acid sequences highly conserved in the C-terminal portions of DGKs α and β (Kai *et al.* 1994; D26135).

■ Gene and sequences

A partial genomic clone encoding human DGKα has been characterized (Fujikawa *et al.* 1993; D16440). Despite the cell-type specific and developmental-stage dependent modes of DGKα expression, this gene can be classified as a housekeeping gene as judged from the absence of canonical TATA and CAAT sequences in the 5′-flanking region. The first EF-hand motif is encoded by three exons (exons 5–7) and the second by a single exon (exon 8). The positions of introns in the EF-hand motifs are different from those found in other EF-hand proteins such as calmodulin.

■ Protein

As depicted in Fig.1, the three mammalian DGKs so far sequenced share four highly conserved regions. The function of these regions, except for the EF-hand motifs, remains unknown. The sequence of zinc fingers is basically the same as those occurring in phosphatidylserine-dependent phorbol ester binding proteins like protein kinase C (Kanoh *et al.* 1993). The zinc finger of DGKα, however, did not bind phorbol esters (Ahmed *et al.* 1991). The most highly conserved region at the C-terminal portion of DGKs may be a catalytic region, since this region is also conserved in the *Drosophila* DGK homologue (Masai *et al.* 1993). The sequences of EF-hand motifs of the three DGKs completely fulfil the conditions required for Ca^{2+}-binding. A truncated DGKγ with an internal deletion of 25 amino acids (Ile451–Gly475) is expressed in most human cells. The truncated enzyme is catalytically inactive as demonstrated by cDNA expression experiments (Kai *et al.* 1994).

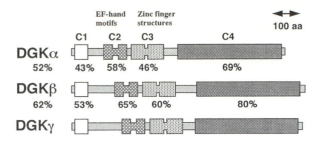

Figure 1. A linear representation of the three DGKs sequenced. The sequences of DGKs α (porcine), β (rat), and γ (human) are aligned and the conserved regions (C1–C4) are indicated by boxes. The extents of amino acid identities compared with DGKγ are shown as percentages (taken from Kai *et al.* 1994).

Localization

DGK isozymes, despite their similar structures, are known to be expressed in a markedly cell-type-dependent manner. DGKα is typically expressed in oligodendroglial cells (Goto *et al.* 1992) and T lymphocytes (Kanoh *et al.* 1990), but to undetectable extents in other cells such as neurons and hepatocytes. This isozyme also shows a development-stage dependent expression in rat brain and becomes maximally expressed at postnatal week 3, coinciding with the maturation process of myelin sheaths (Goto *et al.* 1992). The expression of rat DGKβ, on the other hand, is limited to neurons of restricted brain areas such as those located in the caudate-putamen (Goto and Kondo 1993). DGKγ, although initially cloned from the human hepatoma cell line, HepG2, mRNA, turned out to be expressed in human retina most abundantly and to a much lesser extent in the brain. Other human tissues, including the liver and HepG2 cells, contain very low levels of DGKγ mRNA (Kai *et al.* 1994).

Biological regulation

The DGK inhibitor, R59022 (de Chaffoy de Courcelles *et al.* 1985; available from Boehringer) has been used repeatedly to assess the role of this enzyme in signal transduction. Although the inhibitor has been suggested to attenuate the metabolic processing of the second messenger, diacylglycerol, little is known of the role of DGK isozymes in the cellular functions. DGKα is dependent on both Ca^{2+} and phosphatidylserine for its activity (Sakane *et al.* 1991a,b). Under Ca^{2+}-free conditions, the EF-hand motifs appear to interfere with the enzyme interaction with membrane phospholipids. The activity of DGKβ was also enhanced by Ca^{2+}. However, the effect of Ca^{2+} on DGK activity seems to be variable, depending on the isozymes, since DGKγ does not require Ca^{2+} for its activity (Kai *et al.* 1994). The 58 kDa testis enzyme was also shown to be independent of Ca^{2+} (Walsh *et al.* 1994). The phosphorylation of DGKα by several protein kinases (Kanoh *et al.* 1993; Schaap *et al.* 1993) has also been

noted. *In vivo* DGK phosphorylates diacylglycerol generated by the receptor-linked phospholipase C but not diacylglycerol randomly accumulated by exogenous phospholipase C (van der Bend *et al.* 1994).

References

Ahmed, S., Kozma, R., Lee, J., Monfries, C., Harden, N., and Lim, L. (1991) The cysteine-rich domain of human proteins, neuronal chimaerin, protein kinase C and diacylglycerol kinase binds zinc. Biochem. J. **280**, 233–241.

De Chaffoy de Courcelles, D., Roevens, P., and Van Belle, H. (1985) J. Biol. Chem. **260**, 15762–15770.

Fujikawa, K., Imai, S., Sakane, F., and Kanoh, H. (1993) Isolation and characterization of the human diacylglycerol kinase gene. Biochem. J. **294**, 443–449.

Goto, K. and Kondo, H. (1993) Molecular cloning and expression of a 90-kDa diacylglycerol kinase that predominantly localizes in neurons. Proc. Natl. Acad. Sci. USA **90**, 7598–7602.

*Goto, K., Watanabe, M., Kondo, H., Yuasa, H., Sakane, F., and Kanoh, H. (1992) Gene cloning, sequence, expression and *in situ* localization of 80 kDa diacylglycerol kinase specific to oligodendrocyte of rat brain. Mol. Brain Res. **16**, 75–87.

*Kai, M., Sakane, F., Imai, S., Wada, I., and Kanoh, H. (1994) Molecular cloning of a diacylglycerol kinase isozyme predominantly expressed in human retina with a truncated and inactive enzyme expression in most other human cells. J. Biol. Chem. **269**, 18492–18498.

Kanoh, H., Yamada, K., and Sakane, F. (1990) Diacylglycerol kinase: a key modulator of signal transduction? Trends Biochem. Sci. **15**, 47–50.

Kanoh, H., Sakane, F., and Yamada, K. (1992) Diacylglycerol kinase isozymes from brain and lymphoid tissues. Methods Enzymol. **209**, 162–172.

Kanoh, H., Sakane, F., Imai, S., and Wada, I. (1993) Diacylglycerol kinase and phosphatidic acid phosphatase. Enzymes metabolizing lipid second messengers. Cell. Signalling **5**, 495–503.

Kato, M. and Takenawa, T. (1990) Purification and characterization of membrane-bound and cytosolic forms of diacylglycerol kinase from rat brain. J. Biol. Chem. **265**, 794–800.

Masai, I., Okazaki, A., Hosoya, T., and Hotta, Y. (1993) *Drosophila* retinal degeneration A gene encodes an eye-specific diacylglycerol kinase with cysteine-rich zinc finger motifs and ankyrin repeats. Proc. Natl. Acad. Sci. USA **90**, 11157–11161.

Payrastre, B., van Bergen en Henegouwen, P.M.P., Breton, M., den Hartigh, J.C., Plantavid, M., Verkleij, A.J., and Boonstra, J. (1991) Phosphoinositide kinase, diacylglycerol kinase, and phospholipase C activities associated to the cytoskeleton: Effect of epidermal growth factor. J. Cell Biol. **115**, 121–128.

Payrastre, B., Nievers, M., Boonstra, J., Breton, M., Verkleij, A.J., and Van Bergen en Henegouwen, P.M.P. (1992) A differential location of phosphoinositide kinases, diacylglycerol kinase, and phospholipase C in the nuclear matrix. J. Biol. Chem. **267**, 5078–5084.

*Sakane, F., Yamada, K., Kanoh, H., Yokoyama, C., and Tanabe, T. (1990) Porcine diacylglycerol kinase sequence has zinc finger and E-F hand motifs. Nature **344**, 345–348.

Sakane, F., Yamada, K., Imai, S., and Kanoh, H. (1991a) Porcine 80-kDa diacylglycerol kinase is a calcium-binding and calcium/phospholipid dependent enzyme and undergoes calcium-dependent translocation. J. Biol. Chem. **266**, 7096–7100.

Sakane, F., Imai, S., Yamada, K., and Kanoh, H. (1991b) The regulatory role of EF-hand motifs of pig 80K diacylglycerol kinase as assessed using truncation and deletion mutants. Biochem. Biophys. Res. Commun. **181**, 1015–1021.

Schaap, D., de Widt, J., van der Val, J., Vandekerckhove, J., van Damme, J., Gussow, D., Ploegh, H.L., van Blitterswijk, W.J., and van der Bend, R.L. (1990) Purification, cDNA-cloning and expression of human diacylglycerol kinase, FEBS Lett. **275**, 151–158.

Schaap, D., van der Val, J., van Blitterswijk, W.J., van der Bend, R.L., and Ploegh, H.L. (1993) Diacylglycerol kinase is phosphorylated *in vivo* upon stimulation of the epidermal growth factor receptor and serine/threonine kinases, including protein kinase C-e. Biochem. J. **289**, 875–881.

Van der Bend, R.L., de Widt, J., Hilkmann, H., and van Blitterswijk, W.J. (1994) Diacylglycerol kinase in receptor-stimulated cells converts its substrate in a topologically restricted manner. J. Biol. Chem. **269**, 4098–4102.

Walsh, J.P., Suen, R., Lemaitre, R.N., and Glomset, J.A. (1994) Arachidonoyl-diacylglycerol kinase from bovine testis. J. Biol. Chem. **269**, 21155–21164.

Yada, Y., Ozeki, T., Kanoh, H., and Nozawa, Y. (1990) Purification and characterization of cytosolic diacylglycerol kinases of human platelets. J. Biol. Chem. **265**, 19237–19243.

■ *Hideo Kanoh, Masahiro Kai, and Fumio Sakane:*
Department of Biochemistry,
Sapporo Medical University School of Medicine,
West-17, South-1, Sapporo 060, Japan
Tel.: 011 611 2111
Fax: 81 11 612 5861

ERC-55

ERC-55 is a human Ca^{2+}-binding protein localized to the lumen of the endoplasmic reticulum. The protein sequence comprises six copies of the EF-hand Ca^{2+}-binding motif. It is retained in the endoplasmic reticulum via a carboxyterminal HDEL (His-Asp-Glu-Leu) motif. The mRNA for ERC-55 is ubiquitously expressed in human tissue.

Human ERC-55 (Weis *et al.* 1994), has a calculated molecular mass of 36,877 Da and a calculated isoelectric point of 4.05. It migrates on SDS-PAGE with an apparent molecular mass of 55 kDa. It has an amino terminal signal sequence which targets it to the endoplasmic reticulum. Its name thus reflects its identification as an **ER**-localized Calcium binding protein which migrates on SDS-PAGE at **55** kDa. Its localization in the endoplasmic reticulum has been confirmed by both biochemical fractionation studies and by immuno-fluorescence and immuno-electron microscopy using antibodies specific for ERC-55 (see Fig. 1). It is retained in the endoplasmic reticulum via a carboxy terminal HDEL (His-Asp-Glu-Leu) motif. ERC-55 is the first example of an endogenous human protein that is retained by an HDEL rather than KDEL motif. Northern blotting data show that ERC-55 is encoded by a single mRNA of approximately 1900 nucleotides that is ubiquitously expressed in human tissues.

The ERC-55 protein sequence is mainly comprised of six copies of the EF-hand motif. It was shown to bind Ca^{2+} *in vitro* using the ^{45}Ca^{2+} overlay technique. Sequence comparisons with other EF-hand-containing Ca^{2+}-binding proteins showed that ERC-55 has highest amino acid sequence identity with the subfamily of calmodulins (25% over its full length) and to a unique mouse protein called reticulocalbin (35% over its full length; Ozawa and Muramatsu 1993). It has been proposed that ERC-55 and reticulocalbin represent a distinct subclass of EF-hand proteins that are characterized by having six EF-hand motifs and which localize to the endoplasmic reticulum (Weis *et al.* 1994).

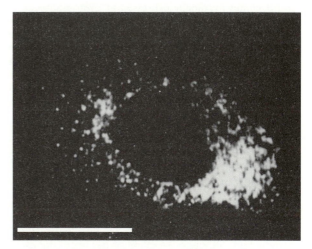

Figure 1. Confocal laser scanning fluorescence micrograph of HeLa cells stained with a polyclonal rabbit antiserum that specifically recognizes ERC-55. The staining is detected by secondary labelling with a goat anti-rabbit antiserum coupled to the fluorochrome Texas red. The typical reticular staining of the endoplasmic reticulum is observed in all cells. The bar indicates 20 µm.

■ Identification

ERC-55 was identified through the isolation of human cDNA clones obtained by screening a HeLa cDNA expression library with patient autoimmune sera (Weis *et al.* 1994). Specific antisera were raised against ERC-55 and used to identify the endogenous protein on Western blots after separation of HeLa cell extracts on one- and two-dimensional gel systems. ERC-55 was also shown to cofractionate with other marker proteins known to localize to the endoplasmic reticulum.

Gene and sequence

Full-length human cDNA clones encoding ERC-55 were isolated from a HeLa cDNA plasmid library and the sequence was deposited in the EMBL sequence databank (accession number X78669). Genomic clones were isolated from a human genomic library and sequence analysis showed that they encoded the promoter region of ERC-55 and the 5' teminus of the gene, including an intron of 375 base pairs. The genomic sequence was deposited in the EMBL sequence databank (accession number X78670).

Protein

ERC-55 has an amino-terminal signal leader peptide that targets it to the endoplasmic reticulum. It is retained in the endoplasmic reticulum via a carboxy-terminal HDEL motif. The internal protein sequence comprises six copies of the EF-hand motif. ERC-55 binds Ca^{2+} *in vitro*.

Antibodies

Polyclonal rabbit antibodies (Weis *et al.* 1994) are available from the authors.

Localization

ERC-55 is an intracellular protein that specifically localizes to the endoplasmic reticulum (Fig. 1; Weis *et al.* 1994).

The mRNA for ERC-55 is ubiquitously expressed in human tissues.

Biological activities

The ERC-55 protein is known to bind Ca^{2+} *in vitro* (Weis *et al.* 1994). As yet its biological function *in vivo* remains unknown.

Mutagenesis studies

Deletion of the carboxy-terminal HDEL motif was shown to result in a slow secretion of ERC-55 into the extracellular medium (Weis *et al.* 1994).

References

Ozawa, M. and Muramatsu, T. (1993) Reticulocalbin, a novel endoplasmic reticulum resident Ca^{2+}-binding protein with multiple EF-hand motifs and a carboxyl-terminal HDEL sequence. J. Biol. Chem. **268**, 699–705.

Weis, K., Griffiths, G., and Lamond, A.I. (1994) The endoplasmic reticulum calcium-binding protein of 55êkDa is a novel EF-hand protein retained in the endoplasmic reticulum by a carboxy-terminal His-Asp-Glu-Leu motif. J. Biol. Chem. **269**, 19142–19150.

■ *Angus I. Lamond[1] and Karsten Weis[2]:*
[1]Department of Biochemistry,
University of Dundee, Dundee, DD1 4HN,
Scotland, UK.
Tel.: +44 1382 345 473,
Fax: +44 1382 200 894,
E-mail: ailamond@bad.dundee.ac.uk.
[2]EMBL, Meyerhofstrasse 1, Postfach 102209,
D-69017 Heidelberg, Germany
Tel.: 49 6221 387 328
Fax: 49 6221 387 518
E-mail: weis@embl-heidelberg.de

Grancalcin

Grancalcin is a 28 kDa EF-hand Ca^{2+}-binding protein abundant in neutrophils and monocytes, and also present in B and T lymphocytes and the promyelocytic cell line HL60s. It is a cytosolic protein, but displays a Ca^{2+}-dependent translocation to the granules and plasma membrane of neutrophils, suggesting that it might play an effector role in the specialized function of these cells.

Human grancalcin has a calculated molecular mass of 24,010 Da. The apparent molecular weight is 28,000 Da on SDS-PAGE. The isoelectric point is 4.9. It contains four EF-hand Ca^{2+}-binding motifs and exhibits strong homology to sorcin, a Ca^{2+}-binding protein overexpressed in multidrug-resistant CHO cell lines (Van der Bliek *et al.*

1986), abundant in heart, and detectable in kidney, brain, and skeletal muscle (Meyers 1989). Grancalcin also shares considerable identity with both the large catalytic and small regulatory subunits of calpain. One phosphorylation and two glycosylation sites are predicted.

■ Isolation/identification

Grancalcin was initially identified as a 28 kDa protein which reacted with antiserum raised to membranes from neutrophils activated with phorbol myristate (PMA), a potent activator of the NADPH oxidase of neutrophils (Babior 1987; Segal 1989) and of degranulation (Repine et al. 1974). A partial grancalcin cDNA clone was obtained by screening a HL60 λgt11 library with antiserum against grancalcin. This was used to obtain a full-length 1.65kb clone from an induced HL60 λgt10 library (Boyhan et al. 1992). Grancalcin was prepared from neutrophil cytosol by 15% $(NH_4)_2SO_4$ precipitation, followed by anion exchange chromatography on a Mono Q column (Teahan et al. 1992). The protein eluted between 0.24 and 0.28 M NaCl, and was then purified to homogeneity by gel filtration on a Superdex 75 column. The apparent molecular mass on gel filtration was 55 kDa, indicating that the native protein exists as a homodimer.

■ Gene and sequence

The human cDNA sequence has been submitted to the GenBank/EMBL Data Bank with accession number M81637.

■ Protein

Grancalcin contains four EF-hand Ca^{2+}-binding motifs. It shares 58% identity over 192 residues with sorcin (Fig. 1) and 30% identity over 180 residues with the Ca^{2+}-binding domains of the calpain subunits. Two of the EF-hand motifs (I and II) are more highly conserved than the other two (III and IV) and probably have a higher affinity for Ca^{2+}. Evidence for Ca^{2+} binding was found in the difference in migration between the Ca^{2+}-loaded and Ca^{2+}-depleted preparations of grancalcin on SDS-PAGE, and by the binding of ^{45}Ca to slot blots of the native protein (Teahan et al. 1992).

■ Antibodies

Affinity purified antibodies to grancalcin were prepared from antisera to PMA-activated neutrophil membranes as described in Boyhan et al. (1992). Polyclonal antibodies were raised to pure grancalcin as described by Teahan et al. (1992).

■ Localization

Western blotting of cytosol from a variety of tissues and cell lines with antibody to the purified protein revealed that grancalcin is most abundant in neutrophils and macrophages, and is present at lower concentrations in B- and T-cell lymphocytes (Fig. 2). It is expressed in uninduced HL60 cells, and its expression is found to increase following induction with DMSO and interferon-γ

```
grancalcin  MAYPGYGGGFGNFSIQVPGMQMGQPVPET
            |||||  |  |          |   |  |
   sorcin   MAYPGHPGAGGGYYPGGYGGAPGGPSFPG


            GPAILLDGYSGPAYSDTYSSAGDSVYTYFSAV
               |  ||                      |  |
            QTQDPLYGY------------------FASV


            AGQDGEVDAEELQRCLTQSGINGTYSPFSLET
            |||||  || |||||||||  |  | || |||
            AGQDGQIDADELQRCLTQSGIAGGYKPFNLET
                           I
            CRIMIAML DRDHTGKMGFNA FKELWAALNA
            ||  ||   ||| |  | |||| |||||| ||
            CRLMVSML DRDMSGTMGFNE FKELWAVLNG
                           II
            WKENFMTV DQDGSGTVEHHE LRQAIGLMGYRLSPQ
            |   |    | | ||||  | |        |  || ||
            WRQHFISF DSDRSGTVDPQE LQKALTTMGFRLNPQ
                           III
            TLTTIVKR YSK-NGRIFFDD YVACCVKLRALT
            |  | ||  ||| |  || |||| |||||||||||
            TVNSIAKR YST-SGKITFDD YIACCVKLRALT
                           IV
            DFFRKRDH LQQGSANFIYDD FLQGTMAI*
            |  ||||  |||  || ||| |  | | |
            DSFRKRDS AQQGMVNFSYDD FIQCVMTV*
```

Figure 1. Amino acid homology between grancalcin and sorcin. Identical residues are indicated by connecting lines. Residues corresponding to the calcium-binding loop of the EF-hands predicted from the homology of this family of calcium-binding proteins are underlined (I–IV).

(IFN-γ) (Fig. 2). Northern blot analysis of human polymorphonuclear neutrophils (PMNs) revealed a transcript of 1.65 kb for grancalcin. This was also present in HL60s and two EBV-transformed B-cell lines, and was extremely abundant in bone marrow. The subcellular distribution of grancalcin in PMNs is dependent on both Ca^{2+} and Mg^{2+}. When the cells were broken in the absence of Ca^{2+} and Mg^{2+}, the protein was located mainly in the cytosol. This effect was accentuated in the presence of EDTA. However, more of this protein became associated with the granules in the presence of Mg^{2+} alone. When the cells were disrupted in the presence of Mg^{2+} and Ca^{2+}, the location of grancalcin shifted from the cytosol to the granules, and to a lesser extent, the membranes, in a Ca^{2+}-dependent fashion.

■ Biological activites

The function of grancalcin has not yet been ascertained, but its association with membranes and granules makes it a candidate for involvement in granule aggregation and degranulation.

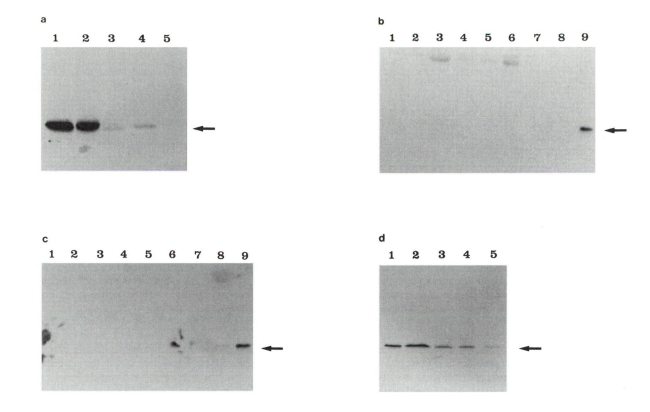

Figure 2. Cell and tissue distribution of grancalcin. Western blot analysis of grancalcin with polyclonal antibodies was conducted against the following: (a) leucocytes. Lane 1, PMNs; lane 2, macrophages/monocytes; lane 3, T cells; lane 4, B cells; lane 5, mast cells. Each lane contained 2×10^6 cells, except for lane 5 which contained 1×10^6 cells. (b) Tissues. Lane 1, endothelial cells; lane 2, mesothelial cells; lane 3, lymph node; lane 4, spleen; lane 5, liver; lane 6, kidney; lane 7, platelets; lane 8, erythrocytes; lane 9, PMNs. (c) Cell lines. Lane 1, EJ; lane 2, HeLa; lane 3, HEP G2 (liver); lane 4, HBF1 (B cell); lane 5, LICR (B cell); lane 6, K 562 (erythroblastoid); lane 7, MOLT 4 (T cell); lane 8, HUT 78 (T cell); lane 9, PMNs. (d) HL60 cells. Lane 1, dimethyl sulfoxide (1%) induced; lane 2, dimethyl sulfoxide + IFN-γ (200 IU/ml) induced; lanes 3 and 4, IFN- (200 IU/ml) treated; lane 5, uninduced. Equal amounts (50 μg) of protein were loaded in each lane.

■ References

Babior, B.M. (1987) The respiratory burst oxidase. Trends Biochem. Sci. **12**, 241–243.

*Boyhan, A., Casimir, C.M., French, J.K., Teahan, C.G., and Segal, A.W. (1992) Molecular cloning and characterisation of grancalcin, a novel EF-hand calcium-binding protein abundant in neutrophils and monocytes. J. Biol. Chem. **267**, 2928–2933.

Meyers, M.B. (1989) Sorcin is a cardiac calcium-binding protein. Proc. Am. Assoc. Cancer Res. **30**, 505 (Abstr. 2007).

Repine, J. E., White, J.G., Clawson, C.C., and Holmes, B.M. (1974) Effects of phorbol myristate acetate on the metabolism and ultrastructure of neutrophils in chronic granulomatous disease. J. Clin. Invest. **54**, 83–90.

*Segal, A.W. (1989) The electron transport chain of the micro-bicidal oxidase of phagocytic cells and its involvement in the molecular pathology of chronic granulomatous disease. *J. Clin. Invest.* **83**, 1785–1793.

*Teahan, C.G., Totty, N.F., and Segal, A.W. (1992) Isolation and characterisation of grancalcin, a novel 28 kDa EF-hand calcium-binding protein from human neutrophils. Biochem J. **286**, 549–554.

Van der Bliek, A. M., Meyers, M.B., Biedler, J.L., Hes, E., and Borst, P. (1986) A 22-kd protein (sorcin/V19) encoded by an amplified gene in multidrug-resistant cells, is homologous to the calcium-binding light chain of calpain. EMBO J **5**, 3201–3208.

■ *Angela Boyhan and Anthony W. Segal:*
Glaxo Wellcome Res. and Dev.
Medicines Research Center,
Gunnels Wood Road,
Stevenage, Hertfordshire
SG1 2NY, UK.
Tel.: +44 1438 764106
Fax: +44 1438 764488
E-mail: ab11372@ggR.co.uk.

Invertebrate, plant, and lower organism calcium-binding proteins

EF-hand containing proteins are present in prokaryotes and show a very high diversity; 23 subfamilies of unique Ca^{2+}-binding proteins (CaBPs) in lower organisms, plants, and invertebrates. The complexity of these unique invertebrate CaBPs often outdoes that of CaBPs in vertebrates. For most of them the biological function is not known, although it is often possible to discriminate between buffers, activators, and enzymes.

■ Introduction

Ca^{2+}-binding proteins (CaBPs) are important relay elements in the Ca^{2+} signal–response coupling. Most of them possess a recurrent structural motif, i.e. the paired EF-hand Ca^{2+}-binding domain (Kretsinger 1987). The interpreters of the Ca^{2+} signal in invertebrate animals are to a large extent the same as in the vertebrates, and include calmodulin, troponin C, essential and regulatory myosin light chains, calcineurin B, α-actinin, calpain, and neuronal CaBPs. Most of these proteins are already present in protista and fungi, and their presence extends up the evolutionary tree to plants and invertebrates. In contrast, no members of some well-known subfamilies, such as parvalbumin, S100 protein, or calbindin, have been reported outside the vertebrate animal kingdom; hence they seem to be unique to vertebrates. Invertebrates, plants, fungi, protista, and even prokaryotes contain in turn some unique CaBPs, not yet found in vertebrates. The latter proteins, which are the subject of this chapter, are listed in Table 1. A caveat about uniqueness is warranted since classical detection strategies may fail for lack of immunoreactivity, of low amount, or of transient expression. A good example is the caltractin and CDC31 subfamily which is present in the microtubule organizing centers of *Chlamydomonas* and of yeast, but whose homologs have recently been identified in vertebrates and cloned at the DNA level from human and mouse (Lee and Huang 1993; Errabolu *et al.* 1994). It is interesting to make the parallel here with the numerous actin-binding proteins which also are much more ubiquitous than initially thought (Pollard 1993).

When examining Table 1 one may question what kind of classification can be applied to the invertebrate CaBPs. On the basis of sequence information, 21 out of the 23 subclasses of CaBPs are very different except in their Ca^{2+}-binding segments (Kawasaki and Kretsinger 1994). However, an intriguing grouping of the functionally unrelated subclasses 1, 2, and 3 is meaningful in spite of the fact that sarcoplasmic CaBPs (SCP) are soluble buffering proteins (Wnuk *et al.* 1982) in invertebrates, aequorin and luciferin-binding protein are directly involved in light emission (Shimomura 1985), and calerythrin is a prokaryotic CaBP of unknown function (Swan *et al.* 1987). These three subclasses display a characteristic register in the partition of the four EF-hands over the polypeptide length. The resemblance of the photoproteins and the prokaryotic CaBP with *Nereis* SCP is particulary striking due the presence of an unusual site I and of an inactive site II, as well as a very similar pronounced positive cooperativity (Cox 1990). Thus there are structural classes, but the majority of the CaBPs unique to non-vertebrates are structurally not related.

■ Function: buffers, activators, enzymes, or light emitters?

Functionally, a distinction can be made between three types of CaBPs: first, those that buffer the Ca^{2+} and Mg^{2+} concentrations inside the cell; secondly, those that convey the Ca^{2+} signal to a specific response system through conformational changes and activation of the target protein, and, thirdly, the chimaeric proteins consisting of a Ca^{2+}-binding segment fused to a domain endowed with enzymatic activity.

The soluble sarcoplasmic Ca^{2+}-binding proteins (SCPs), functionally resemble vertebrate parvalbumins and are most likely involved in the regulation of Ca^{2+}/Mg^{2+} homeostasis (Cox 1990). An appealing hypothesis is that these Ca^{2+}–Mg^{2+}-binding proteins protect the cell and its compartments against high cytotoxic Ca^{2+} concentrations. In addition, since 1981 we have put forward the hypothesis (Wnuk *et al.* 1982) that in stimulated cells SCPs favor the increase of free Mg^{2+}, an important ion for modulation of the energy supply. A parallel can be drawn between these Ca^{2+}–Mg^{2+}-binding proteins, which protect against Ca^{2+} and energize cells, and the mitochondria which also protect against Ca^{2+} and, through influx of Ca^{2+}, stimulate ATP production (Gunter *et al.* 1994). In line with this hypothesis, the rather simple Ca^{2+}–Mg^{2+}-binding proteins and the complex mitochondria are complementary in different muscles: parvalbumins and SCPs are abundant in fast contracting muscle where the mitochondrial content is low, and vice versa. The Spec and Spec-like proteins may play a similar role of Ca^{2+}-buffering in nuclei of echinoderms (Klein *et al.* 1991), whereas 1F8 and TB17 may play this role in the flagellum of *Trypanosoma* (Engman *et al.* 1989). PFS in *Plasmodium* (Rawlings and Kaslow 1992) and ARP in *Euglena* (Gumpel and Smith 1992) associate to plasma membranes and may interfere there with the Ca^{2+} fluxes.

Table 1. CaBPs of invertebrates, plants, protozoa and prokaryotes

Name	No. of res.	Phylum	Common name	No. of sequ.	No. of EF-hands	Ca²⁺/ prot.	Interactive properties	Putative role
1. SCP	182	*Branchio. l.*	amphioxus	7	4	3	no	B
		Peneaus s.	shrimp	3	4	?	no	B
		Astacus p.	crayfish	1	4	3	no	B
		Drosoph. m.	fruit fly	1	4	?	no	B
		Nereis d.	sandworm	2	4	3	no	B
		Palinop. y.	scallop	1	4	2	no	B
2. Calerythrin	177	*Sacchar. e.*	streptomyces	1	4	3	no	B
3. Aequorin	189	*Aequora v.*	sea pansy	2	4	3	luciferin	E
		Clytia g.	hydroid	1	4	?	luciferin	E
LBP	184	*Renilla r.*	jellyfish	1	4	3	luciferin	S
4. Spec	150	*Strongylo. p. Hemicent. p.*	sea urchin	4	4	?	no	B
5. Spec- like	377	*Lytechinus p.*	sea urchin	3	8	not charact.		
6. 1F8 &	211	*Trypano. c.*	flagellate	1	4	2	?	B
TB17	233	*Trypano. b.*	flagellate	1	4	?	?	B
7. EFH5	190	*Trypano. b.*	flagellate	3	4	3	?	B
8. PFS	374	*Plasmod. f.*	slime mold	1	5	?	membranes	B
9. LAV1	355	*Physarum p.*	slime mold	1	4	not charact.		
10. Cal1	161	*Caenorh. e.*	roundworm	1	4	not charact.		
11. TCH2 & TCH3	frag.	*Arabidop. t.*	plant	1	2	not charact.		
12. YLJ5	178	*Caenorh. e.*	roundworm	1	4	not charact.		
13. CABP	69	*Schistos. m.*	blood fluke	1	2	not charact.		
14. SM20	frag.	*Schistos. m.*	blood fluke	1	2	not charact.		
15. ARP	646	*Euglena g.*	flagellate	1	30	?	membrane	B
16. CaVP	161	*Branchio. l.*	amphioxus	1	4	2	melittin & 26 kDa	A
17. Squidulin	149	*Lologo p.*	squid	1	4	4	melittin & chlorpromazin	
18. TCBP	218	*Tetrahym. p.*	ciliate	2	4	?	phenyl-Sepharose	A
19. Caltractin	169	*Chlamyd. r.*	flagellate	2	4	?	phenyl-Sepha-	
CDC31	161	*Saccharo. c.*	yeast				rose & MTOCs	A
20. PFPK	524	*Plasmod. f.*	sporozoa	1	4	?	fused kinase	E
21. CDPK	508	*Glycine m.*	soybean	3	4	?	fused kinase	E
		Daucus c.	carrot					
	624	*Arabidop. t.*	plant					
22. PPTS	661	*Drosoph. m.*	fruit fly	1	3	?	fused phosphatase	E
23. CBPA	467	*Dictyos. d.*	slime mold	1	2	?	fused to Pro-rich	?
24. Calsensin	83	*Hirudinea*	leech	1	2	not charact.		

Legend to the table: No. of res: number of residues; No. of sequ.: number of sequences published; Ca²⁺/prot.: Ca²⁺ bound per protein; not charact.: only the cDNA sequence is known, the protein was not characterized; frag.: the sequence of a fragment of the protein is known; B: buffering function; E: enzymatic activity; S: substrate activity; A: activator. Sequence information to the above-mentioned proteins is found in the references listed at the end of this article.

None of the above-cited proteins seems to be involved in high affinity protein–protein interactions. But other unique invertebrate CaBPs are endowed with this capability: they comprise CaVP in amphioxus (Cox 1986), squidulin in octopus (Head 1989), caltractin in the basal bodies of *Chlamydomonas* (Huang *et al.* 1988) and TCBP-25 in *Tetrahymena* (Takemasa *et al.* 1989). All these proteins can interact in a Ca²⁺-dependent manner with phenyl-Sepharose and thus possess the potential to regulate biochemical processes, although their real function is not known (but see later for caltractin).

The third category, that of the chimaeric proteins with a Ca^{2+}-binding domain and a domain for enzymatic activity, comprises at this moment three CaBPs: a protein phosphatase of *Drosophila* with three EF hands at the C-terminal end (Steele *et al.* 1992), and two types of protein kinases, one in *Plasmodium* with four EF hands at the C-terminal end (Zhao *et al.* 1993) and one in plants (Harper *et al.* 1991). They are evolutionarily not related and, unfortunately, none of them has been characterized at the protein level.

A special place is taken by the photoproteins aequorin and luciferin-binding protein which display a well-defined function. They clearly co-evolved with the SCPs (see above), but only the photoproteins acquired additional potentials: binding of a luciferin chromophore for the anthozoan luciferin-binding protein (LBP) and, even more performant in the case of aequorin, binding of coelenterazine and molecular oxygen (Shimomura 1985). Moreover, aequorin is intrinsically able to catalyse the breakdown of coelenterazine with concomittant emission of light, whereas luciferin-binding protein renders the bioluminescent reaction Ca^{2+}-dependently.

How old are the EF-hand CaBPs?

The importance of Ca^{2+} in the regulation of many molecular events in eukaryotic cells is exemplified by calmodulin which is found from the most organized animals to the lowest eukaryotes. Its distribution in at least 10 Protista belonging to different phyla (ciliates, flagellates, sporozoa, euglena, entamoeba, and stylonychia) (Kawasaki and Kretsinger 1994) suggests that the presence of calmodulin in Protista is not the beginning of the story, but that a calmodulin-like protein may be present in prokaryotes as well. In *Bacillus cereus* (Shyu and Foegeding 1991), *B. subtilis* (Fry *et al.* 1991), *Anabaena* (Petterson and Bergman 1990) and *Nostoc* (Onek and Smith 1992) calmodulin-like activity was reported. Heat shock proteins of *E. coli* contain an authentic calmodulin-binding domain (Stevenson and Calderwood 1990), also suggesting the presence of this activator protein. But, for lack of the amino acid sequence data it can not be concluded that a calmodulin is at work in these bacteria. An alternative hypothesis is that prokaryotes do not use CaBPs for regulation of cellular processes, but only to keep the toxic Ca^{2+} levels low, in other words that Ca^{2+} buffering evolved in prokaryotes before the controlled use of Ca^{2+} in eukaryotes. Indeed the intracellular Ca^{2+} concentration of *E. coli* is regulated at 100 nM, a level similar to that in resting eukaryotes (Knight *et al.* 1991). Interestingly, calerythrin, the only well-documented prokaryotic CaBP, bears more resemblance to buffering proteins, especially to SCPs and aequorin, than to calmodulin, and does not show calmodulin activity (Bylsma *et al.* 1992). The fact that a EF hand is present in prokaryotes is very intriguing since the actin system started to evolve only at the emergence of the eukaryotes (Pollard 1993). However, the hypothesis that the presence of calerythrin

in a prokaryote is the result of a recent gene transfer can not yet be excluded.

Research challenges for the future; learning from invertebrate CaBPs

Despite the numerous biophysical and functional studies on CaBPs, many questions remain unsolved and it is anticipated that invertebrate CaBPs may help to find new clues. For instance, SCPs have very interesting Ca^{2+}- and Mg^{2+}-interactive properties, which may lead to more insight into the molecular chemistry of sequential binding and positive cooperativity. The crystal structures of *Nereis* SCP and amphioxus SCP show also the first cases of a paired two Ca^{2+}-binding-sites domain with a functional site paired to a non-functional one. This may stand as a model for CaBPs in higher animals where the same pairing of a functional to a non-functional site has been reported. The three-dimensional structure of aequorin with bound luciferin and oxygen seems close to elucidation (Hannick *et al.* 1993). Soon we expect to understand the exciting intramolecular process of allosteric Ca^{2+}-binding leading to rearrangements that allow oxygen to break coelenterazine with concomitant emission of light. Aequorin and its targeted recombinant variants offer unique tools to study the homeostasis of Ca^{2+} in all the compartments of a cell. As indicated above, aequorin contains in one molecule the complete arsenal of ligands to function as a Ca^{2+}-controlled light emitter. It can been expressed without harm in the cytoplasm of most cells, and takes up coelenterazine from outside. The Ca^{2+} signal can be monitored by bioluminescence provided the cells are appropriately stimulated. Recently, aequorin cDNA was endowed with a segment that codes for a recognition peptide so that the newly expressed photoprotein directs itself to subcellular compartments. Moreover, site-directed mutagenesis is employed to change the affinity and kinetics of the mutant proteins for Ca^{2+}, so that they can monitor the Ca^{2+}-transient changes in each of these compartments (Kendall *et al.* 1992).

Prokaryotes have no CaM gene but have calmodulin activity. On the other hand the heat shock proteins of *E. coli* contain a canonical calmodulin-binding domain. Is there a Ca^{2+} signal in prokaryotes and, if so, which CaBPs are in charge here to relay the signal and what processes exactly are controlled by Ca^{2+}?

As shown in the last column of Table 1, different invertebrate CaBPs are only known at the gene or cDNA level and not at all at the protein level. Several of the proteins expressed seem to be interactive, meaning that they can interact with non-specific hydrophobic matrices, or with more selective compounds, which were already used in the calmodulin research. It is now an important challenge to determine the immediate targets of these proteins and to pinpoint the physiological systems which are regulated by these proteins. The tools for studying protein–protein interaction are developing rapidly and will soon be used for target identification in the Ca^{2+}-signaling field.

References

Bylsma, N., Drakenberg, T., Anderson, I., Leadlay, P.F., and Försen, S. (1992) Prokaryotic calcium-binding protein of the calmodulin superfamily. Calcium binding to a *Saccharopolyspora erythraea* 20 kDa protein. FEBS Lett. **299**, 44–47.

Cox, J.A. (1986) Isolation and characterization of a new M, 18,000 protein with calcium vector properties in amphioxus muscle and identification of its endogenous target protein. J. Biol. Chem. **261**, 13173–13178.

*Cox, J.A. (1990) Calcium vector protein and sarcoplasmic calcium-binding proteins from invertebrate muscle. In *Stimulus response coupling* (ed. V.L. Smith and J.R. Dedman), pp. 83–107. CRC Press, Boca Raton.

Engman, D.M., Krause, K.-H., Blumin, J.H., Kim, K.S., Kirchhoff, L.V., and Donelson, J.E. (1989) A novel flagellar Ca^{2+}-binding protein in Trypanosomes. J. Biol. Chem. **264**, 18627–18631.

Errabolu, R., Sanders, M.A., and Salisbury, J.L. (1994) Cloning of a cDNA encoding human centrin, an EF-hand protein of centrosomes and mitotic spindle poles. J. Cell Sci. **107**, 9–16.

Fry, I.J., Becker-Hapak, M., and Hageman, J.H. (1991) Purification and properties of an intracellular calmodulin-like protein from *Bacillus subtilis* cells. J. Bacteriol. **173**, 2506–2513.

Gumpel, N.J. and Smith, A.G. (1992) A novel calcium-binding protein from *Euglena gracilis*. Characterisation of a cDNA encoding a 74–kDa acid-repeat protein targeted across the endoplasmic reticulum. Eur. J. Biochem. **210**, 721–727.

Gunter, T.E., Gunter, K.K., Sheu, S.-S., and Gavin, C.E. (1994) Mitochondrial calcium transport: physiological and pathological relevance. Am. J. Physiol. **267**, C313–C339.

Hannick, L.I., Prasher, D.C., Schultz, L.W., Descamps, J.R., and Ward, K.B. (1993) Preparation and initial characterization of crystals of the photoprotein aequorin from *Aequorea victoria*. Proteins **15**, 103–107.

Harper, J.F., Sussman, M.R., Schaller, G.E., Putman Evans, C., Charbonneau, H., and Harmon, A.C. (1991) A calcium-dependent protein linase with a regulatory domain similar to calmodulin. Science **252**, 951–954.

Head, J.F. (1989) Amino acid sequence of a low molecular weight, high affinity calcium-binding protein from the optic lobe of the squid *Loligo pealei*. J. Biol. Chem. **264**, 7202–7206.

Huang, B., Watterson, D.M., Lee, V.D., and Schibler, M.J. (1988) Purification and characterization of a basal body-associated Ca^{2+}-binding protein. J. Cell Biol. **107**, 121–131.

*Kawasaki, H. and Kretsinger, R. (1994) Calcium binding proteins I: EF-hands. Protein Profile **1**, 343–517.

Kendall, J.M., Sala-Newly, G., Ghalaut, V., Dormer, R.L., and Campbell, A.K. (1992) Engineering the Ca^{2+}-activated photoprotein aequorin with reduced affinity for calcium. Biochim. Biophys. Res. Commun. **187**, 1091–1097.

*Klein, W.H., Xiang, M., and Wessel, G.M. (1991) Spec proteins: calcium-binding proteins in the embryonic ectoderm of sea urchins. In *Novel calcium-binding proteins, fundamentals and clinical implications* (ed. C.W. Heizmann), pp. 466–479. Springer-Verlag, Berlin.

Knight, M.R., Campbell, A.K., Smith, S.M., and Trewavas, A.J. (1991) Recombinant aequorin as a probe for cytosolic Ca^{2+} in *Escherichia coli*. FEBS Lett. **282**, 405–408.

Kretsinger, R.H. (1987) Calcium coordination and the calmodulin fold: divergent versus convergent evolution. Cold Spring Harbor Symp. Quant. Biol. **52**, 499–510.

Lee, V.D. and Huang, B. (1993) Molecular cloning and centrosomal localization of human caltractin. Proc. Natl. Acad. Sci. USA **90**, 11039–11043.

Onek, L.A. and Smith, R.J. (1992) Calmodulin and calcium mediated regulation in prokaryotes. J. Gen. Microbiol. **138**, 1039–1049.

Pettersson, A. and Bergman, B. (1990) Calmodulin in heterocystous cyanobacteria: biochemical and immunological evidence. FEMS Microbiol. Lett. **60**, 95–100.

Pollard, T.D. (1993) Actin and actin-binding proteins. In *Guidebook to the cytoskeletal and motor proteins* (ed. T. Kreis and R. Vale), pp. 3–11. Oxford University Press.

Rawlings, D.J. and Kaslow, D.C. (1992) A novel 40-kDa membrane-associated EF-hand calcium-binding protein in *Plasmodium falciparum*. J. Biol. Chem. **267**, 3976–3982.

*Shimomura, O. (1985) Bioluminescence in the sea: photoprotein systems. Symp. Soc. Exp. Biol. **39**, 351–372.

Shyu, Y.-T. and Foegeding, P.M. (1991) Purification and some characteristics of a calcium-binding protein from *Bacillus cereus* spores. J. Gen. Microbiol. **137**, 1611–1623.

Spang, A., Courtney, I., Fackler, U., Matzner, M., and Schiebel, E. (1993) The calcium-binding protein cell division cycle 31 of *Saccharomyces cerevisiae* is a component of the half bridge of the spindle pole body. J. Cell Biol. **123**, 405–416.

Steele, F.R., Washburn, R.T., Rieger, R., and O'Tousa, J.E. (1992) *Drosophila* retinal degeneration C (rdgC) encodes a novel serine/threonine protein phosphatase. Cell **69**, 669–676.

Stevenson, M.A. and Calderwood, S.K. (1990) Members of the 70-kilodalton heat shock protein family contain a highly conserved calmodulin-binding domain. Mol. Cell. Biol. **10**, 1234–1238.

Swan, D.G., Hale, R.S., Dhillon, N., and Leadlay, P.F. (1987) A bacterial calcium-binding protein homologous to calmodulin. Nature **329**, 84–85.

Takemasa, T., Ohnishi, K., Kobayashi, T., Takagi, T., Konishi, K., and Wanatabe, Y. (1989) Cloning and sequencing of the gene for *Tetrahymena* calcium-binding 25-kDa protein (TCBP-25). J. Biol. Chem. **264**, 19293–19301.

Weber, C., Lee, V.D., Chazin, W.J., and Huang, B. (1994) High level expression in *Escherichia coli* and characterization of the EF-hand calcium-binding protein caltractin. J. Biol. Chem. **269**, 15795–15802.

Wnuk, W., Cox, J.A., and Stein, E.A. (1982) Parvalbumin and other soluble sarcoplasmic Ca-binding proteins. In *Calcium and cell function*, Vol. II (ed. W.Y. Cheung), pp. 243–278. Academic Press Inc.

Zhao, Y., Kappes, B., and Franklin, R.M. (1993) Gene structure and expression of an unusual protein kinase from *Plasmodium falciparum* homologous at its carboxyl terminus with the EF-hand calcium-binding proteins. J. Biol. Chem. **268**, 4347–4354.

References to sequences of proteins in Table 1

Branchiost. SCP: Takagi, T. and Cox, J.A. (1990) Eur. J. Biochem. **192**, 387–399.

Peneaus SCP: Takagi, T. and Konishi, K. (1984) J. Biochem. **95**, 1603–1615.

Astacus SCP: Jauregui-Adell, J., Wnuk, W., and Cox, J.A. (1989) FEBS Lett. **243**, 209–212.

Drosophila SCP: Kelly, L.E. (1990) Biochem. J. **271**, 661–666.

Nereis SCP: Collins, J.A., Cox, J.A., and Theibert, J.L. (1988) J. Biol. Chem. **263**, 15378–15385.

Patinop. SCP: Takagi, T., Kobayashi, T., and Konishi, K. (1984) Biochim. Biophys. Acta **787**, 252–257.

Calerythrin: Swan, D.G., Hale, R.S., Dhillon, N., and Leadlay, P.F., (1987) Nature **329**, 84–85.

Aequorin: Charbonneau, H., Walsh, K.A., McCann, R.O., Prendergast, F.G., Cormier, M.J., and Vanaman, T.C. (1985) Biochemistry **24**, 6762–6771.

LBP: Kumar, S., Harrylock, M., Walsh, K.A., Cormier, M.J., and Charbonneau, H. (1990) FEBS Lett. **268**, 287–290.

Strongylo. p. Spec: Carpenter, C.D., Bruskin, A.M., Hardin, P.E., Keast, M.J., Anstrom, J., Tyner, A.L., Brandhorst, B.P., and Klein, W.H. (1984) Cell **36**, 663–671.

Hemicent. Spec: Hosoya, H., Takagi, T., Mabuchi, H., Isawa, H., Sakai, H., Hiramoto, Y., and Konishi, K. (1988) Cell Struct. Funct. **13**, 525–532.

Spec-like: Xiang, M.Q., Bedard, P.A., Wessel, G., Filion, M., Brandhorst, B.P., and Klein, W.H. (1988) J. Biol. Chem **263**, 17173–17180.

1F8: Engman, D.M., Krause, K.H., Blumin, J.H., Kim, K.S., Kirchhoff, L.V., and Donelson, J.E. (1989) J. Biol. Chem. **264**, 18627–18631.

TB17: Lee, M.G., Chen J.F., Ho, A.W., D'Alesandro, P.A., and Vander Ploeg, L.H. (1990) Nucl. Acids Res. **18**, 4252.

EFH5: Wong, S., Kretsinger, R.H., and Campbell, D.A. (1992) Mol. Gen. Genetics-Mgg **233**, 225–230.

PFS, Rawlings, D.J. and Kaslow, D.C. (1992) J. Biol Chem. **267**, 3976–3982.

LAV1: Laroche, A., Lemieux, G., and Pellotta, D. (1989) Nucleic Acids Res. **17**, 10502.

Cal1: Salvato, M., Sulston, J., Albertson, D., and Brenner, S. (1986) J. Mol. Biol. **190**, 281–289.

TCH2 & TCH3: Braam, J. and Davis, R.W. (1990) Cell **60**, 357–364.

YLJ5: Wilson, R. *et al.* (1994) Nature **368**, 32–38.

CABP: Ram, D., Grossman, Z., Markovics, A., Avivi, A., Ziv, E., Lantner, F., and Schlechter, I. (1989) Mol. Biochem. Parasitol. **34**, 167–175.

SM20: Havercroft, J.C., Huggins, M.C., Dunne, D.W., and Taylor, D.W. (1990) Mol. Biochem. Parasitol, **38**, 211–220.

ARP: Gumpel, N.J. and Smith, A.G. (1992) Europ. J. Biochem. **210**, 721–727.

CaVP: Kobayashi, T., Takagi, T., Konishi, K., and Cox, J.A. (1987) J. Biol. Chem. **262**, 2613–2623.

Squidulin: Head, J.F. (1989) J. Biol. Chem. **264**, 7202–7209.

TCBP: Takesama, T. Takagi, T., Kobayashi, T., Konishi, K., and Watanabe, Y. (1990) J. Biol. Chem. **265**, 2514–2517.

Caltractin: Huang, B., Mengersen, A., and Lee, V.D. (1988) J. Cell Biol. **107**, 133–140.

PFPK: Zhao, Y., Kapper, B., and Franklin, R.M. (1993) J. Biol. Chem. **268**, 4347–4354.

Glycine CDPK: Harper, J.F:, Sussman, M.R., Schaller, G.E., Putnam Evans, C., Charbonneau, H., and Harmon, A.C. (1991) Science **252**, 951–954.

Daucus CDPK; Suen, K.L., and Choi, J.H. (1991) Plant Mol. Biol. **17**, 581–590.

Arabidop. CDPK: Harper, J.F., Binder, B.M., and Sussman, M.R. (1993) Biochemistry **32**, 3282–3290.

PPTS: Steele, F.R., Washburn, T., Rieger, R., and O'Tousa, J.E. (1992) Cell **69**, 669–676.

CBPA: Wennington, R., Greenwood, M., and Tsang, A. (1993), submitted.

Calsensin: Lin, C-S., Shen. W., Chen, Z.P., Tu, Y-H., and Matsudaira, P. (1994). Mol. Cell Biol. **14**, 2457–2567.

■ *J.A. Cox:*
Department of Biochemistry,
University of Geneva,
1211, Geneva 4, Switzerland
Tel.: (022) 702 64 91
Fax: (022) 702 64 83
E-mail: cox@sc2a.unige.ch

Aequorin and luciferin-binding protein

The photoproteins of the aequorin type are remarkable by the fact that the whole bioluminescent machinery is confined in one single protein. They bind molecular oxygen and luciferin (= coelenterazine) in proximal sites. Upon the binding of Ca^{2+} to the three allosterically coupled EF-hands I, III and IV the protein becomes a luciferase by oxidizing the luciferin with emission of blue light. The homologous luciferin-binding protein (LBP) in anthozoa fulfils only two of these functions: binding of three Ca^{2+} liberates the protein-bound luciferin for oxidation by an extrinsic luciferase. The photoproteins are increasingly used for monitoring free Ca^{2+} in subcellular compartments in living cells.

Ca^{2+}-binding proteins are key elements in bioluminescence in coelenterates and ctenophores. In the hydrozoa the Ca^{2+}-triggered bioluminescence reaction is carried out by a single photoprotein, the best known being aequorin. In the Anthozoa two distinct proteins are involved, a calcium- and luciferin-binding protein (LBP) and the enzyme luciferase. Aequorin represents an unusually complex mixture of closely related isotypes, whereas LBP shows no polymorphism. Although the photoproteins and LBP have many physical characteristics in common, such as the molecular mass (18.5 to 22 kDa),

isoelectric point (4.2 to 4.9), three Ca^{2+}-binding sites with similar affinity (K_d = 0.14 to 0.2 mM) and strong positive cooperativity ($n_H > 2$), the optical properties are very different, since aequorin is rich in Trp and His, whereas LBP is devoid of Trp and possesses only one His. In coelenterates the bioluminescent blue light at 470 nm is absorbed by a green-fluorescent protein and emitted at 510 nm. Aequorin and the five related photoproteins halistaurin, obelin, mneniopsin, berovin and clytin (Shimomura 1986) contain in one single protein all the elements for the bioluminescent reaction: tightly bound luciferin and

Alignments of amino acid sequences in the SCP*AEQ family

```
Domains I and II:

                 En**nn**nD*D*DG**ID**En***n                                  24                       En***nn**nD*D*DG**ID**En***nn**n

 1. Calerythrin   MTTAIASD       RLKKRFDRWDFDGNGALLERADFEKEAQHI   AEAF-GKDAGAAEVQTLKNAFGG   LFDYLAKEAGVGSDGSLTEEQFIRVTENL   IFEQGE-
 2. Clytin        VKLRPNFDNPKWVN  RHKFMFNFLDINGDGKITLDEIVSKASDD   ICAKLGATPEQTKRHQDAVEAFF   KKIGM--DYGKEVEFPAFVDGWKELANYD   LKLWS
 3. Aequor1      +VKLTPDFDNPKWIG  RHKHMFNFLDVNHNGRISLDEMVYKASDI   VINNLGATPEQAKRHKDAVEAFF   GGAGM--KYGVETEWPEYIEGWKRLASEE   LKRYS
 4. Aequor2      +VKLTSDFDNPRWIG  RHKHMFNFLDVNHNGKISLDEMVYKASDI   VINNLGATPEQAKRHKDAVEAFF   GGAGM--KYGVETDWPAYIEGWKKLATDE   LEKYA
 5. Lucif.BP      PEVTASERAYHLR   KMKTRMKRVDVTGDGFISREDYELIAVRI   AKIAKLSAEKAEETRQEFLRVAD   QLGLAPGVRISVEEAAVNATDSLLKMKAE   EK---N-
 6. Nereis        SDLWVQ         KMKTYFNRIDFDKDGATRMDFESMAERF   AKESE--MKAEHAKVLMDSLTG    VW-DNFLTAVAGGKG-IDETTFINSMKEM   VK--N-
 7. Perinereis    SDLWVQ         KMKTYFNRIDFDKDGATRKDFESMATRF   AKESE--MKPEHAKVLMDSLTG    VW-DKFLANVAGGKG-IDQATFISSMKEK   VK--D-
 8. Scallop       TDYLVS         KWKIWYKSLDVNHDGIISIENVEESRNKF   TDLH---LVGDKSTGVKVDMQK    WW-DTYIFLTPGA--EISETQFVENLGNS   FKK--D-
 9. Crayfish      AYSWDNR        VKYVVRYMYDIDNNGFLDKNDFECLALRN   TLIEGRGEFNEAAYANNQKIMSN   LWNEIAELADFNKDGEVTIDEFKKAVQNV   CVGKAF-
10. Shrimp α1     AYS-DNR        VKYVVRYMYDIDDDGFLDKNDFECIVARN   TLIEGRGEFSAADYANNQKIMRN   L-NEIAELADFNKDGEVTVDEFKMAVQKH   CQGKKY-
11. Shrimp α2     AYSWDNR        VKYVVRYMYDIDDDGFLDKNDFECLAVRN   TLIEGRGEFSAADYANNQKIMRN   LWNEIAELADFNKDGEVTVDEFKMAVQKH   CQGKKY-
12. Shrimp β      AYSWDNR        VKYVVRYMYDIDNDGFLDKNDFECLAVRN   TLIEGRGEFSPEGYAKNKEIMAN   LWNEIAELADFNKDGEVTVDEFKQAVQKN   CKGKAF-
13. Amphiox.I     GLNDFQKQK      IKFTDFFLDYNKDGSIQWEDFEEMIKEY   KEVNK-GSLSDADYKSMQASLED   QWRDLKGRADINKDDVVSWEEYLAMWEKT   IATCKSV
14. Amphiox.II    GLNDFQKQK      IKFTDFFLDMNHDGSIQDNDFEDMMTEY   KEVNK-GSLSDADYKSMQASLED   QWRDLKGRADINKDDVVSWEEYLAMWEKT   IATCKSV


Domains III and IV:

                 En**nn**nD*D*DG**ID**En***nn**n   16                               7           En**nn**nD*D*DG**ID**En***n

 1. Calerythrin   ASFNRVLGP   VVKGTWGMCDKNADGQINADEFAAWLTAL   GMSK---AEA   AEAFNQV--DTNGNGELSLDELLT-AVRD   FHPGRLDVELLG
 2. Clytin        QNKKSLIRD   WGEAVFDIFDKDGSGSISLDEWKAYGRIS   GICS---SDE   DAEKTFKHCDLDNSGKLDVDEMTRQHLGF   WTTLD-PNADGLYGNFVP
 3. Aequor1       KNQITLIRL   WGDALFDIIDKDQNGAISLDEWKAYTKSD   GIIQ---SSE   DCEETFRVCDIDESGQLDVDEMTRQHLGF   WYTMD-PACEKLYGGAVP
 4. Aequor2       KNEPTLIRI   WGDALFDIVDKDQNGAITLDEWKAYTKAA   GIIQ---SSE   DCEETFRVCDIDESGQLDVDEMTRQHLGF   WYTMD-PACEKLYGGAVP
 5. Luciferin BP  ----AMAVI   QSLIMYDCIDTDKDGYVSLPEFKAFLQAV   GPDI---TDD   KAITCFNTLDFNKNGQISRDEFLVTVNDF   LFGLDETALANAPYGDLL
 6. Nereis        PEAKSVVEG   PLPLFFRAVDTNEDNNISRDEYGIFFGML   GLDKT---MA   PASFDAI--DTNNDGLLSLEEFVI-AGSD   FFMNDGDSTNKVFWGPLV
 7. Periner.      PNAKAVVEG   PLPLFFRAVDTNEDNNISRDEYGIFFNML   GLNPD---MA   PASFDAI--DTNNDGLLSQEEFVT-AGSD   FFINDQDSPNKVFWGPLV
 8. Scallop       KAFLATMTA   CFNMIFDVIDTDKDRSIDLNEFIYAFAAF   GHENE---SVV  RTAFALLKPDDDNTVPLRTVVDAWLS--F   VTCEDASKTDVIKSAFES
 9. Crayfish      ATPPAAFKV   FIANQFKTVDVNGDGLVGVDEYRLDCISR   SAFANVKEID  DAYNKLATDADKRAGGISLARYQCISRSA   FANVELYAQFISNPDESANAVYLFGPLKEVQ
10. Shrimp α1     GEFPGAFKV   FIADQFKAIDVNGDGKVGLDEYRLDCITR   SAFAEVKEID  DAYDKLTTEDDRKAGGLTLERYQCITRSA   FAEVDLYAQFISNPNESCSACFLFGPLKVVQ
11. Shrimp α2     SEFPGAFKV   FIANQFKAIDVNGDGKVGLDEYRLDCITR   SAFAEVKEID  DAYDKLTTEDDRKAGGLTLERYQCITRSA   FAEVDLYAQFISNPNESCSACFLFGPLKVVQ
12. Shrimp β      ANFPNAFKV   FIGNQFKTIDVDGDMVGVDEYRLDCITR   SAFADVKEID  DAYDKLCTEEDKAGGINLARYQCITRSA   FADVELYAQFISNEDEKNNACYLFGPLKEVQ
13. Amphiox.I     ADLPAWCQN   RIPFLFKGMDEDGDGIVDLEEFQNYCLNF   -----QLQCA  DVPAVYNVITDGGKVTFDLNRYKELYYRL   LTSPAADAGNTLMGQKP
14. Amphiox.II    ADLPAWCQN   RIPFLFKGMDEDGDGIVDLEEFQNYCLNF   -----QLQCA  DVPAVYNVITDGGKVTFDLNRYKELYYRL   LTSPAADAGNTLMGQKP
```

Figure 1. Alignment of amino acid sequences of the photoproteins, luciferin-binding protein, calerythrin and SCPs. The consensus sequences for canonical EF-hands are indicated above each segment. Functional (i.e. Ca^{2+}-binding) EF-hands are indicated by thin characters. The sequences of amphioxus isoforms III to VII are not shown.

oxygen as well as binding sites for Ca^{2+}. The binding of Ca^{2+} converts the protein to a luciferase, which catalyzes the oxidation of coelenterazine by the bound oxygen to produce CO_2 and coelenteramide, which remains associated to the protein yielding a "blue-fluorescent protein". Upon removal of bound Ca^{2+} the coelenteramide dissociates to form apoaequorin and new coelenterazine is taken up by the protein so as to regenerate the bioluminescent machinery. In Anthozoa the bioluminescent mechanism is different (Charbonneau and Cormier 1979): metal-free LBP sequesters the coelenterazine substrate so that its oxidation by freely dissolved oxygen can not be catalyzed by an extrinsic luciferase. Upon binding of Ca^{2+} to the three EF-hand sites this inhibition is released.

Identification/isolation

After mechanical isolation of photogenic particles classical gel filtration and ion exchange (DEAE), chromatograpy is performed to obtain electrophoretically pure aequorin or LBP (Blinks et al. 1978; Charbonneau and Cormier 1979). The activity of aequorin is monitored by its luminescence after injection of Ca^{2+} in the protein solution; that of LBP needs in addition the presence of a luciferase.

Gene and sequence

The photoproteins aequorin and LBP were discovered and sequenced by techniques of protein purification and chemistry. Cloning and expression of aequorin was

reported by Inouye et al. (1986), cloning of clytin by Inouye and Tsuji (1993). A marked homology exists between the photoproteins aequorin (Swiss Prot P02592), clytin, LBP (Swiss Prot P05938), SCPs and the prokaryotic calerythrin (Fig. 1). Three active EF hands are present in sites I, III and IV. Intriguingly, besides the sequence homology in the Ca^{2+}-binding sites and the characteristic spacing of the EF hands, the primary structure of LBP is very different from that of the photoproteins.

Protein structure

Recently, well-diffracting crystals of recombinant metal-free aequorin have been obtained; as expected they luminesce and then slowly degrade when exposed to Ca^{2+} (Hannick et al. 1993).

Antibodies

No antibodies against aequorin or LBP have been reported.

Biological application of photoproteins

Aequorin and its targeted recombinant variants offer unique tools to study the homeostasis of Ca^{2+} in all the compartments of a cell. As indicated above, aequorin contains in one molecule the complete arsenal of ligands to function as a Ca^{2+}-controlled light emitter. It can be expressed without harm in the cytoplasm of most cells (Inouye et al. 1986), and takes up coelenterazine from

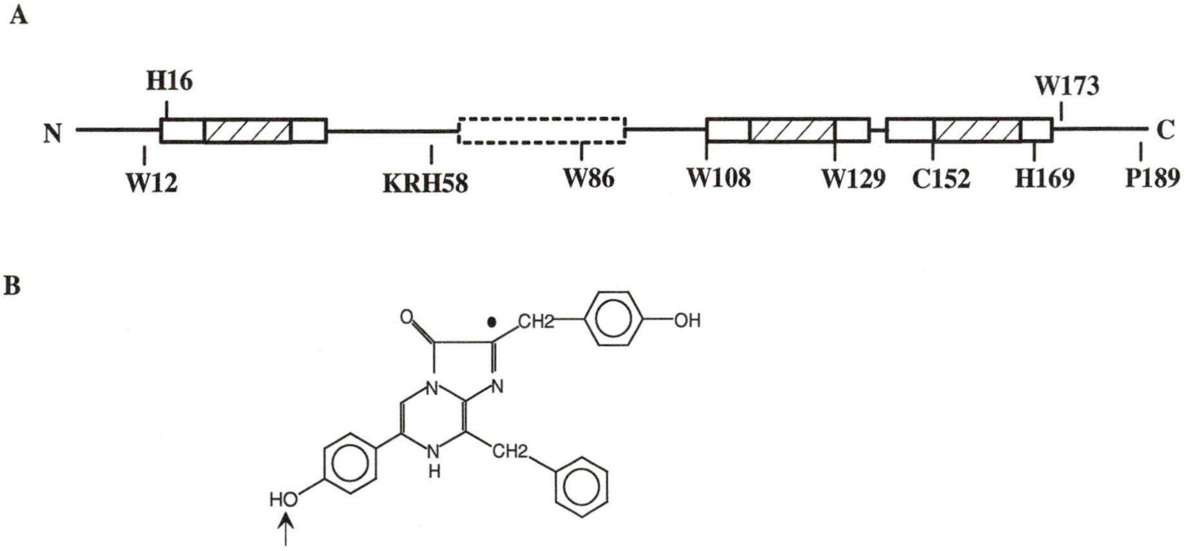

A

B

Figure 2. (A) Domain structure and characteristic features of aequorin. The rectangles correspond to the EF-hands and their Ca^{2+}-binding loops (hatched rectangles). Conserved and functionally important residues in all photoproteins are displayed. (B) Luciferin or coelenterazine. The dot is the site of attachment to molecular oxygen; the arrow the attachment site to a basic region of the protein.

outside. The Ca^{2+} signal can be monitored by biolumines-cence provided the cells are appropriately stimulated (Blinks *et al.* 1976). Recently, recombinant DNA coding for aequorin was endowed with a segment that codes for a recognition peptide so that the newly expressed photo-protein directs itself to either the nucleus (Brini *et al.* 1993), the endoplasmic reticulum (Kendall *et al.* 1992*a*) or to the mitochondria (Rizutto *et al.* 1992). Moreover, site-directed mutagenesis is employed to change the affinity and kinetics for Ca^{2+} of the mutant proteins, so that the Ca^{2+}-transient changes in each of these com-partments can be monitored (Kendall *et al.* 1992*b*). Incubation of these cells with the permeant luciferin allows the measurement of Ca^{2+} changes in real time during and after stimulation of the cell.

■ Mutagenesis studies

Aequorin has been the subject of extensive site-directed mutagenesis in order to unravel the biologically import-ant structural elements (Fig. 2). The binding of molecular oxygen seems directly related to His169; coelenterazine is bound both to the molecular oxygen and to (a) positive amino acid residue(s) of the protein, most likely in the non-functional site II. The luciferase activity can not yet be localized, but seven Trp- and His-containing segments are very well conserved in the photoproteins only. The C-terminal Pro is required for bioluminescence activity (Nomura *et al.* 1991) and Cys152 for the fast re-uptake of coelenterazine by the protein (Kurose *et al.* 1989).

■ References

*Blinks, J.R., Prendergast, F.G., and Allen, D.G. (1976) Photoproteins as biological calcium indicators. Pharmac. Rev. **28**, 1–93.

Blinks, J.R., Mattingly, P.H., Jewell, B.R., van Leeuwen, M., Harrer, G.C., and Allen, D.G. (1978) Practical aspects of the use of aequorin as a calcium indicator: assay, preparation, microinjection, and interpretation of signals. Methods Enzymol. **57**, 292–328.

Brini, M., Murgia, M., Pasti, L., Picard, D., Pozzan, T, and Rizzuto, R. (1993) Nuclear Ca^{2+} concentration measured with specifically targeted recombinant aequorin. EMBO. J. **12**, 4813–4819.

Charbonneau, H. and Cormier, M.J. (1979) Ca^{2+}-induced bioluminescence *in Renilla reniformis*. J. Biol. Chem. **254**, 769–780.

Hannick, L.I., Prasher, D.C., Schultz, L.W., Descamps, J.R., and Ward, K.B. (1993) Preparation and initial characterization of crystals of the photoprotein aequorin from *Aequorea victoria*. Proteins **15**, 103–107.

Inouye, S. and Tsuji, F.I. (1993) Cloning and sequence analysis of cDNA for the Ca^{2+}-activated photoprotein, clytin. FEBS Lett. **325**, 343–346.

Inouye, S., Sakaki, Y., Goto, T., and Tsuji, F.I. (1986) Expression of apoaequorin complementary DNA in *Escherichia coli*. Proc. Natl. Acad. Sci. USA **25**, 8425–8429.

*Kendall, J.M., Dormer, R.L., and Campbell, A.K. (1992*a*) Targeting aequorin to the endoplasmic reticulum of living cells. Biochim. Biophys. Res. Commun. **189**, 1008–1016.

*Kendall, J.M., Sala-Newby, G., Ghalaut, V., Dormer, R.L., and Campbell, A.K. (1992*b*) Engineering the Ca^{2+}-activated photoprotein aequorin with reduced affinity for calcium. Biochem. Biophys. Res. Commun. **187**, 1091–1097.

Kurose, K., Inouye, S., Sakaki, Y., and Tsuji, F.I. (1989) Bioluminescence of the Ca^{2+}-binding photoprotein aequorin after cysteine modification. Proc. Natl. Acad. Sci. USA **86**, 80–84.

Nomura, M., Inouye, S., Ohmiya, Y, and Tsuji, F.I. (1991) A C-terminal proline is required for bioluminescence of the Ca^{2+}-binding photoprotein, aequorin. FEBS Lett. **295**, 63–66.

*Rizzuto, R., Simpson, A.W.M., Brini, M., and Pozzan, T. (1992) Rapid changes of mitochondrial Ca^{2+} revealed by specifically targeted recombinant aequorin. Nature **358**, 325–327.

*Shimomura, O. (1986) Bioluminescence in the sea: photoprotein systems. Symp. Soc. Exp. Biol. **39**, 351–372.

■ *J.A. Cox:*
Department of Biochemistry,
University of Geneva,
1211, Geneva 4, Switzerland
Tel.: (022) 702 64 91
Fax: (022) 702 64 83
E-mail: cox@sc2a.unige.ch

Calcium vector protein

Calcium vector protein (CaVP) is a cytosolic calcium-binding protein abundant in the muscle of amphioxus. It is associated in vivo with a 26 kDa target protein (CaVPT). The latter displays a multidomain structure, including two IgC2-like domains and an IQ-motif. The exact function of both proteins is still unknown but their abundance in amphioxus points to a major regulatory role in motility or cytoskeleton dynamics.

Calcium vector protein (CaVP) was originally identified as an abundant acidic Ca^{2+}-binding protein in the muscle of amphioxus, having a calculated molecular mass of 18.3 kDa and an isoelectric point of 4.9 (Cox 1986). Upon gel filtration it migrates with an apparent molecular mass of 28 kDa which is indicative of an asymmetric shape. *In vivo*, CaVP forms a complex with a 26 kDa target protein (CaVPT). In the absence of Ca^{2+}, the complex

CaVP–CaVPT is stable under physiological conditions, but Ca^{2+}-binding to CaVP reinforces the affinity between the proteins 70-fold (Petrova *et al.* 1995). The cellular concentrations of CaVP and CaVPT are approximately 100 and 50 µM, respectively, which is about 10 times higher than the concentration of CaM and comparable to that of TnC in rabbit skeletal muscle (Cox *et al.* 1981).

Identification/isolation

CaVP can be isolated from physiological ionic strength extracts of amphioxus muscle, both as a complex with CaVPT and as an individual protein. The purification procedure includes a passage through a DEAE-cellulose column in the presence of Ca^{2+}, followed by gel filtration. Treatment with 2 M urea in the presence of 1 mM EDTA dissociates CaVP from CaVPT. Further separation of the components is achieved by ion-exchange chromatography (Cox 1986; Petrova *et al.* 1995).

Sequence

CaVP (Kobayashi *et al.* 1987: Swiss Prot. P04573) contains four EF-hand sites and displays from 20 to 30% amino acid sequence identity with TnC and CaM. However, phylogenetically CaVP can not be classified in one of the 32 subfamilies of EF-hand Ca^{2+}-binding proteins and is considered as unique (Kawasaki and Kretsinger 1994). The two N-terminal sites of CaVP are non-functional whereas the C-terminal sites bind Ca^{2+} specifically (Kobayashi *et al.* 1987; Petrova *et al.* 1995). The protein is acetylated at the N-terminus and contains two ε-*N*-trimethyllysine residues in the α-helices flanking the Ca^{2+}-binding loop III (Fig.1).

Protein

Two cysteine residues, situated in the N-terminal half of CaVP, are able to form a disulfide bridge. The oxidized and reduced forms of CaVP have different electrophoretic mobilities and can be easily transformed from one into the other. In the freshly isolated CaVP–CaVPT complex these thiols are free, but react slowly with thiol reagents (Petrova *et al.* 1995). All Trp and Tyr residues are located in the N-terminus of CaVP and are not disturbed by Ca^{2+}-binding to the protein (Cox 1986). The two C-terminal sites of CaVP bind Ca^{2+} specifically with the intrinsic affinity constants $K'_{Ca1} = 4.9 \times 10^6$ M^{-1} and $K'_{Ca2} = 7.3 \times 10^3$ M^{-1}. The complex also binds two Ca^{2+}, but with strong positive cooperativity and with distinctly higher affinity $K'_{Ca1} = 2.4 \times 10^5$ M^{-1} and $K'_{Ca2} = 1.0 \times 10^8$ M^{-1} (Petrova *et al.* 1995). The ratio of the product ($K'_{Ca1} \times K'_{Ca2}$) is 80-fold higher in the complex than in the isolated protein, which represents also the Ca^{2+}-induced increase in the affinity of CaVP for CaVPT.

Antibodies

Polyclonal antibodies against CaVP and CaVPT have been raised in rabbits and affinity purified (Valette-Talbi *et al.* 1993). An antibody against the CaVP-binding domain of CaVPT is also available (T. Petrova and J.A. Cox, unpublished results). No cross-reactivity has been observed in other animals.

Anatomical localization

CaVP and CaVPT are abundant both in striated muscle and in other tissues such as gonad and spinal chord. In muscle CaVP is enriched in the Z-line and I-band of the sarcomere (periodicity of approximately 2 µM). CaVPT shows striations at the Z and M lines with a periodicity of 1 µm (Valette-Talbi *et al.* 1993).

Biological activities

Biophysical studies indicate that isolated CaVP and CaVPT show the characteristics of highly dynamic interactive proteins, whereas their complex most likely represents a non-interactive end product. CaVP seems to regulate the availability of CaVPT which is a multidomain protein (Takagi and Cox 1991: Swiss Prot. P05548), containing a site for the binding of CaVP and two immunoglobulin-like folds type C2 (IgC2) (Fig. 2). IgC2 domains, often in multiple copies, have been found in myosin light chain kinase, twitchin, titin, and telokin, i.e. proteins believed to interact with the myosin rod (Trinick 1991). The CaVP binding site displays a high degree of homology to the IQ-motifs defined as Ca^{2+}-independent calmodulin-binding sites in neuromodulin and neurogranin (Apel *et al.* 1990; Baudier *et al.* 1991). In these proteins the regulation of the interaction with CaM is achieved through serine phosphorylation by protein kinase C. Isolated CaVPT can be

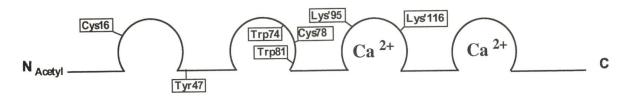

Figure 1. Domain structure and characteristic features of CaVP. ε-Trimethyllysine residues are designated as Lys'.

A

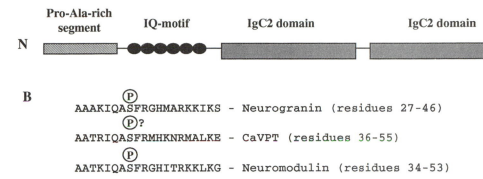

B

```
          Ⓟ
AAAKIQASFRGHMARKKIKS - Neurogranin (residues 27-46)
          Ⓟ?
AATRIQASFRMHKNRMALKE - CaVPT (residues 36-55)
          Ⓟ
AATKIQASFRGHITRKKLKG - Neuromodulin (residues 34-53)
```

Figure 2. (A) Domain structure of CaVPT. (B) Sequence comparison of calmodulin-binding domains in neuro-modulin and neurogranin and CaVP-binding domain in CaVPT. The question mark indicates the site which is likely to be phosphorylated by protein kinase C.

phosphorylated by protein kinase C to a 1:1 protein/phosphate ratio, whereas the addition of CaVP prevents the phosphorylation and the phosphorylation of CaVPT abolishes its interaction with CaVP (T. Petrova and J.A. Cox, unpublished results). This might represent a critical point in the regulation of the interaction between CaVP and CaVPT allowing dissociation and interaction of CaVPT with other target molecules in amphioxus muscle.

■ References

Apel, E.D., Byford, M.F., Au, D., Walsh, K., and Storm, D. (1990) Identification of the protein kinase C phosphorylation site in neuromodulin. Biochemistry **29**, 2330–2335.

Baudier, J., Deloulme, J.C., Van Dorsselaer, A., Black, D., and Matthes, H.W.D. (1991) Purification and characterization of a brain-specific protein kinase C substrate, neurogranin (p17). J. Biol. Chem. **266**, 229–237.

Cox, J.A. (1986) Isolation and characterization of a new Mr 18,000 protein with calcium vector properties in amphioxus muscle and identification of its endogenous target protein. J. Biol. Chem. **261**, 13173–1378.

Cox, J.A., Comte, M., and Stein, E.A. (1981) Calmodulin-free troponin C prepared in the absence of urea. Biochem. J. **195**, 205–211.

Kawasaki, H. and Kretsinger, R.H. (1994) Calcium-binding proteins 1: EF-hands. Protein Profile **1**, 344.

Kobayashi, T., Takagi, T., Konishi, K., and Cox, J.A. (1987) The primary structure of a New Mr 18,000 calcium vector protein from amphioxus. J. Biol. Chem. **262**, 2613–2623.

Kretsinger, R., Moncrief, N.D., Goodman, M., and Czelusniak, J. (1988) Homology of calcium-modulated proteins: Their evolutionary and functional relationships. In *The calcium channel: structure, function and implications* (ed. M. Morad, W. Nayler, S. Kazda, and M. Schramm), pp. 16-38. Springer-Verlag, Berlin.

*Petrova, T.V., Comte, M., Takagi, T., and Cox, J.A. (1995) Thermodynamic and molecular properties of the interaction between amphioxus calcium vector protein and its 26 kDa target. Biochemistry **34**, 312–318.

*Takagi, T. and Cox, J.A (1991) Primary structure of CaVPT, the target of calcium vector protein of amphioxus. J. Biol. Chem. **265**, 652–656.

Trinick, J. (1991) Elastic filaments and giant proteins in muscle. Curr. Opin. Cell Biol. **3**, 112–119.

*Valette-Talbi, L., Chaponnier, C., and Cox, J.A. (1993) Immunolocalization of calcium vector protein of amphioxus and its target in amphioxus. Histochemistry **100**, 73–81.

■ *T.V. Petrova and J.A. Cox:*
Department of Biochemistry,
University of Geneva,
1211, Geneva 4, Switzerland.
Tel.: (022) 702 64 91
Fax: (022) 702 64 83
E-mails: tanya@sc2a.unige.ch and cox@sc2a.unige.ch

Calsensin

Calsensin is an invertebrate, nervous system specific, cytosolic Ca^{2+}-binding protein which is expressed in only a small subset of leech neurons. It is a small 9 kDa protein with two EF-hand binding domains which binds $^{45}Ca^{2+}$ in vitro.

Calsensin has a calculated molecular mass of 9.1 kDa, migrates on SDS gels with an apparent molecular mass of 10 kDa and has a projected isoelectric point of 8.6. It consists of 83 residues which contain two EF-hand domains (Briggs *et al.* 1995). The Ca^{2+}-binding domains are likely to be functional since a fusion protein derived from the calsensin clone binds $^{45}Ca^{2+}$ after SDS-PAGE and transfer to nitrocellulose paper (Briggs *et al.* 1995). The limited homology of calsensin to other Ca^{2+}-binding proteins suggests that it may be a member of a novel subfamily. Calsensin is selectively expressed in the leech nervous system by a small subset of neurons (Fig. 1; Briggs *et al.* 1991, 1993).

Alternative names

Before its cloning calsensin was referred to as the lan3-6 antigen (Briggs *et al.* 1993).

Identification/isolation

Calsensin was originally defined as the antigen for the monoclonal antibody lan3-6 (Zipser and McKay 1981). This antibody was used to screen a leech expression vector library from which a full length clone was isolated (Briggs *et al.* 1995). That the identified clone corresponds to the lan3-6 antigen was verified by *in situ* hybridizations to leech embryos using a calsensin sequence as a probe, the labeling of which exactly matches the lan3-6 antibody staining pattern (Briggs *et al.* 1995).

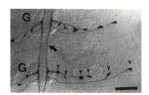

Figure 1. Calsensin localization to a subset of peripheral sensory neurons (arrows) in an E10 *Macrobdella* leech embryo. The sensory neurons extend their growth cones and axons into the ganglia (G) and connectives of the CNS where they fasciculate in a single axon tract (curved arrow). The preparation, which shows two hemisegments, was labeled with the lan3-6 antibody. Scale bar, 50 μm.

Gene and sequences

The sequence of calsensin (accession number U22066) contains a 249 nt open reading frame with 408 nt of 3′ and 153 nt of 5′ noncoding sequence. The open reading frame contains a 5′ ATG initiation codon, which has a favorable A_{-3}/G_{+4} context for initiation just downstream from an in-frame TGA stop codon. The sequence was assembled from three independent cDNA clones of 820, 777, and 754 nt, from ampliFINDER-RACE extension, and from a 15 kb genomic clone. There are no introns present in the genomic coding sequence.

Protein

Calsensin consists of 83 residues which comprise two EF-hand Ca^{2+}-binding domains. The highest homology of calsensin (38%) is to the EF-hand domain of I-plastin (Lin *et al.* 1994). Calsensin has cysteine residues located at position 3 and 80 suggesting that under some conditions the conformation of the protein may involve the formation of intra- or intermolecular disulfide bridges. The protein, which is basic, contains 15 lysines which account for 18% of the molecular weight. No prolines, arginines, histidines, or tryptophans are present.

Antibodies

A monoclonal antibody, lan3-6 (Zipser and McKay 1981), as well as two rabbit polyclonal antisera (Briggs *et al.* 1995) specific to calsensin exist. None are available from commercial sources.

Localization

The lan3-6 antibody has been used to study the localization and developmental expression of calsensin in various leech species (Briggs *et al.* 1991, 1993). In all hirudinid leeches calsensin is expressed in the axons and growth cones of a subpopulation of peripheral neurons whose afferents segregate into a single axon fascicle in the developing leech CNS (Fig. 1). This very restricted expression of calsensin has led to the hypothesis that calsensin may be involved in the formation or maintenance of specific axonal tracts (Briggs *et al.* 1995). In some leech species a small number of central neurons, in addition to the peripheral neurons, also contain calsensin (Briggs *et al.* 1991).

References

Briggs K.K., Johansen, K.M., and Johansen, J. (1991) Development and distribution of peripheral and central neurons labeled by the monoclonal antibody lan 3-6 in leech. Soc. Neurosci. Abstr. **17**, 740.

Briggs K.K., Johansen, K.M., and Johansen, J. (1993) Selective pathway choice of a single central axonal fascicle by a subset of peripheral neurons during leech development. Dev. Biol. **158**, 380–389.

Briggs K.K., Silvers, A.J., Johansen, K.M., and Johansen, J. (1995) Calsensin: a novel invertebrate calcium-binding protein expressed in a subset of peripheral leech neurons fasciculating in a single axon tract. J. Cell. Biol. **129**, 1355–1362.

Lin, C.-S., Shen, W., Chen, Z.P., Tu, Y-H., and Matsudaira, P. (1994) Identification of I-plastin, a human fimbrin isoform expressed in intestine and kidney. Mol. Cell. Biol. **14**, 2457–2467.

Zipser, B. and McKay, R. (1981) Monoclonal antibodies distinguish identifiable neurons in the leech. Nature **289**, 549–554.

■ *Jørgen Johansen, Kristen K. Briggs, and Kristen M. Johansen:*
Department of Zoology and Genetics,
Iowa State University,
Ames, A 50011, USA
Tel.: +1 515 294 2358
Fax: +1 515 294 0345
E-mail: jorgen@iastate.edu

Flagellar calcium-binding protein of *Trypanosoma cruzi*

Flagellar calcium-binding protein (FCaBP) is a 24 kDa, EF-hand Ca^{2+}-binding protein found in the American trypanosome, Trypanosoma cruzi. *The abundance and specific localization of FCaBP differs among the three life-cycle stages of this parasite; however, the protein is most highly concentrated in the flagellum of all stages, suggesting that it functions in motility or some other aspect of flagellar structure or function. FCaBP is an immunogenic protein that elicits humoral and cell-mediated immune responses in* T. cruzi-*infected individuals and experimental animals.*

The first report on FCaBP described the cloning of the 940 bp gene sequence and the analysis of its genomic organization and expression (Gonzalez *et al.* 1985). There are at least 40 *FCaBP* genes in *T. cruzi*, organized as two allelic direct tandem arrays of identical or nearly identical copies (Gonzalez *et al.* 1985; Godsel *et al.* 1995a). In a later study, the amino acid sequence of FCaBP was analyzed and EF-hand Ca^{2+}-binding motifs were observed. In a $^{45}Ca^{2+}$ overlay analysis a β-galactosidase-FCaBP fusion protein was found to bind one Ca^{2+} ion with an apparent K_d of approximately 50 μM. FCaBP-specific antiserum was produced and used in immunoblots and immunofluorescence assays of the epimastigote life-cycle stage of *T. cruzi*. These studies demonstrate that FCaBP is a 24 kDa protein with a calculated p*I* of 4.5 that is found exclusively in the parasite flagellum (Engman *et al.* 1989; see Fig. 1). More recent results from our laboratory and other laboratories demonstrate that FCaBP is more diffusely localized throughout the cell in the other two life-cycle stages; however, it is still most highly concentrated in the flagellum in all three of the stages (Ouaissi *et al.* 1992; Godsel *et al.* manuscript in preparation). Interestingly, FCaBP is highly immunogenic and *T. cruzi*-infected individuals and experimental animals mount strong humoral and cell-mediated immune responses to the protein (Engman *et al.* 1989; Taibi *et al.* 1993, Godsel *et al.* 1995b). Recently,

homologues of FCaBP have been discovered in the African trypanosome, *T. brucei*; these include Tb44, Tb24, and Tb17 (Lee *et al.* 1990; Wu *et al.* 1994). The *T. brucei* proteins were initially purified through anion exchange chromatography followed by Ca^{2+}-dependent hydrophobic interaction chromatography, and also were found to localize to the flagellum (Wu *et al.* 1992).

■ Protein homologues

Tb44, Tb24, and Tb17 of *Trypanosoma brucei* (Lee *et al.* 1990; Wu *et al.* 1994); Tl-17 of *Trypanosoma lewisi* (Lee *et al.* 1990).

■ Identification/isolation

FCaBP was identified by virtue of its high immunogenicity in *T. cruzi*-infected humans and experimental animals and the relative abundance of FCaBP cDNAs in *T. cruzi* expression libraries. Several groups have identified FCaBP clones by screening cDNA expression libraries with infected human and mouse sera. The reader is referred to several papers that report on the cloning of FCaBP from *T. cruzi* expression libraries (Lizardi *et al.* 1985; Engman *et al.* 1989; Ouaissi *et al.* 1992; Godsel *et al.* 1995a).

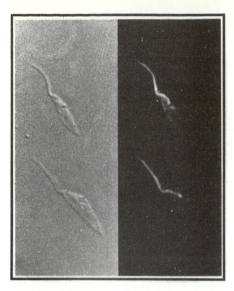

Figure 1. Subcellular localization of *T. cruzi* FCaBP. Methanol fixed parasites were stained with FCaBP-specific mouse serum and visualized by fluorescence microscopy (*right*) and by Nomarski direct interference contrast microscopy (*left*).

Gene and sequence

The *T. cruzi* FCaBP genes are organized in a tandem array of 20 or more copies (Gonzalez *et al.* 1985) on each of two allelic chromosomes (Godsel *et al.* 1995a). The FCaBP coding region is 633 base pairs in size and encodes a protein of 211 amino acids; the FCaBP mRNA is 900 bases in size (Gonzalez *et al.* 1985; Taibi *et al.* 1993; Godsel *et al.* 1995a). FCaBP sequences were compared by Wu *et al.* (1994) and it was calculated that the amino acid sequences of the *T. brucei* homologs are 50–55% identical to the *T. cruzi* protein, while the *T. lewisi* sequence is 70% identical. The FCaBP amino acid sequences of the Y and PBOL strains of *T. cruzi* were compared by Godsel *et al.* (1995a) and found to be 97–98% identical.

Accession numbers for *T. cruzi* sequences are: IF8 (Y strain), X02838; FCaBP (PBOL strain), L26971; 24 kDa antigen (Y strain), S43664. *T. brucei* sequences: Tb44, U06463; Tb24, U06644; Tb17, X53464.

Protein

FCaBP is a 24 kDa Ca^{2+}-binding protein that contains four canonical EF-hand Ca^{2+}-binding motifs (Wong *et al.* 1992) as well as distinct N- and C- termini. $^{45}Ca^{2+}$ overlay analysis of recombinant FCaBP indicates that the protein binds approximately one mol. of Ca^{2+} with a K_d of 50 μM (Engman *et al.* 1989).

Antibodies

Small amounts of polyclonal mouse sera specific for recombinant FCaBP are available from the authors' laboratories (Engman *et al.* 1989). A monoclonal antibody has also been described: however, it may not be specific for FCaBP alone (Ouaissi *et al.* 1992).

Anatomical localization

T. cruzi FCaBP is found throughout the cell, but is highly concentrated in the flagellum of all three life cycle stages of the parasite (Engman *et al.* 1989; Taibi *et al.* 1993; Godsel *et al.* manuscript in preparation; see Fig. 1).

References

*Engman, D.M., Krause, K.H., Blumin, J.H., Kim, K.S., Kirchhoff, L.V., and Donelson, J.E. (1989) A novel flagellar Ca^{2+}-binding protein in trypanosomes. J. Biol. Chem. **264**, 18627–18631.

*Godsel, L.M., Olson, C.L., Lacava, Z.G.M., and Engman, D.M. (1995a) Comparison of the 24 kDa flagellar calcium-binding protein cDNAs of two strains of *Trypanosoma cruzi*. J. Euk. Microbiol. **42**, 320–321.

Godsel, L.M., Tibbetts, R.S., Olson, C.L., Chaudoir, B.M., and Engman, D.M. (1995b) Utility of recombinant flagellar calcium-binding protein for the serodiagnosis of *Trypanosoma cruzi* infection. J. Clin. Microbiol. **33**, 2082–2085.

Gonzalez A., Lerner, T.J., Huecas, M., Sosa-Pineda, B., Nogueira, N., and Lizardi, P.M. (1985) Apparent generation of a segmented mRNA from two separate tandem gene families in *Trypanosoma cruzi*. Nucleic Acids Res. **13**, 5789–5804.

Haghighat, N.G. and Ruben, L. (1992) Purification of novel calcium-binding proteins from *Trypanosoma brucei*: properties of 22-, 24- and 38-kilodalton proteins. Mol. Biochem. Parasitol. **51**, 99–110.

Lee, M.G.S., Chen, J., Ho, A.W.M., DõAlesandro, P.A., and Van der Ploeg, L.H.T. (1990) A putative flagellar Ca^{2+}-binding protein of the flagellum of trypanosomatid protozoan parasites. Nucleic Acids Res. **18**, 4252.

Lizardi, P., Lerner, T.J., Gonzalez, A., and Nogueira, N. (1985) Expression in *Escherichia coli* of a cDNA clone encoding a hypothetical calcium-binding protein from *Trypanosma cruzi* epimastigotes. In *Cold Spring Harbor Vaccines 85* (ed. R.A. Lerner, R.M. Chanock, and F. Brown), pp. 67–70. Cold Spring Harbor Laboratory, New York.

Ouaissi, A., Aguirre, T., Plumas-Marty, B., Piras, M., Schoneck, R., Gras-Masse, H., Taibi, A., Loyens, M., Tartar, A., Capron, A., and Piras, R. (1992) Cloning and sequencing of a 24-kDa *Trypanosoma cruzi* specific antigen released in association with membrane vesicles and defined by a monoclonal antibody. Biol. Cell. **75**, 11–17.

Taibi, A., Plumas-Marty, B., Guevara-Espinoza, A., Schoneck, R., Pessoa, H., Loyens, M., Piras, R., Aguirre, T., Gras-Masse, H., Bossus, M., Tartar, A., Capron, A., and Ouaissi, A. (1993) *Trypanosoma cruzi*: immunity-induced in mice and rats by trypomastigote excretory-secretory antigens and identification of a peptide sequence containing a T cell epitope with protective activity. J. Immunol. **151**, 2676–2689.

Wong, S., Kretsinger, R.H., and Campbell, D.A. (1992) Identification of a new EF-hand superfamily member from *Trypanosoma brucei*. Mol. Gen. Genet. **233**, 225–230.

*Wu, Y., Haghighat, N.G., and Ruben, L. (1992) The predominant calcimedins from *Trypanosoma brucei* comprise a family of flagellar EF-hand calcium-binding proteins. Biochem. J. **287**, 187–193.

Wu, Y., Deford, J., Benjamin, R., Lee, M.G.S., and Ruben, L. (1994) The gene family of EF-hand calcium-binding proteins from the flagellum of *Trypanosoma brucei*. Biochem. J. **304**, 833–841.

■ *Lisa M. Godsel, John E. Donelson*, and David M. Engman:*

Departments of Pathology and Microbiology-Immunology,
Northwestern University Medical School,
Chicago, IL 60611, USA
Tel.: +1 312 503 1267
Fax: +1 312 503 1265
E-mail: dengman@casbah.acns.nwu.edu

*Department of Biochemistry,
Howard Hughes Medical Institute,
University of Iowa,
Iowa City, IA 52242, USA

Troponin (nonvertebrate)

Troponin (Tn), which lies on the actin–tropomyosin filament of muscle, is a Ca^{2+}-dependent regulatory protein complex, active in muscle contraction. Troponin consists of three components; TnC which binds Ca^{2+}, TnI which is able to bind not only to TnC but also to actin and inhibits actomyosin ATPase activity, and TnT which binds to tropomyosin and is required for Ca^{2+}-dependent regulatory function of the Tn complex. Apart from vertebrate skeletal and cardiac muscle, the presence of Tn has been described in arthropod, mollusc, and protochordate muscle (e.g. Endo and Obinata 1981; Wnuk et al., 1984; Ojima and Nishita 1986; Nishita and Ojima 1990).

Nonvertebrate Tn, like vertebrate Tn, consists of three components. The molecular weight of each component differs from species to species. Generally, the smallest (M_r = 16,000–18,000) component corresponds to TnC. The middle (M_r = 24,000–31,000) and the largest (M_r = 33,000–45,000) correspond to TnI and TnT, respectively, as in vertebrates. One exception has been found in scallop muscle; the largest (M_r = 52,000) component possesses the inhibitory activity of actomyosin ATPase activity (Ojima and Nishita 1986). From the indirect flight muscle of the waterbug, a heavy component with apparent M_r = 80,000 has been detected (Bullard *et al.* 1988). Isoelectric points of Tn components vary from species to species. Generally, TnC is acidic (pI = 4–5), as is typical for EF-hand type Ca^{2+}-binding proteins, and TnI is basic (pI = 9–10). The most remarkable differences between vertebrate and nonvertebrate Tns are their molecular weights and their Ca^{2+}-binding properties. Nonvertebrate Tn, particularly TnT, has a higher molecular weight than its vertebrate counterpart. So far only Ca^{2+}-specific binding sites have been identified in nonvertebrate Tn, whereas vertebrate Tn contains in addition Ca^{2+}/Mg^{2+}-mixed binding sites.

■ Isolation

Nonvertebrate Tn can be isolated from muscle with the same methods as described for vertebrate skeletal muscle Tn.

■ Gene and sequences

Nonvertebrate TnC, like vertebrate, is a member of the EF-hand type of Ca^{2+}-binding proteins and has four putative EF-hands. Amino acid sequences of two major isoforms from crayfish (Kobayashi *et al.* 1989c; Swissprot accession numbers P06707 and P06708), three isoforms from lobster (Garone *et al.* 1991; P29289, P29290, and P29291), two isoforms from barnacle (Collins *et al.* 1991; P21797 and P21798), horseshoe crab (Kobayashi *et al.* 1989a; P15159), ascidian (Takagi and Konishi 1983; P06706), amphioxus (Takagi *et al.* 1994), and scallop (Nishita *et al.* 1994) have been determined. The N-termini of these TnCs are acetylated. Amphioxus TnC possesses either methyllysine or dimethyllysine in the A-helix. A cDNA sequence of Akazara scallop TnC was also reported (Ojima *et al.* 1994; EMBL S70002). Among four Ca^{2+}-binding sites of nonvertebrate TnCs, the predicted functional sites, based on the amino acid sequences and Ca^{2+}-binding measurements described below, are summarized in Table 1. The amino acid sequence of crayfish TnI was determined by protein sequence analysis and the presence of trimethyllysine residues among the "inhibitory region" was revealed (Kobayashi *et al.* 1989b; Swissprot P05547). The sequences of *Drosophila* TnI (Barbas *et al.* 1991 EMBL X58188; Beall and Fryberg 1991 EMBL X59376) were determined from cDNA. Although the nonvertebrate TnIs show rather low (20–25%) sequence identity with vertebrate TnI, the "inhibitory region" displays almost 60% sequence identity. The consensus sequence of this region is as follows: D L R G K F X

R* P X L R* R+ V, where R* and R+ stand for Arg or trimethyllysine and Lys or Arg, respectively, and X stands for any amino acid residue. The *Drosophila* TnT gene was described by Fyrberg *et al.* (1990; EMBL X54504). *Drosophila* TnT, encoded in 9 exons, is significantly larger than vertebrate TnT due to a highly acidic C-terminal extension (the C-terminal 51 residues consist of 43 Glu, 5 Asp, and 3 Val). The extension of acidic residues at the C-terminus was also found in lobster TnT (Kobayashi *et al.*, manuscript in preparation).

■ Protein

The Ca^{2+}-binding properties of nonvertebrate TnCs are strikingly different from those of vertebrate TnCs. In vertebrate TnC, the two N-terminal Ca^{2+}-binding sites bind Ca^{2+} specifically with association constants $K_a \cong 3 \times 10^5$ M^{-1}, and are responsible for regulation, while the two C-terminal sites bind both Ca^{2+} and Mg^{2+} ($K_{a.Ca} \cong 2 \times 10^7$ M^{-1}, $K_{a.Mg} \cong 2 \times 10^3$ M^{-1}) and play a structural role. So far, Ca^{2+}-binding experiments have been carried out for amphioxus TnC (Takagi *et al.* 1994), crayfish TnCs (Wnuk 1989), barnacle TnCs (Collins *et al.* 1991), and scallop TnCs (Ojima and Nishita 1986). Although the binding constants vary (10^6 M^{-1} to 10^4 M^{-1}), all of these TnCs bind Ca^{2+} specifically. Thus, Ca^{2+}/Mg^{2+}-mixed binding sites have not yet been identified in nonvertebrate TnC. This indicates that the interactions of nonvertebrate TnCs, particularly between their C-domain and other Tn components, are different from those of vertebrate TnCs.

■ Antibodies

Antibodies specific for *Drosophila* TnT and TnH were produced by Bullard *et al.* (1988).

■ Anatomical localization

Tn is localized on the thin filaments of striated muscle. The only smooth muscle that contains Tn is found in ascidians.

■ Biological activity

The effect of TnC substitution on myofibrillar ATPase activity has been investigated (Nakamura *et al.* 1994). TnC from vertebrate sources (i.e. rabbit fast skeletal and bovine cardiac muscle) did not activate the TnC-depleted crustacean striated myofibrils. On the other hand, crustacean TnC (crayfish and lobster) did not activate the TnC-depleted vertebrate myofibrils. Scallop TnC did not activate either TnC-depleted vertebrate or TnC-depleted crustacean myofibrils.

Some of the nonvertebrate muscles are regulated by both the myosin-linked regulatory system and the actin-linked regulatory system, i.e. Tn. Scallop striated muscle is known to be regulated by direct Ca^{2+}-binding to myosin. But, as mentioned above, Tn complex was isolated and has been revealed to be functional like other Tn, although scallop Tn binds only one mol Ca^{2+}/mol of protein (Ojima and Nishita 1986). In the case of the striated muscle from horseshoe crab, Tn acts as a Ca^{2+}-dependent regulator only when myosin regulatory light chain is phosphorylated by myosin light chain kinase (Wang *et al.* 1993).

So far no study of site-directed mutagenesis of nonvertebrate Tn has been done. In *Drosophila*, abnormal embryogenesis with structural defects in the nervous system and muscle abnormalities are caused by TnI or TnT mutations (Fyrberg *et al.* 1990; Barbas *et al.* 1991; Beall and Fyrberg 1991)

■ References

Barbas, J., Garcera, J., Krah-Jentgens, I., de la Pompa, J.L., Canal, I., Pongs, O., and Ferrus, A. (1991) Troponin I is encoded in

Table 1. Topography of Ca^{2+}-binding sites on TnCs

Protein/site	I	II	III	IV
RsTnC[1]	Ca-specific	Ca-specific	Ca/Mg	Ca/Mg
BcTnC	n[2]	Ca-specific	Ca/Mg	Ca/Mg
AsTnC	n	F[3]	n	F
AmTnC[4]	Ca-specific	Ca-specific	Ca-specific	n?
CrTnC	n	Ca-specific	n	Ca-specific
LoTnC	n	F	n	F
BaTnC	n	Ca-specific	n	Ca-specific
HsTnC	n	F	?	F
ScTnC	n	n	n	Ca-specific

[1]Abbreviations: RsTnC, TnC from rabbit fast skeletal muscle; BcTnC, TnC from bovine cardiac muscle; AsTnC, TnC from ascidian; AmTnC, TnC from amphioxus; CrTnC, TnC from crayfish; LoTnC, TnC from lobster; BaTnC, TnC from barnacle; HsTnC, TnC from horseshoe crab; ScTnC, TnC from scallop.
[2]n stands for nonfunctional site.
[3]F stands for functional site; affinity for Ca^{2+} not determined.
[4]Amphioxus TnC binds 3 mol/mol of Ca^{2+} specifically. Although from the amino acid sequence all 4 Ca^{2+}-binding sites seem to be functional, the replacement of one hydrophobic residue in site IV can be crucial (see discussion in Takagi *et al.* 1994).

the haplolethal region of the *Shaker* gene complex of *Drosophila*. Genes and Develop. **5**, 132–140.

Beall, C. and Fyrberg, E. (1991) Muscle abnormalities in *Drosophila melanogaster heldup* mutants are caused by missing or aberrant troponin-I isoforms. J. Cell Biol. **114**, 941–951.

Bullard, B., Leonard, K., Larkins, A., Butcher, G., Karlik, C., and Fyrberg, E. (1988) Troponin of asynchronous flight muscle. J. Mol. Biol. **204**, 621–637.

Collins, J.H., Theibert, J.L., Francois, J.-M., Ashley, C.C., and Potter, J.D. (1991) Amino acid sequences and Ca²⁺-binding properties of two isoforms of barnacle troponin C. Biochemistry **30**, 702–707.

Endo, T. and Obinata, T. (1981) Troponin and its components from ascidian smooth muscle. J. Biochem. **89**, 1599–1608.

Fyrberg, E., Fyrberg, C.C., Beall, C., and Saville, D.L. (1990) *Drosophila melanogaster* troponin-T mutants engender three distinct syndromes of myofibrillar abnormalities. J. Mol. Biol. **216**, 657–675.

Garone, L., Theibert, J.L., Miegel, A., Maeda, Y., Murphy, C., and Collins, J.H. (1991) Lobster troponin C: amino acid sequences of three isoforms. Arch. Biochem. Biophys. **291**, 89–91.

Kobayashi, T., Kagami, O., Takagi, T., and Konishi, K. (1989a) Amino acid sequence of horseshoe crab, *Tachypleus tridentatus*, striated muscle troponin C. J. Biochem. **105**, 823–828.

Kobayashi, T., Takagi, T., Konishi, K., and Cox, J.A. (1989b) Amino acid sequence of crayfish troponin I. J. Biol. Chem. **264**, 1551–1557.

Kobayashi, T., Takagi, T., Konishi, K., and Wnuk, W. (1989c) Amino acid sequences of the two major isoforms of troponin C from crayfish. J. Biol. Chem. **264**, 18247–18259.

Nakamura, Y., Shiraishi, F., and Ohtsuki, I. (1994) The effect of troponin C substitution on the Ca²⁺-sensitive ATPase activity of vertebrate and invertebrate myofibrils by troponin Cs with various numbers of Ca²⁺-binding sites. Comp. Biochem. Physiol. **108B**, 121–133.

Nishita, K. and Ojima, T. (1990) American lobster troponin. J. Biochem. **108**, 677–683.

Nishita, K., Tanaka, H., and Ojima, T. (1994) Amino acid sequence of troponin C from scallop striated adductor muscle. J. Biol. Chem. **269**, 3464–3468.

Ojima, T. and Nishita, K. (1986) Troponin from Akazara scallop striated adductor muscles. J. Biol. Chem. **261**, 16749–16754.

Ojima, T., Tanaka, H., and Nishita, K. (1994) Cloning and sequence of a cDNA encoding Akazara scallop troponin C. Arch. Biochem. Biophys. **311**, 272–276.

Takagi, T. and Konishi, K. (1983) Amino acid sequence of troponin C obtained from ascidian (*Halocynthia roretzi*) body wall muscle. J. Biochem. **94**, 1753–1760.

Takagi, T., Petrova,T., Comte, M., Kuster, T., Heizmann, C.W., and Cox, J.A. (1994) Characterization and primary structure of amphioxus troponin C. Eur. J. Biochem. **221**, 537–546.

Wang, F., Martin, B.M., and Sellers, J.R. (1993) Regulation of actomyosin interactions in *Limulus* muscle proteins. J. Biol. Chem. **268**, 3776–3780.

Wnuk, W. (1989) Resolution and calcium-binding properties of the two major isoforms of troponin C from crayfish. J. Biol. Chem. **264**, 18240–18246.

Wnuk, W., Schoechlin, M., and Stein, E.A. (1984) Regulation of actomyosin ATPase by a single calcium-binding site on troponin C from crayfish. J. Biol. Chem. **259**, 9017–9023.

■ *Tomoyoshi Kobayashi:*
International Institute for Advanced Research,
Matsushita Electric Industrial Co.,
3–4 Hikaridai, Seika, Kyoto 619–02,
Japan
Tel.: +81 774 98 2543
Fax: +81 774 98 2575
E-mail: tomo@crl.mei.co.jp

Plasmodium falciparum calcium-dependent protein kinase (PfCPK)

PfCPK, Plasmodium falciparum calcium-dependent protein kinase, is the first malarial member of the Ca²⁺-dependent protein kinase subfamily. As typical for all Ca²⁺-dependent protein kinases, PfCPK contains two functional domains, the catalytic kinase domain, which is located in the N-terminal part of the protein, and a calmodulin-like Ca²⁺-binding domain consisting of four EF-hands and functioning as a regulatory Ca²⁺ sensor. PfCPK preferentially phosphorylates proteins of the host erythrocyte membrane, is activated in the presence of red blood cells, and may be involved in the invasion of the red blood cell by merozoites.

PfCPK is one of the two Ca²⁺-dependent protein kinases we have cloned from *Plasmodium falciparum* libraries. A number of Ca²⁺-dependent protein kinases have been identified in other unicellular organisms and in plants (for review see Roberts 1993). The recombinant PfCPK has a native molecular mass of 62 kDa and four Ca²⁺-binding sites of the EF-hand type. The kinase undergoes autophosphorylation upon expression in bacteria, giving rise to differentially phosphorylated forms of the protein. These can be separated by isoelectric focusing into several spots lying in a p*I* range from 5 to 6. PfCPK is most abundant in the earliest and the latest stage of parasitic development within the red blood cell and is mainly localized in the parasitic membrane and the organelle fraction. Under *in vitro* conditions, PfCPK kinase activity is regulated by Ca²⁺ levels, phosphatidylserine, and auto-phosphorylation. These regulation mechanisms may also be involved in the *in vivo* control of PfCPK enzyme activity. As is true of several other Ca²⁺-regulated enzymes, PfCPK may have multiple functions. One of its roles may be an involvement in the invasion process.

■ Identification/isolation

The PfCPK gene was isolated from cDNA and genomic libraries of *Plasmodium falciparum* using a degenerate oligonucleotide probe directed against a conserved sub-domain of serine-threonine protein kinases. The protein was expressed in bacteria as a histidine fusion protein (Zhao *et al.* 1993; EMBL data bank accession number: X67288). The recombinant protein kinase was purified to homogeneity by affinity chromatography using a nickel-NTA column and further fractionation by gel filtration on a Sephacryl S-300 column (Zhao *et al.* 1994a).

■ Genes and sequences

PfCPK contains two functional domains. The 524 amino acid protein is divided into an amino terminal protein kinase domain stretching from 1 to 325, followed by a linker of unknown function (325–342), a junction domain (342–370), and a calmodulin-like domain (370–524) containing four EF-hand motifs.

The protein kinase domain has highest homology to several serine-threonine kinase subfamilies, including *Zea mays* calcium-dependent protein kinase (Genbank accession number: L15390), ribosomal S6 protein kinase (M28489), SNF1 protein kinase (M13971), and rat calcium/calmodulin dependent protein kinase II (CaM kinase II) (J04063). The homologies range from 40–42% amino acid sequence identity. The linker domain is not found in any of the kinases in the protein sequence databank. The junction domain, which is involved in autoinhibition, is homologous with comparable domains from *Arabidopsis* calcium-dependent protein kinase (AK1) (L14771), soybean calcium-dependent protein kinase (M64987), and CaM kinase II. The homology is about 30% amino acid sequence identity. The calmodulin domain has highest amino acid sequence identity (35–38%) with human calmodulin (J04046) and the *Plasmodium falciparum* calmodulin (M59770) (Zhao *et al.* 1993).

■ Protein

The purified recombinant protein kinase is activated by Ca²⁺ in the presence of Mg²⁺ or Mn²⁺, with half-maximal activation at a free Ca²⁺ concentration of 15 µM (Zhao *et al.* 1994b). The activation by Ca²⁺ could be partially replaced by Mn²⁺, but not by Zn²⁺ or Mg²⁺. PfCPK preferentially phosphorylates casein and histone H1 as exogenous substrates. The K_m and V_{max} for ATP were 26 µM and 70 nmol min⁻¹ mg⁻¹ with casein as substrate, and 34 µM and 143 nmol min⁻¹ n⁻¹ mg⁻¹ with histone H1 as substrate (Zhao *et al.* 1994a).

As predicted from the cDNA sequence, the kinase binds four Ca²⁺ ions under saturation conditions. The mean $K_d(Ca^{2+})$ for PfCPK is 80 µM, which is significantly higher than the mean K_d for calmodulin $K_d(Ca^{2+}) = 4$ µM; Kilhoffer *et al.* 1992). To understand the roles of the individual Ca²⁺-binding sites, two series of mutations were generated at the individual EF-hand motifs. The highly conserved glutamic acid residue at position 12 in each Ca²⁺-binding loop was mutated to either lysine or glutamine. Either of these mutations (to lysine or glutamine) is sufficient to eliminate Ca²⁺ binding at the mutated site. Sites I and II appear to be crucial for both Ca²⁺-induced conformational change and enzymatic activation. Whereas mutations at site II almost completely abolish kinase activity, mutations at site I are also deleterious and dramatically reduce the sensitivity of Ca²⁺-induced conformational change and the Ca²⁺-dependent activation. Mutations at sites III and IV have minor effects (Zhao *et al.* 1994b).

Calmodulin antagonists (calmidazolium, trifluoperazine, *N*-[6-aminohexyl]-5-chloro-naphatalene-sulfonamide, and ophiobolin A) can inhibit the kinase activation, but much higher concentrations of the antagonists are needed than required to inhibit calmodulin-mediated effects (Zhao *et al.* 1994a).

The junction domain of PfCPK is homologous to the regulatory domain of CaM kinase II. The regulatory domain of CaM kinase II comprises an autoinhibitory and a CaM-binding domain. The autoinhibitory segment is positioned in the active site of the kinase, blocking access to its substrates by steric hindrance. In a model put forward by Schulman, binding of Ca²⁺-activated CaM displaces this segment and thereby activates the enzyme (Schulman 1993). A similar control mechanism for kinase activation may exist for PfCPK with the difference that the CaM-like structure is part of the protein. Therefore the effect of six overlapping peptides, deduced from the sequence of the junction domain of the kinase, on PfCPK

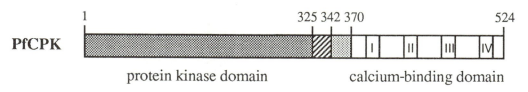

Figure 1. Schematic representation of the protein structure of PfCPK. See text for further details.

kinase activity and parasite growth was investigated. One of these peptides inhibited PfCPK kinase acitivity with an IC_{50} of 15–20 μM. Addition of the same peptide to parasitic cultures resulted in an inhibition of parasitic growth with an IC_{50} of 87 μM (Weyrauch et al. 1995).

■ Antibodies

Polyclonal antibodies were raised against the purified recombinant protein as described in Zhao et al. 1994a.

■ Anatomical localization

PfCPK is most abundant in ring and schizont stages, the earliest and latest stage of the intraerythrocytic development of the parasite. PfCPK is mainly found in the parasitic membrane and organelle fraction, and to a small extent in the membrane fraction of infected erythrocytes. In the latter fraction it is only found in significant amounts in the ring stage (Zhao et al. 1994a). Further details of PfCPK localization were obtained by immunogold electron microscopy. In younger stages of parasitic development the antigen was mainly found in the parasitophorous vacuole, in older stages between newly formed merozoites. In the invasive form of the blood stage parasite, the merozoite, PfCPK seems to be surface located (Kappes et al. unpublished observations).

■ Biological activities

Several lines of evidence have allowed us to hypothesize on a possible involvement of the enzyme in the invasion process of the red blood cell: (1) iodination experiments and co-localization studies with MSP-1, one of the main merozoite surface proteins, suggest a localization of PfCPK on the surface of merozoites (Kappes et al. unpublished observations); (2) the recombinant enzyme phosphorylates proteins of the inner surface of the host erythrocytic membrane under in vitro conditions. The proteins prominently phosphorylated by PfCPK are β spectrin, band 4.1, and band 4.9 (Zhao et al. 1994a); (3) PfCPK is transformed into a more active enzyme in the presence of red blood cells (Kappes et al. unpublished observations). A further function of PfCPK could be a contribution to the altered membrane properties of the erythrocyte observed after infection of the red blood cell by the parasite.

■ Biological regulation

The kinase activity is strongly Ca^{2+}-dependent and saturates at a Ca^{2+} concentration of about 150 μM, corresponding to two calcium ions bound per mole of PfCPK (Zhao et al. 1994b). In the presence of Ca^{2+}, PfCPK kinase activity can be further stimulated by phosphatidylserine.

Therefore, the selectivity of the phosphorylation of native substrates may be partially controlled by this phospholipid (Zhao et al. 1994a).

Besides Ca^{2+}, as an effector which is absolutely required for PfCPK substrate phosphorylation activity, autophosphorylation is another tool for the regulation of PfCPK enzyme activity. Studies with the recombinant enzyme suggest an intermolecular mode of autophosphorylation, although we cannot completely exclude intramolecular autophosphorylation as a second mode. In contrast to the findings that Ca^{2+}/calmodulin-stimulated autophosphorylation of CaM kinase II enables this enzyme to phosphorylate substrates in a Ca^{2+}/calmodulin-independent manner, autophosphorylation of PfCPK does not seem to lead to a Ca^{2+}-independent substrate phosphorylation activity of PfCPK (Zhao et al. 1994a). Incubation of the recombinant PfCPK with intact red blood cells leads to an approximately ninefold higher autophosphorylation activity of the enzyme, which is associated with a roughly twofold higher substrate phosphorylation activity.

■ References

Kilhoffer, M.C., Kubina, M., Travers, F., and Haiech, J. (1992) Use of engineered proteins with internal tryptophan reporter groups and pertubation techniques to probe the mechanism of ligand-protein interactions: investigation of the mechanism of calcium binding to calmodulin. Biochemistry **31**, 8098–8106.

Roberts, D.M. (1993) Protein kinases with calmodulin-like domains: novel targets of calcium signals in plants. Curr. Opin. Cell Biol. **5**, 242–246.

Schulman, H. (1993) The multifunctional Ca^{2+}/calmodulin-dependent protein kinases. Curr. Opin. Cell Biol. **5**, 247–253.

Weyrauch, G., Zhao, Y., Bell, A., Franklin, R.M. and Kappes, B. (1995) Characterization of the junction domain of a calcium-dependent protein kinase from Plasmodium falciparum. Annals of Trop. Med. Parasitol. **89**, 216.

*Zhao, Y., Kappes, B., and Franklin, R.M. (1993) Gene structure and expression of an unusual protein kinase from Plasmodium falciparum homologous at its carboxyl terminus with EF hand calcium-binding proteins. J. Biol. Chem. **268**, 4347–4354.

*Zhao, Y., Franklin, R.M., and Kappes, B. (1994a) Plasmodium falciparum calcium-dependent protein kinase phosphorylates proteins of the host erythrocytic membrane. Mol. Biochem. Parasitol. **66**, 329–343.

*Zhao, Y., Pokutta, S., Maurer, P., Lindt, M., Franklin, R.M., and Kappes, B. (1994b) Calcium-binding properties of a calcium-dependent protein kinase from Plasmodium falciparum and the significance of the individual calcium-binding site for kinase activation. Biochemistry **33**, 3714–3721.

■ Barbara Kappes:
Dept. of Structural Biology,
Biozentrum, University of Basel,
Klingelbergstrasse 70,
CH-4056 Basel, Switzerland
Tel.: +41 61 267 2101 or -267 2107
Fax: +41 61 267-2109
E-mail: KAPPES@UBACLU.UNIBAS.CH

rdgC serine/threonine protein phosphatase

The rdgC serine/threonine protein phosphatase was identified as the gene product responsible for causing inherited retinal degeneration in Drosophila *rdgC mutants. The rdgC protein is classified as a serine/threonine protein phosphatase because it contains a domain with significant sequence identity with the catalytic domains of the protein phosphatase 1, 2A and 2B family of enzymes. This protein contains multiple Ca²⁺-binding motifs and is thought to be directly regulated by Ca²⁺ levels.*

This serine/threonine protein phosphatase is called rdgC because it is the third *Drosophila* gene named for a retinal degeneration (rdg) mutant phenotype. The rdgC protein contains two domains: a domain sharing sequence identity with an extended family of serine/threonine protein phosphatases and a Ca^{2+}-binding domain with multiple EF-hand motifs. It is the only known phosphatase possessing a Ca^{2+}-binding domain. The rdgC protein is expressed predominantly in retinal tissue but is also found in specific central brain structures. It is predominantely recovered in the cytosolic fractions of retinal tissues. No posttranslational modifications are known. RdgC is a 661 amino acid containing protein with an expected molecular mass of 75.5 kDa and p*I* of 6.8.

Isolation/identification

The rdgC gene was located within the 77B1 region of the *Drosophila* salivary chromosome and cloned via chromosome walking. Identification was confirmed by the ability of the cloned gene to rescue the mutant phenotype in transgenic animals (Steele *et al.* 1992).

Gene and sequence

The gene has 12 exons and 11 introns, as shown in Fig. 1. The DNA sequence accession number is M89628.

Protein

The rdgC protein has not been purified. The protein contains a phosphatase catalytic domain, and also multiple calmodulin-like EF-hand Ca^{2+}-binding motifs in the carboxyl end of the protein (Steele *et al.* 1992). The location of these motifs is shown in Fig. 1.

Antibodies

Polyclonal antibodies raised against fusion proteins containing two different internal domains of the rdgC protein react with both native and denatured rdgC protein. Production of these reagents is described by Steele *et al.* (1992).

Anatomical localization

As suggested by the genetic information, rdgC protein is expressed in the photoreceptors of both the compound eye and the ocelli. The protein is also expressed in discrete structures of the central brain, notably in all aspects of the mushroom bodies (Steele *et al.* 1992).

Biological activities

Genetic data suggested that *rdgC* function is required to prevent light-triggered retinal degeneration (Steele and

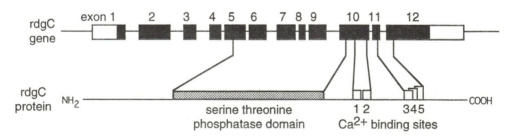

Figure 1. Organization of the *rdgC* gene and protein (from Steele *et al.* 1992). In the *rdgC* gene, the 5′ and 3′ untranslated regions are shown as open boxes, coding regions as black boxes, and introns as horizontal lines. The relative positions of the phosphatase catalytic domain and the five EF-hand Ca^{2+}-binding motifs in the gene and the protein are indicated. The Ca^{2+}-binding motifs are labeled 1–5. The order of these sites, from the best to the worst match to the consensus EF-hand sequence, is 3–1–5–4–2.

O'Tousa 1990). A phosphatase activity using phosphorylated rhodopsin as a substrate has been attributed to the rdgC protein because this activity is present in homogenates of rdgC+ (wildtype) eyes, but missing in rdgC mutant eyes (Byk et al. 1993). No other substrates have been identified.

Biological regulation

A major substrate of the rdgC phosphatase is phosphorylated rhodopsin. Rhodopsin, labeled by endogenous kinases, is dephosphorylated by retinal extracts of rdgC+ flies, but is poorly dephosphorylated by rdgC mutant extracts. This phosphatase activity is dependent on Ca^{2+}. Calmodulin is unlikely to mediate the Ca^{2+} dependence, as this phosphatase activity is not inhibited by M5, the peptide inhibitor of calmodulin (Byk et al. 1993). These results are consistent with expectations from molecular characterization of rdgC, that the presence of Ca^{2+}-binding sites allows the enzyme to be directly regulated by Ca^{2+}.

Mutagenesis studies

Rescue of mutant animals with the cloned rdgC+ gene shows that mutations in the gene described here are responsible for light-induced retinal degeneration. Degeneration can be prevented in genetic backgrounds with low rhodopsin protein (Steele et al. 1992; Kurada and O'Tousa 1995), consistent with a role of phosphory-

lated rhodopsin in causing retinal degeneration. Photoreceptors failing to increase cytosolic Ca^{2+} levels during the light response also show retinal degeneration. This result suggested that without high Ca^{2+} levels in vivo, the rdgC phosphatase does not dephosphorylate rhodopsin, thereby leading to retinal degeneration (Byk et al. 1993).

References

*Byk, T., Bar-Yaacov, M., Doza, Y.N., Minke, B., and Selinger, Z. (1993) Regulatory arrestin cycle secures the fidelity and maintenance of the fly photoreceptor cell. Proc. Natl. Acad. Sci. USA **90**, 1907–1911.
*Kurada, P. and O'Tousa, J.E. (1995) Retinal degeneration caused by dominant rhodopsin mutants in Drosophila. Neuron **14**, 571–579.
Steele, F. and O'Tousa, J.E. (1990) Rhodopsin activation triggers retinal degeneration in Drosophila rdgC mutant. Neuron **4**, 883–890.
*Steele, F.T.W., Rieger, R., and O'Tousa, J. E. (1992) Drosophila rdgC encodes a novel protein phosphatase. Cell **69**, 669–676.

■ Joseph E. O'Tousa:
Dept. Biological Sciences,
University of Notre Dame,
Notre Dame, IN 46556-0369, USA
Tel.: 219 631 6093
Fax: 219 631 7413
E-mail: "o'tousa.1"@nd.edu

Sarcoplasmic calcium-binding proteins and calerythrin

Sarcoplasmic Ca^{2+}-binding proteins (SCPs) are acidic cytosolic proteins of 20 kDa found only in invertebrates, where they are abundant in muscle and neurons. They exhibit strong polymorphism and the three-dimensional structure of two forms is known. They bind 2–3 Ca^{2+} ions, and Mg^{2+} antagonizes Ca^{2+} binding in a complex way. SCPs apparently fulfill no specific activator function, but seem to interfere strongly with the cytoplasmic Ca^{2+} fluxes and regulate Mg^{2+} ion concentrations. The unique prokaryotic Ca^{2+}-binding protein calerythrin shows a marked homology to the SCPs, especially that of annelids.

SCPs possess molecular weights of c. 20,000 and a pI of c. 5. Only crustacean SCPs occur naturally in dimeric form. They bind three Ca^{2+} ions and Mg^{2+} antagonizes Ca^{2+} binding in a complex manner, including pronounced positive cooperativity, which is re-enforced in the presence of Mg^{2+} (Table 1). Calerythrin (Swan et al. 1987), a Ca^{2+}-binding protein from Saccharopolyspora erythraea, formerly Streptomyces erythraeus, also belongs to this subfamily, as deduced from the sequence homology with its typical site-spacing discussed below. The prokaryotic

protein possesses a molecular weight of 20,090 and three Ca^{2+}-binding sites, two of which are strongly cooperative, and one of lower affinity, a property quite reminiscent of crayfish SCP (Bylsma et al. 1992).

Identification/isolation

SCPs were discovered during the search for parvalbumin in different phyla of the invertebrate kingdom, i.e. in

Table 1. Intrinsic Ca^{2+}-binding constants of SCPs and calerythrin

	Crustacea (crayfish)		Annelids (sandworm)		Calerythrin
Mg^{2+} (mM)	0	1	0	1	0
K'_1 (M^{-1})	1.3×10^8	5.8×10^6	1.7×10^8	1.8×10^6	1.2×10^8
K'_2 (M^{-1})	3.5×10^8	2.2×10^7	1.7×10^8	9.0×10^6	1.3×10^9
K'_3 (M^{-1})	2.0×10^7	1.1×10^6	1.7×10^8	2.7×10^7	3.7×10^7

crustaceans, mollusks, protochordates, and in insects (Wnuk *et al.* 1982; Cox 1990). The animal phyla where SCPs are distributed are depicted in a simplified evolutionary tree shown in Fig. 1. They are very soluble and abundant and, therefore, quite easy to purify from invertebrate muscles. Moreover, most of them are thermostable and show reversible precipitation with 3% trichloroacetic acid, properties which can be exploited during the extraction. Classical DEAE and gel filtration chromatography allowed the purification of the SCPs to homogeneity. In our laboratory a particular Ca^{2+}-binding

protein detection method is very often successful: after chromatography the eluants are screened for the Ca^{2+} content by atomic absorption spectrometry (Cox 1990). Kelly (1990) described a purification of *Drosophila m.* SCP based on affigel-phenothiazine chromatography. Recombinant calerythrin has also been purified by classical chromatographic procedures (Bylsma *et al.* 1992).

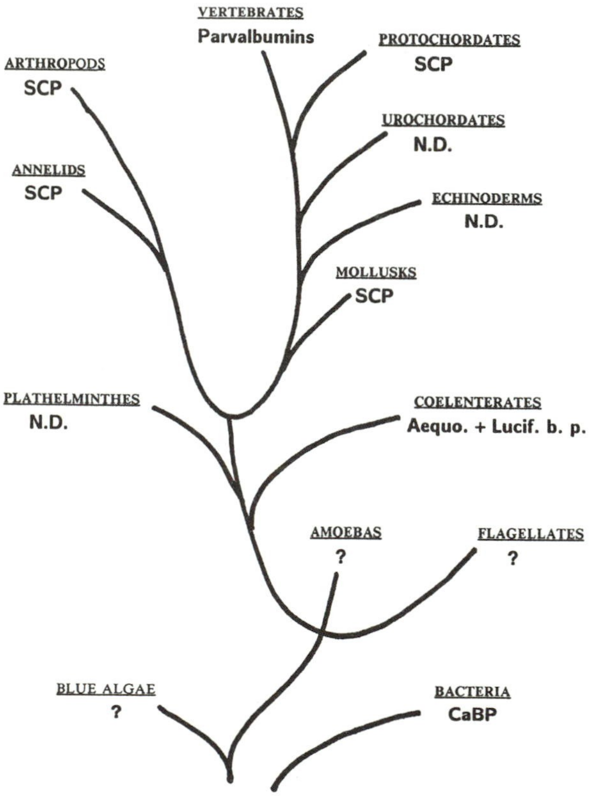

■ Gene and sequence

All the SCPs were first discovered by protein isolation technology, but recently a reconstructed gene system with appropriate cleavage sites was developed for *Nereis* SCP and the protein was expressed as a fusion protein (Dekeyser *et al.* 1994). The calerythrin gene has been cloned (Swan *et al.* 1987: Swiss Prot P06495) and expressed in *E. coli*.

The sequences of nine SCPs (referenced in Cox *et al.* 1991: Swiss Prot P05946, P04569, P04570, P02636, P02635; P04571, P02637) show a restricted sequence identity to each other (15 to 20% between different phyla) and to the coelenterate photoproteins and the unique prokaryotic Ca^{2+}-binding protein, calerythrin (see Fig. 1 in the chapter on aequorin and luciferin-binding protein). But all the proteins enumerated above clearly display a comon fingerprint: the particular spacing of the EF-hands over the polypeptide with a $(EF_1)-x_{21-24}-(EF_2)-x_{12-16}-(EF_3)-x_{4-7}-(EF_4)$ register, x_n being the lengths (in amino acid residues) of the linkers (Cox 1990). This asymmetric disposition of the sites is not encountered in any other Ca^{2+}-binding protein subfamily. Sites I and III have canonical consensus sequences in all SCPs; site II is inactive in mollusk and annelid SCP and in the photoproteins and prokaryote Ca^{2+}-binding protein; site IV is inactive in crustaceans, insects, and protochordates. SCPs exhibit a high degree of polymorphism and evolutionary drift between different phyla. In amphioxus up to seven isoforms of SCP have so far been sequenced; they vary only in a 17 residue-long segment from residue 20 to 36, but this leads to important changes in the physicochemical properties (Takagi and Cox 1990; Takagi *et al.* 1992).

■ Protein structure

Recently, the three-dimensional structures of two SCPs have been reported: that of the annelid *Nereis* (Cook *et al.* 1991) and that of the isoform II of amphioxus (Cook *et al.* 1993). Both structures display the typical paired EF-hands in each of the N- and C-terminal moieties of the

Figure 1. Distribution of SCPs and SCP-like Ca^{2+}-binding proteins on a simplified evolutionary tree. CaBP stands for calerythrin; N.D. means that no SCP has been detected; ? means that the phylum has not been investigated.

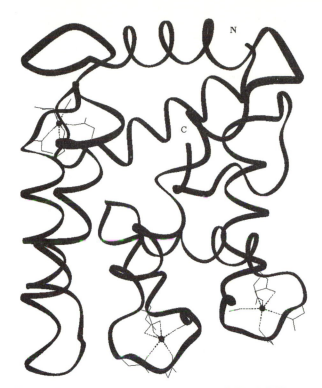

Figure 2. Three-dimensional structure of *Nereis* SCP. The Ca²⁺ atoms in the functional binding sites I, III, and IV are represented by spheres, linked to the seven respective ligands.

molecule Fig. 2). But in contrast to the activator proteins CaM and TnC, SCPs display a very compact structure with the N- and C-terminal paired domains strongly "glued" together (Durussel *et al.* 1993). The presence of an extensive contact surface between the N- and C-terminal domains is unique to SCPs; whereas the other typical buffering protein, parvalbumin, has a much smaller contact surface. This probably explains why pronounced positive cooperativity in ion binding is only found in SCPs. Activator proteins are elongated and possess metastable, solvent-accessible hydrophobic surfaces. SCPs are very stable by themselves, thus explaining why they are not able to act as activator proteins.

Antibodies

Polyclonal antibodies have been raised against crayfish (Benzonana *et al.* 1977), sandworm (unpublished), and two types (forms I and II) of amphioxus SCP (Valette-Talbi *et al.* 1993). They do not cross-react with each other, but the antibody against crustacean SCP recognizes the one in *Drosophila* (by Western analysis, unpublished). An affinity-purified antibody against *Drosophila* SCP was raised by Kelly (1990). No antibody has been described for calerythrin.

Anatomical localization

Immunolocalization studies indicate that SCPs have been found only in invertebrates, predominantly in muscle and neurons. In crayfish (Benzonana *et al.* 1977) and amphioxus muscle (Valette-Talbi *et al.* 1993) the protein appears associated with the isotropic bands in muscle, a region rich in sarcoplasmic reticulum and in glycogen. Antibodies against amphioxus SCP isoforms I and II distinguish between muscle and nervous tissues of *Aplysia* (Pauls *et al.* 1993) and *Helix pomatia* (Kerschbaum *et al.* 1993), SCP I-like material being exclusively present in neurons, SCP II-like protein in muscle. In *Drosophila* the antibody against amphioxus SCP II stained few neurons very specifically (Buchner *et al.* 1988). This antigen was isolated and characterized by two groups (Kelly 1990; Kiehl and D'Haese 1992). Contradictory reports exist on its tissue distribution: whereas Kelly (1990) found it to be widespread, but absent in muscle, Kiehl and D'Haese (1992) found it to be abundant in leg and extracoxal depressor muscle, but not in power muscles.

Biological activities

SCPs do not interact with hydrophobic matrices, amphiphilic peptides, or immobilized calmodulin inhibitors, suggesting that they do not fulfill any specific activatory function. Nevertheless, they are very abundant (over 1 mM binding sites in the cytosol) and efficient Ca²⁺ sinks. The fact that these proteins respond rather slowly to Ca²⁺ and Mg²⁺ changes in the cell allows fast Ca²⁺-mediated events to occur in the presence of a safety device against long lasting Ca²⁺ overshoots. Interestingly, SCPs usually are abundant in cells with a low content of mitochondria, another protecting device against massive Ca²⁺ influx. A plausible hypothesis concerning the Ca²⁺/Mg²⁺ antagonism is that the important amounts of Mg²⁺ released from SCPs during prolonged stimulation of muscle (Cox 1990) stimulate the glycogenolytic and glycolytic enzymes enriched at the I band. But SCPs can show highly specific localizations in other tissues in different invertebrates. This array of properties indicates that the SCPs probably have evolved to satisfy cell-specific needs in the invertebrate tissues in order to cope with the Ca²⁺ signal, known to be characteristic for each type of cell and even for different parts of an individual cell.

Calerythrin also does not possess calmodulin-like activity and probably buffers the Ca²⁺ concentration in *S. erythraea*, where it can be overexpressed without harm at levels of 30% of total cell protein (Swan *et al.* 1989).

References

Benzonana, G., Wnuk, W., Cox, J.A., and Gabbiani, G. (1977) Cellular distribution of sarcoplasmic calcium-binding protein by immuno-fluorescence. Histochemistry **51**, 335–341.

Buchner, E., Bader, R., Buchner, S., Cox, J.A., Emson, P.C., Flory, E., Heizmann, C.W., Hemmm, S., Hofbauer, A., and Oertel,

W.H. (1988) Cell-specific immuno-probes for the brain of normal and mutant *Drosophila melanogaster*. Part I: Wildtype visual system. Cell Tissue Res. **253**, 357–370.

Bylsma, N., Drakenberg, T., Andersson, I., Leadlay, P.F., and Forsén, S (1992) Prokaryotic calcium-binding protein of the calmodulin superfamily. Calcium binding to a *Saccharopolyspora erythraea* 20 kDa protein. FEBS Lett. **299**, 44–47.

Cook, W.J., Ealick, Y.S., Babu, Y.S., Cox, J.A., and Vijay-Kumar, S. (1991) Three-dimensional structure of a sarcoplasmic calcium binding protein. J. Biol. Chem. **266**, 652–656.

Cook, W.J., Jeffrey, L.C., Cox, J.A., and Vijay-Kumar, S. (1993) Structure of a sarcoplasmic calcium-binding protein from amphioxus refined at 2.4 Å resolution. J. Mol. Biol. **229**, 461–471.

Cox, J.A. (1990) Calcium vector protein and sarcoplasmic calcium-binding proteins from invertebrate muscle. In *Stimulus-response coupling: the role of intracellular calcium* (ed. J.R. Dedman and V.L. Smith), pp. 83–1070. CRC Press, Boca Raton, Florida.

Cox, J.A., Luan-Rilliet, Y., and Takagi, T. (1991) Unique Ca^{2+}-binding proteins in metazoan invertebrates. In *Novel calcium-binding proteins* (ed. C.W. Heizmann), pp. 447–463. Springer-Verlag, Berlin.

Dekeyzer, N., Engelborghs, Y., and Volckaert, G. (1994) Cloning, expression and purification of a sarcoplasmic calcium-binding protein from the sandworm *Nereis diversicolor* via a fusion product with chloramphenicol acetyltransferase. Prot. Eng. **7**, 125–130.

Durussel, I., Luan-Rilliet, Y., Petrova, T., Takagi. T., and Cox, J.A. (1993) Cation binding and conformation of tryptic fragments of *Nereis* sarcoplasmic calcium-binding protein: Calcium-induced homo- and heterodimerization. Biochemistry **32**, 2394–2400.

Kelly, L.E. (1990) Purification and properties of a 23 kDa Ca^{2+}-binding protein from *Drosophila melanogaster*. Biochem. J. **271**, 661–666.

Kerschbaum, H.H., Kainz, V., and Hermann, A. (1993) Sarcoplasmic calcium-binding protein-immunoreactive material in the central nervous system of the snail, *Helix pomatia*. Brain. Res. **597**, 339–342.

Kiehl, E. and D'Haese, J.D. (1992) A soluble calcium-binding protein (SCBP) present in *Drosophila melanogaster* and *Calliphora erythrocephala* muscle cells. Comp. Biochem. Physiol. **102B**, 475–482.

Pauls, T.L., Cox, J.A., Heizmann, C.W., and Hermann, A. (1993) Sarcoplasmic calcium-binding proteins in *Aplysia* nerve and muscle cells. Eur. J. Neurosci. **5**, 549–559.

Swan, D.G., Hale, R.S., Dhillon, D., and Leadlay, P.F. (1987) A bacterial calcium-binding protein homologous to calmodulin. Nature **329**, 84–85.

*Swan, D.G., Cortes, J., Hale, R.S., and Leadlay, P.F. (1989) Cloning, characterization, and heterologous expression of *Saccharopolyspora erythraea* (*Streptomyces erythraeus*) gene encoding a EF-hand calcium-binding protein. J. Bacteriol. **171**, 5614–5619.

Takagi, T. and Cox J.A. (1990) Amino acid sequences of four isoforms of amphioxus sarcoplasmic calcium-binding proteins. Eur. J. Biochem. **192**, 387–399.

Takagi, T., Valette-Talbi, L., and Cox, J.A (1992) Primary structure of three minor isoforms of Amphioxus sarcoplasmic calcium-binding proteins. FEBS Lett. **302**, 159–160.

Valette-Talbi, L., Comte, M., Chaponnier, C., and Cox, J.A. (1993). Immunolocalization of calcium vector protein and its target in amphioxus. Histochemistry **100**, 73–81.

*Wnuk, W., Cox, J.A., and Stein, E.A. (1982) Parvalbumin and other soluble sarcoplasmic Ca-binding proteins. In *Calcium and Cell Function*, (ed. W.Y. Cheung) Vol. II pp. 243–278. Academic Press Inc.

■ *J.A. Cox and Tanya V. Petrova:*
Department of Biochemistry,
University of Geneva,
1211, Geneva 4, Switzerland
Tel.: (022) 702 64 91
Fax: (022) 702 64 83
E-mail: cox@sc2a.unige.ch and tanya@sc2a.unige.ch

Spec and LpS1 proteins from sea urchins

The Spec protein family of Strongylocentrotus purpuratus *and the related LpS1 proteins of* Lytechinus pictus *are cytosolic Ca^{2+}-binding proteins found exclusively in ectoderm-derived cells of sea urchin embryos. They are likely to function as calcium buffers, mediating the transport of calcium from the sea water to the blastocoel where calcium is required for skeleton formation.*

Eight related genes encode the *S. purpuratus* Spec proteins. Their molecular masses are 16–18 kDa and each protein contains four EF-hand domains (Klein *et al.* 1991). Spec genes are activated at the late cleavage stage of development and Spec mRNAs and proteins accumulate specifically in the aboral ectoderm, a squamous ciliated epithelium covering the external surface of the embryo. Spec proteins are the major Ca^{2+}-binding proteins in the embryo. Spec1 is the most abundant, existing in the cytoplasm as a monomer. The other family members, the Spec2 proteins, are more closely related to each other than to Spec1 but have the same expression patterns as

Spec1. The Spec genes have served as models for cell type-specific gene activation during embryogenesis (Brandhorst and Klein 1992).

There are two LpS1 genes in *L. pictus* that are only distantly related to the Spec genes. The LpS1 proteins have molecular masses of 34 kDa with eight EF-hands, seven of which appear to bind Ca^{2+}. Comparisons of the Spec and LpS1 genes indicate that the LpS1 genes arose through an exon duplication some time after *S. purpuratus* and *L. pictus* lineages diverged. Beyond limited similarity in their EF-hands, little sequence conservation exists between the LpS1 and Spec genes (Moncrief *et al.* 1990). The LpS1 genes are also activated at the late cleavage stage and LpS1 mRNAs and proteins accumulate exclusively in aboral ectoderm cells.

The fact that Spec and LpS1 proteins accumulate in an epithelial layer separating the sea water from the blastocoel suggests these proteins function as Ca^{2+} buffers, perhaps leading to increased Ca^{2+} flux from the sea water to the blastocoel (Klein *et al.* 1991). This is similar to the vertebrate calbindins which apparently assist in the transport of Ca^{2+} across the intestinal epithelium.

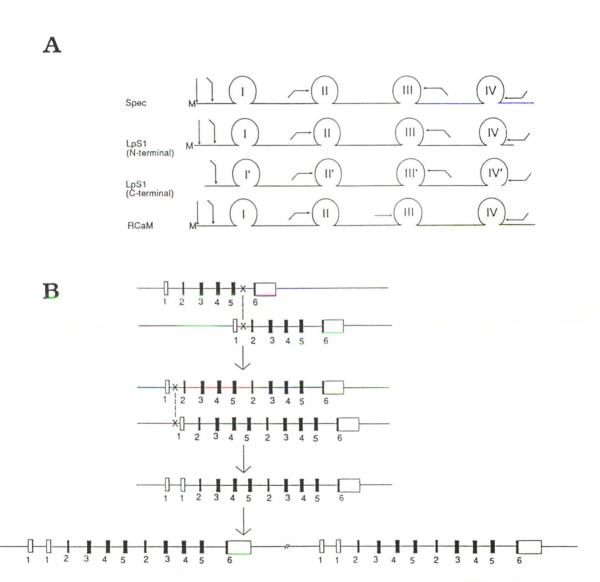

Figure 1. Spec/LpS1 structure and evolution. (A) Comparison of intron position in relation to EF-hand domains. Each EF-hand domain is represented by a Ca^{2+}-binding loop flanked by two straight lines indicating the two α-helices. The EF-hand domains are numbered I-IV or I'-IV'. Arrows indicate intron positions. RCaM, rat calmodulin. (B) A duplication model of the LpS1 genes. The two LpS1 genes are hypothesized to have arisen from two internal duplications and one external duplication of an ancestral Spec-like gene.

■ Identification/isolation

Spec cDNA clones were isolated in a differential hybridization screen using RNA from *S. purpuratus* ectoderm and endoderm cells (Brandhorst and Klein 1992). LpS1 cDNA clones were selected from an *L. pictus* library using an oligonucleotide probe representing a consensus EF-hand (Brandhorst and Klein 1992). Spec/LpS1 proteins can be purified by phenyl-Sepharose affinity chromatography in the presence of Ca^{2+} followed by elution from SDS-PAGE (Keast 1987).

■ Gene and sequences

The *S. purpuratus* Spec genes (GenBank accession numbers M32446, X14530, X14535) contain six exons and, based on the placement of introns, appear to derive from a duplication of a calmodulin gene, which shares about 30% amino acid sequence similarity with the Spec genes (S.H. Hardin *et al.* 1985; P.E. Hardin *et al.* 1988). The Spec gene subfamily then arose from a series of duplications of an ancestral Spec gene. As with many genes in this superfamily, there is no correlation between the placement of introns and EF-hand domains (Fig. 1).

The two *L. pictus* LpS1 genes (GenBank accession number M62848) have virtually identical sequences, implying a recent gene duplication (Xiang *et al.* 1991). These genes apparently arose from a duplication of a Spec-like ancestral gene where the coding exons were duplicated to give rise to a gene with eleven exons (Fig. 1).

■ Protein

Comparison of the Ca^{2+}-binding domains with those of other EF-hand proteins suggests that Spec/LpS1 proteins can bind Ca^{2+} with high affinity (Moncrief *et al.* 1990). By this analysis, Spec1 has four strong binding domains, Spec2a and Spec2c have three, and LpS1 has seven. Although affinity constants have not been measured, Spec1 and LpS1 have been shown to bind Ca^{2+} with high affinity based on SDS-PAGE mobility shifts in the presence and absence of Ca^{2+} and on their ability to bind to phenyl-Sepharose in the presence but not in the absence of Ca^{2+} (Muesing *et al.* 1984; Keast 1987). Spec1 and, by inference, the other Spec/LpS1 proteins are present as monomers in the cytosolic fraction of embryo extracts (Keast 1987). The most striking aspect of these proteins is the unusually high rate of sequence divergence, particularly outside of the EF-hand domains. The relationship of the Spec/LpS1 proteins to other proteins in the calmodulin superfamily has been described by Moncrief *et al.* (1990).

■ Antibodies

Rabbit antibodies against a recombinant Spec1/maltose-binding fusion protein are available upon request. The antibodies are specific for Spec1, although there may be some cross-reaction with the less abundant Spec2 proteins (Wikramanayake *et al.* 1995).

■ Anatomical localization

Spec/LpS1 mRNAs and proteins are highly specific to the embryonic aboral ectoderm cells of sea urchins as determined by *in situ* hybridization and immunofluorescence (Fig. 2; Carpenter *et al.* 1984; Hardin *et al.* 1988).

■ Biological activities

Other than Ca^{2+} binding, no biological activities have been reported for the Spec/LpS1 proteins.

■ Biological regulation

The Spec genes are under the control of both transcriptional and post-transcriptional regulation. In early embryonic stages, Spec genes are transcriptionally activated in all cells but Spec mRNAs and proteins accumulate only in aboral ectoderm cells (Gagnon *et al.* 1992). At

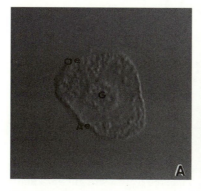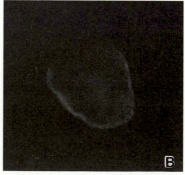

Figure 2. Immunolocalization of Spec1 in *S. purpuratus* embryos. (A) Differential interference contrast image of a three day embryo. Oe represents oral ectoderm; Ae, aboral ectoderm; and G, gut. (B) Epifluorescent image showing Spec1 staining in the aboral ectoderm.

later stages, transcription is restricted to aboral ectoderm cells. An enhancer located 440 bases from the Spec2a transcriptional start site confers aboral ectoderm and mesenchyme cell expression to reporter genes (Mao *et al.* 1994). Aboral ectoderm specificity results when a mesenchyme repressor element which exists within 1100 bases upstream of the enhancer is added to the enhancer-reporter gene construction. The enhancer contains four redundant DNA-regulatory elements which bind the orthodenticle-related protein SpOtx. SpOtx is a homeobox-containing transcription factor involved in the activation of the Spec2a gene but its role in spatial control is unknown (Gan *et al.* 1995).

Less is known about the regulation of the LpS1 genes, but the DNA-regulatory elements important for the transcriptional control of LpS1 are distinct from those of the Spec genes (Brandhorst and Klein 1992).

■ Interactions

Biochemical fractionation studies have failed to demonstrate any interaction of the Spec1 protein with other proteins, including homo-oligomeric forms (Keast 1987).

■ References

Brandhorst, B.P. and Klein, W.H. (1992) Territorial specification and control of gene expression in the sea urchin embryo. Seminars in Developmental Biology **3**, 175–186.

Carpenter, C.D., Bruskin, A.M., Hardin, P.E., Keast, M.J., Anstrom, J., Tyner, A.L., Brandhorst, B.P., and Klein, W.H. (1984) Novel proteins belonging to the troponin C superfamily are encoded by a set of mRNAs in sea urchin embryos. Cell **36**, 663–671.

Gagnon, M.L., Angerer, L.M., and Angerer, R.C. (1992) Posttranscriptional regulation of ectoderm-specific gene expression in early sea urchin embryos. Development **114**, 457–467.

*Gan, L., Mao, C.-A., Wikramanayake, A., Angerer, L.M., Angerer, R.C., and Klein, W.H. (1995) An orthodenticle-related protein from *Strongylocentrotus purpuratus*. Dev. Biol. **167**, 517–528.

Hardin, P.E., Angerer, L.M., Hardin, S.H., Angerer, R.C., and Klein, W.H. (1988) The Spec2 genes of *Strongylocentrotus purpuratus*: Structure and differential expression in embryonic aboral ectoderm cells. J. Mol. Biol. **202**, 417–431.

Hardin, S.H., Carpenter, C.D., Hardin, P.E., Bruskin, A.M., and Klein, W.H. (1985) Structure of the Spec1 gene encoding a major calcium-binding protein in the embryonic ectoderm of the sea urchin, *Strongylocentrotus purpuratus*. J. Mol. Biol. **186**, 243–255.

Keast, M. J. (1987) Studies regarding the characterization of a sea urchin calcium-binding protein. Masters Thesis Dissertation, Indiana University, Bloomington, IN.

*Klein, W.H., Xiang, M., and Wessel, G.M. (1991) Spec proteins: Calcium-binding proteins in the embryonic ectoderm of sea urchins. In *Novel calcium-binding proteins: structures, principles and chemical relevance* (ed. C.W. Heizmann), pp.465–479. Springer Verlag, Heidelberg.

Mao, C.-A., Gan, L., and Klein, W.H. (1994) Multiple Otx-binding sites required for expression of the *Strongylocentrotus purpuratus* Spec2a gene. Dev. Biol. **165**, 229–242.

*Moncrief, N.D., Kretsinger, R.H., and Goodman, M. (1990) Evolution of EF-hand calcium-modulated proteins: (I) Relationships based on amino acid sequences. J. Mol. Evol. **30**, 522–562.

Muesing, M.A., Carpenter, C.D., Klein, W.H., and Polisky, B. (1984) High level expression in *E. coli* of calcium-binding domains of an embryonic sea urchin protein. Gene **31**, 155–164.

Wikramanayake, A.H., Brandhorst, B.P., and Klein, W.H. (1995) Autonomous and non-autonomous differentiationof ectoderm in different sea urchin species. Development **121**, 1497–1505.

Xiang, M., Tong, G., Tomlinson, C.R., and Klein, W.H. (1991) Structure and promoter activity of the LpS1 genes of *Lytechinus pictus*: Duplicated exons account for LpS1 proteins with eight calcium-binding domains. J. Biol. Chem. **266**, 10524–10533.

■ *William H. Klein and Athula H. Wikramanayake: Department of Biochemistry and Molecular Biology, University of Texas M.D. Anderson Cancer Center, 1515 Holcombe Blvd., Houston, Texas 77030, USA*
Tel.: 713–792–3646
Fax: 713–790–0329
E-mail: wklein@utmdacc.mda.uth.tmc.edu

Squidulin

Squidulin is a high affinity Ca^{2+}-binding protein found principally in the cytosol of the cells of squid nervous tissues, including cerebral ganglion, optic lobe, visceral ganglion, stellate ganglion, and giant axon. It is present in these tissues in amounts comparable to calmodulin with which it shares 68% sequence identity. While a similar immunocross-reactive protein is found in the nervous tissues of other cephalopods, octopus, and cuttlefish, no such immunocross-reacting protein has been found in vertebrates. Squidulin is able to activate a number of calmodulin-dependent enzymes.

Squidulin, consisting of 149 amino acids, with a sequence very similar to that of calmodulin, has a calculated molecular weight of 16,894. The isoelectric point is 4.5. Squidulin and calmodulin coexist in the cytoplasm of the cells of the squid nervous system in similar amounts. However, squidulin is restricted to the nervous system and the pancreas, whereas calmodulin is found in all cells. Squidulin binds four Ca^{2+} ions per mol with macroscopic dissociation constants, K_d of 0.9, 0.4, 4.1, and 10.3 × 10^{-6} M. Binding of Ca^{2+} produces changes in the conformation of the molecule, as monitored by changes in the absorption spectra of two tyrosines, one in each half of the molecule (Sheldon and Head 1988). Small angle X-ray scattering measurements of squidulin in the presence of Ca^{2+} show that this molecule, like calmodulin, exists in solution as a dumb-bell-shaped structure (M. Kataoka and J.F. Head, unpublished observation).

■ Alternative names

SCaBP, squid calcium-binding protein (Sheldon and Head 1988).

■ Proteins

Squidulin includes four EF-hand domains, all of which bind Ca^{2+} with high affinity, having macroscopic dissociation constants, K_d of 0.9, 0.4, 4.1, and 10.3 × 10^{-6} M (Sheldon and Head 1988).

Measurements of UV absorption spectra of squidulin on titrating with Ca^{2+}, show that the binding of Ca^{2+} induces conformational changes altering the environment of tyrosine residues which are located one in each half of the molecule. The intrinsic tyrosine chromophores also undergo some change in environment when mM Mg^{2+} is added to the metal-free protein, indicative of a weak interaction with Mg^{2+}, although the spectral change is qualitatively different from that induced by Ca^{2+}. No effect of Mg^{2+} is observed when it is added to the Ca^{2+}-loaded form of squidulin.

Small angle X-ray scattering measurements of squidulin in the presence of Ca^{2+} show that this molecule, like calmodulin, exists in solution as a dumb-bell-shaped structure (M. Kataoka and J.F. Head, unpublished observation).

■ Antibodies

Polyclonal antibodies raised to squidulin immunocross-react with similar proteins in the nervous tissue of other cephalopods, octopus, and cuttlefish, but show no cross-reactivity with components of vertebrate nervous tissue (S. Sarin and J.F. Head, unpublished observation).

■ Gene and sequence

The amino acid sequence of squidulin was determined by Edman degradation methods (Head 1989) and subsequently confirmed by sequencing the cDNA (H. Lucero, D. McDermot, and J.F. Head, unpublished observation). The sequence shows the protein to consist of 149 amino acids with an acetylated N-terminus. The sequence aligns with calmodulin but for a single insertion in squidulin between domains III and IV. There is a lysine at the equivalent position to Lys116 of calmodulin, but it is not trimethylated in squidulin. The sequence of squidulin is 68% identical with calmodulin and many of the remaining differences are conservative substitutions. Significant differences in the sequence include the presence of a tyrosine residue in domain II, as well as IV, at the equivalent position in the Ca^{2+}-binding loop to Tyr138 of calmodulin. This Tyr65 can act as an intrinsic chromophore in the N-terminal lobe of the protein. In the center of the linker region of squidulin are a glycine and two proline residues (residues 77, 78, and 81, respectively). Because of the constraints placed by prolines on peptide backbone conformation, the presence of the two prolines in this location may produce a modification of the flexibilty of the linker region.

■ Identification/isolation

Squidulin was originally identified on gels as a band migrating close to calmodulin in samples of squid axoplasm (Head and Kaminer 1980). It initially copurified with calmodulin from squid optic lobe, but could be separated from calmodulin on DEAE cellulose chromatography using shallow salt gradients (Head et al. 1983). Subsequent studies showed calmodulin and squidulin could be more readily separated on fluphenazine-sepharose (or phenyl Sepharose) by elution with carefully controlled decreasing levels of free Ca^{2+} (Sheldon and Head 1988). Under the conditions used, squidulin eluted at a pCa of approximately 5.9 whereas calmodulin eluted close to pCa 5.5.

■ Localization

Polyclonal antibodies have been used to study the tissue distribution of squidulin. It is found in all components of the nervous system, including cerebral ganglion, optic lobe, visceral ganglion, stellate ganglion, and giant axon, and in reduced amounts in the pancreas. No detectable amounts were found in other squid tissues.

■ Biological activities

Squidulin was found to activate both calmodulin-dependent adenylate cyclase and calmodulin-dependent cyclic nucleotide phosphodiesterase from mammalian brain, although approximately 1.5 to 2 times as much squidulin was required to produce maximal stimulation when compared to mammalian or squid calmodulin. Only calmodulin-dependent cyclic nucleotide phosphodiesterase activity was assayed from squid nervous tissue with similar results (A. Sheldon and J.F. Head, unpublished observation).

■ Interactions

Squidulin appears to bind to a number of proteins in a Ca^{2+}-dependent manner. However, no specific target for squidulin has been identified. Affinity chromatography experiments using immobilized squidulin and calmodulin to identify proteins of squid nervous tissue which bind in a Ca^{2+}-dependent manner, showed that the same proteins bind to squidulin and calmodulin. Many bands of different intensities and molecular weights were apparent on gels of samples from both columns with no apparent differences between the two sets (A. Sheldon and J.F. Head, unpublished observation). Since the sequences of calmodulin and squidulin are so similar (68% identity with many of the remaining differences conservative substitutions), distinctions in their functional interactions *in vivo* may be too subtle for ready resolution using these *in vitro* techniques.

■ References

*Head, J.F. (1989) Amino acid sequence of a low molecular weight, high affinity calcium-binding protein from the optic lobe of the squid *Loligo pealei*. J. Biol. Chem. **264**, 7202–7209.

Head, J.F. and Kaminer, B. (1980) Calmodulin from the axoplasm of the squid. Biol. Bull. Woods Hole. **159**, 485.

*Head, J.F., Spielberg, S., and Kaminer, B. (1983) Two low-molecular weight, high affinity calcium-binding proteins isolated from squid optic lobe by phenothiazine-sepharose chromatography. Biochem J. **209**, 797–802.

*Sheldon, A. and Head, J.F. (1988) Calcium-binding properties of two high affinity calcium-binding proteins from squid optic lobe. J. Biol. Chem. **263**, 14384–14389.

■ *James F. Head:*
Structural Biology Group,
Department of Physiology,
Boston University School of Medicine,
80 E. Concord St.,
Boston, MA 02118,
USA
Tel.: 1 617 638 4396
Fax: 1 617 638 4273
E-mail: jfh@medxtal.bu.edu

TCBP-25

TCBP-25 (Tetrahymena Ca^{2+}-binding protein of 25 kDa) is one of three proteins of the calmodulin family (calmodulin, TCBP-25, and TCBP-23) present in the ciliated protozoan Tetrahymena. TCBP-25 may play crucial roles in the regulation of intracellular Ca^{2+} concentration and in a Ca^{2+}-dependent pronuclear exchange process during conjugation.

The apparent molecular mass of TCBP-25 is 25 kDa on SDS-PAGE, hence its name. From the analysis of cDNA, TCBP-25 is composed of 218 amino acids and its M_r is calculated to be 24,702. The protein contains four EF-hand Ca^{2+}-binding domains, but has little sequence homology with other proteins, except for the EF-hand regions of *Tetrahymena's* third calmodulin family protein TCBP-23 (Takemasa *et al.* 1991), as has been shown by computer search. During various growth phases of *Tetrahymena* cells, TCBP-25 is localized in alveoli, composed of a mosaic of flattened membrane-bounded sacs close to the inner surface of plasma membranes. These alveoli are considered to be a Ca^{2+}-storage compartment resembling the muscle sarcoplasmic reticulum (Hanyu et al. 1995). TCBP-25 is also localized around gametic nuclei during conjugation, suggesting a Ca^{2+}-dependent action in the fertilization process (Hanyu et al. 1995).

■ Alternative names

The protein first reported as TCBP-10 (Ohnishi and Watanabe 1983) was found to be a proteolytic C-terminal fragment of TCBP-25

■ Isolation/identification

A cDNA for TCBP-25 was cloned from a Tetrahymena cDNA library (Takemasa et al. 1989) with synthetic oligonucleotide probes corresponding to the amino acid sequence of TCBP-10 (Kobayashi et al. 1988). Since in Tetrahymena, the universal stop codons, TAA and TAG, are used as glutamine codons, the five TAA codons included in the open reading frame had to be changed to CAAs (Gln89, Gln105, Gln147, Gln181, Gln214) by site-

```
-45    AATTC ATAAAATTCA AAAAACAACA AACAAACAAT    -11

       AAATAAATAA ATG GCT CAA TAC TCT CAA ACT CTC AGA TCT TCT GGT TTC ACT TCC ACT    48
              Met Ala Gln Tyr Ser Gln Thr Leu Arg Ser Ser Gly Phe Thr Ser Thr
                  1                               10

       GTT GGT CTC ACC GAT ATT GAA▼GGT GCT AAG ACT GTC GCT AGA AGA ATC TTC GAA AAC TAC    108
       Val Gly Leu Thr Asp Ile Glu Gly Ala Lys Thr Val Ala Arg Arg Ile Phe Glu Asn Tyr
                  20                              30

       GAC AAG GGC AGA AAG GGC AGA ATC GAA AAC ACC GAC TGT GTT CCC ATG ATT ACT GAA GCC    168
       Asp Lys Gly Arg Lys Gly Arg Ile Gln Asn Thr Asp Cys Val Pro Met Ile Thr Glu Ala
                  40                              50

       TAC AAG TCC TTC AAC TCC TTC TTT GCC CCC TCT TCT GAT GAC ATC AAG GCC TAC CAC AGA    228
       Tyr Lys Ser Phe Asn Ser Phe Phe Ala Pro Ser Ser Asp Asp Ile Lys Ala Tyr His Arg
                  60                              70

       GTC CTC GAC AGA AAC GGT GAC GGT ATT GTT ACT TAC TAA GAT ATT GAA GAA CTT TGC ATC    288
       Val Leu Asp Arg Asn Gly Asp Gly Ile Val Thr Tyr Gln Asp Ile Glu Glu Leu Cys Ile
                  80                              90

       AGA TAC CTC ACT GGT ACC ACT GTC TAA AGA ACT ATC GTC ACT GAA GAA AAG GTT AAG AAG    348
       Arg Tyr Leu Thr Gly Thr Thr Val Gln Arg Thr Ile Val Thr Glu Glu Lys Val Lys Lys
                  100                             110

       TCC AGC AAG CCC AAA TAC AAC AAT GAA GTT GAA GCT AAG CTC GAC GTC▼GCT AGA AGA CTC    408
       Ser Ser Lys Pro Lys Tyr Asn Asn Glu Val Glu Ala Lys Leu Asp Val Ala Arg Arg Leu
                  120                             130

       TTC AAG AGA TAC GAC AAG GAC GGT TCT GGT TAA TTA CAA GAT GAC GAA ATC GCT GGC TTA    468
       Phe Lys Arg Tyr Asp Lys Asp Gly Ser Gly Gln Leu Gln Asp Asp Glu Ile Ala Gly Leu
                  140                             150

       TTA AAG GAC ACC TAT GCT GAA ATG GGT ATG TCC AAC TTC ACC CCT ACT AAG GAA GAC GTT    528
       Leu Lys Asp Thr Tyr Ala Glu Met Gly Met Ser Asn Phr Thr Pro Thr Lys Glu Asp Val
                  160                             170

       AAG ATC TGG TTA TAA ATG GCT GAC ACC AAC TCT GAT GGT TCA GTC TCC CTT GAA GAA TAC    588
       Lys Ile Trp Leu Gln Met Ala Asp Thr Asn Ser Asp Gly Ser Val Ser Leu Glu Glu Tyr
                  180                             190

       GAA GAC CTC ATT ATC AAG TCT CTC CAA AAG GCT GGT ATT AGA GTC GAA AAG TAA TCC TTA    648
       Glu Asp Leu Ile Ile Lys Ser Leu Gln Lys Ala Gly Ile Arg Val Glu Lys Gln Ser Leu
                  200                             210

       GTT TTC TGA   GCAAAATAAT AACCAATTTC TTTAACAAAT CAATACACAC TAATATTAAT TTGTCCTAAC    717
       Val Phe ***
                  218

          TAATATGAAA ATAACATATA ACACTGTACA GAGAAATTTT ATGTATGCTT TGTATTTGAG ACATTTTTA    787

          ACTTTTCTTT ATAAAATCAT TAAAAAAAAA    817
```

Figure 1. The nucleotide sequence and its deduced amino acid sequence of TCBP-25. The amino acid sequence underlined corresponds to that of TCBP-10. Ca^{2+}-binding loops are boxed and positions of introns are indicated by arrows.

directed mutagenesis before cloning into pGEX-2T in order to express TCBP-25 in *E. coli*, strain JM109. The expressed fusion protein was purified on glutathion Sepharose 4B and then TCBP-25 was recovered by thrombin digestion (Hanyu *et al.* 1995). About 1.5 mg of TCBP-25 was produced from 1 liter of bacterial culture. Purified TCBP-25 produced in *E. coli* showed the characteristic Ca^{2+}-dependent mobility shift in alkali glycerol gel electrophoresis that is seen with other proteins of the calmodulin family (Hanyu *et al.* 1995).

Gene and sequences

From the analysis of genomic DNA (accession number J05109) and cDNA (accession number J05110) for TCBP-25, the nucleotide sequence and its deduced amino acid sequence have been derived (Fig. 1; Takemasa *et al.* 1989). Two introns are situated at short distances before the Ca^{2+}-binding domains I and III (arrows), implying gene duplication in genealogy.

Protein

TCBP-25 consists of four EF-hand Ca^{2+}-binding domains. Two special features of TCBP-25 are worth considering: first, the distance between domains II and III is extraordinarily long as compared with calmodulin, the B subunit of calcineurin, and troponin C (Takemasa *et al.* 1989). Second, the domain I (residues 37–48) might be unable to bind Ca^{2+}, since the apparently essential serine, threonine, aspartic acid, asparagine, glutamic acid, or glutamine in the ligand positions Y and Z are replaced by glycine 39 and lysine 41, respectively (Takemasa *et al.* 1989; Watanabe *et al.* 1990; Takemasa *et al.* 1991).

Antibodies

Polyclonal antibodies specific for TCBP-25, which do not crossreact with any other *Tetrahymena* proteins including

calmodulin and TCBP-23, are available (Hanyu *et al.* 1995). The antibodies are raised in rabbits, using purified recombinant TCBP-25 as an antigen.

Localization

The localization of TCBP-25 by immunofluorescence is shown in Fig. 2. TCBP-25 exists in all the cell cortex except for a linear punctate array in 4% paraformaldehyde-fixed cells. Centers of the punctate areas correspond exactly to ciliary basal bodies, so that TCBP-25 seems to be a structural component of cortical alveoli which are important in the regulation of the intracellular Ca^{2+} concentration (Fig. 2A; Hanyu *et al.* 1995). In addition to the cortical localization, TCBP-25 exists around gametic pronuclei at a certain stage of conjugation (Fig. 2B; Hanyu *et al.* 1995). The localizations of TCBP-25 in *Tetrahymena* are quite different from those of calmodulin (Suzuki *et al.* 1982; Watanabe and Nozawa 1982), so that TCBP-25 and calmodulin may not function cooperatively but may share some *in vivo* functions (Hanyu *et al.* 1995).

Biological activities

Possible biological roles for TCBP-25 would be the regulation of the intracellular Ca^{2+} concentration and Ca^{2+}-dependent involvement in pronuclear exchange processes during conjugation. Purification procedures for TCBP-25, TCBP-23, and calmodulin have already been established, but biochemical interactions between them have not yet been investigated. The Ca^{2+}-binding affinity (K_d) and Ca^{2+}-dependent target (counterpart) protein(s), are now under investigation.

References

Hanyu, K., Takemasa, T., Numata, O., Takahashi, M., and Watanabe, Y. (1995) Immunofluorescence localization of a 25-kDa *Tetrahymena* EF-hand Ca^{2+}-binding protein, TCBP-25,

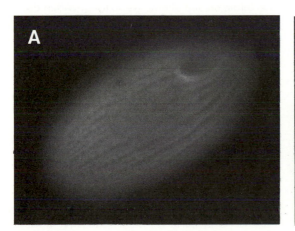
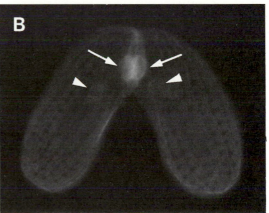

Figure 2. Localization of TCBP-25 by immunofluorescence. A log-phase cell (A) and a conjugating pair (B) are shown. Arrows and arrowheads represent migratory and stationary gametic pronuclei, respectively.

in the cell cortex and possible involvement in conjugation. Exp. Cell Res. **219**, 487–493.

Kobayashi, T., Takagi, T., Konishi, K., Ohnishi, K., and Watanabe, Y. (1988) Amino acid sequence of a calcium-binding protein (TCBP-10) from *Tetrahymena*. Eur. J. Biochem. **174**, 579–584.

Ohnishi, K. and Watanabe, Y. (1983) Purification and some properties of a new Ca^{2+}-binding protein (TCBP-10) present in *Tetrahymena* cilium. J. Biol. Chem. **258**, 13978–13985.

Suzuki, Y., Ohnishi, K., Hirabayashi, T., and Watanabe, Y. (1982) *Tetrahymena* calmodulin. Characterization of an anti-*Tetrahymena* calmodulin and the immunofluorescent localization in *Tetrahymena*. Exp. Cell Res. **137**, 1–14.

Takemasa, T., Ohnishi, K., Kobayashi, T., Takagi, T., Konishi, K., and Watanabe, Y. (1989) Cloning and sequencing of the gene for *Tetrahymena* calcium-binding 25 kDa protein (TCBP-25). J. Biol. Chem. **264**, 19293–19301.

Takemasa, T., Takagi, T., and Watanabe, Y. (1991) Calcium-binding proteins from *Tetrahymena*. In *Novel calcium-binding proteins* (ed. C. W. Heizmann), pp. 481–495. Springer-Verlag Berlin.

Watanabe, Y. and Nozawa, Y. (1982) Possible roles of calmodulin in a ciliated protozoan *Tetrahymena*. In *Calcium and cell function*, (ed. W. Y. Cheung), Vol. II, pp. 297–323. Academic Press, New York.

Watanabe, Y., Hirano-Ohnishi, J., and Takemasa, T. (1990) Calcium-binding proteins and ciliary movement regulation in *Tetrahymena*. In *Calcium as an intracellular messenger in eucaryotic microbes* (ed. D. H. O'Day), pp. 343–361. American Society for Microbiology, Washington, DC.

■ *Yoshio Watanabe*, Kazuko Hanyu, Tohru Takemasa**, and Osamu Numata, Institute of Biological Sciences, The University of Tsukuba, Tsukuba, Ibaraki 305, Japan Tel.: +81 298 53 6648 Fax: +81 298 53 6614 E-mail: numata@sakura.cc.tsukuba.ac.jp*

■ **Present address: University of Joubu, Toyatsuka 634, Isesaki, Gumma 372, Japan Tel.: +81 270 32 1011 Fax: +81 270 32 1021*

■ ***Present address: Department of Anatomy I, Nippon Medical School, Bunkyo-ku, Tokyo 113, Japan Tel.: +81 3 3822 2131, ext. 285 Fax: +81 3 5685 3052 E-mail: takemasa@nms.ac.jp*

Myosin essential light chain

Myosin essential light chain (ELC) is a subunit of conventional myosin-II in muscle and non-muscle tissues with cell- and tissue-specific isoforms. It contains four EF-hand domains, has lost the ability to bind Ca^{2+} and is required for efficient conversion of chemical energy into movement.

Conventional myosin-II consists of two heavy chains (MHC) and four light chains (LC). MHC and LC occur in tissue- and species-specific isoforms. LC exist in two sub-families: essential LC (ELC) and regulatory LC (RLC) (see chapter on myosin regulatory light chain). Both belong to the superfamily of intracellular Ca^{2+}-binding proteins containing four EF-hand (helix–loop–helix) domains (Fig.1). The molecular masses of ELC isoforms range between 16 and 22 KDa, and those of RLC isoforms between 17 and 20 kDa. One of each LC-type is non-covalently associated with an α-helical portion of the MHC near the globular head of muscular (skeletal, cardiac, and smooth muscles) and non-muscular myosin. ELC and RLC are thought to stabilize the α-helical portion of the myosin head region before the two MHC join together to form the C-terminal rod portion which, in the case of muscles, is anchored in the myosin filament (Rayment *et al.* 1993). During evolution all four EF-hand domains of ELC have lost the ability to bind Ca^{2+}. In RLC the first EF-hand domain can bind either Ca^{2+} or Mg^{2+}.

In fast skeletal muscle fibres ELC exists in two isoforms (ELCf1 and ELCf2) resulting from one gene by differential initiation and alternative splicing. Within the myosin hexamer both MHC have either bound ELCf1 or ELCf2. Only a few molecules have bound a mixture of the two ELCf isoforms. ELC has no direct effect on myosin ATPase activity, but ELCf1 seems to affect the myosin actin interaction and to modulate the speed of contraction in mammalian skeletal muscles (Schiaffino and Reggiani 1994). ELC isolated from molluscan striated muscles does not bind Ca^{2+} but forms with its first EF-hand domain in myosin, together with RLC and MHC, an unusual specific Ca^{2+}-binding site which is involved in myosin regulation of contraction (Xie *et al.* 1994).

■ Alternative names

Alkaline or alkali LC (can be removed from myosin under alkaline conditions); catalytic, enzymatic, or essential LC (was thought to be involved in the enzymatic function of myosin) (Matsuda 1983).

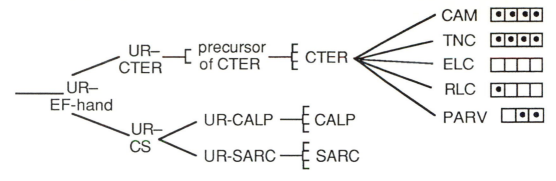

Figure.1. Evolution of EF-hand protein families. Calmodulin (CAM), troponin-C (TNC), ELC and RLC are congruent and form the CTER family. Parvalbumin (PARV) is probably congruent with CTER with subsequent deletion of EF-hand domain-1. An UR-EF-hand domain duplicated without fusion to form the domain of UR-CTER and of UR-CS. UR-CTER then duplicated by fusion to form the common two-domain precursor of CTER which duplicated again by fusion to form the common four-domain precursor of CTER. Subsequent gene duplications without fusion in orgaisms ancestral to animals, plants, fungi, and protists, produced the genes for the subfamilies CAM, TNC, ELC, RLC, and PARV. UR-CS which duplicated first without fusion was followed by several cycles of gene duplication and fusion to produce the precursor genes for the subfamilies of calpain (CALP) and sarcoplasmic Ca^{2+}-binding protein (SARC). (Adapted from Collins 1991; Kawasaki and Kretsinger 1994.) The number of EF-hand domains (squares) and those of them that have retained the ability to bind Ca^{2+} (dots) are indicated for contemporary proteins.

■ Isolation/identification

ELC is prepared from myosin. Myosin (EC 3.6.1.3) is prepared from striated (skeletal and heart muscles) or smooth muscles by extraction with 0.3 M KCl, 0.15 M KH(PO4), pH 6.8 (including some EDTA, MgCl2, dithiothreitol, and ATP or pyrophosphate) and purified by repeated cycles of dilution and precipitation (Margossian and Lowey 1982). Mixed LC are either removed from myosin in 4 M urea or in 5 M guanidine-HCl at pH 8.0 and 4°C. After precipitation of MHC with cold water or with ethanol, the LC are collected by freeze drying or by precipitation. ELC is separated from RLC by ethanol fractionation and/or ion exchange chromatography on DEAE-cellulose (Wagner 1982). The various isoforms of ELC are identified by SDS-PAGE and by two-dimensional gel electrophoresis.

■ Gene and sequence

Approximately 30 protein sequences of both ELC and RLC have been derived, mostly for animals (two fungi), from genomic DNA or cDNA and from protein sequencing. Evolutionary dendrograms based on exon sequences are nearly identical to those based on protein sequences (Collins 1991; Nakayama and Kretsinger 1993). No linkage of genes nor chromosomal clustering is apparent in the CTER subfamilies (Berchtold 1993). Chromosomal translocations must have occurred before divergence of the species. The two LC subfamilies are not more similar to each other (~25% identical amino acid residues) than to the TnC and CaM subfamilies. This may reflect functional pressure inducing a faster rate of gene divergence of ELC and RLC in comparison to TnC and CaM.

All ELC genes in vertebrates have seven exons except for fast skeletal muscle ELC (ELCf) which has nine exons (GenBank at NCBI, 1994). The gene for ELCf is transcribed from two different promoters with differential splicing giving rise to ELCf1 and ELCf2 (mouse, rat, chicken). The mRNA for ELCf1 derives from exons 1, 4, 5, 6, 7, 8, and 9 while that for ELCf2 derives from exons 2, 3, 5, 6, 7, 8, and 9. So most ELC mRNAs are derived from seven exons of which the last is not translated. The exons 2 (4), 3 (5), 4 (6), 5 (7), and 6 (8) (being different in size) are almost identical in length among all ELC isogenes (in brackets the corresponding exons of the ELCf1 genes). The other exons are more variable among different genes. ELCf1 is about 190 amino acid residues long while ELCf2 contains only about 150 residues. ELCf2 lacks about 40 residues rich in Ala and Pro at its N-terminus. Smooth muscle and non-muscle ELC are encoded by a single gene (with seven exons) by differential splicing (human). Their mRNA comprises exons 1, 2, 3, 4, 5, and 6, or 1, 2, 3, 4, 5, and 7, respectively. In these two cases all exons are used for translation. In mammals, atrial ELC (ALC1) and skeletal embryonic ELC (ELCemb) are identical and come from one gene. The same holds for ventricular ELC (VLC1) and slow skeletal muscle ELC (ELCs1b). Slow skeletal muscle ELCs1a is more closely related to the smooth muscle and non-muscle ELC (human) than to any other muscle ELC (protein data).

Gene accession numbers for different ELC isoforms in various databases are in most cases only given for individual exons (e.g. for rat ELCf1 and ELCf2 the accession numbers are M12017, M12018, M12019, M12020, and M12021 at Genome Sequence Data Base). All protein sequences are to be found in Kawasaki and Kretsinger (1994).

Protein and interactions

Absorption coefficients A280 (1%, 1 cm) are for ELC 2.0, and for RLC 5.5 (rabbit); in solution the RLC (rabbit, scallop) exists as a compact ellipsoidal structure of 100 Å length and with a Stokes' radius of 26 (Stafford and Szent-Györgyi 1978). ELC and RLC have a dumb-bell-like fold similar to that of CaM (EF-hand domains 1 and 2 in the N-terminal lobe with EF-hand domains 3 and 4 in the C-terminal lobe, connected by a helix linker). The two LC associate non-covalently, mainly by van der Waals contacts, with a hydrophobic stretch on the MHC α-helix at the base of the myosin head portion. In this region conventional myosin contains two IQ motifs in tandem which are characteristic for CaM-binding domains in general, with the extended consensus sequence: Ile-Gln-X-X-X-Arg-Gly-X-X-X-Arg-X-X-Tyr/Trp (Cheney and Mooseker 1992; Xie et al. 1994). Both LCs are located in series on the MHC, running anti-parallel to it and being wrapped around the MHC, with ELC binding from Leu783 to Met806 and RLC from Glu808 to Leu842 (numbering according to the chicken sequence) (Rayment et al. 1993).

Antibodies

The monoclonal antibody (mAB) F109.8H7 (mouse IgG1) recognizes residues 71–74 of human ventricular myosin ELC1; it also reacts with the ventricular ELC1 of chicken, ox, rabbit, and mouse. A second mAB, F109.12A8 (mouse IgG1) recognizes the first 8 residues of both ventricular myosin ELC1 and RLC of human, chicken, ox, rabbit, and mouse. Both mABs are available from Alexis Corp..

Biological activities and regulation

The extended N-terminus rich in Ala and Pro of ELCf1 can, in actomyosin, interact with actin and thereby increase the maximum turnover rate (V_{max}) and Michaelis constant (K_m) for the actin-activated myosin-ATPase to the level of those observed with myosin containing ELCf2 (Hayashibara and Miyanishi 1994). In principle, ELC hardly affects the actomyosin ATPase activity. But both ELC and RLC are required for physiological speed of movement (~9 μm/s for fast skeletal muscle and ~0.5 μm/s for smooth muscle myosin) as assessed by the in vitro motility assay (Lowey et al. 1993). LC thus plays an important role in conversion of chemical energy into movement.

In vertebrate and arthropod striated muscle Ca^{2+} regulates contraction by binding to TnC in the actin filaments. In molluscan muscle contraction is monitored by myosin regulation. Isolated ELC does not bind Ca^{2+}. In scallop myosin the first EF-hand domain of ELC forms, together with RLC and MHC, an unusual Ca^{2+}-specific binding site (Xie et al. 1994). For this the EF-hand domain-1 of ELC interacts with the third EF-hand domain of RLC and, in the presence of near physiological Mg^{2+}, binds one Ca^{2+} ion per myosin head with a K_d of 10-7 (Kwon et al. 1990).

ELC from Physarum is able to bind Ca^{2+} with a K_d of 10^{-6} in the presence of Mg^{2+} in myosin or when isolated. It seems to function as a Ca^{2+}-receptive myosin subunit; the mode of regulation of contraction is not clear (Kohama et al. 1991).

The expression of isoforms of ELC and RLC is mainly regulated by transcriptional mechanisms (Wade and Kedes 1989). Interaction between positive and negative cis-acting elements and trans-acting factors in various combinations seems to be operative for cell- and tissue-specific expression programs. LC isoform expression is regulated developmentally, hormonally, and by changes in physiological demands (mechanical parameters).

Mutagenesis studies

Functional domain mapping with chimaeras from ELCf1, ELCf2, and non-muscle ELC indicates the location of a basal MHC-binding region in the more conserved C-terminus, and the direction of interaction to specific MHC isoforms by the central part of ELC (Soldati and Perriard 1991). The C-terminal portion of ELC seems not to be involved in governing interaction with myosin.

References

Berchtold, M.W. (1993) Evolution of EF-hand calcium-modulated proteins. V. The genes encoding EF-hand proteins are not clustered in mammalian genomes. J. Mol. Evol. **36**, 489–496.

Cheney, R.E. and Mooseker, M.S. (1992) Unconventional myosins. Curr. Opin. Cell Biol. **4**, 27–35.

Collins, J.H. (1991) Myosin light chains and troponin C: structural and evolutionary relationships revealed by amino acid sequence comparisons. J. Muscle Res. Cell Motil. **12**, 3–25.

Hayashibara, T. and Miyanishi, T. (1994) Binding of the amino-terminal region of myosin alkali 1 light chain to actin and its effect on actin-myosin interaction. Biochemistry **33**, 12821–12827.

Kawasaki, H. and Kretsinger, R. (1994) Calcium-binding proteins 1: EF-hands. Protein Profile **1**, 343–517.

Kohama, K., Okagaki, T., Takano-Ohmuro, H., and Ishikawa, R. (1991) Characterization of calcium-binding light chain as a Ca^{2+}-receptive subunit of Physarum myosin. J. Biochem. **110**, 566–570.

Kwon, H., Goodwin, E.B., Nyitray, L., Berliner, E., O'Neall-Hennessey, E., Melandri, F.D., and Szent-Györgyi, A.G. (1990) Isolation of the regulatory domain of scallop myosin: Role of the essential light chain in calcium binding. Proc. Natl. Acad. Sci. USA **87**, 4771–4775.

Lowey, S., Waller, G.S., and Trybus, K.M. (1993) Skeletal muscle myosin light chains are essential for physiological speeds of shortening. Nature **365**, 454–456.

Margossian, S.S. and Lowey, S. (1982) Preparation of myosin and its subfragments from rabbit skeletal muscle. Methods in Enzymology **85**, 55–71.

Matsuda, G. (1983) The light chains of muscle myosin: its structure, function, and evolution. Adv. Biophys. **16**, 185–218.

Nakayama, S. and Kretsinger, R.H. (1993) Evolution of EF-hand calcium-modulated proteins. III. Exon sequences confirm most dendrograms based on protein sequences: Calmodulin dendrograms show significant lack of parallelism. J. Mol. Evol. **36**, 458–476.

Rayment, I., Rypniewski, W.R., Schmidt-Bäse, K., Smith, R., Tomchick, D.R., Benning, M.M., Winkelmann, D.A., Wesenberg, G., and Holden, H.M. (1993) Three-dimensional structure of myosin subfragment-1: A molecular motor. Science **261**, 50–58.

Schiaffino, S. and Reggiani, C. (1994) Myosin isoforms in mammalian skeletal muscle. J. Appl. Physiol. **77**, 493–501.

Soldati, T. and Perriard, J.-C. (1991) Intracompartmental sorting of essential myosin light chains: Molecular dissection and *in vivo* monitoring by epitope tagging. Cell **66**, 277–289.

Stafford, W.F. and Szent-Györgyi, A.G. (1978) Physical characterization of myosin light chains. Biochemistry **17**, 607–614.

Wade, R. and Kedes, L. (1989) Developmental regulation of contractile protein genes. Ann. Rev. Physiol. **51**, 179–188.

Wagner, P.D. (1982) Preparation and fractionation of myosin light chains and exchange of the essential light chains. Methods in Enzymology **85**, 72–81.

Xie, X., Harrison, D.H., Schlichting, I., Sweet, R.M., Kalabokis, V.N., Szent-Györgyi, A.G., and Cohen, C. (1994) Structure of the regulatory domain of scallop myosin at 2.8 Å resolution. Nature **368**, 306–312.

■ *Marcus C. Schaub and Daniel Koch:*
Institute of Pharmacology, University of Zürich,
Winterthurerstrasse 190,
CH-8057 Zürich, Switzerland
Tel.: +41-1-257 59 19
Fax: +41-1-257 57 08
E-mail: schaub@pharma.unizh.ch

Myosin regulatory light chain

Myosin regulatory light chain (RLC) is a subunit of conventional myosin-II, with cell- and tissue-specific isoforms in muscle and non-muscle tissues. It contains four EF-hand domains of which the first is able to bind either Ca^{2+} or Mg^{2+}. In vertebrates reversible phosphorylation of RLC regulates contraction in smooth muscle and non-muscle cells.

Regulatory light chain (RLC) and essential light chain (ELC) are congruent and belong both to the CTER family comprising the subfamilies of troponin C (TnC), calmodulin (CaM), and probably also of parvalbumin (PARV) (see chapter on myosin essential light chain). In general, the structure and organization of RLC is similar to that of ELC. Both light chains (LC) are non-covalently associated with the heavy chains (MHC) of conventional myosin-II at the base of the head part where the C-terminal rod portion begins (Fig.1). In the scallop the first EF-hand domain of ELC interacts with the third EF-hand domain of RLC, forming, together with the MHC, an unusual Ca^{2+}-binding site for myosin-based regulation of contraction in molluscs (Fig. 2) (Xie *et al.* 1994). While most of the recent ELC isoforms have lost the ability to bind Ca^{2+}, RLC is able to bind one Ca^{2+} in the first EF-hand domain. Like ELC, RLC also occurs in cell- and tissue-specific isoforms. Unlike ELC, RLC can be reversibly phosphorylated. This is the basis for myosin-linked regulation of contraction in vertebrate smooth muscle and non-muscle cells. Phosphorylation of myosin RLC is catalysed by CAM-dependent myosin light chain kinase (MLCK). Dephosphorylation of RLC by myosin light chain phosphatase (MLCP) induces relaxation. Further modulation of contraction in smooth muscle is effected by the caldesmon and calponin systems, both located on the actin filaments (Marston and Redwood 1991; Allen and Walsh 1994).

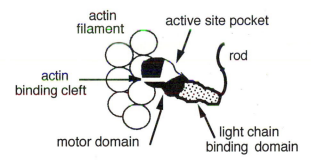

Figure. 1. Conceptual rigor state interaction of myosin with actin (only one head shown). Motor domain (black) contains the actin binding cleft and the active site pocket. Light chain binding domain (shadowed). Actin is represented as a sphere. (Adapted from Rayment *et al.* 1993.)

■ Alternative names

DTNB light chain (RLC can be removed from myosin in the presence of 5,5'-dithiobis(2-nitrobenzoic acid = DTNB); light chain-2 (based on electrophoretic mobilities of mixed LC from vertebrate striated muscles in SDS-PAGE), when LC2 is used for RLC, the two splice products of fast skeletal muscle ELC are called LC1 and LC3 (Matsuda 1983).

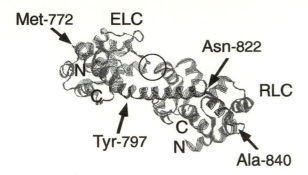

Figure. 2. Structure of light chain binding domain of scallop myosin. The MHC runs from Met772 to Ala840 (molluscan numbering). MHC lies approximately in the plane of view showing two bendings, 40° at Tyr797 and 60° at Asn822 (adapted from Xie *et al.* 1994). Circle indicates region of contact between ELC and RLC.

Identification/isolation

RLC can be selectively dissociated from myosin by treatment with millimolar concentrations of DTNB in the presence of EDTA at pH 8.5 and at high ionic strength. After precipitation of myosin by dilution with cold water, RLC can be collected from the supernatant by freeze-drying or by precipitation with ammonium sulfate and further purified by ion exchange chromatography on DEAE-cellulose (Wagner 1982). Identification is by SDS-PAGE and by two-dimensional gel electrophoresis (2D-gel). The degree of phosphorylation can be assessed electrophoretically based on charge differences in 8 M urea polyacrylamide gels at pH 8.6 without SDS (Perrie and Perry 1970) or in 2D-gels.

For scallop RLC, actomyosin is prepared first, followed by dissociation of myosin from actin by Mg-ATP at pH 7.0. RLC is extracted from myosin in 10 mM EDTA at pH 7.0 and low ionic strength at 23°C (Szent-Györgyi and Nibieski 1982). Myosin is centrifuged off and RLC precipitated from the supernatant. Scallop ELC can be prepared from the myosin devoid of RLC by the guanidine-HCl method (Wagner 1982). Identification of scallop RLC is by 8 M urea gel electrophoresis at pH 8.6 (Perrie and Perry 1970).

Antibodies

Monoclonal antibody (mAB) F109.17C5 (mouse IgG2b) recognizes residues 60–80 of human ventricular myosin RLC; it also reacts with the ventricular RLC of chicken, ox, and rabbit. A second mAB, F109.12A8 (mouse IgG1) recognizes the first 8 residues of both ventricular myosin ELC1 and RLC of human, chicken, ox, rabbit, and mouse. Both mAB are available from Alexis Corp.

Gene and sequence

The branching order and lengths of evolutionary trees for RLC and ELC are similar (Collins 1991; Kawasaki and Kretsinger 1994). In mammals ventricular and skeletal muscle RLC genes contain seven exons which are all used for transcription and translation (GenBank at NCBI, 1994). Among the isogenes, exons 2, 3, 4, 5, and 6 (being different in size) are of almost identical length, as is the case for ELC. Protein data indicate that cardiac ventricular RLC and slow skeletal muscle RLC are products from the same gene. For ELC also the products of two genes occur in both cardiac and skeletal muscles. So the cardiac isoforms are closely related to those of skeletal muscles in both LC subfamilies (Kawasaki and Kretsinger 1994). In chicken, RLC and ELC isoforms are identical in atrial and ventricular muscles whereas, they are different in mammals. Duplication into two genes in mammals can only have occurred after divergence from birds (Kurabayashi *et al.* 1988). The gene for smooth muscle RLC-A (rat) contains only four exons of which the first is not used for translation (Grant *et al.* 1990). RLC-B is predominantly a non-muscle isoform generated from a separate gene closely linked to the RLC-A gene. So the gene organization of RLC from smooth muscle and non-muscle has diverged more from that of striated muscles than has that of ELC. Protein data indicate, in general, that in vertebrate RLC and ELC subfamilies, smooth and non-muscle isoforms are closely related but distant from the striated muscle isoforms. Differentiation into smooth and non-muscle isoforms has occurred after separation of birds and mammals.

Gene accession numbers for different RLC isoforms in various databases are in most cases only given for individual exons (for rat skeletal muscle myosin RLC the complete gene is accessible under X00975 at EMBL). All protein sequences are to be found in Kawasaki and Kretsinger (1994).

Protein and interactions

For molecular mass, overall structure in solution, and absorption coefficient, see chapter on myosin essential light chain. The region at the end of MHC of the head portion where the RLC is located undergoes conformational changes connected with movement (spin label probe experiments) (Cooke 1987). RLC is running anti-parallel on the MHC from Glu808 to Leu842 (numbering according to the chicken sequence) (Rayment *et al.* 1993). The corresponding scallop RLC binding region on MHC runs from Asp802 to Leu836 (numbering according to the scallop sequence). The 60-degree bend in scallop MHC at Asn822 followed downstream by the characteristic Trp–Gln–Trp (Fig. 2) corresponds in chicken MHC to His828 followed by Trp–Pro–Trp. MHC contains within the binding region with RLC its second IQ motif (characteristic binding site for CaM; Cheney and Mooseker 1992) running from Ile816 to Trp829 (chicken) or from Ile810 to Trp823 (scallop). The distance between Cys815 (directly preceding the IQ motif) of MHC to Cys128 in the C-terminal part of RLC is 8 Å (crosslinking experiments, rabbit) (Schaub *et al.* 1995). In the scallop key contacts between Phe20 and Arg24 in the first EF-hand domain of ELC and with Gly117 in the third EF-hand domain of RLC, are crucial for the unusual but functional Ca^{2+}-binding site. This Gly117 is only conserved in molluscan and vertebrate smooth muscle RLC (Xie *et al.* 1994).

Biological activities and regulation

All RLC isoforms bind Ca^{2+} or Mg^{2+} in the first EF-hand domain. Ca^{2+}-specific sites for regulation have an intrinsic affinity for Ca^{2+} $K_d \sim 10^{-8}$ M. In the presence of millimolar Mg^{2+} the apparent affinity for Ca^{2+} is $K_d \sim 10^{-6}$ M. Mg^{2+} has an intrinsic affinity of K_d between 10^{-4} and 10^{-3}. At rest these sites are occupied by Mg^{2+} (e.g. CaM, TnC). The divalent metal ion binding site of RLC is not Ca^{2+}-specific, but belongs to the Ca^{2+}–Mg^{2+} mixed type. The intrinsic affinity for Ca^{2+} of RLC (fast skeletal muscle, rabbit) is K_d $\sim 10^{-8}$, but the intrinsic affinity for Mg^{2+} is $K_d \sim 10^{-7}$, so in presence of millimolar Mg^{2+} the apparent affinity for Ca^{2+} is $K_d \sim 10^{-5}$ (Watterson *et al.* 1979). These sites are not involved in regulation of contraction and remain occupied by Mg^{2+} during a muscle twitch. These sites may become occupied in part by Ca^{2+} during muscle tetanus, with sustained elevation of cytosolic free Ca^{2+} ions. No function can be assigned to the Ca^{2+} or Mg^{2+} bound state at present.

In vertebrate smooth muscle and non-muscle cells reversible phosphorylation of Ser19 (chicken gizzard), preceding the first EF-hand domain, regulates myosin assembly into filaments, and contraction (Allen and Walsh 1994; Trybus 1994). The degree of RLC phosphorylation correlates directly with the magnitude of contraction and ATPase activity. Dephosphorylation of RLC by MLCP precedes relaxation. MLCK has a narrow substrate specificity (RLC is the only known substrate). Eight of the first 16 amino acid residues of chicken gizzard smooth muscle RLC are basic. Positions P-3, P-6, P-7, P-8, and P-11 upstream from the phosphorylatable Ser19 are basic residues, decisive for substrate recognition (Knighton *et al.* 1992). Cardiac RLC (chicken, bovine) has Gly instead of Arg in P-3 position and is phosphorylated by a striated muscle specific MLCK isoform.

In striated muscles (including cardiac and skeletal muscle) Ser16 (rabbit fast skeletal muscle) can also be reversibly phosphorylated. Phosphorylation increases force production at low levels of Ca^{2+} activation (Sweeney *et al.* 1993). In striated muscles RLC is not involved in contraction triggering but only in modulation of contractile properties.

Mutagenesis studies

In chicken gizzard, smooth muscle RLC phosphorylation of Thr18 alone instead of Ser19, also induces contraction. Chimaeric RLC, with chicken N-terminal skeletal and C-terminal smooth RLC regulates smooth muscle myosin

by phosphorylation at Ser13 (Trybus 1994). Relatively non-specific phosphorylation in the N-terminus of RLC is sufficient for regulation of smooth muscle myosin as long as the C-terminus is smooth and not skeletal muscle RLC. Chimaeric constructs of smooth and skeletal muscle RLC, or of scallop and skeletal muscle RLC, are regulatory in scallop myosin only if the critical Gly residue is present in the third EF-hand domain (see above). Mutation of Gly117 in scallop RLC to either Cys or Ala abolishes Ca^{2+} binding. Conversely, Ca^{2+} regulation can be rescued by incorporating skeletal muscle RLC after mutation of its critical Cys into Gly.

Mutations that decrease the net negative charge in the basic N-terminal region of skeletal muscle RLC, mimic the force potentiation induced by phosphorylation of Ser16. *Drosophila* insect flight muscle RLC has a long extension, placing the phosphorylation site far away from the N-terminus. Flies whose phosphorylatable Ser66 and Ser67 in the RLC are mutated to Ala show reduced flight ability and decreased mechanical performance.

References

Allen, B.G. and Walsh, M.P. (1994) The biochemical basis of the regulation of smooth-muscle contraction. TIBS **19**, 362–368.

Cheney, R.E. and Mooseker, M.S. (1992) Unconventional myosins. Curr. Opin. Cell Biol. **4**, 27–35.

Collins, J.H. (1991) Myosin light chains and troponin C: structural and evolutionary relationships revealed by amino acid sequence comparisons. J. Muscle Res. Cell Motil. **12**, 3–25.

Cooke, R. (1987) The mechanism of muscle contraction. CRC Crit. Rev. Biochem. **21**, 53–118.

Grant, J.W., Taubman, M.B., Church, S.L., Johnson, R.L., and Nadal-Ginard, B. (1990) Mammalian nonsarcomeric myosin regulatory light chains are encoded by two differentially regulated and linked genes. J. Cell Biol. **111**, 1127–1135.

Kawasaki, H. and Kretsinger, R. (1994) Calcium-binding proteins 1: EF-hands. Protein Profile **1**, 343–517.

Knighton, D.R., Pearson, R.B., Sowadski, J.M., Means, A.R., Ten Eyck, L.F., Taylor, S.S., and Kemp, B.E. (1992) Structural basis of the intrasteric regulation of myosin light chain kinases. Science **258**, 130–135.

Kurabayashi, M., Komuro, I., Tshuchimochi, H., and Yazaki, Y. (1988) Molecular cloning and characterization of human atrial and ventricular myosin alkali light chain cDNAs. J. Biol. Chem. **263**, 13930–13936.

Marston, S.B. and Redwood, C.S. (1991) The molecular anatomy of caldesmon. Biochem. J. **279**, 1–16.

Matsuda, G. (1983) The light chains of muscle myosin: its structure, function, and evolution. Adv. Biophys. **16**, 185–218.

Perrie, W.T. and Perry, S.V. (1970) An electrophoretic study of the low-molecular-weight components of myosin. Biochem. J. **119**, 31–38.

Rayment, I., Holden, H.M., Whittaker, M., Yohn, C.B., Lorenz, M., Holmes, K.C., and Milligan, R.A. (1993) Structure of the actin–myosin complex and its implications for muscle contraction. Science **261**, 58–65.

Schaub, M.C., Frank, G., and Koch, D. (1995) Crosslinking of the regulatory light chain to Cys-815 of skeletal myosin heavy chain. Biophys. J. **68**, 3295.

Sweeney, H.L., Bowman, B.F., and Stull, J.T. (1993) Myosin light chain phosphorylation in vertebrate striated muscle: regulation and function. Am. J. Physiol. **264**, C1085–C1095.

Szent-Györgyi, A.G. and Nibieski, R. (1982) Preparation of light chains from scallop myosin. Methods in Enzymology **85**, 81–84.

Trybus, K.M. (1994) Role of myosin light chains. J. Musc. Res. Cell Motil. **15**, 587–594.

Wagner, P.D. (1982) Preparation and fractionation of myosin light chains and exchange of the essential light chains. Methods in Enzymology **85**, 72–81.

Watterson, J.G., Kohler, L., and Schaub, M.C. (1979) Evidence for two distinct affinities in the binding of divalent metal ions to myosin. J. Biol. Chem. **254**, 6470–6477.

Xie, X., Harrison, D.H., Schlichting, I., Sweet, R.M., Kalabokis, V.N., Szent-Györgyi, A.G., and Cohen, C. (1994) Structure of the regulatory domain of scallop myosin at 2.8 Å resolution. Nature **368**, 306–312.

■ *Marcus C. Schaub and Daniel Koch:*
Institute of Pharmacology, University of Zürich,
Winterthurerstrasse 190,
CH-8057 Zürich, Switzerland
Tel. +41-1-257 59 19
Fax +41-1-257 57 08
E-mail: schaub@pharma.unizh.ch

Neuron specific calcium sensors (the NCS subfamily)

Neurotransmitters, photons, hormones, odorants, or electrical activity can increase levels of Ca^{2+} within neuronal cells, either by the release of Ca^{2+} from internal stores or through influx from outside the cell across the plasma membrane. Ca^{2+}, once released in the cytosol, functions as a second messenger that regulates cell cycle progression, transformation, proliferation, contraction, exocytosis, membrane potential, synaptic plasticity, enzyme activation, and proteins such as calmodulin, troponin C, or recoverin. In many cases, the function of Ca^{2+} depends on the interaction with specific intracellular Ca^{2+}-binding proteins (CaBPs) which may, for example, mediate the effects of Ca^{2+} on enzyme activities or control the effective concentration of the ion. In neurons, CaBPs can usually be divided into two distinct groups: (a) CaBPs with Ca^{2+}-buffer activity, such as calbindin D9k, calbindin D28k, or parvalbumin, which are thought to limit the concentration of free Ca^{2+} in the cytosol; (b) CaBPs with calcium sensor activity, such as calmodulin or recoverin, which are involved in the fine regulation of Ca^{2+}-dependent specific pathways. The binding of Ca^{2+} to calcium sensors induces conformational changes that expose hydrophobic surfaces. Determination of the crystal structures of several CaBPs has permitted the elucidation of the structure responsible for the binding of the Ca^{2+} ion by a canonical domain of 29 residues arranged in a helix–loop–helix conformation, a structure named "EF-hand" (Moews and Kretsinger 1975). To date, >900 EF-hands from >250 CaBP homologs have been characterized (Kretsinger and Nakayama 1993).

Ca^{2+} is also an essential second messenger in neurons and plays a critical role in the regulation of synaptic efficacy and in transmitter release. Secretion of neurotransmitter can be effectively turned on by rapid increases in cytosolic Ca^{2+} concentrations. It is generally admitted that the entry of Ca^{2+} into presynaptic terminals with nerve impulses is the trigger for the release of transmitter. This short-lived event is followed, in most synapses, by a much longer period of facilitation during which a second nerve impulse is much more effective than the first in releasing transmitter. Such a use-dependent increase in synaptic efficacy is significant for optimizing the operation of synapses under a variety of physiological situations. Synaptic plasticity such as long-term potentiation (LTP) in the hippocampus and neocortex or long-term depression (LTD) in the cerebellum and hippocampus are induced by a postsynaptic increase in Ca^{2+} concentration (Bliss and Collingridge 1993). Neuronal calcium sensor (NCS) proteins in their calci-bound forms could be active, like calmodulin, as enzymes or as regulators of potential postsynaptic targets, such as membrane ion channels, key enzymes such as CaM kinase II, C kinase, phospholipase A, calpain, nitric oxide synthetase, calcineurin, and protein phosphatases PP1 or PP2A, that could contribute to the regulation of synaptic efficacy.

Recently, a new subfamily of neuron-specific Ca^{2+}-binding proteins designated as the recoverin family and composed of species homologs that modulate light-induced signal transduction, was discovered. Each retina-specific CaBP contains four EF-hands, which allows the protein to bind Ca^{2+} selectively and with a high affinity. They seem to act as Ca^{2+}-sensitive regulators that are activated through a cooperative interaction with Ca^{2+} and that, at submicromolar concentrations, function as an on/off switch.

Additional members of this subfamily were also found in several neurons of various brain regions. Together with the retina-specific CaBP, they form a novel and large subfamily of neuron-specific Ca^{2+}-binding proteins, termed the neuronal calcium sensors (NCS) subfamily (De Castro et al. 1995). The growing NCS subfamily is, today, composed of 18 amino acid sequences (Fig. 1) which probably evolved from a common precursor gene. Members of the NCS subfamily have been isolated in several species such as yeast, *C. elegans*, *Drosophila*, frog, chick, rat, mouse, bovine, and human. It includes visinin (Yamagata et al. 1990), S-modulin (Kawamura et al. 1993), recoverin (Dizhoor et al. 1991), NCS-1 (Nef et al. 1995), Ce-NCS-1 (De Castro et al. 1995), frequenin (Pongs et al. 1993), neurocalcin (Okazaki et al. 1992), hippocalcin (Kobayashi et al. 1992), vilip1 (Lenz et al. 1992), vilip2 (Kajimoto et al. 1993), vilip3 (Kajimoto et al. 1993), hLP2 (Kobayashi et al. 1994), and Ce-NCS-2 (De Castro et al. 1995). The

main characteristics and the potential functions of several NCS members are described in the following sections.

Structurally, the 18 members of the NCS subfamily possess a high degree of homology, showing about 37–100% of amino acid identity. They all are globular proteins of 190–200 amino acids with a molecular mass of about 22–24 kDa. They all contain four putative EF-hands (Fig. 1), although some binding sites are clearly

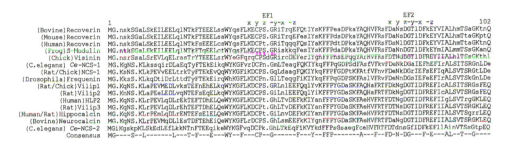

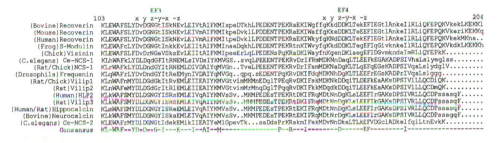

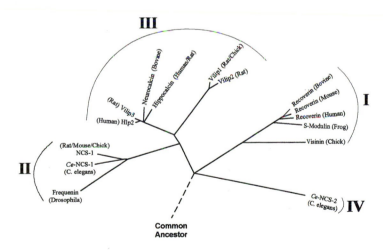

Figure 1. Alignment of the 18 members and phylogenetic tree analysis of the NCS subfamily. Two members of the first three branches have an identical primary amino acid sequence: NCS-1 from chick and rat; vilip1 from chick and rat; and hippocalcin from rat and human. x, y, z and -x, -y, -z represent the positions of amino acids binding to Ca^{2+} in EF-hands. EF1 is an ancestral site and is quite divergent from the consensus sequence for EF-hand. EF2, EF3, and EF4 are likely to bind Ca^{2+} with some exceptions. For every position (vertical row), the most frequent amino acid is shown in upper case, whereas less abundant or unique amino acid positions are shown in lower case. The consensus line indicates the identical amino acid in 14 out of the 18 sequences.

degenerated and probably do not bind Ca^{2+}. The degree of homology between NCS proteins can be estimated using a phylogenetic tree analysis (Fig. 1) which allows a classification of the NCS subfamily. The general topology of the tree gives information on how the sequences should be grouped. Four main branches (I to IV) are observed. Retina-specific NCS are on branch I. Highly homologous NCS from rat, chick, *Drosophila*, and *C. elegans* are on branch II. Other homologous sequences are grouped on branch III. The most distant sequence of the NCS family computed in this analysis, is *Ce*-NCS-2 from *C. elegans* (branch IV).

Members of the NCS family can be considered as species homologs (orthologs) if their phylogenetic distances are short, their amino acid sequence comparison scores high, and their gene structures (exon/intron border) comparable. Branch I orthologs are: frog S-modulin, bovine/mouse/human recoverins, and chick visinin; branch II orthologs are: chick/rat NCS-1, *Ce*-NCS-1, and *Drosophila* frequenin; branch III orthologs are: chick/rat vilip1; human/rat hippocalcin; rat vilip3 and human HLP2.

Functional features of selected NCS proteins

◼ Branch I: S-modulin and recoverin

S-modulin (sensitivity-modulating protein) was purified from frog rod outer segment (ROS) and its deduced amino acid sequence showed that S-modulin is highly related to visinin and recoverin, two other retina-specific NCS proteins. Its concentration in intact frog ROS was estimated to be ~40 mM (Kawamura and Murakami 1991) and shown to prolong the lifetime and activity of frog rod cGMP-phosphodiesterase through the inhibition of rhodopsin phosphorylation (named the S-modulin effect) (Kawamura 1993). Recoverin itself was purified from bovine retinas and crystallized (Flaherty *et al*. 1993). Recoverin is a compact protein made of two domains separated by a narrow cleft. In solution, two Ca^{2+} molecules bind to a molecule of recoverin. In the crystal form, Ca^{2+} is bound to EF3 but not to the other EF hands. The ancestral EF1 is distorted from a favorable Ca^{2+}-binding geometry by the ro residue between the X and Y position of the Ca^{2+}-binding loop (Fig. 1). Moreover, the EF4 loop (Gly160 and Lys162) cannot bind Ca^{2+}. In contrast, EF2 in the crystal structure is devoid of Ca^{2+}, but binds samarium, despite having a sequence that matches the consensus for strong Ca^{2+} binding. Recoverin has an exposed array of nonpolar residues that could form a binding site for a target protein. Recoverin is present in retina homogenates and in pineal homogenates (Korf

et al. 1992), but is not detectable in brain, heart, liver, lung, and kidney, nor in spleen, muscle, or adrenal tissues. Recoverin also exhibits the S-modulin effect, and, in human, is implicated in an autoimmune disease (Polans *et al*. 1991), named cancer-associated retinopathy (CAR) which is characterized by the degeneration of retinal photoreceptors under conditions where the tumor and its metastases have not invaded the eye.

◼ Branch II: Frequenin, NCS-1 and *Ce*-NCS-1

The modulation of synaptic efficacy is a cornerstone of neural physiology and, thereby, of behavior. If one of the many elements that compose the finely tuned machinery at the synaptic terminal is altered, changes in the probability or the amount of neurotransmitter release are likely to occur. These changes affect, for example, motor activity of simple organisms, and in the case of *Drosophila*, several mutants have been described for their abnormal motor phenotype. Electrophysiological analysis of these mutants has shown altered action potential duration and/or frequencies as well as abnormal neurotransmitter release at neuromuscular junctions. In some mutants, the molecular basis of an altered motor activity has been discovered. In *Drosophila* V7 mutants, enhanced potentiation of transmitter release at neuromuscular junctions in response to repetitive nerve stimulation is observed. The V7 mutant shows an altered expression of a gene that encode frequenin, a member of the NCS family.

Frequenin shares only 41% identity with recoverin. Frequenin mRNA is expressed throughout embryonic, larval, pupal, and adult stages. In adult flies frequenin mRNA is expressed predominantly in the adult nervous system and appears to be concentrated in synaptic regions. The concentration of immunoreactivity is particularly intense in the synapses of motor nerves innervating larval or adult muscle. In V7 mutant flies, the amount of frequenin RNA is approximately three- to fourfold higher than in wildtype flies. Thus, the V7 phenotype may result from a deregulated expression of frequenin. Pongs *et al*. (1993) produced transgenic flies, which expressed a higher amount (7–14 times) of frequenin than normal flies. The electrophysiological consequences of elevated frequenin protein levels are a four- to fivefold increase in the magnitude of facilitation of neurotransmitter release at motor nerve endings (Rivosecchi *et al*. 1994).

NCS-1 from rat and chick shares 72% identity with frequenin, and can be considered as species orthologs. In addition, the *Ce*-NCS-1 protein, from *C. elegans*, shares 75% identity with frequenin and 72% with NCS-1. NCS-1 is specifically expressed in postmitotic neurons, and the protein is enriched in postsynaptic densities of several synapses in the central nervous system, including the CA3 dendrites in the hippocampus (De Castro *et al*. 1995). Moreover, NCS-1, like frequenin, is present in the presynaptic motor nerve terminals. NCS-1 exhibits the S-modulin-like effect.

■ Branch III: Vilip1 and hippocalcin

Vilip1 and hippocalcin possess the S-modulin activity (inhibition of rhodopsin phosphorylation in a Ca^{2+}-dependent manner).

■ Branch IV: *Ce*-NCS-2

Ce-NCS-2, from *C. elegans* is, to date, the most divergent protein of the NCS family since it shares only 37–49% of identity with other members. *Ce*-NCS-2 also has S-modulin activity.

■ What are the functional roles of NCS proteins?

Since amino acid sequence homologies are very high among the members of the NCS subfamily, it is of interest to know whether each member of the NCS family shares the same function(s). Various functional roles have been proposed for several NCS proteins: (1) based on *in vivo* experiments, it has been observed that visinin and recoverin prolong the rising phase of light-induced photoresponses; (2) based on *in vitro* assays, a Ca^{2+}-dependent inhibition of rhodopsin phosphorylation (the S-modulin effect) has been shown to occur with native S-modulin and recoverin, as well as with recombinant NCS-1, *Ce*-NCS-1, *Ce*-NCS-2, vilip1, and hippocalcin; (3) based on studies of the *Drosophila* V7 mutant, it has been observed that the overexpression of frequenin could be responsible for an enhanced release of neurotransmitter at neuromuscular junctions, which suggests a role for frequenin in synaptic facilitation; (4) based on a binding study, it has been observed that actin is one of the intracellular binding partners for vilip1, which suggests a role for vilip1 in the regulation of the dynamics of the actin-based cytoskeleton. Since 12 members of the NCS subfamily show the S-modulin effect by inhibiting rhodopsin phosphorylation in a Ca^{2+}-dependent manner, a conserved region must be present in the structure of these proteins for the regulation of receptor phosphorylation. It also suggests that a potential NCS target could be either rhodopsin itself, or the kinase associated with rhodopsin. However, *in vivo*, the potential functions and targets of individual NCS proteins are not yet known, although it is likely that NCS proteins regulate Ca^{2+}-dependent signal transduction and vesicle secretion mechanisms, perhaps by modulating phosphorylation reactions in neuronal cells. Clearly, more work is needed to shed some light on the molecular function(s) of the neuron-specific Ca^{2+}-binding proteins of the NCS family.

■ References

Bliss, T.V. and Collingridge, G.L. (1993) A synaptic model of memory: long-term potentiation in the hippocampus. Nature **361**, 31–39.

De Castro, E., Nef, S., Fiumelli, H., Lenz, E.S., Kawamura, S., and Nef, P. (1995) Regulation of rhodopsin phosphorylation by a family of neuronal calcium sensors. Biochem. Biophys. Res. Commun. **216**, 133–140.

Dizhoor, A.M., Ray, S., Kumar, S., Niemi, G., Spencer, M., Brolley, D., Walsh, K.A., Philipov,.P.P., Hurley, J.B., and Stryer, L. (1991) Recoverin: a calcium sensitive activator of retinal rod guanylate cyclase. Science **251**, 915–918.

Flaherty, K.M., Zozulya, S., Stryer, L., and McKay, D.B. (1993) Three-dimensional structure of recoverin, a calcium sensor in vision. Cell **75**, 709–716.

Kajimoto, Y., Shirai, Y., Mukai, H., Kuno, T., and Tanaka, C. (1993) Molecular cloning of two additional members of the neural visinin- like Ca($^{2+}$)-binding protein gene family. J. Neurochem. **61**, 1091–1096.

Kawamura, S. and Murakami, M. (1991) Calcium-dependent regulation of cyclic GMP phosphodiesterase by a protein from frog retinal rods. Nature **349**, 420–423.

Kawamura, S. (1993) Rhodopsin phosphorylation as a mechanism of cyclic GMP phosphodiesterase regulation by S-modulin. Nature **362**, 855–857.

Kawamura, S., Hisatomi, O., Kayada, S., Tokunaga, F., and Kuo, C. H. (1993) Recoverin has S-modulin activity in frog rods. J. Biol. Chem. **268**, 14579–14582.

Kobayashi, M., Takamatsu, K., Saitoh, S., Miura, M., and Noguchi, T. (1992) Molecular cloning of hippocalcin, a novel calcium-binding protein of the recoverin family exclusively expressed in hippocampus. Biochem. Biophys. Res. Commun. **189**, 511–517.

Kobayashi, M., Takamatsu, K., Fujishiro, M., Saitoh, S., and Noguchi, T. (1994) Molecular cloning of a novel calcium-binding protein structurally related to hippocalcin from human brain and chromosomal mapping of its gene. Biochimica et Biophysica Acta **1222**, 515–518.

Korf, H.W., White, B.H., Schaad, N.C., and Klein, D.C. (1992) Recoverin in pineal organs and retinae of various vertebrate species including man. Brain Research **595**, 57–66.

Kretsinger, R.H. and Nakayama, S. (1993) Evolution of EF-hand calcium-modulated proteins. IV. Exon shuffling did not determine the domain compositions of EF-hand proteins. J. Mol. Evol. **36**, 477–488.

Lenz, S.E., Henschel, Y., Zopf, D., Voss, B., and Gundelfinger, E.D. (1992) vilip, a cognate protein of the retinal calcium binding proteins visinin and recoverin, is expressed in the developing chicken brain. Brain Res. Mol. Brain Res. **15**, 133–140.

Lenz, S.E., Braun, K., Braunewell, K.-H., and Gundelfinger, E.D. (1994) vilip–Ca^{2+}-dependent interaction with cell membrane and cytoskeleton. J. Neurochem. **63**, 72.

Moews, P.G., and Kretsinger, R.H. (1975) Refinement of the structure of carp muscle calcium-binding parvalbumin by model building and difference Fourier analysis. J. Mol. Biol. **91**, 201–228.

Nef, S., Fiumelli, H., De Castro, E., Raes, M.-B., and Nef, P. (1995) Identification of a neuronal calcium sensor (NCS-1) possibly involved in the regulation of receptor phosphorylation. J. Recept. Res. **15**, 365–378.

Okazaki, K., Watanabe, M., Ando, Y., Hagiwara, M., Terasawa, M., and Hidaka, H. (1992) Full sequence of neurocalcin, a novel calcium-binding protein abundant in central nervous system. Biochem. Biophys. Res. Commun. **185**, 147–153.

Polans, A.S., Buczylko, J., Crabb, J., and Palczewski, K. (1991) A photoreceptor calcium binding protein is recognized by autoantibodies obtained from patients with cancer-associated retinopathy. J. Cell Biol. **112**, 981–989.

Pongs, O., Lindemeier, J., Zhu, X.R., Theil, T., Engelkamp, D., Krah-Jentgens, I., Lambrecht, H.G., Koch, K.W., Schwemer, J., Rivosecchi, R., Mallart, A., Galceran, J., Canal, I., Barbas, J.A., and Ferrus, A. (1993) Frequenin, a novel calcium-binding protein that modulates synaptic efficacy in the *Drosophila* nervous system. Neuron **11**, 15–28.

Rivosecchi, R., Pongs, O., Theil, T., and Mallart, A. (1994) Implication of frequenin in the facilitation of transmitter release in *Drosophila*. J. of Physiol. **474**, 223–232.

Yamagata, K., Goto, K., Kuo, C.H., Kondo, H., and Miki, N. (1990) Visinin: a novel calcium binding protein expressed in retinal cone cells. Neuron **4**, 469–476.

■ *Patrick Nef:*
Biochemistry Dept., Sciences II, University of Geneva, 30, quai Ernest Ansermet, CH-1211 Geneva 4, Switzerland
Tel : +41 22 702 64 81
Fax: +41 22 702 64 83
E-mail: Patrick.Nef@biochem.UNIGE.CH

Neurocalcin

Neurocalcin, a three EF-hand type protein purified from mammalian brain, has a unique and specific distribution in the nervous system. Interactions between neurocalcin δ and target proteins are apparent.

Bovine neurocalcin exists as different isoforms with molecular mass of 23 kDa, or 24 kDa on SDS-PAGE (Hidaka and Okazaki 1993). It consists of three functional EF-hand domains with high sequence homology to recoverin and visinin. There are at least six isoforms of bovine neurocalcin and their distribution seems to be restricted to the nervous system. In the adult rat, neurocalcin δ-like immunoreactivity was found in the cytosol of neurons and nerve terminals (Fig. 1). Neurocalcin δ-like immunoreactivity was identified in the cytosol of glial cells in the spinal cord and in the nucleus of neurons in the dorsal root ganglia (Okazaki *et al.* 1994).

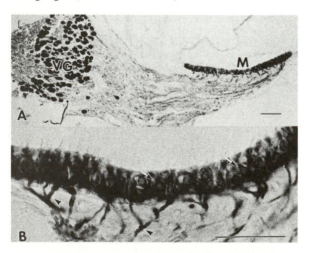

Figure 1. Neurocalcin-like immunoreactivity in the vestibular system. (A) Macula (M) and vestibular ganglion (VG) are intensely immunostained. Bar = 50 μm. (B) Hair cells in the macula are immunonegative, while nerve fibers (arrowhead) and nerve calices (arrow) are immunopositive. (The immunohistochemistry was carried out by S. Iino, Department of Anatomy, Nagoya University School of Medicine.)

■ Related proteins

NVP-3 (Kajimoto *et al.* 1993) is closely related to neurocalcin and may be a member of the neurocalcin family.

■ Isolation/identification

Neurocalcin was purified from bovine brain using an affinity column and the calmodulin antagonist, W77 as an affinity ligand (Terasawa *et al.* 1992). The proteins which eluted from the W-77 affinity column in a calcium-dependent manner, were identified as 23 kDa and 24 kDa neurocalcin, by Tricine-SDS-PAGE. Two isoforms of neurocalcin, α and β, were separated from the 23 kDa protein fraction on a C18 reverse phase column of the HPLC system (Terasawa *et al.* 1992). The 24 kDa protein fraction was subdivided into two components designated neurocalcin γ1 and γ2 (Hidaka and Okazaki 1993).

■ Gene and sequences

A partial clone (N3) and a complete clone (plasmid pCalN, containing the cDNA of neurocalcin δ; accession number D10884) were obtained from bovine brain cDNA library (Okazaki *et al.* 1992). The sequence of neurocalcin δ, one of the six bovine neurocalcin isoforms, contains the open reading frame of the 193 amino acids, with a calculated molecular mass of 22,284 Da. The amino terminal sequence of neurocalcin δ meets the criteria for myristoylation, a post-translational modification which is involved in interactions with membranes (Zozulya and Stryer 1992). The deduced amino acid sequences of N3 and of neurocalcin δ have a high homology but no apparent identity with the other four native isoforms.

■ Protein

At least six members of the neurocalcin family have been identified in the bovine brain. The amino acid sequences of the isoforms are highly conserved within the EF-hand domains as well as in the regions connecting the domains. Domain III is aberrant and in the case of neurocalcin δ, it does not bind ions. Recombinant neurocalcin δ was used in equilibrium dialysis *in vitro* to identify Ca^{2+}-binding sites (2 mol/molecule) and to measure Ca^{2+}-binding affinity (K_d = 2.2 μM) (Nakano *et al*. 1993). Neurocalcin is homologous with recoverin (46.5%) and visinin (51.6%), three EF-hand calcium-binding proteins exclusively expressed in retina. Neurocalcin δ has more than 90% homology with hippocalcin.

■ Antibodies

Antibodies specific to W77-purified bovine-brain neurocalcin as well as antibodies against recombinant neurocalcin δ, were raised in rabbits. Neither of the antibodies are commercially available.

■ Localization

The presence of neurocalcin-like immunoreactivity was observed in brain, cerebellum, adrenal gland, retina (Nakano *et al*. 1992, 1993), olfactory bulb (Bastianelli *et al*. 1993), cranial motoneurons (Junttila *et al*. 1995), spinal cord (Okazaki *et al*. 1994), and inner ear (Iino *et al*. 1995).

In electron microscopy, immunoreactive product was found diffusely in the matrix of the cytoplasm of the spiral and vestibular ganglion cells, nerve fibers, and nerve terminals (Iino *et al*. 1995). A preferential association with microtubules, outer mitochondrial membrane, synaptic vesicles, and synaptic membranes was observed.

■ Biological activities

By equilibrium dialysis, recombinant neurocalcin δ was found to bind two Ca^{2+} ions per molecule (Nakano *et al*. 1993) with a K_d value of 2.2 μM. By the ultrafiltration method, both unmyristoylated and myristoylated neurocalcin δ bound three Ca^{2+} per molecule (Landant 1995). The unmyristoylated protein bound Ca^{2+} with a higher affinity than the myristoylated protein (1.7×10^7 versus 2.8×10^5). Neurocalcin δ and calmodulin bind to W-77 Sepharose in 10^{-5} M Ca^{2+} while only neurocalcin binds to W-77 Sepharose in 10^{-6} M Ca^{2+}. Thus, compared to calmodulin, neurocalcin δ has a higher affinity to W-77 at low Ca^{2+} concentration. Neurocalcin was not phosphorylated by PKC, cAMP-dependent protein kinase, or Ca^{2+}/calmodulin-dependent protein kinase. No other

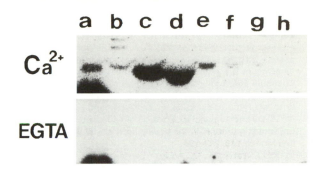

Figure 2. Calcium-dependent binding of ^{125}I-neurocalcin δ to various Ca^{2+}-binding proteins. Fifty μg of the homogenate from bovine brain (a), one μg of purified proteins (b–h) were subjected to SDS-PAGE and incubated with ^{125}I-neurocalcin δ in the presence of Ca^{2+} or EGTA. b, Semi-purified neurocalcin δ; c, S100β (10 kDa); d, S100β (9 kDa, could represent a degraded form); e, S100A6; f, S100C; g, S100A4; h, calmodulin.

biochemical or biological studies on the function of neurocalcin have been published.

■ Interactions

In studies using neurocalcin δ-affinity chromatography and ^{125}I-neurocalcin δ gel overlay, neurocalcin δ bound to S100β protein in a calcium-dependent manner (Fig. 2) and also to S100A6 (Okazaki *et al*. 1995). Neurocalcin did not bind to calmodulin and other members of the S100 family, including S100C or S100A4 (Okazaki *et al*. 1994).

■ References

Bastianelli, E., Okazaki, K., Hidaka, H., and Pochet, R. (1993) Neurocalcin immunoreactivity in rat olfactory bulb. Neurosci. Lett. **161**, 165–168.

*Hidaka, H. and Okazaki, K. (1993) Neurocalcin family: a novel calcium-binding protein abundant in bovine central nervous system. Neurosci. Res. **16**, 73–77.

Iino, S., Kobayashi, S., Okazaki, K., and Hidaka, H. (1995) Immunohistochemical localization of neurocalcin in the rat inner ear. Brain Res. **680**, 128–134.

Junttila, T., Koistinaho, J., Rechardt, L., Hidaka, H., Okazaki K., and Pelto-Huikko, M. (1995) Localization of neurocalcin-like immunoreactivity in rat cranial motoneurons and spinal cord interneurons. Neurosci. Lett. **183**, 100–103.

Kajimoto, Y., Shirai, Y., Mukai, H., Kuno, T., and Tanaka, C. (1993) Molecular cloning of two additional members of the neural visinin-like Ca^{2+}-binding protein gene family. J. Neurochem. **61**, 1091–1096.

Ladant, D. (1995) Calcium and membrane binding properties of bovine neurocalcin δ expressed in *Escherichia coli*. J. Biol. Chem. **270**, 3179–3185.

Nakano, A., Terasawa, M., Watanabe, M., Usuda, N., Morita, T., and Hidaka, H. (1992) Neurocalcin, a novel calcium binding protein with three EF-hand domains, expressed in retinal amacrine cells and ganglion cells. Biochem. Biophys. Res. Commun. **186**, 1207–1211.

Nakano, A., Terasawa, M., Watanabe, M., Okazaki, K., Inoue, S., Kato, M., Nimura, Y., Usuda, N., Morita, T., and Hidaka, H. (1993) Distinct regional localization of neurocalcin, a Ca^{2+}-binding protein, in the bovine adrenal gland. J. Endocrinol. **138**, 283–290.

Okazaki, K., Watanabe, M., Ando, Y., Hagiwara, M., Terasawa, M., and Hidaka, H. (1992) Full sequence of neurocalcin, a novel calcium-binding protein abundant in central nervous system. Biochem. Biophys. Res. Commun. **185**, 147–153.

* Okazaki, K., Iino, S., Inoue, S., Kobayashi, S., and Hidaka, H. (1994) Differential distribution of neurocalcin isoforms in rat spinal cord, dorsal root ganglia and muscle spindle. Biochim. Biophys. Acta **1223**, 311–317.

Okazaki, K., Obata, N.H., Inoue, S., and Hidaka, H. (1995) S100β is a target protein of neurocalcin δ, an isoform abundant in the glial cells. Biochem. J. **306**, 551–555.

* Terasawa, M., Nakano, A., Kobayashi, R., and Hidaka, H.(1992) Neurocalcin, a novel calcium-binding protein from bovine brain. J. Biol. Chem. **267**, 19596–19599.

Zozulya, S. and Stryer, L. (1992) Calcium-myristoyl protein switch. Proc. Natl. Acad. Sci. USA **89**, 11569–11573.

■ *Hiroyoshi Hidaka and Katsuo Okazaki:*
Department of Pharmacology, Nagaya University School of Medicine,
65 Tsurumai Cho, Showa-ku, Nagoya 466, Aichi, Japan
Tel.: +81 52 741 2111
Fax: +81 52 744 2083
E-mail address: hhidaka@tsuru.med.nagoya-u.ac.jp

Hippocalcin

Hippocalcin is a cytosolic Ca^{2+}-binding protein abundant in hippocampal pyramidal cells and is also expressed in considerable amounts in the dentate granule cells, cortical pyramidal cells, and cerebellar Purkinje cells. Physiological functions in nerve cells, have not been elucidated.

Hippocalcin is a cytosolic Ca^{2+}-binding protein with a calculated molecular mass of 22.4 kDa and an isoelectric point of 4.7. It migrates on SDS gels with an apparent M_r of 21,000 in the presence of Ca^{2+}, or of 23,000 in the absence of Ca^{2+}. Hippocalcin comprises three functional EF-hand domains and the NH$_2$-terminus of the mature protein is myristoylated. It is a cytosolic protein and has Ca^{2+}-dependent membrane-binding properties. Recombinant hippocalcin suppressed light-induced rhodopsin phosphorylation by rhodopsin kinase at Ca^{2+} concentrations of 10 μM in rod outer segment membrane preparations. Physiological functions of hippocalcin are not known yet; however, hippocalcin may act as a Ca^{2+}-sensitive regulator of synaptic function in its host cells.

In the adult rat, hippocalcin is expressed abundantly in the hippocampal pyramidal cells, and moderately in the dentate granule cells, cortical pyramidal cells, and cerebellar Purkinje cells (Fig. 1, Saitoh *et al.* 1993). During rat development, hippocalcin expression in the cortical pyramidal cells and cerebellar Purkinje cells attains high levels early in development but decreases in the adult animal (Saitoh *et al.* 1994).

■ Alternative names

P23K (Takamatsu and Uyemura 1992; Takamatsu *et al.* 1992).

■ Isolation/identification

During a survey of recoverin-like immunoreactivity in various tissues by immunoblot analysis, a 23 kDa Ca^{2+}-binding protein (P23k) was found in mouse and rat brain. It was labeled with an antiserum raised against the NH$_2$-terminus of recoverin but it could not be detected by an antiserum raised against the COOH-terminus of recoverin (Takamatsu and Uyemura 1992; Takamatsu *et al.* 1992). Blots with ^{45}Ca demonstrated that P23k bound Ca^{2+}. P23k was purified by Ca^{2+}-dependent hydrophobic interaction and ion-exchange chromatography. Based on partial amino acid sequences, several different cDNA clones were isolated from a rat brain cDNA library. One of these clones which encodes a novel Ca^{2+}-binding protein, was found to be expressed abundantly in the hippocampus (Kobayashi *et al.* 1992). This protein was therefore designated hippocalcin.

■ Gene and sequences

The sequences of rat (Kobayashi *et al.* 1992; DDBJ accession number: D12573) and human hippocalcin cDNAs (Takamatsu *et al.* 1994; D16593) are highly homologous. Rat (Kobayashi *et al.*, unpublished observation) and human hippocalcin genes have recently been cloned (Saitoh *et al.*, unpublished observation). The hippocalcin genes consist of three exons spanning 13 kb and

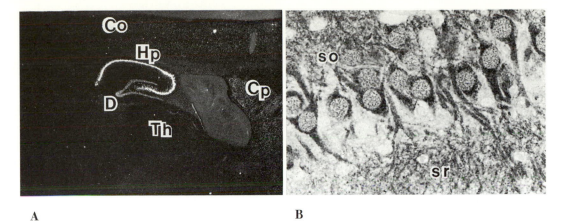

A   B

Figure 1. (A) Dark-field photomicrograph of *in situ* hybridization of a sagittal section of rat brain. The most intense expression of hippocalcin mRNA is seen in the pyramidal cell layer of Ammon's horn (Co, neocortex; CP, caudate-putamen; D, dentate gyrus; Hp, hippocampus; Th, thalamus; taken from Saitoh *et al.* 1993).
(B) Immunohistochemical staining of pyramidal cells in the CA1 region of rat hippocampus. Intense immuno-reactivity is seen in cell bodies and dendrites of pyramidal cells (so, stratum oriens; sr, stratum radiatum; taken from Saitoh *et al.* 1993).

exist as a single copy in the haploid genome. The three exons contain the entire coding sequence. The intron positions of the rat and human hippocalcin genes are in exactly the same positions, and are not consistently placed with respect to the coding regions of the tandemly repeated EF-hand domains (Fig. 2, Kobayashi *et al.*, un-published observations). The human hippocalcin gene is located on chromosome 1 (Takamatsu *et al.* 1994).

■ Protein

The deduced amino acid sequences of rat and human hippocalcin consist of 193 amino acid residues and are 100% identical. Hippocalcin originally contains four EF-hand domains, but the NH$_2$-terminal domain is aber-rant and does not bind Ca^{2+}. The NH$_2$-terminal glycine residue of the mature protein is acylated with myristic acid (Kobayashi *et al.* 1993).

■ Antibodies

A rabbit antibody was raised against a recombinant hippocalcin/maltose-binding fusion protein and affinity purified using the fusion protein-coupled cellulofine. The antibody specifically recognizes hippocalcin and does not cross-react with other homologous proteins, such as recoverin, S-modulin, and vilip2 on immunoblot analysis (Saitoh *et al.* 1993).

■ Localization

Immunohistochemical and *in situ* hybridization analyses have been carried out using, respectively, an antibody against recombinant hippocalcin and a specific cRNA probe. In the adult rat, hippocalcin is expressed abun-dantly in the hippocampal pyramidal cells, and moder-ately in the dentate granule cells, cortical pyramidal cells,

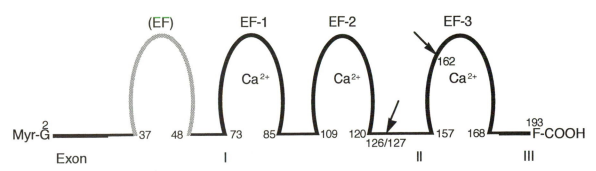

Figure 2. EF-hand structure of hippocalcin. The presumed intron/exon junctions are marked by arrows. Amino acid residues are numbered beginning with the initiator methionine.

and cerebellar Purkinje cells (Saitoh *et al.* 1993). In most cell types, hippocalcin immunoreactivity is localized in the cytoplasm and plasma membrane of the cell bodies and dendrites. During rat development, hippocalcin expression in the cortical pyramidal cells and cerebellar Purkinje cells attains transiently high levels but decreases in the adult (Saitoh *et al.* 1994).

■ Biological activities

Hippocalcin binds to the membrane fraction prepared from rat brain in a Ca^{2+}-dependent manner. The maximal membrane binding was observed at about 30 µM $[Ca^{2+}]$, and half the maximal binding at about 5 µM $[Ca^{2+}]$. NH_2-terminal myristoylation of hippocalcin was essential to its Ca^{2+}-dependent membrane-binding properties (Kobayashi *et al.* 1993).

Recombinant hippocalcin suppressed light-induced rhodopsin phosphorylation by rhodopsin kinase at high concentrations of Ca^{2+} (10 µM) (Kawamura and Takamatsu, unpublished observation). NH_2-terminal myristoylation is not essential for the inhibition of rhodopsin phosphorylation. Although the mechanism regulating receptor phosphorylation in neurons is different from that of photoreceptors, Hippocalcin may act as a Ca^{2+}-sensitive regulator of synaptic function.

■ References

*Kobayashi, M., Takamatsu, K., Saitoh, S., Miura, M., and Noguchi, T. (1992) Molecular cloning of hippocalcin, a novel calcium-binding protein of the recoverin family exclusively expressed in hippocampus. Biochem. Biophys. Res. Commun. **189**, 511–517.

*Kobayashi, M., Takamatsu, K., Saitoh, S., and Noguchi, T. (1993) Myristoylation of hippocalcin is linked to its calcium-dependent membrane association properties. J. Biol. Chem. **268**, 18898–18904.

*Saitoh, S., Takamatsu, K., Kobayashi, M., and Noguchi, T. (1993) Distribution of hippocalcin mRNA and immunoreactivity in rat brain. Neurosci. Lett. **157**, 107–110.

Saitoh, S., Takamatsu, K., Kobayashi, M., and Noguchi, T. (1994) Expression of hippocalcin in the developing rat brain. Dev. Brain Res. **80**, 199–200.

Takamatsu, K. and Uyemura, K. (1992) Identification of recoverin-like immunoreactivity in mouse brain. Brain Res. **571**, 350–353.

Takamatsu, K., Kitamura, K., and Noguchi, T. (1992) Isolation and characterization of recoverin-like Ca^{2+}-binding protein from rat brain. Biochem. Biophys. Res. Commun. **183**, 245–251.

Takamatsu, K., Kobayashi, M., Saitoh, S., Fujishiro, M., and Noguchi, T. (1994) Molecular cloning of human hippocalcin cDNA and chromosomal mapping of its gene. Biochem. Biophys. Res. Commun. **200**, 606–611.

■ *Ken Takamatsu, Shigeharu Saitoh, and Masaaki Kobayashi:*
Department of Physiology,
Toho University School of Medicine,
Ohta-ku, Tokyo 143, Japan
Tel.: +81 3 3762 4151
Fax: +81 3 3762 8225
E-mail: physiken@med.toho-u.ac.jp

Frequenin

Drosophila *frequenin (d-frq) is a Ca^{2+}-binding protein that modulates synaptic efficacy in the nervous system of* Drosophila melanogaster. *Overexpression of d-frq either in mutant or transgenic flies leads to an enhanced, frequency-dependent facilitation of neurotransmitter release at neuromuscular junctions of third instar larvae.*

Drosophila frequenin has a calculated molecular mass (M_r) of 21.7 kDa, migrates on SDS gels with an apparent M_r of 22 kDa and has an isoelectric point of 5.2. The protein sequence contains four EF-hand domains. The first motif misses three potential Ca^{2+}-coordinating amino acids and therefore might not be functional.

Drosophila frequenin is expressed through all developmental stages with predominant localization in the nervous system. The highest densities are present in synaptic regions.

■ Isolation/identification

The characterization of frq was obtained by genetic and electrophysiological analysis of T(X;Y)*V7* mutants of *Drosophila melanogaster* (Tanouye *et al.* 1981; Mallart *et al.* 1991).

Genomic DNA was cloned by "chromosomal walking" of the *Shaker* complex (*ShC*) and subsequent characterization of the transcription unit affected by the chromosomal rearrangement T(1;Y)*V7* (Ferrus *et al.* 1990). Frq-cDNA clones were isolated from *Drosophila* head libraries (λgt 11) using genomic DNA probes from the distal *V7* region (Pongs *et al.* 1993). For biochemical studies recombinant frq was produced and purified from *E.coli*.

■ Gene and sequence

The frq gene is located on the X-chromosome of *Drosophila melanogaster* at 16F 5-8. Frq derives from two

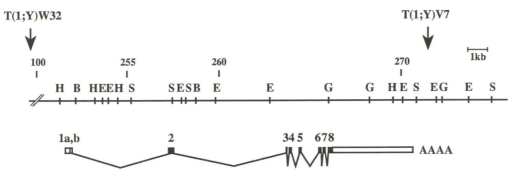

Figure 1. Physical map of the frq-gene and deduced frq amino acid sequence. Physical map of the genomic DNA of the proximal limit of the *Sh* complex. Centromere is to the right. Arrows indicate the location of chromosomal rearrangements associated with a Sh phenotype. The coordinates of the maps are as defined by Baumann *et al.* (1987). Bar indicates calibration. B, *Bam*H I; G, *Bgl* II; E, *Eco*R I; H, *Hin*d III; S, *Sst* I. Below, alignment map of exons of frq-RNA with genomic DNA is shown. Numbered boxes represent exons, which are numbered from left to right in the direction of transcription. Empty boxes correspond to untranslated sequences; closed boxes to the open reading frame.

alternatively spliced transcripts (see Fig. 1). Both transcripts consist of eight exons. Exon 1 has 264 nucleotides in one transcript; in the other, exon 1 is extended 3' by 98 nucleotides. The longest open reading frame extends from exon 2 to exon 8 and is identical for both transcripts. The reading frame is followed by a ~4600 bp 3' untranslated region which is AU rich and contains several UUUUNU motifs which might be important for mRNA stability. The cDNA sequence has been deposited with GenBank (accession number L08064).

Protein

The predicted frequenin protein sequence is 187 amino acids long with a calculated M_r of 21.7 kDa. The protein shares homologies to the proteins of the "neuronal

specific Ca^{2+} sensors(NCS) (classification by P. Nef, this book). The greatest number of homologies exist to the flup-proteins (71% identity) (Lindemeier *et al.*, see next chapter). The sequence possesses four EF-hands. The first domain contains two amino acid replacements at position x and -z (amino acids K36 and G47) important for binding Ca^{2+}. Therefore, this might not be a functional Ca^{2+}-binding site. The sequence also contains potential consensus sequences for phosphorylation (protein kinase C and A) and N-myristoylation (MGKKSS in frequenin).

Antibodies

Antibodies are available from the authors.

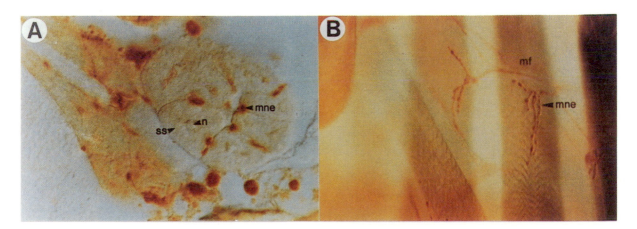

Figure 2. Localization of frq-protein in the nervous system of *Drosophila melanogaster* from Pongs *et al.* 1993. Magnification × 63. (a) View of a 10 μm horizontal section of adult *Drosophila* thorax showing trochanter muscle: n, nucleus of muscle cell; ss, sarcostyles; mne, motor nerve ending. (b) Neuromuscular preparation of third-instar larvae: mf, muscle fiber; mne, motor nerve ending.

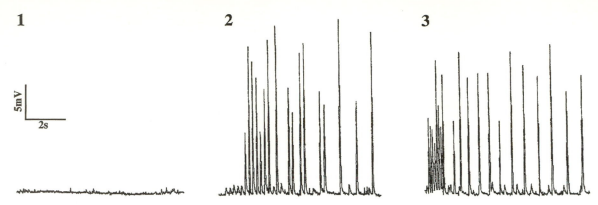

1

2

3

5mV

2s

Figure 3. Frequency dependence of facilitated postsynaptic responses at the neuromuscular junctions of third-instar larvae of T(X;Y)$V7$ *Drosophila* mutants. Intracellular EJP (excitatory junctional potential) recordings from muscle fibers during trains of 1 Hz (1), 5 Hz (2) and 10Hz (3) stimulations of $V7$ motor nerve endings. EJP recordings from wildtype muscle fibers during trains of 1 Hz, 5 Hz or 10Hz stimulations of wild type motor nerve endings showed no increase facilitation and were similar to that of the mutant. (taken from Pongs *et al.* 1993)

■ Anatomical localization

In situ hybridizations and immunocytochemical analyses of frequenin tissue distribution indicate that frq-protein is concentrated predominantly in the *Drosophila* nervous system. In late embryos anti-frq-antibodies stain discrete groups of cells in the central nervous system and some neurons in the peripheral nervous sytem. Frequenin seems to be concentrated in synaptic regions, since antibodies stain neuropil areas heavily. This is especially visible in the adult brain but also in larval and adult neuromuscular junctions. Immunostain is particularly intense in motor end plates of larval and adult muscles (Fig. 2).

■ Biological activities

Ca^{2+}-binding capability of frq was confirmed by $^{45}Ca^{2+}$-blots and with Ca^{2+}-mobility shift assays using recombinant protein. *In vitro* studies showed the ability of recombinant frq to stimulate guanylyl cyclase (GC) in bovine rod outer segment (ROS) preparations in a Ca^{2+}-sensitive manner (Pongs *et al.* 1993). Electrophysiological recordings at larval *Drosophila* neuromuscular junctions might indicate a modulation of the Na^+-Ca^{2+} exchanger by d-frq (Rivosecchi *et al.* 1994)

■ Mutagenesis studies

The *Drosophila* mutant T(X;Y)$V7$ shows abnormally high levels of neurotransmitter release in a time- and frequency-dependent manner upon repetitive stimulation of motor nerve endings (Mallart *et al.* 1991). It was shown that this enhanced facilitation could be adressed to an overexpression of frq-protein in *Drosophila* (Pongs *et al.* 1993). This result was confirmed by transgenic flies which

overexpressed d-frq-protein after heat shock (Fig. 3; Pongs *et al.* 1993).

■ References

Baumann, A., Krah-Jentgens, I., Muller-Holtkamp, F., Seidel, R., Keckskemethy, N., Casal, J., Ferrus, A., and Pongs, O. (1987) Molecular characterisation of the maternal effect region of the *Shaker* complex of *Drosophila*: characterisation of an I(A) channel transcript with homology to vertebrate Na channel. EMBO J. **6**, 34, 3419–3429.

Ferrus, A., Llamazares, S., de la Pompa, J.L., Tanouye, M.A., and Pongs, O. (1990) Genetic analysis of the *Shaker* gene complex of *Drosophila melanogaster*. Genetics **125**, 383–398.

Mallart, A., Angaut-Petit, D., Bourret-Poulain, C., and Ferrus, A. (1991) Nerve terminal excitability and neuromuscular transmission in T(X;Y)$V7$ mutants of *Drosohila melanogaster*. J. Neurogen. **7**, 7–84.

*Pongs, O., Lindemeier, J., Zhu, X.R., Theil, T., Engelkamp, D., Krah-Jentgens, I., Lambrecht, H.-G., Koch, K.W., Schwemer, J., Rivosecchi, R., Mallart, A., Calceran, J., Canal, I., Barbas, J.A., and Ferrus, A. (1993) Frequenin-a novel calcium-binding protein that modulates synaptic efficacy in the *Drosophila* nervous system. Neuron **11**, 15–28.

*Rivosecchi, R., Pongs, O., Theil, T., and Mallart, A. (1994). Implication of frequenin in the facilitation of transmitter release in *Drosophila*. J. Physiol. **474.2**, 223–232.

Tanouye, M.A., Ferrus, A., and Fujita, S.C. (1981) Abnormal action potentials associated with the *Shaker* complex locus of *Drosophila*. Proc. Natl. Sci. USA **78**, 6548–6552.

■ *Jürgen Lindemeier and Olaf Pongs:*
Zentrum für Molekulare Neurobiologie,
Institut für Neurale Signalverarbeitung,
Martinistr. 52,
D-20246 Hamburg, Germany
Tel.: +49 040 4717 4811
Fax: +49 040 4717 5102
E-mail: lindemeier@zmnh.zmnh.uni-hamburg.de

Frequenin-like ubiquitous protein (flup)

Rat-flup is widely expressed in the rat nervous system and several other tissues. This Ca^{2+}-binding protein may be a Ca^{2+}-sensitive regulator of calcineurin activity. It has been shown to be involved in rapid inactivation of an A-type voltage-gated potassium channel (K_v 1.4). Therefore, flup may represent a novel type of Ca^{2+}-signalling molecule which couples calcineurin activity with cellular targets controlling excitability.

Rat-flup (r-flup) has a calculated molecular mass of 21.9 kDa. On SDS gels it migrates with an apparent molecular mass of 22 kDa. The human homolog (h-flup) has a M_r of 21.9 and is 98% identical to r-flup. Both proteins share 71% identity to *Drosophila* frequenin (d-frq). Like d-frq the flup-sequences contain four EF-hands but in the first Ca^{2+}-binding domain two potential Ca^{2+}-coordinating amino acids of the EF-hand at the position x, and -z are exchanged.

Rat-flup is most prominently expressed in rat brain and markedly in heart, skeletal muscle, and kidney. Transcripts are also detectable in spleen, lung, and testis. Flup protein seems to be translocated to cellular membranes in a Ca^{2+}-dependent manner. Human-flup was detected in HEK 293 cells by cross-immunoreactivity with anti-r-flup antibodies.

■ Identification/isolation

Rat-flup cDNA was isolated by screening a rat cerebellar cDNA library (λ-ZAPII) with a d-frq probe under low stringency conditions. The human flup cDNA was obtained from nested PCR reactions employing rat-flup-derived degenerated primers and HEK 293 (human embryonic kidney cell line 293) cDNA as templates. The amplified PCR fragment was then used for isolation of h-flup cDNA from a human adult cDNA library. For biochemical studies recombinant r-flup was expressed in *E. coli*. The protein was expressed as a fusion protein using the pGEX-2T plasmid (Pharmacia), chromatographed over a glutathione-agarose column and cleaved by thrombin.

■ Gene and sequence

The r-flup cDNA sequence has been deposited with GenBank (accession number X82188, available after publication (Lindemeier *et al.* in preparation)).

■ Protein

Both flup sequences consist of four EF-hands (Fig. 1). The first of the four domains misses three potential Ca^{2+}-coordinating amino acids at the x, y and -z position (K36, C38, and G47). Therefore, these EF-hands may not bind Ca^{2+}. Metal binding was confirmed by $^{45}Ca^{2+}$-blots and

```
                                                                 Ca I
                              ▲                  △             ┌─────────────┐
                                                              │x  y  z -y -x  -z│
r-flup   MGKSNSKLKPEVVEELTRKTYFTEKEVQQWYKGFIKDCPSGQLDAAGFQK   50
h-flup   --------------------------------------------------   50
d-frq    ---KS----QDTIDR--TD-------IR--H---L----N-L-TEQ--I-   50
                                  Ca II
                       ┌─────────────┐              △
                       │x  y  z -y -x  -z│
r-flup   IYKQFFPFEDPTKFATRVFNVVDENKDGRIEFSEFIQALSVTSRGTLDEK  100
h-flup   -------------P------------------------------------  100
d-frq    ------QG--S---SL--R-F---N--S---E---R------K-N----  100
              Ca III
           ┌─────────────┐
           │x  y  z -y  -z│
r-flup   LRWAFKLYDLDNDGYITRNEMLDIVDAIYQMVGNTVELPEEENTPEKRVD  150
h-flup   ----L--------------------------------------------  150
d-frq    -Q---R---V--------E--YN----------QQPQ•S-D----Q----  149
              Ca IV
           ┌─────────────┐
           │x  y  z -y -x  -z│
r-flup   RIFAMMDKNADGKLTLQEFQEGSKADPSIVQALSLYDGLL            190
h-flup   ---------------------------------------            190
d-frq    K--DQ----H------E--R-------R-------GG-              187
```

Figure 1. Deduced protein sequences of the flup-proteins. Amino acid sequences are given for the open reading frame of the cloned r-flup and h-flup. The sequences are compared to *Drosophila* frequenin (d-frq)(Pongs *et al.*, 1993). Identical amino acids are indicated by vertical bars. For optimal alignment, one gap indicated by a (•) was introduced into the d-frq sequence. EF-hands are indicated by brackets with a Roman numeral (I-IV) above the amino acid sequences. The predicted Ca^{2+}-contact-sites are marked by x, y, z, -x, -y, and -z. Open triangles mark protein kinase C, and closed triangles protein kinase A, consensus phosphorylation sites.

mobility shift assays with recombinant expressed proteins. The protein sequences show consensus sequences for phosphorylation and for *N*-myristoylation (MGKSNS in flup proteins). The fatty acids are probably responsible for membrane association of the proteins in a Ca^{2+}-dependent manner. In rat synaptosome preparations r-flup was detected in the membrane fraction (P2) when Ca^{2+} was present. In preparation with Ca^{2+}-free conditions r-flup was found in the soluble fraction (S2). The same result was obtained with h-flup in HEK 293 cell homogenates.

Antibodies

Antibodies are available from the authors.

Anatomical localization

In situ hybridizations (IHS) and immunocytochemical analysis of r-flup indicated widespread occurrence in embryonic rat tissue. The most intense hybridization signals were obtained in the spinal ganglia and the developing brain. The expression seems to be specific for neurons with no detectable staining in glial cells. The most intense signals were found in retina, neocortical layers, thalamic nuclei, inferior colliculus, cerebellum, and hippocampus (stratum moleculare, dentate gyrus). High resolution IHS analysis of this area revealed a dendritic localization of the transcript.

Biological activities

In HEK 293 cells h-flup is involved in the phosphatase/kinase dependent regulation of the activity of a voltage

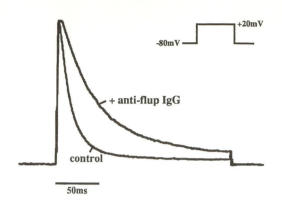

Figure 3. Rapid A-type K_v channel inactivation depends on flup activity. Microinjected anti-flup IgGs slow the inactivation of K_v 1.4 (RCK4) stably expressed in HEK 293 cells. (1) anti-flup-IgG (300 ng/ml); (2) control (preimmune IgGs, 1 mg/ml). HEK cells were plated on cellocates® (Eppendorf, Germany) and whole-cell patch recordings were performed 1–2 h after injection.

activated, rapidly inactivating (A-type) potassium (K_v 1.4) channel (Stümer *et al.* 1989). A rise in the intracellular Ca^{2+}-concentration (from 20 to 200 nM) leads to activation of calcineurin which modulates the inactivation behavior of K_v 1.4. When calcineurin activity is blocked by a specific inhibitor peptide, the rapid inactivation is slowed down. This effect can by mimicked by injecting anti-flup antibodies into K_v 1.4 expressing HEK 293 cells, suggesting a close interaction of flup with the Ca^{2+}-sensitive phosphatase 2B, calcineurin (Fig. 3).

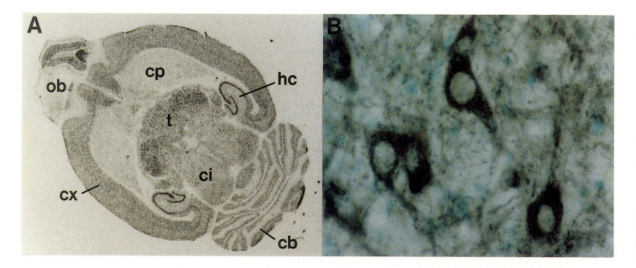

Figure 2. Localization of r-flup RNA and protein in rat brain. (A) *In situ* hybridization of flup transcripts in horizontal sections of P30 rat brain probed with ^{33}P-endlabeled antisense oligonucleotides: ob, olfactory bulb; ci, inferior colliculus; cp, caudate putamen; cx, neocortex; hc, hippocampus; t, thalamic nuclei. (B) Anti-r-flup staining of thalamic neurons, × 400.

References

Lindemeier, J., Röper J., Hauenschild, A., and Pongs, O. (1995) Frequenin-like Ca²⁺-binding protein (flup) modulates fast inactivation of mammalian presynaptic A-type K-channel. Neuron (submitted).

Pongs, O., Lindemeier, J., Zhu, X.R., Theil, T., Engelkamp, D., Krah-Jentgens, I., Lambrecht, H.-G., Koch, K.W., Schwemer, J., Rivosecchi, R., Mallart, A., Calceran, J., Canal, I., Barbas, J.A. and Ferrus, A., (1993) Frequenin-a novel calcium-binding protein that modulates synaptic efficacy in the *Drosophila* nervous system. Neuron **11**, 15–28.

Stühmer, W., Ruppersberg, P., Schröter, K., Sakmann B., Stocker M., Giese, K.P., Persckke, A., Baumann, A., and Pongs, O. (1989) Molecular basis of functional diversity of voltage-gated potassium channels in mammalian brain. EMBO J., **8**, 3235–3244.

■ *Jürgen Lindemeier, Jochen Röper, Alexander Hauenschild, and Olaf Pongs:*
Zentrum für Molekulare Neurobiologie,
Institut für Neurale Signalverarbeitung,
Martinistr. 52,
D-20246 Hamburg, Germany
Tel.: +49 40 4717 4811
Fax: +49 40 4717 5102
E-mail: lindemeier@zmnh.uni-hamburg.de

Vilip 1

Vilip 1 (Visinin-Like-Protein)1 is a neuronal Ca²⁺-binding protein expressed in a subpopulation of neurons in all parts of the brain and in the retina, starting from the onset of their terminal differentiation. Vilip interacts with cell membranes and, in a Ca²⁺-dependent manner, with components of the cortical cytoskeleton. One of the intracellular binding partners is actin. Vilip is hypothesized to be involved in the functional interaction of G protein-coupled receptors and the actin-based cytoskeleton.

The neuronal Ca²⁺-binding protein vilip has a molecular mass of about 22 kDa and a calculated isoelectric point of 4.9. The protein belongs to the visinin/recoverin sub-family of neuron-specific Ca²⁺-binding proteins (Yamagata *et al.* 1990; Dizhoor *et al.* 1991; Lenz *et al.* 1992) . Vilip is expressed by a subset of neurons of the chick brain and the retina (Lenz *et al.* 1992). Two of the four EF-hand Ca²⁺-binding motifs of vilip are able to bind either Ca²⁺ or Mg²⁺ in a non-cooperative manner. Binding of Ca²⁺, but not of Mg²⁺, to vilip leads to specific conformational changes in the protein. This may regulate the interaction of vilip with intracellular target molecules (Cox *et al.* 1994). Cell fractionation experiments in the presence or absence of Ca²⁺ have shown that vilip translocates from the cytoplasm to the particulate membrane fraction in the presence of Ca²⁺. This is partly due to the Ca²⁺-dependent interaction of vilip with the membrane-associated cytoskeleton. One of the binding partners of vilip has been identified as actin, a main component of the cortical cytoskeleton (Lenz *et al.* 1994).

■ Alternative names

The rat homolog of vilip displays 100% sequence identity with the chicken protein. It has been named NVP-1, for neural visinin-like protein 1 (Kuno *et al.* 1992; Kajimoto *et al.* 1993).

■ Isolation/identification

The vilip cDNA was isolated from a differentiation-specific cDNA library enriched for transcripts that are newly expressed in the chicken optic tectum during synaptic connection and terminal differentiation of the visual system, i.e. between day 7 of embryogenesis and the day of hatching (Lenz *et al.* 1992). NVP-1 was originally isolated from bovine brain by Ca²⁺-dependent hydrophobic-interaction chromatography and described as a 21 kDa CaBP (Walsh *et al.* 1984). Later, the complete amino acid sequence of its rat homolog was deduced from cloned cDNA obtained by screening with oligonucleotides that were based on partial amino acid sequences (Kuno *et al.* 1992).

■ Gene and sequences

Two transcripts of 2.9 kb and 1.6 kb derived from the *vilip*-gene only differ in the length of the 3′-untranslated region and the level of expression (Lenz *et al.* 1992). The vilip cDNA clone corresponds to the 1.6 kb transcript which has an open reading frame of 191 amino acids. The deduced protein has a calculated molecular mass of 22,144 Da and contains four internal repeats of 36–38 amino acids, each containing a potential EF-hand domain. Vilip/NVP-1 displays 40% amino acid sequence identity with visinin (Yamagata *et al.* 1990) and 46% identity with recoverin/S-modulin (Dizhoor *et al.* 1991; Kawamura *et al.* 1992). Vilip and NVP-1 sequences are

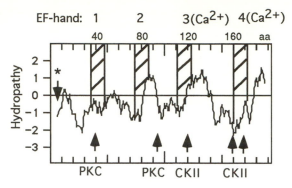

Figure 1. Hydropathy blot according to Kyte–Doolittle and EF-hand distribution of vilip. Putative sites for myristoylation (asterisk) and phosphorylation (upwards arrows) are indicated.

accessible in the EMBL/GenBank/DDBJ Nucleotide Sequence Databases under the accession numbers X63530 and D10666, respectively.

■ Protein

Vilip possesses four EF-hand motifs. The motif of EF-hand 1 is degenerated and most likely does not bind Ca^{2+}. Two of the motifs (most likely EF-hands 3 and 4) are capable of binding Ca^{2+}-ions in a non-cooperative manner with affinity constants of about 1.0 μM (Cox et al. 1994). Like other members of the visinin/recoverin sub-family, vilip has a potential N-terminal myristoylation site. Several potential phosphorylation sites for protein kinase C (PKC) and casein kinase II (CKII) are located within or in the vicinity of the EF-hands (Fig. 1).

■ Antibodies

Polyclonal antibodies against bacterially expressed vilip have been raised in rats and rabbits (DeRaad et al. 1995; Lenz et al. in preparation). Commercial antibodies are not available.

■ Localization

In situ hybridization has shown that vilip transcripts are widely distributed throughout the brain (Lenz et al. 1992). Vilip is expressed only in a sub-population of brain and retinal neurons. Immunohistochemical studies, e.g. of the cerebellum (Fig. 2), have revealed that a subset of granule cells, but not Purkinje cells, contain vilip.

Immunoreactivity is detected in all parts of the neurons including cell bodies, axons, and dendrites as well as presynaptic and post-synaptic structures (Lenz et al. 1994). In the retina vilip transcripts are present in neurons of the ganglion cell layer and the inner nuclear

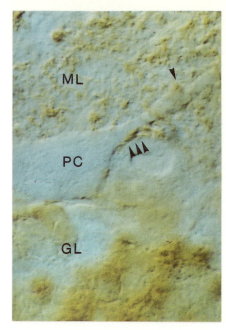

Figure 2. Immunohistochemical localization of vilip in climbing fiber synapses projecting on to Purkinje cell (PC) dendrites in the chick cerebellum (arrowheads). Purkinje cells themselves do not express vilip. Granule cell layer (GL) and molecular layer (ML) are indicated.

layer, but not in photoreceptor cells (Lenz et al. 1992; DeRaad et al. 1995).

■ Biological activities

Flow dialysis for Ca^{2+} binding, and equilibrium gel filtration for Mg^{2+}-binding have shown that bacterially expressed vilip has only two active Ca^{2+}/Mg^{2+}-binding sites (Cox et al. 1994). Recombinant vilip binds Ca^{2+} and Mg^{2+} with affinity constants K'_{Ca} of 1×10^6 M^{-1} and K'_{Mg} of 4.8×10^{-3} M^{-1}, respectively. The Ca^{2+}-bound, but not the metal-free, form of vilip is able to interact with hydrophobic matrices such as phenyl-Sepharose, indicating that exposure of hydrophobic amino acids to the surface occurs upon Ca^{2+} binding. This switch may regulate the interaction of vilip with intracellular target molecules (Cox et al. 1994). Ca^{2+}-dependent interaction with a hydrophobic matrix has also been shown for the bovine and rat homologs NVP-1 (Kuno et al. 1992; Walsh et al. 1984).

■ Interactions and possible functions

Using the overlay technique, vilip has been shown to interact in a Ca^{2+}-dependent manner with several binding partners in cytosolic and particulate membrane fractions of chicken brain. Further fractionation has revealed binding of vilip to the cortical cytoskeleton. One of the binding partners has been identified as actin (Lenz et al. 1994). In addition, though vilip is not expressed in retinal photoreceptor cells (Lenz et al. 1992), it displays an S-modulin-like activity in vitro, i.e. it inhibits rhodopsin phosphorylation at high but not at low Ca^{2+} concentrations (chapter on the NCS sub-family). These results suggest that vilip may play a functional role in the modulation of the interaction of G protein-coupled receptors with the cortical cytoskeleton.

■ References

*Cox, J.A., Isabelle, D., Compte, M., Nef, P., Lenz, S.E., and Gundelfinger, E.D. (1994) Cation binding and conformational changes in vilip and NCS-1, two neuron-specific calcium-binding proteins. J. Biol. Chem. **269**, 32807–32813.

DeRaad S., Compte M., Nef P., Lenz S.E., Gundelfinger E.D., and Cox J.A. (1995) Distribution pattern of three neural calcium-binding proteins-NCS1, vilip and recoverin-in chicken, bovine and rat retinas. Histochem. J. **27**, 524–535.

Dizhoor, A.M., Ray, S., Kumar, S., Niemi, G., Spencer, M., Brolley, D., Walsh, K.A., Philipov, P.P., Hurlay, J.B., and Stryer, L. (1991) Recoverin: a calcium sensitive activator of retinal rod guanylate cyclase. Science **251**, 915–918.

Kajimoto, Y., Shirai, Y., Mukai, H., Kuno, T., and Tanaka, C. (1993) Molecular cloning of two additional members of the neural visinin-like Ca^{2+}-binding protein gene family. J. Neurochem. **61**, 1091–1096.

Kawamura, S., Takamatsu, K., and Kitamura, K. (1992) Purification and characterization of S-modulin, a calcium-dependent regulator on cGMP phosphodiesterase in frog rod photoreceptors. Biochem. Biophys. Res. Commun. **186**, 411–417.

*Kuno, T., Kajimoto, Y., Hashimoto, T., Mukai, H., Shirai, Y., Saheki, S., and Tanaka, C. (1992) cDNA cloning of a neural visinin-like Ca^{2+}-binding protein. Biochem. Biophys. Res. Commun. **184**, 1219–1225.

Lenz, S.E., Henschel, Y., Zopf, D., Voss, B., and Gundelfinger, E.D. (1992) Vilip, a cognate protein of the retinal calcium binding proteins visinin and recoverin, is expressed in the developing chicken brain. Mol. Brain Res. **15**, 133–140.

*Lenz, S.E., Braun, K., Braunewell, K.-H., and Gundelfinger, E.D. (1994) Vilip–Ca^{2+}-dependent interaction with cell membrane and cytoskeleton. J. Neurochem. **63**, Suppl. 1, p. 72.

Walsh, M.P., Valentine, K.A., Ngai, P.K., Carruthers, C.A., and Hollenberg, M.D. (1984) Ca^{2+}-dependent hydrophobic-interaction chromatography: Isolation of a novel Ca^{2+}-binding protein and protein kinase C from bovine brain. Biochem. J. **224**, 117–127.

Yamagata, K., Goto, K., Kuo, C.H., Kondo, H., and Miki, N. (1990) Visinin: A novel calcium binding protein expressed in retinal cone cells. Neuron **2**, 469–476.

■ *Karl-Heinz Braunewell, Stefan E. Lenz, and Eckart D. Gundelfinger:*
Department of Neurochemistry and Molecular Biology,
Federal Institute for Neurobiology,
P.O. Box 1860, D-39008 Magdeburg, Germany
Tel.: + 49 391 6263 228
Fax: + 49 391 6263 229
E-mail: braunew@jupiter.ifn-magdeburg.de or gundelfinger@ifn-magdeburg.de

Vilip2

Vilip2, from rat, is a member of a large family of neuronal Ca^{2+}-binding proteins (named the NCS subfamily) composed of eighteen related amino acid sequences, including visinin, S-modulin, recoverin, NCS-1, Ce-NCS-1, Ce-NCS-2, vilip1, vilip3, hippocalcin, neurocalcin, hlp2, and frequenin. Vilip2 has 89% of identity with vilip1, and the lowest score of identity within the NCS family is with visinin (40%). In brain, two abundant mRNA species of 6.5 and 1.6 kb hybridize to a vilip2 probe. Vilip2 is not detected in other tissues, except in the testis, although at a lower level, where a 2.4 kb mRNA hybridizes to vilip2. The highest amount of vilip2 mRNA is observed in the hippocampus. Only a small amount is detected in the cerebellum and pons plus medulla oblongata.

A general description of the subfamily of neuronal calcium sensors (NCS) is presented in the introductory chapter. Vilip2 is a member of the NCS subfamily shown to be expressed in the rat brain and, at a lower level, in rat testis (Kajimoto et al. 1993). As shown in Table 1, vilip2 has 40–89% of homology with the other members of the NCS family. By evolutionary tree analysis (see the NCS tree, introduction chapter), vilip2 is found on branch III of the NCS family tree, in close association with vilip1 from rat/chick. Homologs of the vilip2 gene have not yet been found.

Vilip2 has a calculated molecular mass of 22,245 Da and a theoretical isolectric point of 4.75.

■ Alternative names

Neural visinin-like Ca^{2+}-binding protein 2, NVP-2 (Kajimoto et al. 1993); Vilip2 (De Castro et al. 1995)

Table 1. Comparison of the vilip2 amino acid (a.a.) sequence (in % of identity) with other members of the NCS subfamily

% of a.a. identity	Chick visinin	Human recoverin	*C. elegans* Ce-NCS-2	Chick/rat NCS-1	Human hlp2	Bovine neurocalcin	Rat vilip3	Chick/rat vilip1
Vilip2	40	46	47	55	66	66	67	89

Identification/isolation

The full-length vilip2 cDNA clone (named pK329) was obtained by screening a λgt10 rat brain cDNA library at low stringency with the rat vilip1 (or NVP-1) probe (Kuno *et al.* 1992).

Gene and sequence

Vilip2 accession numbers are D13125 (GenBank) and P35332 (SwissProt).

Protein

Vilip2 consists of 191 amino acids with four potential EF-hand domains. The first site is ancestral and probably not functional since a lysine residue and a cysteine residue are found at positions X and Y, respectively, of the Ca^{2+}-binding loop. The other EF-hand sites are predicted by the pattern recognition program Prosite to represent three potential Ca^{2+}-binding sites. Unlike recoverin, S-modulin, and visinin, a myristoylation consensus site at the amino terminus of vilip2 is not detected with the pattern recognition program Prosite.

Anatomical localization

The tissue and gross regional distributions of vilip2 were determined by Northern blot analysis. Vilip2 mRNA is abundant, and found in many regions of the brain including cortex, hippocampus, hypothalamus, thalamus, midbrain, olfactory bulb, and caudate putamen. However, low amounts of vilip2 mRNA are present in the cerebellum and pons plus medulla oblongata.

References

De Castro, E., Nef, S., Fiumelli, H., Lenz, E.S., Kawamura, S., and Nef, P. (1995) Regulation of rhodopsin phosphorylation by a family of neuronal calcium sensors. Biochem. Biophys. Res. Commun. **216**, 133–140.

Kajimoto, Y., Shirai, Y., Mukai, H., Kuno, T., and Tanaka, C. (1993) Molecular cloning of two additional members of the neural visinin- like Ca^{2+}-binding protein gene family. J. Neurochem. **61**, 1091–1096.

Kuno, T., Kajimoto, Y., Hashimoto, T., Mukai, H., Shirai, Y., Saheki, S., and Tanaka, C. (1992) cDNA cloning of a neural visinin-like Ca^{2+}-binding protein. Biochem. Biophys. Res. Commun. **184**, 1219–1225.

■ *Patrick Nef:*
Biochemistry Dept., Sciences II,
University of Geneva,
30 quai Ernest Ansermet,
CH-1211 Geneva 4, Switzerland
Tel.: +41 22 702 64 81
Fax: +41 22 702 64 83
E-mail: Patrick.Nef@biochem.unige.ch

Vilip3

Vilip3, from rat, is a member of a large family of neuronal Ca²⁺-binding proteins (named the NCS subfamily) composed of eighteen related amino acid sequences, including visinin, S-modulin, recoverin, NCS-1, Ce-NCS-1, Ce-NCS-2, vilip1, vilip2, hippocalcin, neurocalcin, hlp2, and frequenin. Rat vilip3 has 97% of amino acid identity with its human homologue, hlp2. The lowest score of identity within the NCS family is with S-modulin (48%) and Ce-NCS-2 (49%). In brain, an abundant mRNA species of 1.6 kb hybridizes to a vilip3 probe. Vilip3 is not detected in other tissues, although barely detectable levels of vilip3 mRNA are detected in the lung, spleen, and skeletal muscle. The highest amounts of vilip3 mRNA are observed in the cerebellum and in pons plus medulla oblongata. In other brain regions, vilip3 gene expression is not detected, except at a low level in the hypothalamus and thalamus.

A general description of the family of neuronal calcium sensors (NCS) is presented in the introductory chapter. Vilip3 is a member of the NCS family, and is specifically expressed in the rat brain. Barely detectable levels are observed in the lung, spleen, and skeletal muscle (Kajimoto *et al.* 1993). As shown in Table 1, vilip3 has 49–97% of homology with the other members of the NCS family. By evolutionary tree analysis (see the NCS family tree, introduction chapter), vilip3 is located on branch III of the NCS tree, in close association with human hlp2, its homologue.

Vilip3 has a calculated molecular mass of 22,063 Da and a theoretical isolectric point of 5.45. Human hlp2 has a calculated molecular mass of 22,312 Da and an isolectric point of 5.07.

Alternative names

Neural visinin-like Ca²⁺-binding protein 3, NVP-3 (Kajimoto *et al.* 1993); vilip3 (De Castro *et al.* 1995); human hlp2 or bdr-1 (Kobayashi *et al.* 1994).

Identification/isolation

The full-length vilip3 cDNA clone (named pK395) was obtained by screening a λgt10 rat brain cDNA library at low stringency with the rat vilip1 (or NVP-1) probe (Kuno *et al.* 1992). The human hlp2 cDNA, the homolog of rat vilip3, was isolated from a human hippocampus cDNA library using a rat hippocalcin probe under low stringency conditions.

Gene and sequence

Vilip3 accession numbers are D13126 (GenBank) and P35332 (SwissProt). Human hlp2 accession numbers are D16227 (GenBank) and P37235 (SwissProt). Using the genomic DNA panel (Bios Lab.) composed of 18 human–hamster somatic cell hybrids, the hlp2 gene was mapped on human chromosome 2 (Kobayashi *et al.* 1994).

Protein

Vilip3 and hlp2 consist of 193 amino acids with four potential EF-hand domains. The first site is ancestral and probably not functional since a lysine residue and a cysteine residue are found at positions X and Y, respectively, of the Ca²⁺-binding loop. The other EF-hand sites are predicted by the pattern recognition program Prosite to represent three potential Ca²⁺-binding sites. Unlike recoverin, S-modulin, and visinin, a myristoylation consensus site at the amino terminus of vilip3 or hlp2 is not detected with the pattern recognition program Prosite.

Anatomical localization

The tissue and gross regional distributions of vilip3 were determined by Northern blot analysis. Vilip3 mRNA is only abundant in the cerebellum; it is also found in the pons plus medulla oblongata. Other regions of the brain, including cortex, hippocampus, hypothalamus, thalamus, midbrain, olfactory bulb, and caudate putamen, are not positive for villip3. Hlp2 gene expression in human was also determined by Northern analysis; hlp2 mRNA was found only in the brain. No hlp2 signal was detected in

Table 1. Comparison of the vilip3 amino acid (a.a.) sequence (in % of identity) with other members of the NCS family

% of a.a. identity	*C. elegans* Ce-NCS-2	Chick visinin	Human recoverin	Chick/rat NCS-1	Bovine neurocalcin	Rat vilip3	Chick/rat vilip1	Human hlp2
Vilip3	49	49	50	59	67	67	69	97

the human heart, placenta, lung, liver, skeletal muscle, kidney, or pancreas.

References

De Castro, E., Nef, S., Fiumelli, H., Lenz, E.S., Kawamura, S., and Nef, P. (1995) Regulation of rhodopsin phosphorylation by a family of neuronal calcium sensors. Biochem. Biophys. Res. Commun. **216**, 133–140.

Kajimoto, Y., Shirai, Y., Mukai, H., Kuno, T., and Tanaka, C. (1993) Molecular cloning of two additional members of the neural visinin- like Ca^{2+}-binding protein gene family. J. Neurochem. **61**, 1091–1096.

Kobayashi, M., Takamatsu, K., Fujishiro, M., Saitoh, S., and Noguchi, T. (1994) Molecular cloning of a novel calcium-binding protein structurally related to hippocalcin from human brain and chromosomal mapping of its gene. Biochemica et Biophysica Acta **1222**, 515–518.

Kuno, T., Kajimoto, Y., Hashimoto, T., Mukai, H., Shirai, Y., Saheki, S., and Tanaka, C. (1992) cDNA cloning of a neural visinin-like Ca^{2+}-binding protein. Biochem. Biophys. Res. Commun. **184**, 1219–1225.

■ *Patrick Nef:*
Biochemistry Dept., Sciences II,
University of Geneva,
30 quai Ernest Ansermet,
CH-1211 Geneva 4, Switzerland
Tel.: +41 22 702 64 81
Fax: +41 22 702 64 83
E-mail: Patrick.Nef@biochem.unige.ch

NCS-1

NCS-1 is a neuronal calcium sensor which regulates receptor phosphorylation in a Ca^{2+}-dependent manner. It is a member of a large family of neuronal Ca^{2+}-binding proteins (named the NCS subfamily) composed of 18 related amino acid sequences, including visinin, S-modulin, recoverin, Ce-NCS-2, vilip1, vilip2, vilip3, hippocalcin, neurocalcin, hlp2, frequenin. NCS-1 is highly conserved during evolution, because chick, rat, and mouse NCS-1 proteins possess 100% of amino acid identity, and because NCS-1 orthologs from C. elegans (Ce-NCS-1, 75%) and Drosophila (frequenin, 72%) have been isolated. NCS-1 proteins are specifically expressed in postmitotic neurons in several regions of the entire nervous system. NCS-1, as a regulator of G-protein-coupled receptor desensitization, may, in turn, participate in the regulation of signal transduction and of Ca^{2+}-dependent synaptic efficacy.

A general description of the family of neuronal calcium sensors (NCS) is presented in the introductory chapter. The NCS-1 subfamily is composed of four highly homologous sequences that have been isolated in species including chick NCS-1 (De Castro *et al.* 1995); rat and mouse NCS-1 (De Castro *et al.* 1995), C. elegans (named Ce-NCS-1, De Castro *et al.* 1995a), and Drosophila (named frequenin, Pongs *et al.* 1993). As shown in Table 1, rodent and avian NCS-1 have identical amino acid sequences, whereas C. elegans and Drosophila orthologs exhibit a very high score of homology (72–75%) with rat, chick, or mouse NCS-1.

Chick (or rat) NCS-1 has a calculated molecular mass of 21,878 Daltons and a theoretical isolectric point of 4.53.

Table 1. Comparison of amino acid (a.a.) sequence identity (in %) among four NCS-1 homologs

% of a.a. identity	Chick NCS-1	C. elegans Ce-NCS-1	Drosophila frequenin
Rat/mouse NCS-1	100	75	72
Chick NCS-1	–	75	72
C. elegans Ce-NCS-1		–	72

NCS-1 mRNA and protein expressions are detected in postmitotic neurons of several regions of the nervous system throughout the entire development (Nef *et al.* 1995). NCS-1 gene expression is turned on at very early stages during embryogenesis (~E3 in the chick) and persists in newborn and adult animals. In the adult rat, NCS-1 labeling is concentrated in neuronal cell bodies and axons throughout the brain. NCS-1 labeling is not detected in glial cells. The most intense labeling is seen in cell bodies of retina neurons, brainstem neurons in the pons and medulla, and also in myelinated axons of the corpus callosum, internal capsule, anterior commissure, pyramidal tract, and cerebellar white matter (Nef *et al.* unpublished). Some non-myelinated axons are also labeled including the axons of basket cells in the cerebellum. Purkinje neurons and dendrites are lightly labeled. In the forebrain, labeling is observed in cell bodies and dendrites of hippocampal neurons in the dentate gyrus and pyramidal cell layers. Pyramidal neurons in the cerebral cortex as well as neurons in the neostriatum, olfactory bulb, and basal forebrain are also NCS-1 positive. Axon terminals in the central nervous system are not labeled for NCS-1, whereas presynaptic NCS-1 labeling is observed at neuromuscular junctions. By EM, the subcellular distribution of NCS-1 labeling is observed in cell bodies, dendrites, and axons. NCS-1 is present in several postsynaptic densities in dendrites from brain regions including CA1, CA3 hippocampal neurons and brainstem neurons (Nef *et al.*, unpublished).

Consistent with its subcellular distribution, NCS-1 regulates the phosphorylation of G-protein-coupled receptors in a Ca^{2+}-dependent manner. *In vitro*, NCS-1 from rat, chick, mouse and *C. elegans* (De Castro *et al.* 1995a). inhibit the phosphorylation of rhodopsin at high physiological Ca^{2+} concentrations (~10 μM). However, at low physiological Ca^{2+} concentration (~10 nM), rhodopsin desensitization is not affected by NCS-1. The subcellular distributions and the "*in vitro*" function suggest a potential role for NCS-1 in Ca^{2+}-triggered synapses. NCS-1, through the regulation of receptor desensitization, may modulate synaptic efficacy such as facilitation.

Alternative names

The *C. elegans* ortholog of chick/rat NCS-1 displays 75% of amino acid identity. It has been named Ce-NCS-1. Another likely ortholog of NCS-1 is frequenin from *Drosophila*, with 75% of amino acid identity.

Identification/isolation

Degenerated primers were designed to code for conserved regions of three members of the NCS subfamily (vilip1, visinin, and recoverin) and were used in a RT-PCR experiment to amplify chick brain cDNA (Nef *et al.* 1995). The RT-PCR product contained several members of the NCS family, among them NCS-1. The full-length NCS-1 clone (named RL25) was obtained by screening a chick brain cDNA library at high stringency (Nef *et al.* 1995). NCS-1 homologous genes in other species were isolated by screening cDNA librairies from rat brain, mouse brain, and *C. elegans* at low stringency with the chick NCS-1 full-length probe (De Castro *et al.* 1995). The entire open reading frame of the chick NCS-1 cDNA was inserted in the pET 8c vector for overexpression in *E. coli*, and NCS-1 was purified by affinity chromatography on a phenyl sepharose column.

Gene and sequence

Chick and rat NCS-1 accession numbers are P36610 (SwissProt) and L27420-L27421 (GenBank). Ce-NCS-1 accession number is L33680 (GenBank), and *Drosophila* frequenin is L08064 (GenBank). A genomic phage encoding the mouse NCS-1 gene has been partially sequenced (De Castro *et al.* 1995a). It possesses an exon (encoding residues 31–76) which has 5′ and 3′ exon borders which are identical to the 5′ end of exon 5 and the 3′ end of exon 6 of frequenin, the *Drosophila* homolog of NCS-1.

Protein

NCS-1 amino acid sequence has been highly conserved throughout evolution (Fig. 1) and consists of 190 amino acids with four potential EF-hand domains. The first site is ancestral and probably not functional since a lysine residue and a cysteine residue are found at positions X and Y, respectively, of the Ca^{2+}-binding loop. The other EF-hand sites are predicted by the pattern recognition program Prosite to represent three potential Ca^{2+}-binding sites. There is 59% of amino acid identity between the chick or rat NCS-1 and vilip3, 58% with neurocalcin, 57% with hippocalcin, 57% with vilip1, 55% with vilip2, 46% with recoverin, 45% with Ce-NCS-2, 43% with S-modulin, and 40% with visinin.

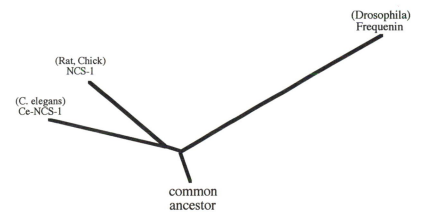

Figure 1. Phylogenetic tree analysis of NCS-1 homologs (Branch II). NCS-1 amino acid sequences from distant species including rat, chick, *Drosophila*, and *C. elegans* have been analysed with the program TREE developed by R.F. Doolittle, UCSD, La Jolla, USA. The minimum mutation matrix of Dayhoff was used to determine the distance scores between each pair of aligned sequences.

On SDS-PAGE gels, the native forms of NCS-1 purified from different nervous tissues or the recombinant NCS-1 purified from *E. coli* migrate with the same apparent molecular mass of 22 kDa. By mass spectroscopic analysis, the molecular mass of NCS-1 produced by overexpression in *E. coli* is 21,755 +/- 3.5 Da, suggesting that the first methionine is removed from the recombinant protein. The recombinant form of NCS-1 crystallizes and its structure is being analyzed by X-ray diffraction (Sygusch and Nef, unpublished). In contrast to recoverin, S-modulin, visinin, and *Ce*-NCS-2, a myristoylation consensus site at the amino terminus of NCS-1 was not detected with the pattern recognition program Prosite. This observation suggests that when NCS-1 is associated with membranes, it is probably not via a *N*-myristoylated amino terminus (Kawamura *et al.* 1994).

■ Antibodies

Polyclonal antibodies specific for NCS-1 that do not cross-react with recoverin, vilip1, or other members of the NCS subfamily, are available from the author.

■ Anatomical localization

Antibodies against NCS-1 are excellent markers for post-mitotic neurons in several regions (retina, brain, neuromuscular junction) of the central and peripheral nervous systems. NCS-1 labeled regions consist of cell body, dendrites, and axons of several neuronal cell types. By EM, NCS-1 labeling is also detected in postsynaptic densities of central neurons, and in presynaptic nerve terminals at neuromuscular junctions (Nef *et al.*, unpublished).

■ Biological activites

In vitro, NCS-1 inhibits the phosphorylation of a G-protein-coupled receptor, rhodopsin, only at high physiological Ca^{2+} concentrations. At low physiological Ca^{2+} concentration, rhodopsin phosphorylation is not affected by NCS-1. A similar function was observed with the majority of the members of the NCS subfamily, including native S-modulin and recoverin, as well as recombinant *Ce*-NCS-1, *Ce*-NCS-2, recoverin, vilip1, and hippocalcin (Kawamura 1994). In such an assay, calmodulin and ovalbumin have no effect on rhodopsin phosphorylation (Kawamura *et al.* 1994).

■ Biological regulation

Similarly to calmodulin, the binding of Ca^{2+} to NCS-1 induced allosteric changes and the exposure of hydrophobic surfaces. Only the Ca^{2+}- and the Ca^{2+}/Mg^{2+}-loaded forms possess strong solvent-exposed hydrophobic patches which are likely to represent the sites of interaction with potential targets.

■ Interaction

Although the target(s) of NCS-1 are not yet identified, it is quite possible that rhodopsin kinase, and perhaps other members of the G-protein-coupled receptor kinase (GRK) subfamily, are modulated by NCS-1. Surprisingly, NCS-1 co-localizes with neurofilament in myelinated axons.

■ References

De Castro, E., Nef, S., Fiumelli, H., Lenz, E.S., Kawamura, S., and Nef, P. (1995) Regulation of rhodopsin phosphorylation by a family of neuronal calcium sensors. Biochem. Biophys. Res. Commun. **216**, 133–140.

Kawamura, S. (1994) Photoreceptor light-adaptation mediated by S-modulin, a member of a possible regulatory protein family of protein phosphorylation in signal transduction. Neurosci. Res. **20**, 293–298.

Kawamura, S., Cox, J.A., and Nef, P. (1994) Inhibition of rhodopsin phosphorylation by non-myristoylated recombinant recoverin. Biochem. Biophys. Res. Commun. **203**, 121–127.

Nef, S., Fiumelli, H., De Castro, E., Raes, M.-B., and Nef, P. (1995) Identification of a neuronal calcium sensor (NCS-1) possibly involved in the regulation of receptor phosphorylation. J. Recept. Res. **15**, 365–378.

Pongs, O., Lindemeier, J., Zhu, X.R., Theil, T., Engelkamp, D., Krah-Jentgens, I., Lambrecht, H.G., Koch, K.W., Schwemer, J., Rivosecchi, R., Mallart, A., Galceran, J., Canal, I., Barbas, J.A., and Ferrus, A. (1993) Frequenin, a novel calcium-binding protein that modulates synaptic efficacy in the *Drosophila* nervous system. Neuron **11**, 15–28.

■ *Patrick Nef:*
Biochemistry Dept., Sciences II, University of Geneva, 30 quai Ernest Ansermet, CH-1211 Geneva 4, Switzerland
Tel.: +41 22 702 64 81
Fax: +41 22 702 64 83
E-mail: Patrick.Nef@biochem.unige.ch

S-modulin

S-modulin (sensitivity-modulating protein) is a Ca^{2+}-binding protein found in frog retinal photoreceptors. It inhibits phosphorylation of a photoreceptive molecule, rhodopsin, at high Ca^{2+} concentrations and thereby increases the light-sensitivity of photoreceptor cells during dark adaptation.

S-modulin was found in frog retinal rod photoreceptors (Kawamura and Murakami 1991) and is composed of 201 amino acids; its calculated molecular mass is 23 kDa; the apparent molecular mass on an SDS gel is 26 kDa; the isoelectric point is 5.8. It has four putative EF-hand structures but probably only two of them (EF 2 and 3) are occupied. At the N-terminus, S-modulin has a consensus *N*-myristoylation site (Kawamura *et al.*, 1993) and therefore the N-terminal glycine is probably lipidated as has been shown for a bovine homolog, recoverin (Dizhoor *et al.*, 1992). At high Ca^{2+} concentrations, S-modulin inhibits phosphorylation of a photoactivated rhodopsin (Kawamura 1993). Recently many S-modulin-like proteins were found in neurons and they have been grouped into a new protein family (Nef *et al.* 1995). According to their amino acid sequences, they are classified into four sub-families. All members from each sub-family so far tested (S-modulin, recoverin, NCS-1 or RL25, vilip1, hippocalcin) inhibited the phosphorylation reaction at 10 μM Ca^{2+} (Kawamura 1994). This result suggests that the role of the proteins in this family is to regulate the phosphorylation reaction in their host cells.

Alternative names

Recoverin (which is the bovine homolog to S-modulin; Dizhoor *et al.*, 1991; Kawamura *et al.*, 1993).

Isolation

S-Modulin can be purified by two-step column chromatography (Kawamura *et al.*, 1992). S-Modulin binds to membranes at high Ca^{2+} concentrations, but its binding is weak (half-binding; ~10 μM Ca^{2+}). For isolation, firstly S-modulin should be extracted into an aqueous phase by homogenization of fragmented rod outer segments at low Ca^{2+} concentrations. After centrifugation, the concentration of Ca^{2+} in the supernatant is increased by adding $CaCl_2$ and it is applied to a phenyl-sepharose column equilibrated with the same buffer solution. The Ca^{2+}-bound form of S-modulin binds to the column and is eluted by reducing the Ca^{2+} concentration. Before elution, the column must be washed extensively with a high Ca^{2+} buffer. S-modulin is eluted by applying a low Ca^{2+} and low salt solution, for example, a solution containing 10 mM HEPES, 30 mM NaCl, 3 mM EGTA (pH 7.5). Then the eluate is applied to a DEAE column. S-Modulin is obtained and purified in a pass-through fraction from the DEAE column. Approximately 5 μg of S-modulin can be obtained per frog.

Since S-modulin is sticky, it is highly recommended to coat tubes, etc. with ovalbumin to avoid a loss of S-modulin during purification. We do not use BSA as the coating material because BSA has effects on some enzyme reactions; for example, cGMP phosphodiesterase activation in photoreceptors. The irreversible binding to plastics and glasswares is more pronounced at high Ca^{2+} concentrations. For this reason, addition of a small amount of EGTA is recommended during storage. The addition of EGTA also prevents aggregation of S-modulin.

Gene and sequence

The amino acid sequence of S-modulin is deduced from its cDNA (Kawamura *et al.*, 1993; accession number: Swiss Prot. P31227). Its amino acid identity to recoverins (human, bovine and mouse) is 79–83% and to visinin (chick) is 62%.

Protein

The binding of Ca^{2+} to S-modulin has been shown with the protein blotted on a nylon membrane. S-modulin shows Ca^{2+}-dependent binding to disk membranes. However, the binding target has not been identified: Ca^{2+}/S-modulin complex binds to disk membranes treated with proteolytic enzyme and does not bind to liposomes constructed by commercially available various phospholipids (Kawamura *et al.*, 1992).

Antibodies

An anti-S-modulin antibody (from rabbit) is now available through the author.

Anatomical localization

So far, no histochemical attempts have been made to localize S-modulin in the retina. However, S-modulin was obtained from an isolated rod outer segment preparation (Kawamura and Murakami 1991). The bovine homolog, recoverin has been shown to be present in photoreceptor inner and outer segments by immunohistochemistry (Dizhoor *et al.*, 1991).

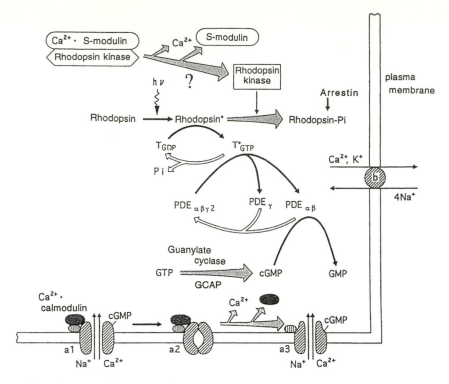

Figure 1. A scheme of the phototransduction and the adaptation mechanisms in a rod. Filled arrows indicate the reactions activated in the presence of light. Open arrows indicate the inactivation processes. Gray arrows indicate the reactions activated at low [Ca^{2+}] during light-adaptation. Symbols are: Rhodopsin*, light-activated rhodopsin; Rhodopsin-Pi, phosphorylated rhodopsin; T_{GDP}, inactive transducin; T_{GTP}*, active transducin; $PDE_{\alpha\beta\gamma2}$, inactive cGMP phosphodiesterase; $PD_{\alpha\beta}$, active PDE; GCAP, guanylate cyclase activating protein; a1, activated cGMP-gated channel desensitized by Ca^{2+}/calmodulin; a2, inactive cGMP-gated channel; a3, active cGMP-gated channel sensitized by dissociation of Ca^{2+}/calmodulin; b, Na^+-Ca^{2+}/K^+ exchanger. The inhibition of the rhodopsin kinase by the direct binding of Ca^{2+}/S-modulin has not been established, but is indicated in this figure as one of the possibilities. (Modified from Kawamura 1994.)

■ Biological activity

In rod photoreceptors, rhodopsin absorbs light and this light detection is converted into an electrical signal. This mechanism, the phototransduction mechanism, is summarized in Fig. 1. Briefly, the absorption of a photon by rhodopsin induces a conformational change of the protein leading to its active form (R*). R* then activates a GTP-binding protein, transducin (T) by replacing bound GDP (T_{GDP}) for GTP (T_{GTP}). The active form of transducin (T_{GTP}) activates a cGMP-hydrolyzing enzyme, the cGMP phosphodiesterase (PDE), which leads to a decrease of the intracellular cGMP concentration as a result of light absorption by rhodopsin.

In the plasma membrane of rods a cGMP-activated channel is present. In the dark Na+ and Ca^{2+} enter the cell through the open channel. When the cGMP concentration decreases in the light, the cGMP dissociates from the channel resulting in a closure of the channel. Since the

steady inward current carried by Na+ and Ca^{2+} is bocked in the light the cell hyperpolarizes.

R* is inactivated by phosphorylation of its C-terminal region. Arrestin binds to the phosphorylated rhodopsin to ensure its inactivation. S-Modulin inhibits this phosphorylation reaction at high Ca^{2+} concentrations and prolongs the lifetime of R* (Kawamura 1993). Since the intracellular Ca^{2+} concentration is high in the dark (Nakatani and Yau 1988), S-modulin prolongs the lifetime of R* and therefore increases the light-sensitivity of a rod in the dark (Kawamura 1993). When a rod is exposed to a steady light, the intracellular Ca^{2+} concentration decreases (Nakatani and Yau 1988). S-Modulin does not inhibit rhodopsin phosphorylation under these conditions, and thus, the lifetime of R* is short, and the light-sensitivity of the cell becomes low. By this mechanism, S-modulin regulates the light sensitivity of the photoreceptor (for details, see Kawamura 1994).

■ References

Dizhoor, A.M., Ray, S., Kumar, S., Niemi, G., Spencer, M., Brolley, D., Walsh, K.A., Philipov, P.P, Hurley, J.B., and Stryer, L. (1991) Recoverin: a calcium sensitive activator of retinal guanylate cyclase. Science **251**, 915–918.

Dizhoor, A.M., Ericsson, L.H., Johnson, R.S., Kumar, S., Olshevskaya, E., Zozulya, S., Neubert, T.A., Stryer, L., Hurley, J.B., and Walsh, K.A. (1992) The NH$_2$ terminus of retinal recoverin is acylated by a small family of fatty acids. J. Biol. Chem. **267**, 16033–16036.

*Kawamura, S. (1993) Rhodopsin phosphorylation as a mechanism of cyclic GMP phosphodiesterase regulation by S-modulin. Nature **362**, 855–857.

*Kawamura, S. (1994) Photoreceptor light-adaptation mediated by S-modulin, a member of a possible regulatory protein family of protein phosphorylation in signal transduction. Neurosci. Res. **20**, 293–298.

*Kawamura, S. and Murakami, M. (1991) Calcium-dependent regulation of cyclic GMP phosphodiesterase by a protein from frog retinal rods. Nature **349**, 420–423.

Kawamura, S., Takamatsu, K., and Kitamura, K. (1992) Purification and characterization of S-modulin, a calcium-dependent regulator on cGMP phosphodiesterase in frog rod photoreceptors. Biochem. Biophys. Res. Commun. **186**, 411–417.

Kawamura, S., Hisatomi, O., Kayada, S., Tokunaga, F., and Kuo, C.-H. (1993) Recoverin has S-modulin activity in frog rods. J. Biol. Chem. **268**, 14579–14582.

Nakatani, K. and Yau, K.-W. (1988) Calcium and light adaptation in retinal rods and cones. Nature **334**, 69–71.

Nef, S., De Castro, E., and Nef, P. (1995) Identification of a neuronal calcium sensor (NCS-1) possibly involved in the regulation of receptor phosphorylation. J. Recep. Sig. Transduc. **15**, 365–378.

■ *Satoru Kawamura*:
Department of Biology,
Faculty of Science,
Osaka University,
Machikane-yama 1-1,
Toyonaka, Osaka 560, Japan
Tel.: +81 6 850 5436
Fax: +81 6 850 5444
Email: kawamura@bio.sci.osaka-u.ac.jp

Ce-NCS-2

Ce-NCS-2, from C. elegans, *is a member of a large family of neuronal Ca^{2+}-binding proteins (named the NCS subfamily) composed of 18 related amino acid sequences, including visinin, S-modulin, recoverin, NCS-1, vilip1, vilip2, vilip3, hippocalcin, neurocalcin, hlp2, and frequenin. Ce-NCS-2 is a neuronal calcium sensor from* C. elegans, *which regulates receptor phosphorylation in a Ca^{2+}-dependent manner, like several members of the NCS subfamily such as S-modulin, NCS-1, Ce-NCS-1, vilip1, or hippocalcin. Ce-NCS-2 is the most divergent sequence of the NCS subfamily, since it possesses only 37–49% of amino acid identity when compared to the other members of the NCS subfamily. As a regulator of G-protein-coupled receptor desensitization, Ce-NCS-2, like Ce-NCS-1, may participate in the regulation of signal transduction and of Ca2+-dependent synaptic plasticity in the worm nervous system.*

A general description of the subfamily of neuronal calcium sensors (NCS) is presented in the introductory chapter. *Ce*-NCS-2, is the second member of the NCS subfamily (with *Ce*-NCS-1) to be expressed in *Caenorhabditis elegans* (De Castro *et al.* 1995), and to date, no homologous gene for NCS-2 has been found in other species. As shown in Table 1, *Ce*-NCS-2 possesses 37–49% amino acid identity compared to the other members of the NCS subfamily.

Ce-NCS-2 has a calculated molecular mass of 21,985 Da and a theoretical isolectric point of 4.92.

Ce-NCS-2 may regulate the phosphorylation of G-protein-coupled receptors in a Ca^{2+}-dependent manner. Indeed, like NCS-1 from rat, chick, mouse (De Castro *et al.* 1995) and *Ce*-NCS-1 from *C. elegans* (De Castro *et al.* 1995), *Ce*-NCS-2 inhibits the phosphorylation of rhodopsin at high physiological Ca^{2+} concentrations (~10 μM) but not at low physiological Ca^{2+} concentration (~10 nM). The *in vitro* function of NCS-2 suggests a potential role for this protein in Ca^{2+}-triggered synapses, and in the regulation of receptor desensitization that may modulate synaptic efficacy in *C. elegans*.

■ Identification/isolation

The full-length *Ce*-NCS-2 cDNA clone was obtained by screening a *C. elegans* cDNA library at low stringency with a *Ce*-NCS-1 probe (Nef *et al.* 1995). The entire open reading frame of *Ce*-NCS-2 was inserted in the pET8c vector for overexpression in *E. coli*, and the corresponding recombinant *Ce*-NCS-2 protein was purified by affinity chromatography on a phenyl sepharose column.

■ Gene and sequence

Ce-NCS-2 accession number is L33681 (GenBank). The gene is represented as a single copy in the *C. elegans* genome, covers ~3 kb in length, and contains several small exons and introns.

Table 1. Comparison of the Ce-NCS-2 amino acid (a.a.) sequence (in % of identity) with other members of the NCS subfamily

% of a.a. identity	Chick visinin	Human recoverin	*C. elegans* Ce-NCS-1	Rat NCS-1	Rat vilip1	Human hlp2	Rat vilip3	Bovine neurocalcin
Ce-NCS-2	37	44	45	45	47	48	49	49

■ Protein

Ce-NCS-2 consists of 190 amino acids with four potential EF-hand domains. The first site is ancestral and probably not functional since a glutamine residue and a cysteine residue are found at positions X and Y, respectively, of the Ca^{2+}-binding loop. The other EF-hand sites are predicted by the pattern recognition program Prosite to represent three potential Ca^{2+}-binding sites. On SDS-PAGE gels, the recombinant Ce-NCS-2 purified from *E. coli* migrates with an apparent molecular mass of 22 kDa. Similarly to recoverin, S-modulin, and visinin, a myristoylation consensus site at the amino terminus of Ce-NCS-2 is detected with the pattern recognition program Prosite. This observation suggests that Ce-NCS-2 could be associated with membranes probably via its N-myristoylated amino terminus (Kawamura et al. 1994).

■ Antibodies

Polyclonal antibodies specific for Ce-NCS-2 and that do not crossreact with Ce-NCS-1 are available from the author.

■ Anatomical localization

Antibodies against Ce-NCS-2 are currently being tested for immunostaining of *C. elegans* neurons.

■ Biological activities

In vitro, Ce-NCS-2 inhibits the phosphorylation of a G protein-coupled receptor, rhodopsin, only at high physiological Ca^{2+} concentrations. At low physiological Ca^{2+} concentration, rhodopsin phosphorylation is not affected by Ce-NCS-2. A similar function was observed with the majority of the members of the NCS subfamily, including native S-modulin and recoverin, as well as recombinant NCS-1, Ce-NCS-1, recoverin, vilip1, and hippocalcin (Kawamura 1994; De Castro et al. 1995). In such an assay, calmodulin and ovalbumin have no effect on rhodopsin phosphorylation (Kawamura et al. 1994).

■ References

De Castro, E., Nef, S., Fiumelli, H., Lenz, E.S., Kawamura, S., and Nef, P. (1995) Regulation of rhodopsin phosphorylation by a family of neuronal calcium sensors. Biochem. Biophys. Res. Commun. **216**, 133–140.

Kawamura, S. (1994) Photoreceptor light-adaptation mediated by S-modulin, a member of a possible regulatory protein family of protein phosphorylation in signal transduction. Neurosci. Res. **20**, 293–298.

Kawamura, S., Cox, JA., and Nef, P. (1994) Inhibition of rhodopsin phosphorylation by non-myristoylated recombinant recoverin. Biochem. Biophys. Res. Commun. **203**, 121–127.

Nef, S., Fiumelli, H., De Castro, E., Raes, M.-B., and Nef, P. (1995) Identification of a neuronal calcium sensor (NCS-1) possibly involved in the regulation of receptor phosphorylation. J. Recept. Res. **15**, 365–378.

■ *Patrick Nef:*
Biochemistry Dept., Sciences II,
University of Geneva,
30 quai Ernest Ansermet,
CH-1211 Geneva 4, Switzerland
Tel.: +41 22 702 64 81
Fax: +41 22 702 64 83
E-mail: Patrick.nef@biochem.unige.ch

Recoverin

Recoverin is a heterogeneously acylated Ca²⁺-binding protein expressed primarily in vertebrate photoreceptor cells. Recoverin prolongs light-stimulated hydrolysis of cyclic GMP (cGMP) in photoreceptors by inhibiting rhodopsin phosphorylation in a Ca²⁺-dependent manner. A specific Ca²⁺-dependent interaction between recoverin and rhodopsin kinase underlies the effect of recoverin on rhodopsin phosphorylation.

Recoverin has an apparent molecular mass of 26 kDa on SDS-PAGE. The calculated M_r of the unmodified recoverin without its N-terminal methionine is 23,203 and its calculated isoelectric point is 5.2. The N-terminus of recoverin purified from bovine retinas is heterogeneously acylated by one of the four fatty acids, C14:0, C14:1, C14:2, or C12:0 (Dizhoor et al. 1992). N-acylation of recoverin plays an essential role in Ca²⁺-dependent membrane targeting (Dizhoor et al. 1993) through a novel Ca²⁺-myristoyl switch mechanism (Zozulya and Stryer 1992). Recoverin represents a recently identified family of neuronal-specific Ca²⁺-binding proteins which includes hippocalcin, neurocalcin, visinin, S-modulin, vilip, frequenin and Guanylyl Cyclase Activating Protein (GCAP). Recoverin was initially described as a Ca²⁺-sensitive activator of guanylyl cyclase, but this function has not been confirmed (Hurley et al. 1993). Its effects in prolonging the photoresponse (Gray-Keller et al. 1993), activating cGMP phosphodiesterase (PDE) (Kawamura et al. 1993), and inhibiting rhodopsin phosphorylation (Kawamura 1993) are widely accepted.

■ Alternative names

p26 (Polans et al. 1991), S-modulin (Kawamura and Murakami, 1991). Recoverin from bovine retinas and S-modulin from frog retinas are 83% identical and are functionally interchangeable (Kawamura et al. 1993).

■ Identification/isolation

Recoverin was first described as a Ca²⁺ sensitive activator of retinal guanylyl cyclase (Dizhoor et al. 1991; Lambrecht and Koch 1991). S-modulin was initially described as a protein that stimulates and prolongs light-stimulated cGMP hydrolysis (Kawamura and Murakami 1991). Recoverin was also recognized as the CAR antigen because it reacts with sera from patients who develop cancer-associated retinopathy (Polans et al. 1991). Due to its abundance in the retina (rhodopsin : recoverin = 20:1) and its Ca²⁺-binding properties, recoverin is readily purified by phenyl Sepharose chromatography (Polans et al. 1991) followed by monoQ FPLC. Bacterial expression of both unmodified and myristoylated recoverin has facilitated the structural and functional studies of recoverin (Ray et al. 1992).

■ Protein

The structure of unmodified recoverin containing a single bound Ca²⁺ has been solved by X-ray crystallography (Flaherty et al. 1993). Recoverin contains 4 EF-hand domains (referred to as EF-1, EF-2, EF-3, EF-4, in the N- to C-terminal direction). The four EF-hand domains are arranged in a compact, linear array in contrast to the dumb-bell arrangement seen in the crystal structures of other Ca²⁺-binding proteins such as calmodulin and troponin C. Ca²⁺ binds only to EF-3 in the crystal form of recoverin; however, Sm³⁺ binds to both EF-2 and EF-3. An unusual concave hydrophobic surface is formed by conserved nonpolar residues from EF-1 and EF-2. This hydrophobic "patch" may be a docking site for the fatty acyl group linked to the N-terminus or for a target protein. Recently the secondary structure of Ca²⁺-free myristoylated recoverin has been determined by multidimensional heteronuclear NMR (Ames et al. 1994). In this structure, the most N-terminal helix of EF-2 is flexible in the myristoylated Ca²⁺-free recoverin, whereas it has a well-defined structure in the unmodified Ca²⁺-bound form. This difference suggests that the binding of Ca²⁺ to EF-3 induces EF-2 to adopt a conformation favorable for the binding of a second Ca²⁺ to recoverin. It has also been shown that the N-terminal helix (K5-E16) in myristoylated Ca²⁺-free recoverin is significantly longer than that in unmyristoylated Ca²⁺-bound recoverin.

■ Localization

Recoverin is present in outer segments, cell bodies, and synaptic region of photoreceptors. It is also present in pineal and certain cone bipolar cells (Milam et al. 1993).

■ Interactions

Three proteins, interphotoreceptor retinoid binding protein (IRBP), tubulin, and rhodopsin kinase (RK), interact with immobilized recoverin in a Ca²⁺-dependent manner (Chen et al. 1995). The interaction of recoverin with RK is highly specific and essential for recoverin's inhibitory effect on rhodopsin phosphorylation. The RK/Rv interaction does not require N-acylation of recoverin. The IRBP/recoverin interaction requires N-acylation of recoverin, but this interaction may not be physiologically relevant because most IRBP is extracellular while recoverin is intracellular. The physiological role of recoverin/tubulin interaction has yet to be determined. Recoverin also interacts with rod outer segment (ROS) membranes in a Ca^{2+}-dependent manner. This interaction requires N-acylation of recoverin. It is not clear if recoverin interacts directly with the phospholipid or if it interacts with a receptor on the membranes (Dizhoor *et al.* 1993).

■ Biological activity

When dialyzed into sealed ROS, recoverin prolonged the photoresponse (Gray-Keller *et al.* 1993). *In vitro*, recoverin inhibits rhodopsin phosphorylation in a Ca^{2+}-dependent manner. There are disparate reports about this Ca^{2+}-dependency of recoverin's action. Original reports indicated that the IC_{50} of both recoverin and S-modulin was 100–200 nM free Ca^{2+} concentration, but recent studies indicate that the IC_{50} may be significantly higher (Klenchin *et al.* 1994; Chen *et al.* 1995).

■ References

Ames, J.B., Tanaka, T., Stryer, L., and Ikura, M. (1994) Secondary structure of myristoylated recoverin determined by three-dimensional heteronuclear NMR: implications for the calcium-myristoyl switch. Biochemistry **33**, 10743–10753.

Chen, C.-K., Inglese, J., Lefkowitz, R.J., and Hurley, J.B. (1994) Ca^{2+}-dependent interaction of recoverin with rhodopsin kinase as a regulator mechanism in rhodopsin signalling, J. Biol. Chem. **270**, 18060–18066.

Dizhoor, A.M., Ray, S., Kumar, S., Niemi, G., Spencer, M., Brolley, D., Walsh, K.A., Philipov, P.P., Hurley, J. B., and Stryer, L. (1991) Recoverin: a calcium sensitive activator of retinal rod guanylate cyclase. Science **251**, 915–918.

Dizhoor, A.M., Ericsson, L.H., Johnson, R.S., Kumar, S., Olshevskaya, E., Zozulya, S., Neubert, T.A., Stryer, L., Hurley, J.B., and Walsh, K.A. (1992) The NH_2 terminus of retinal recoverin is acylated by a small family of fatty acids. J. Biol. Chem. **267**, 16033–16036.

Dizhoor, A.M., Chen, C.-K., Olshevskaya, E., Sinelnikova, V.V., Phillipov, P., and Hurley, J.B. (1993) Role of the acylated amino terminus of recoverin in Ca^{2+}-dependent membrane interaction. Science **259**, 829–832.

Flaherty, K.M., Zozulya, S., Stryer, L., and McKay, D.B. (1993) Three dimensional structure of recoverin, a calcium sensor in vision. Cell **75**, 709–716.

Gray-Keller, M.P., Polans, A.S., Palczewski, K., and Detwiler, P.B. (1993) The effect of recoverin-like calcium-binding proteins on the photoresponse of retinal rods. Neuron **10**, 523–531.

Hurley, J.B., Dizhoor, A.M., Ray, S., and Stryer, L. (1993) Recoverin's role: conclusion withdrawn. Science **260**, 740.

Kawamura, S. (1993) Rhodopsin phosphorylation as a mechanism of cyclic GMP phosphodiesterase regulation by S-modulin. Nature **362**, 855–857.

Kawamura, S. and Murakami, M. (1991) Calcium-dependent regulation of cyclic GMP phosphodiesterase by a protein from frog retinal rods. Nature **349**, 420–423.

Kawamura, S., Hisatomi, O., Kayada, S., Tokunaga, F., and Kuo, C.H. (1993) Recoverin has S-modulin activity in frog rods. J. Biol. Chem. **268**, 14579–14582.

Klenchin, V.A., Calvert, P.D., and Bownds, M.D. (1994) Calcium dependence of rhodopsin phosphorylation in frog photoreceptor outer segments. Biophys. J. **66**, A48.

Lambrecht, H.G. and Koch, K.W. (1991) A 26 kd calcium binding protein from bovine rod outer segments as modulator of photoreceptor guanylage cyclase. EMBO J. **10**, 793–798.

Milam, A.H., Dacey, D.M., and Dizhoor, A.M. (1993) Recoverin immunoreactivity in mammalian cone bipolar cells. Vis. Neurosci. **10**, 1–12.

Polans, A.S., Buczylko, J., Crabb J., and Palczewski, K. (1991) A photoreceptor calcium binding protein is recognized by autoantibodies obtained from patients with cancer-associated retinopahty. J. Cell Biol. **112**, 981–989.

Ray, S., Zozulya, S., Niemi, G.A., Flaherty, K.M., Brolley, D., Dizhoor, A.M., McKay, D.B., Hurley, J.B., and Stryer, L. (1992) Cloning, expression and crystallization of recoverin, a calcium sensor in vision. Proc. Natl. Acad. Sci. USA. **89**, 5705–5709.

Zozulya, S. and Stryer, L. (1992) Calcium-myristoyl protein switch. Proc. Natl. Acad. Sci. USA. **89**, 11569–11573.

■ *Ching-Kang Chen and James B. Hurley:*
Department of Biochemistry, SJ-70 and Howard Hughes Medical Institute, SL-15,
University of Washington, Seattle, WA98195,USA

Visinin

Visinin is a soluble Ca^{2+}-binding protein with three functional EF-hand structures, expressed in cone photoreceptors of various vertebrate retinae. Its putative physiological function is to regulate phototransduction via delaying the termination of phototransduction cascade in cone photoreceptors.

Chicken visinin has a calculated molecular weight of 22,500 and migrates with an apparent molecular mass of 24 kDa on SDS-PAGE. Its isoelectric point is 5.1. Visinin is exclusively expressed in the inner segment and outer nuclear layers of cone photoreceptors of vertebrate retinae.

It consists of three functional EF-hand domains and has a striking homology to other retina-derived (such as recoverin and s-modulin) and brain-derived (neurocalcin, hippocalcin, neural visinin-like proteins, vilips, etc.) members of the neuron specific calcium sensors subfamily (NCS).

The NH_2-terminal sequences of all members of the visinin family meet the criteria for NH_2-terminal myristoylation. This modification has been shown to be related to their association with cell membranes. Recently, recoverin and visinin have been reported to prolong the rising phase of the light response (Gray-Keller *et al.* 1993).

■ Isolation/identification

Visinin was originally identified as a retinal protein that increases in concentration during development (Hatakenaka *et al.* 1983). This protein was purified from soluble fractions of chicken retinae with sequential chromatographic steps including DEAE-cellulose and Sephadex G-75 gel-filtration. Antibodies were raised against the purified protein (Hatakenaka *et al.* 1985) and used to isolate visinin cDNA from a chick retinal expression library (Yamagata *et al.* 1990).

■ Gene and sequences

The sequence of visinin cDNA contains 576 bases of one open reading frame (GenBank accession number M84729). It encodes a 192 amino acid polypeptide.

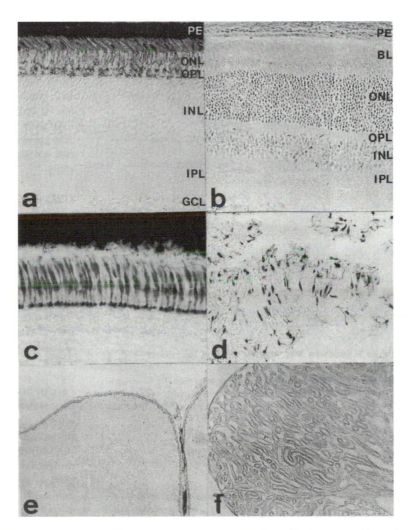

Figure 1. Immunohistochemistry with affinity-purified visinin antibodies. Chick (a), rat (b), and goldfish (c) retinal sections and chick pineal (d), cerebellar (e), and renal (f) sections were stained with affinity-purified visinin antibodies. (a) The inner segments and outer nuclear layers of the chick retina (photoreceptor cell layer) were stained. (b) No immunoreactive cells are seen in the rat retina. (c) Visinin protein is just localized in cone photoreceptors of the goldfish retina. (d) Some pinealocytes were stained. (e) No immunoreactive cells are seen. (f) No immunoreactive cells are observed. Abbreviations; PE, pigment epithelium; IS, inner segments; ONL, outer nuclear layer; OPL, outer plexiform layer; INL, inner nuclear layer; IPL, inner plexiform layer; GCL, ganglion cell layer; BL, photoreceptors layer.

Protein

The predicted amino acid sequence of visinin contains three putative Ca^{2+}-binding domains of the EF-hand type. The molecular weight and isoelectric point are 22,514 and 5.1, respectively. Blots with ^{45}Ca demonstrate that the recombinant visinin protein binds ^{45}Ca. Although the first EF-hand domain does not seem to satisfy the structural criteria for a high-affinity Ca^{2+}-binding site, Kobayashi *et al.* (1993) showed that all of the three EF-hands of hippocalcin, which is a member of NCS-family, had Ca^{2+}-binding activity on ^{45}Ca-blot analysis. This suggests that visinin may also have the ability to bind 3 mol of Ca^{2+} per mol of protein.

Antibodies

Antibodies specific for visinin, which do not crossreact with calbindin D-28k, are available from the authors (Hatakenaka *et al.* 1983).

Localization

The inner segment, the outer nuclear layer of chick cone photoreceptors, and some pinealocytes were stained with affinity-purified visinin antibodies (Fig. 1). These antibodies also reacted with cone photoreceptors of various species including goldfish, carp, frog, and turtle (Yamagata *et al.* 1990 and unpublished data). Rod photoreceptors failed to react with these antibodies. Therefore, visinin is exclusively expressed in cone photoreceptors and represents an excellent marker for them.

Biological activities

Recently, recoverin and visinin have been reported to prolong the rising phase of the light response, while having no effect on the kinetics of response-recovery (Gray-Keller *et al.* 1993). Visinin is thought to delay the termination of the phototransduction cascade rather than affecting the resynthesis of cyclic GMP and recovering of the dark current in cone photoreceptors.

Biological regulation

Continuous environmental light induced an increase in the number of visinin-positive cells in chick pineal body. Furthermore, visinin protein was also induced by direct light stimulation of an explant culture of the pineal body (Goto *et al.* 1990). Visinin seems to be a good marker for investigating direct photosensitivity of the pinealocytes.

References

Hatakenaka, S., Kuo, C.-H., and Miki, N. (1983) Analysis of a distinctive protein in chick retina during development. Dev. Brain Res. **10**, 155–163.

Hatakenaka, S., Kiyama, H., Tohyama, M., and Miki, N. (1985) Immunohistochemical localization of chick retinal 24 kdalton protein (Visinin) in various vertebrate retinae. Brain Res. **331**, 209–215.

*Goto, K., Yamagata, K., Miki, N., and Kondo, H. (1990) Direct photosensitivity of chick pinealocytes as demonstrated by visinin immunoreactivity. Cell Tissue Res. **262**, 501–505.

*Gray-Keller, M.P., Polans, A.S., Palczewski, K., and Detwiler, P.B. (1993) The effect of recoverin-like calcium-binding proteins on the photoresponse of retinal rods. Neuron **10**, 523–531.

Kobayashi, M., Takamatsu, K., Saitoh, S., and Noguchi, T. (1993) Myristoylation of hippocalcin is linked to its calcium-dependent membrane-association properties. J. Biol. Chem. **268**, 18898–18904.

*Yamagata. K., Goto, K., Kuo, C.-H., Kondo, H., and Miki, N. (1990) Visinin: a novel calcium binding protein expressed in retinal cone cells. Neuron **4**, 469–476.

■ *Kanato Yamagata and Naomasa Miki:*
Department of Pharmacology I,
Osaka University School of Medicine,
2–2 Yamadaoka, Suita 565,
Japan
Tel.: +81 6 879 3521
Fax: +81 6 879 3529
E-mail: Kyamagat@pharma1.med.osaka-u.ac.jp

Parvalbumin

Parvalbumin (PV) is a soluble Ca²⁺-binding protein found at highest concentration in fast contracting/relaxing muscle fibers of vertebrates. In the muscle PV is believed to facilitate the transfer of Ca²⁺ from the myofibrils to the sarcoplasmic reticulum. PV is also found in certain neurons and subpopulations of cells in endocrine glands where its function has not been established.

Parvalbumin (PV) is a polypeptide consisting of 107 to 113 amino acids and has an apparent M_r of 12 000 to 14 000 on SDS-PAGE gels. Sequences of PVs from many lower and higher vertebrate species are known from protein and cDNA analysis (Moncrief *et al.* 1990). Based on IEP values, sequences and structural characterization, PVs have been classified into α and β lineages. α PVs consist mostly of 109 amino acids with p/s of approximately 5 and β PVs have mostly 108 amino acids and p/s of around 4. α and β PVs occur in the same species. In mammals β PV is known under the name oncomodulin (see chapter on oncomodulin). In chickens two β PVs have been described (see chapter on avian thymus hormone.).

The three-dimensional structure of carp 4.25 PV (4.25 indicates the IEP) was reported in 1973 (Kretsinger and Nockolds 1973) and serves as a model for high affinity Ca²⁺-binding characteristics since PV was the first Ca²⁺-binding protein to be analysed on the level of its 3D structure. The term EF-hand was deduced from the C-terminal functional Ca²⁺-binding domain (E-helix–loop–F-helix) in carp PV. PV is expressed at high levels in the fast anaerobic IIB muscle fibres which are found most frequently in fast contracting/relaxing muscles. PV exhibits a neuron-specific distribution in the brain and is frequently localized in fast firing nerve cells, especially in GABA-ergic neurons (reviewed in Celio 1986; Berchtold 1989). Literature on the anatomical localization of PV in the nervous system has increased exponentially during recent years since this protein, together with calbindin, has proven to be an excellent neuronal marker, as exemplified in Fig. 1 (Celio 1990).

■ Identification/isolation

Already in 1952 PV had obtained its name from its albumin-like solubility (parv = small) (Henrotte 1952). PV can be isolated in large amounts from muscle tissues by conventional biochemical methods (Strehler *et al.* 1977) or from brain (Berchtold *et al.* 1982). Generally, a heat treatment preceeds an ammonium sulfate precipitation followed by ion exchange chromatography. A detailed method for isolating recombinant PV is described in Pauls and Berchtold (1993). PV is found in the fast skeletal muscle of vertebrates in millimolar concentrations (reviewed in Heizmann 1984) whereas in neurons concentrations generally do not exceed 50 μmolar (Plogmann and Celio 1993).

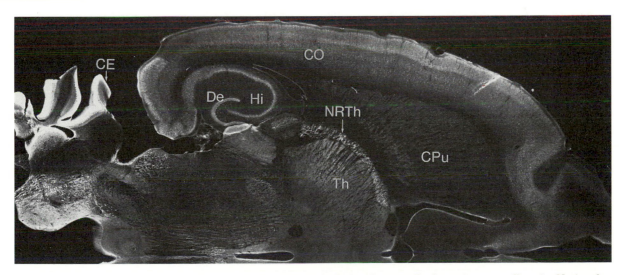

Figure 1. Horizontal section of the adult rat brain immunolabelled with an antibody against parvalbumin. Notice the selective labelling of various brain regions. Ce, cerebellum; De, dentate nucleus; Co, cerebral cortex; Cpu, caudate-putamen; Hi, hippocampus; NRTh, reticular nucleus of the thalamus; Th, thalamus. Modified from Celio (1990).

■ Gene and sequence

PV gene structure of human, mouse and rat are known (reviewed in Berchtold 1989 and Pauls *et al.* 1996).

Accession nos., genes (Genembl, release 40.4/9.94): human, Em_pr: Hsparval1-5; mouse, Em_ro: Mmpvaex1-5; rat, Em_ro: Rnpalb1-5.

Accession nos., cDNAs (Genembl, release 40.0/9.94): human, Em_pr: Hsparval; mouse, Em_ro: Mmpva; rat, Em_ro: Rnpalb; *X. laevis*, Em_ov: x1pal.

The PV gene is located on human chromosome 22 and mouse chromosome 15 (Berchtold 1993).

■ Protein

PV contains three EF-hand domains of which two (CD and EF) are functional high affinity Ca^{2+}-binding sites of the Ca^{2+}/Mg^{2+} mixed type, with metal-binding characteristics as described in Eberhard and Erne (1994) and Pauls *et al.* (1993). In contrast, the N-terminal domain (AB) is non-functional, due to the deletion of two amino acids in the Ca^{2+}-binding loop. In most cases the two functional sites have equivalent binding properties and bind Ca^{2+} in a noncooperative fashion. Accession nos., origin, and length of sequences as well as lineages are listed in Table 1.

■ Antibodies

Monospecific and monoclonal antibodies are available through Sigma and Swant.

Table 1. Accession numbers of parvalbumins

Accession Nos		Lineage	Length (AA)	Species
sequence	3D-structure			
Sw: Prva_Ampme		ALPHA	109	*Amphiuma means* (salamander) (two toed amphiuma)
Sw: Prva_Cypca		ALPHA (A1)	108	*Cypimus carpio* (common carp)
Sw: Prva_Esolu		ALPHA	108	*Esox lucius* (northern pike)
Sw: Prva_Felca		ALPHA	109	*Felis catus* (cat)
Sw: Prva_Gersp		ALPHA	109	*Gebrillus* sp. (gebril)
Sw: Prva_Human		ALPHA	109	*H. sapiens* (human)
Sw: Prva_Latch		ALPHA	111	*Latimeria chalumnae* (latineria coelacanth)
Sw: Prva_Macfu		ALPHA	109	*Macaca fuscata* (Japanese macaque)
Sw: Prva_Mouse		ALPHA	109	*Mus musculus* (mouse)
Sw: Prva_Rabit		ALPHA	109	*Oryctolagus coniculus* (rabbit)
Sw: Prva_Rajcl		ALPHA	109	*Raja clavata* (thornback ray)
Sw: Prva_Ranca		ALPHA	110	*Rana catesbeiana* (bull frog)
Sw: Prva_Ranes		ALPHA	109	*Rana esculenta* (edible frog)
Sw: Prva_Rat	Nrl: 1rtpa	ALPHA	109	*Rattus norvegicus* (rat)
Sw: Prva_Trise	nrl: 5 pal	ALPHA	109	*Triakis semifasciata* (leopard shark)
Pir3: S11054		ALPHA	109	*Rana catesbeiana* (bull frog)
Pir3: S27208		ALPHA	109	*Meriones unguiculatus* (mongolian jiid)
Pir3: S27210		ALPHA	109	*Macaca fuscata* (Japanese macaque)
Sw: Prvm_Chick		ALPHA	109	*Gallus gallus* (chicken)
Sw: Prvb_Ampme		BETA	108	*Amphiuma means* (salamander) (two toed amphiuma)
Sw: Prvb_Boaco		BETA	109	*Boa constrictor* (boa)
Sw: Prvb_Cypca	nrl: 4cpv	BETA	108	*Cyprinus carpio* (common carp)
Sw: Prvb_Esolu	nrl. 1pal.	BETA	107	*Esox lucius* (northern pike)
Sw: Prvb_Gadca		BETA	113	*Gadus callaria* (baltic cod)
Sw: Prvb_Grage		BETA	108	*Graptemys geographica* (map turtle)
Sw: Prvb_Latch		BETA	108	*Latimeria chalumnae* (latimeria) (coelacanth)
Sw: Prvb_Leuce		BETA	106	*Leuciscus cephalus* (chub)
Sw: Prvb_Merme		BETA	108	*Merluccius merluccius* (European hake)
Sw: Prvb_Mermr		BETA	108	*Merlangius merlangus* (whiting)
Sw: Prvb_Opsta		BETA	109	*Opsanus tau* (oyster toadfish)
Sw: Prvb_Ranes		BETA	108	*Rana esculenta* (edible frog)
Sw: Prvb_Xenla		BETA	108	*Xenopus laevis* (africans clawed frog)
Pir 1: Pvcd		BETA	113	*Gadus morhua callarias* (baltic cod)
Pir 1: Pvhk		BETA	108	*Merluccius merluccius* (European hake)

Only full length sequences were considered. Only sequences not present in the Swiss database (release 30.0/10.94) were taken from PIR (release 42.0/10.94). Accession nos. for 3D-information are from nrl_3D database (release 16/9.94). To avoid repetition, accession No. of oncomodulin and chicken thymus parvalbumins are not listed here.

Anatomical localization

Numerous publications exist concerning PV expression in the central and peripheral nervous system. The reader is, therefore, referred to reviews (Celio 1990; Heizmann and Braun, 1990). The distribution in non-neuronal tissues is reviewed in Berchtold and Means (1985) and Heizmann and Berchtold (1987). Except from muscle where PV occurs in high abundance this protein is found in seminal vesicles, the prostate, adipose tissue, testis, ovary, and kidney in decreasing order of levels.

Biological activities and developmental appearance

PV is thought to exert its biological activity through Ca^{2+}-binding with its two Ca^{2+}/Mg^{2+} mixed binding sites. In muscle, PV is proposed to act as a relaxing factor [reviewed in Berchtold (1989) Heizmann (1984) and Pauls et al. (1996)]. Recently, this was directly demonstrated by transfer of PV cDNA into the slow soleus muscle in vivo which caused an increase in relaxation speed (Müntener et al, 1995). PV has been shown to be down-regulated in the ADR (arrested development of righting response) mutant mouse but the PV gene does not directly cause the altered phenotype. PV was found to be overexpressed in fast skeleton muscle of mdx mice (Gailly et al. 1993). It has been hypothesized that PV could act in neurons as a Ca^{2+} buffer which protects cells from Ca^{2+} overload (Sloviter 1989). PV could therefore potentially inhibit Ca^{2+}-dependent apoptosis or modulate gene induction triggered by elevated intracellular Ca^{2+}. Overexpression of PV in C-127 mouse cells shortened the length of their G1 cell cycle phase (Rasmussen and Means 1989). Overexpression in a adenocarcinoma cell line showed a decrease in mitotic rate, changes in morphology from epitheloid to fusiform and an increase in motility of these cells (Andressen et al. 1995).

PV appears prenatally in the brain (Celio 1990). In rodent muscle PV synthesis starts at days 4–6 of postnatal development (Berchtold and Means 1985).

Mutagenesis studies

Site-directed mutagenesis of rat PV was carried out to study molecular mechanisms of metal interaction (Pauls et al. 1993, 1994). In a first step, Phe102 was replaced by a unique Trp in the central core, leading to a mutant, PV_{F102W}, with a suitable optical probe inside the protein and cation binding properties very similar to those of the recombinant wildtype protein, PV_{WT}. Subsequent modifications of PV_{F102W} with the goal to inactivate either the CD or the EF metal-binding domain indicated that the EF domain is dominant in terms of structural stability and thereby influences the metal-binding characteristics of the CD domain.

References

Andressen, C., Gotzos, V., Berchtold, M.W., Pauls, T.L., Schwaller, B., Fellay, B., and Celio, M.R. (1995) Changes in shape and motility of cells transfected with parvalbumin cDNA. Exp. Cell Res. **219**, 420–426.

*Berchtold, M.W. (1989) Structure and expression of genes encoding the three-domain Ca^{2+}-binding proteins parvalbumin and oncomodulin. Biochim. Biophys. Acta **1009**, 201–215.

Berchtold, M.W. (1993) Evolution of EF-hand calcium-modulated proteins. V. The genes encoding EF-hand proteins are not clustered in mammalian genomes. J. Mol. Evol. **36**, 489–496.

Berchtold, M.W. and Means, A.R. (1985) The Ca^{2+}-binding protein parvalbumin: molecular cloning and developmental regulation of mRNA abundance. Proc. Natl. Acad. Sci. USA **82**, 1414–1418.

Berchtold, M.W., Wilson, K.J., and Heizmann, C.W. (1982) Isolation of neuronal parvalbumin by high-performance liquid chromatography. Characterization and comparison with muscle parvalbumin. Biochemistry **21**, 6552–6557.

Celio, M.R. (1986) Parvalbumin in most γ-aminobutyric acid-containing neurons of the rat cerebral cortex. Science **231**, 995–997.

*Celio, M.R. (1990) Calbindin D-28k and parvalbumin in the rat nervous system. Neuroscience **35**, 375–475.

Eberhard, M. and Erne, P. (1994) Calcium and magnesium binding to rat parvalbumin. Eur. J. Biochem. **222**, 21–26.

Gailly, P., Hermans, E., Octave, J.N., and Gillis, J.M. (1993) Specific increase of genetic expression of parvalbumin in fast skeletal muscles of mdx mice. FEBS Lett. **326**, 272–274.

*Heizmann, C.W. (1984) Parvalbumin, an intracellular calcium-binding protein; properties and possible roles in mammalian cells. Experientia **40**, 910–921.

Heizmann, C.W. and Berchtold, M.W. (1987) Expression of parvalbumin and other Ca^{2+}-binding proteins in normal and tumor cells: A topical review. Cell Calcium **8**, 1–41.

Heizmann, C.W. and Braun, K. (1993) Calcium binding proteins: Molecular and functional aspects. In The role of calcium in biological systems ed. L.J. Anghileri, Vol **5**, (pp. 21–66. CRC Press).

Henrotte, J.G. (1952) A crystallin constituent from myogen of carp muscle. Nature **169**, 968–969.

Kretsinger, R.H. and Nockolds, C.E. (1973) Carp muscle calcium-binding protein. II. Structure determination and general description. J. Biol. Chem. **248**, 3313–3326.

Moncrief, N.D., Kretsinger, R.H., and Goodman, M. (1990) Evolution of EF-hand calcium-modulated proteins. I. Relationships based on amino acid sequences. J. Mol. Evol. **30**, 522–562.

Müntener, M., Käser, L., Weber, J., and Berchtold, M.W. (1995) Increase of skeletal muscle relaxation speed by direct injection of parvalbumin cDNA. Proc. Natl. Acad. Sci. USA **92**, 6504–6508.

Pauls, T.L. and Berchtold, M.W. (1993) Efficient complementary DNA amplification and expression using polymerase chain reaction technology. Methods Enzymol., **217**, 102–122.

Pauls, T.L., Cox, J.A., and Berchtold, M.W. (1996) The Ca^{2+}-binding proteins parvalbumin and oncomodulin and their genes: new structural and functional findings. Biochim. Biophys. Acta (in press).

Pauls, T.L., Durussel, I., Cox, J.A., Clark, I.D., Szabo, A.G., Gagné, S.M., Sykes, B.D., and Berchtold, M.W. (1993) Metal binding properties of recombinant rat parvalbumin wild-type and F102W mutant. J. Biol. Chem. **268**, 20897–20903.

Pauls, T.L., Durussel, I., Berchtold, M.W., and Cox, J.A. (1994) Inactivation of individual Ca^{2+}-binding sites in the paired EF-hand domain of parvalbumin reveals asymmetrical metal-binding properties. Biochemistry **33**, 10303–10400.

Plogmann, D. and Celio, M.R. (1993) Intracellular concentrations of parvalbumin in nerve cells. Brain Res. **600**, 273–279.

Rasmussen, C.D. and Means, A.R. (1989) The presence of parvalbumin in a nonmuscle cell line attenuates progression through mitosis. Mol. Endocrinol. **3**, 588–596.

Sloviter, R.S. (1989) Calcium-binding protein (calbindin-D28k) and parvalbumin immunocytochemistry: Localization in the rat hippocampus with specific reference to the selective vulnerability of hippocampal neurons to seizure activity. J. Comp. Neurol. **280**, 183–196.

Strehler, E.E., Eppenberger, H.M., and Heizmann, C.W. (1977) Isolation and characterization of parvalbumin from chicken leg-muscle. FEBS Lett. **78**, 127–133.

■ Martin W. Berchtold:
Institute of Veterinary Biochemistry,
University of Zürich-Irchel,
Winterthurerstr. 190,
CH-8057 Zürich,
Switzerland
Tel.: 0041 1 257 54 73
Fax: 0041 1 362 05 01
E-mail: berchtol@vetbio.unizh.ch

Oncomodulin

Oncomodulin (OM) is a β-parvalbumin expressed during early development in the fetal placenta and in a variety of tumor cells. OM has some calmodulin-like activities with respect to enzyme activation and growth regulation. Its specific biological functions in developing tissues are unknown.

For general biophysical properties see chapter on parvalbumin. OM contains 108 amino acids and has a molecular mass (M_r) of 11 500 Da and an isoelectric point (IEP) of 3.8 to 4.0. In contrast to mammalian parvalbumin, OM contains a Ca^{2+}-specific (modulatory) Ca^{2+}-binding site (CD-domain) and a Ca^{2+}/Mg^{2+} mixed buffering site (EF-domain) (MacManus *et al.* 1984; Pauls *et al.* 1996). OM is localized in pre-implantation embryos in the cytotrophoblast of the placenta and in neoplastic tissues as well as in tumor cell lines, but not in normal fetal or adult tissues (Brewer and MacManus 1985; MacManus *et al.* 1985). Although OM has been shown to be present in tumors of a variety of origins, it is not considered as a general tumor marker (Huber *et al.* 1990). Highest expression is found in tumors of the rat. This is most likely due to the presence of an LTR sequence which is a strong promoter in the rat (reviewed in Berchtold 1989; Pauls *et al.* 1996). The genomic structure of OM is identical to PV concerning splice site positions with respect to the amino acid sequences. The modulatory function of OM is controversial (discussed in Berchtold 1989).

■ Identification/isolation

OM has been isolated from solid tumors of the rat (MacManus and Brewer 1987) as well as from rodent cell lines (Sommer and Heizmann 1989). Recombinant rat OM could be produced in high amounts (Gillen *et al.* 1987).

■ Gene and sequence

The OM genes of rat (Banville and Boie 1989) and mouse (Banville *et al.* 1992) are known. The rat gene contains an endogenous retrovirus-related LTR sequence which is a strong promoter. This LTR sequence is not present in the mouse and human genomes (Banville *et al.* 1992).

Genomic sequences accession numbers (Genembl, release 40/9.94): Human, Em_pr: H somdln01-04; rat, Em_ro: Rnoncmo1-5; mouse, Em_un: S51655-661.

cDNA sequence accession number (Genembl, release 40/9.94): rat, Em_ro: Ruom.

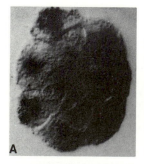 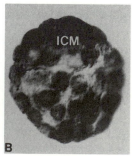 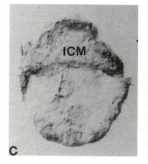 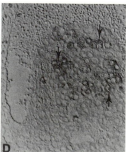

Figure 1. Localization of oncomodulin mRNA and protein during early development. (A) Morula (day 4), immunostaining in all cells. (B) Blastula (day 5), *in situ* hybridization showing oncomodulin mRNA in all cells. (C) Control for (B) using sense probe. (D) Positive immunostaining in ectoplacental cone (day 9). ICM, inner cell mass. (Reproduced from MacManus *et al.* (1990) Adv. Exp. Med. Biol. *269*, 107–110, with permission from authors and publisher.)

The OM gene is localized on human chromosome 7 (Berchtold 1993).

Protein

Rat OM has been sequenced on the protein level and its structure has been determined by X-ray diffraction analysis (Ahmed *et al.* 1990). Accession no. (Swissprot. release 30.0/10.94) for protein sequences: human, SW: onco_human; rat, SW: onco_rat. The protein structure is very similar to parvalbumin. OM may produce dimers through Cys (position 18) linkage.

Accession no (Nrl_3D, release 16/9.94) for 3D-structure: rat, nrl1:1rro.

Antibodies

Monospecific antibodies are commercially available through Swant.

Anatomical localization

Localization in the cytoplasm of cytotrophoblasts and early embryos has been described for rodents and other mammals (Brewer and MacManus 1985; MacManus *et al.* 1990) (Fig. 1).

Biological activities

OM activates cAMP phosphodiesterase (MacManus 1981). Compared to calmodulin, higher activator concentrations are needed. OM in its dimeric form may inhibit glutathione-reductase activity with enhanced efficency (Mutus *et al.* 1988). OM overexpression by a metallothionine promoter in embryos is lethal (Chalifour *et al.* 1989). OM overexpression does not lead to transformation (Mes-Masson *et al.* 1989). Therefore, OM can not be considered as an oncogene.

Biological regulation

The rat OM gene is driven by a retroviral LTR sequence which is a strong promoter (Banville and Boie 1989). The molecular mechanism of tumor cell type specific gene activation is not known. So far no specific interactions with putative target proteins have been described.

Mutagenesis studies

Site-directed mutagenesis has been used to study the metal binding properties of OM (Hapak *et al.* 1989; MacManus *et al.* 1989; Palmisano *et al.* 1990) and Cys18 reactivity (Clayshulte *et al.*, 1990).

References

Ahmed, F.R., Przybyska, M., Rose, D.R., Birnbaum, G.I., Pippy, M.E., and MacManus, J.P. (1990) Structure of oncomodulin refined at 1.85 Å resolution: an example of extensive molecular aggregation via Ca^{2+}. J. Mol. Biol **216**, 127–140.

Banville, D. and Boie, Y. (1989) Retroviral long terminal repeat is the promoter of the gene encoding the tumor associated calcium binding protein oncomodulin in rat. J. Mol. Biol. **207**, 481–490.

Banville, D., Rotaru, M., and Boie, Y. (1992) The intracisternal A particle derived solo LTR promoter of the rat oncomodulin gene is not present in the mouse gene. Genetica **86**, 85–97.

*Berchtold, M.W. (1989) Structure and expression of genes encoding the three-domain Ca-binding proteins parvalbumin and oncomodulin. Biochim. Biophys. Acta **1009**, 201–215.

Berchtold, M.W. (1993) Evolution of EF-hand calcium-modulated proteins. V. The genes encoding EF-hand proteins are not clustered in mammalian genomes. J. Mol. Evol. **36**, 489–496.

Brewer, L.M. and MacManus, J.P. (1985) Localization and synthesis of the tumour protein oncomodulin in extraembryonic tissues of the fetal rat. Dev. Biol. **112**, 49–58.

Chalifour, L.E., Gomes, M.L., and Mes-Masson, A-M. (1989) Microinjection of metallothionein-oncomodulin DNA into fertilized mouse embryos is correlated with fetal lethality. Oncogene **4**, 1241–1246.

Clayshulte, T.M., Taylor, D.F., and Henzl, M.T. (1990) Reactivity of cysteine 18 in oncomodulin. J. Biol. Chem. **265**, 1800–1805.

Gillen, M.F., Banville, D., Rutledge, R.G., Narang, S., Seligy, V.L., Whitfield, J.F., and MacManus, J.P. (1987) A complete complementary DNA for the oncodevelopmental calcium-binding protein, oncomodulin. J. Biol. Chem. **262**, 5308–5312.

Hapak, R.C., Lammers, P.J., Palmisano, W.A., Birmbaum, E.R., and Henzl, M.T. (1989) Site-specific substitutions of glutamate for aspartate at position 59 of rat oncomodulin. J. Biol. Chem. **264**, 18751–18760.

Huber, S., Leuthold, M., Sommer, E.W., and Heizmann, C.W. (1990) Human tumor cell lines express low levels of oncomodulin. Biochem. Biophys. Res. Commun. **169**, 905–909.

MacManus, J.P. (1981) The stimulation of cyclic nucleotide phosphodiesterase by a Mr 11500 calcium binding protein from hepatoma. FEBS Lett. **126**, 245–249.

MacManus, J.P. and Brewer, L.M. (1987) Isolation, localisation and properties of the oncodevelopmental calcium-binding protein oncomodulin. Methods Enzymol. **139**, 156–168.

MacManus, J.P., Szabo, A.G., and Williams, R.E. (1984) Conformational changes induced by binding of bivalent cations to oncomodulin, a parvalbumin-like tumour protein. Biochem. J. **220**, 261–268.

*MacManus, J.P., Brewer, L.M., and Whitfield, J.F. (1985) The widely disstributed tumor-protein, oncomodulin, is a normal costitutent of human and rodent placentas. Cancer Lett., **27**, 145–151.

MacManus, J.P., Hutnik, C.M.L., Sykes, B.D., Szabo, A.G., and Williams, T.C. (1989) Characterization and site-specific mutagenesis of the calcium-binding protein oncomodulin produced by recombinant bacteria. J. Biol. Chem. **264**, 3470–3477.

*MacManus, J.P., Brewer, L.M., and Banville, D. (1990) Oncomodulin in normal and transformed cells. Adv. Exp. Med. Biol. **269**, 107–110.

Mes-Masson, A.M., Masson, S., Banville, D., and Chalifour, L. (1989) Expression of oncomodulin does not lead to the transformation or immortalization of mammalian cells *in vitro*. J. Cell Sci. **94**, 517–525.

Mutus, B., Palmer, E.J., and MacManus, J.P. (1988) Disulphide-linked dimer of oncomodulin: comparison to calmodulin. Biochemistry **27**, 5615–5622.

Palmisano, W.A., Trevino, C.L., and Henzl, M.T. (1990) Site-specific replacement of amino acids residues within the CD binding loop of rat oncomodulin. J. Biol. Chem. **265**, 14450–14456.

Pauls, T.L., Cox, J.A., and Berchtold, M.W. (1996) The Ca²⁺-binding proteins parvalbumin and oncomodulin and their genes: new structural and functional findings. Biochim. Biophys. Acta (in press).

Sommer, E.W., and Heizmann, C.W. (1989) Expression of the tumor-specific and calcium-binding protein oncomodulin during chemical transformation of rat fibroblasts. Cancer Res. **49**, 899–905.

■ Martin W. Berchtold:
Institute of Veterinary Biochemistry,
University of Zürich-Irchel,
Winterthurerstr. 190,
CH-8057 Zürich,
Switzerland
Tel.: 0041 1 257 54 73
Fax: 0041 1 362 05 01
E-mail: berchtol@vetbio.unizh.ch

Avian thymic hormone

Avian thymic hormone (ATH) is an EF-hand helix–loop–helix Ca²⁺-binding protein which belongs to the group of parvalbumins (PVs) with two functional Ca²⁺/Mg²⁺-mixed metal-binding sites. However, due to its specific expression exclusively in thymus glands of birds and its proposed function in promoting immunological maturation of chicken bone marrow cells it deserves a separate discussion when compared to other PVs.

ATH was originally described as a thymus-specific antigen T_1 in the chicken (Pace *et al.* 1978). It has a calculated molecular mass (M_r) of 11.7 kDa and an isoelectric point of 4.35 (Serda and Henzl 1991). The protein contains three EF-hand type helix–loop–helix Ca²⁺-binding sites, two of them being functional and of the Ca²⁺/Mg²⁺-mixed metal-binding type. Due to its high homology in amino acid sequence, and similarity in metal-binding properties, to parvalbumins (PVs) it was assigned to the subfamily of PVs in the superfamily of EF-hand Ca²⁺-binding proteins (Brewer *et al.* 1990; Serda and Henzl 1991). However, in contrast to other PVs it seems to be exclusively expressed in thymus glands of birds, where it is localized in reticuloepithelia-like cells (Murthy *et al.* 1984; Hall *et al.* 1991). Due to its ability to stimulate differentiation of T-cell precursors and to enhance the proliferative activity of certain mitogens, ATH was proposed to be a hormone and therefore renamed "avian thymic hormone" (Murthy and Ragland 1984; Murthy *et al.* 1984).

■ Alternative names

Thymus specific antigen T_1 (Pace *et al.* 1978).

■ Identification/isolation

Two methods for protein purification have been described. In the first method (Barger *et al.* 1991) ATH was isolated from chicken thymus, after enrichment using heat treatment (80°C) and hydrochloric acid precipitation, followed by Sephadex G-75-40 chromatography and affinity chromatography, recovering about 9% of the total ATH from the extracted tissue. The second proce-

dure (Serda and Henzl 1991) involves heat treatment followed by trichloroacetic acid precipitation, DEAE-agarose chromatography and gel filtration, yielding 10–12 mg ATH from 200 g crude chicken thymus (about 3% of total ATH). The concentration of ATH in chicken thymus was estimated to be 1.2–1.8 mg ATH per g thymic tissue using radial immunodiffusion (Murthy *et al.* 1984). Amino acid sequence analysis revealed a high homology to PVs especially to the β-type isoforms from lower vertebrates (Brewer *et al.* 1990, 1991). Recombinant ATH was expressed in *E. coli* and subsequently characterized (Palmisano and Henzl 1991).

■ Gene and sequences

Whereas the ATH gene has not been studied so far, the cDNA has been isolated and the amino acid sequence has been determined (Brewer *et al.* 1990; Palmisano and Henzl 1991) (accession numbers: SW:Prvt_chick; EM_OV:M34330). The ATH mRNA comprises approximately 1050 bp and the translated amino acid sequence consists of 108 amino acids. Of these, 45 positions are different when compared to the 109 amino acid containing PV isoform isolated from chicken muscle (Kuster *et al.* 1991). There is more amino acid sequence homology of ATH to β-type PVs from lower vertebrates than to α- and β-PVs from higher vertebrates (Brewer *et al.* 1991). Southern blot analysis of genomic DNA suggests the presence of a single copy of the ATH gene in the chicken genome. The absence of hybridization between an ATH cDNA fragment and genomic DNA from rat and rabbit indicates that the ATH gene is restricted to avian species (Palmisano and Henzl 1991). It seems that ATH is encoded by a species-specific gene which is expressed in a tissue-specific fashion (see also localization).

■ Protein

ATH was characterized as an acidic protein rich in pheny-lalanine, alanine, and serine, but lacking histidine, trypto-phan, and methionine (Brewer et al. 1990; Palmisano and Henzl 1991). The only post-translational modification is a blocked N-terminal alanine (Brewer et al. 1990). ATH is very stable to extremes of temperature and pH. Like other PVs, it contains three EF-hand type helix–loop–helix Ca^{2+}-binding sites. Only two of these, the CD and the EF sites, are functional, having high affinity for Ca^{2+} ions (dissociation constant K_{Ca} = 8 nM) and moderate affinity for Mg^{2+} ions (dissociation constant K_{Mg} = 68 μM) under physiological conditions (Serda and Henzl 1991). The two metal-binding sites are functionally indistinguishable and belong to the Ca^{2+}/Mg^{2+}-mixed binding type. Due to its amino acid sequence and biochemical characteristics ATH was assigned to be a β-PV, whereas the chicken muscle isoform is an α-PV (Kuster et al. 1991). Nevertheless, the ion-binding properties of ATH (Serda and Henzl 1991) more closely resemble muscle-associated α-PVs of higher vertebrates than mammalian oncomodulin, the only other β-PV described in higher vertebrates, with a pro-posed enzyme modulatory function. Recently however, a third avian PV, called CPV3, has been isolated with two non-equivalent Ca^{2+}-binding sites (Henzl et al. 1991; Hapak et al. 1994) (accession number: EM_OV:U03850). The CPV3 is restricted to the non-lymphoid compartments of the thymus. It contains 108 amino acid residues typical for β-PVs with sequence identities of 52% to the chicken muscle isoform, 58% to ATH, and 68% to rat oncomodulin.

■ Antibodies

Polyclonal antibodies (Murthy et al. 1984; Serda and Henzl 1991) and monoclonal antibodies (Hall et al. 1991) directed against ATH have been generated and show cross-reactivity neither to chicken leg muscle PV nor to other muscle-associated PVs.

■ Localization

In immunohistochemical studies, ATH was localized within large epithelial cells of the thymus and in small thymocytes in the thymic cortex (Murthy et al. 1984; Hall et al. 1991). It was not detected in frozen tissue sections and extracts from other organs including chicken muscle, which suggests that ATH expression is restricted to the thymus gland. ATH was localized in thymus extracts of other avian species but no cross-reactions with mam-malian thymic extracts have been found. However, mono-clonal antibodies directed against the Ca^{2+}-binding loop of the CD site in carp muscle PV also gave immuno-reactivity in the epithelial cells in chicken embryos of day 9 and in the cortical reticular cells in the adult chicken, but the antigen recognized by these antibodies was not further characterized (Kiraly and Celio 1993). There is a report that ATH can circulate in the blood-stream with a periodic variation of its concentration (Hall et al. 1993).

■ Biological activities

ATH is the first PV in non-muscle tissue to be directly con-nected with a specific biological function. In vitro studies have demonstrated that ATH can induce expression of T-cell markers on chicken bone marrow precursor cells in cell culture (Murthy and Rayland 1984). Furthermore, mitogen-triggered proliferation of immature and mature thymocytes seems to be enhanced by ATH in vivo and in vitro (Brewer et al. 1989; Murthy and Ragland 1992). It has been suggested that ATH functions as an extracellular hormone-like protein, triggering immunological matura-tion of immature T lymphocytes. According to this hypothesis, ATH would be secreted by the thymic epithe-lial cells and would interact with peptide receptors on immature T lymphocytes and/or T-cell precursors in bone marrow. A protein–protein interaction between ATH and a target protein has been proposed (Serda and Henzl 1991) and recently, cells with putative receptors for ATH have been localized in spleen and caecal tonsils (Novak et al. 1995).

The finding that ATH is a PV with a postulated hormone-like activity is of particular interest since so far PVs have been considered mainly to constitute an import-ant Ca^{2+}-buffering system within the cell.

■ References

*Barger, B., Pace, J.L., and Ragland, W.L. (1991) Purification and partial characterization of an avian thymic hormone. Thymus **17**, 181–197.

Brewer, J.M., Wunderlich, J.K., Doo-Ha, K., Carr, M.Y., Beach, G.G., Ragland, W.L. (1989) Avian thymic hormone (ATH) is a parvalbumin. Biochem. Biophys. Res. Commun. **160**, 1155–1161.

Brewer, J.M., Wunderlich, J.K., and Ragland, W.L. (1990) The amino acid sequence of avian thymic hormone, a parvalbumin. Biochimie **72**, 653–660.

*Brewer, J.M., Arnold, J., Beach, G.G., Ragland, W.L., and Wunderlich, J.K. (1991) Comparison of the amino acid sequences of tissue-specific parvalbumins from chicken muscle and thymus and possible evolutionary significance. Biochem. Biophys. Res. Commun. **181**, 226–231.

Hall, C.A., Beach, G.G., and Ragland, W.L. (1991) Monoclonal antibody for avian thymic hormone. Hybridoma **10**, 575–582.

Hall, CA., Beach, G.G., & Ragland, W.L. (1993) Serum levels of avian thymic hormone. In: Avian immunology in progress (ed. F. Coudert), Tours (France), August 31–Sept. 2, Colloques de l'INRA, No. 62, pp. 125–130.

Hapak, R.C., Zhao, H., Boschi, J.M., and Henzl, M.T. (1994) Novel avian thymic parvalbumin displays high degree of sequence homology to oncomodulin. J. Biol. Chem. **269**, 5288–5296.

Henzl, M.T., Serda, R.E., and Boschi, J.M. (1991) Identification of a novel parvalbumin in avian thymic tissue. Biochem. Biophys. Res. Commun. **177**, 881–887.

Kiraly, E. and Celio, M. R. (1993) Parvalbumin and calretinin in avian thymus. Anatomy and Embryology **188**, 339–344.

Kuster, T., Staudemann, W., Hughes, G.J., and Heizmann, C.W. (1991) Parvalbumin isoforms in chicken muscle and thymus.

Amino acid sequence analysis of muscle parvalbumin by tandem mass spectroscopy. Biochemistry **30**, 8812–8816.

Murthy, K.K. and Ragland, W.L. (1984) Immunomodulation by thymic hormones: studies with an avian thymic hormone. In: *Chemical regulation of immunity in veterinary medicine* (ed. M. Kinde, J. Gainer, and M. Chirigos) Alan R. Liss, New York.

*Murthy, K.K., Pace, J.L., Barger, B.O., Dawe, D.L., and Ragland, W.L. (1984) Localization and distribution by age and species of an avian thymus-specific antigen. Thymus **6**, 43–55.

Murthy, K.K. and Ragland, W.L. (1992) Effect of thymic extract on blastogenic responses of chickens. Poultry Science **71**, 311–315.

Novak, R., Steffens, W.L., Brewer, J.M., and Ragland, W.L. (1995) Receptor cells for avian thymic hormone in spleen and caecal tonsils. FASEB J. **9**, A818.

Pace, J.L., Barger, B.O., Dawe, D.L., and Ragland, W.L. (1978) Specific antigens of chicken thymus. Eur. J. Immunol. **8**, 671–678.

*Palmisano, W.A. and Henzl, M.T. (1991) Molecular cloning of the thymus-specific parvalbumin known as avian thymic hormone: isolation of a full length cDNA and expression of recombinant protein in *Escherichia coli*. Arch. Biochem. Biophys. **285**, 211–220.

*Serda, R.E. and Henzl, M.T. (1991) Metal ion-binding properties of avian thymic hormone. J. Biol. Chem. **266**, 7291–7299.

■ Thomas L. Pauls:
*Institute of Histology and General Embryology,
University of Fribourg,
CH-1705 Fribourg, Switzerland,
Tel.: 0041-26300 8490
Fax: 0041-26300 9732
E-mail: thomas.pauls@unifr.ch*

Reticulocalbin

Reticulocalbin (RCN) is an endoplasmic reticulum (ER)-resident Ca^{2+}-binding protein with six EF-hand motifs. In mouse and human it shows a ubiquitous expression pattern. Its hypothetical function in cells includes the regulation of Ca^{2+}-dependent activities in the lumen of the ER or post-ER compartment.

Reticulocalbin (RCN) has six repeats of a domain containing the EF-hand motif (Fig. 1; Ozawa and Muramatsu 1993). The overall structure of RCN is similar to that of calbindin D-28k and calretinin, in that all of these proteins have six EF-hand motif domains. RCN, however, has a long amino-terminal extension as well as a short carboxyl-terminal extension. The latter has an His-Asp-Glu-Leu (HDEL) sequence, a variant of the Lys-Asp-Glu-Leu sequence, that serves as part of the retention signal for the protein in the ER. The amino-terminal extension is composed of a leader sequence, which directs the translocation of the protein into the lumen of the ER, and the amino-terminal region of the mature protein (~50 amino acids) of unknown function, which contains a single N-glycosylation site. The amino acid sequence of human RCN shows 95% identity to that of mouse RCN (Ozawa 1995a).

A human protein termed ERC-55 (endoplasmic reticulum calcium-binding protein of 55 kDa) has been described recently (Weis *et al.* 1994). The cDNA of ERC-55 is predicted to encode a protein of 317 amino acids, which is similar to the number of amino acids (331 residues) in human RCN. Like RCN, this protein has six copies of the EF-hand Ca^{2+}-binding motif and also possesses a carboxy-terminal HDEL tetrapeptide sequence. Thus, ERC-55 has many of the structural features found in RCN. However, the amino acid sequence of ERC-55 has a low degree of

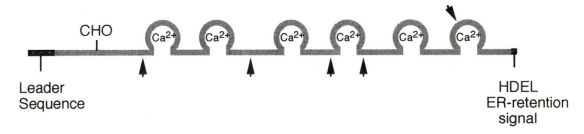

Figure 1. Schematic representation of the RCN-protein. Putative loop structures of the EF-hand domains are shown as circles. Intron break-points are indicated by arrows.

homology with human RCN, with 37% identity (Ozawa 1995a).

Isolation/identification

The mouse RCN cDNA was isolated from a λgt11 expression library constructed from mouse teratocarcinoma OTT6050 cDNA by screening with antibodies against *Dolichos biflorus* agglutinin-binding glycoproteins of the cells (Ozawa and Muramatsu 1993). The human RCN cDNA was isolated from a λgt10 cDNA library derived from a human transitional carcinoma cell line (BOY) using a cDNA probe that had been isolated from cDNAs of the cells by polymerase chain reaction (Ozawa 1995a).

Gene and sequences

The sequences of mouse RCN (Ozawa and Muramatsu 1993 GenBank accession number D13003) and human RCN (Ozawa, 1995a; D42073) are highly homologous. The mouse RCN gene spans over 13 kilobase pairs (Ozawa 1995b; D43952, D43953, D43954, D43955, and D43956). The gene is encoded on six separate exons (Fig. 1), and it thus differs from the cytosolic Ca^{2+}-binding protein calbindin D-28k, which also has six EF-hand motif domains but whose gene is divided into 11 exons. Comparison of the gene organization of reticulocalbin with that of other EF-hand proteins has revealed that reticulocalbin diverged very early from other members of the EF-hand protein superfamily (Ozawa 1995b).

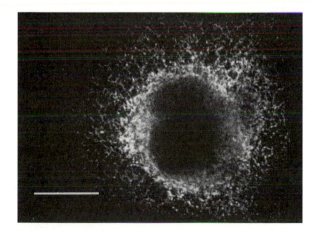

Figure 2. Localization of RCN by immunofluorescence staining. COS cells transfected with RCN cDNA were stained with anti-RCN antibodies, and an image was generated by a confocal scanning laser microscope on a video monitor (taken from Ozawa and Muramatsu 1993). Bar = 25 μm.

Protein

Mouse RCN has a calculated molecular mass of 36.2 kDa, whereas it migrates on SDS-gels as a doublet with an apparent molecular mass of 44 kDa and 46 kDa. The 46 kDa species is produced by N-glycosylation (high mannose type) of the 44 kDa species at a consensus N-glycosylation site (Ozawa and Muramatsu 1993). Human RCN has a calculated molecular mass of 35.9 kDa. Similar or slightly lower molecular weight bands were also detected upon SDS-gel electrophoresis of the human cell line (Ozawa 1995a).

Antibodies

No antibodies against RCN are commercially available. Antibodies specific for RCN, which were raised against recombinant mouse RCN, are available on request. The antibodies also recognize human RCN (Ozawa 1995a).

Localization

Antibodies against mouse RCN were used to localize the protein in the ER by immunofluorescence staining and immunoblotting after subcellular fractionation (Ozawa and Muramatsu 1993)

Biological activities

Recombinant RCN expressed in bacterial cells binds Ca^{2+} in calcium overlay assays (Ozawa and Muramatsu 1993). As yet no other biochemical studies, including equilibrium dialysis analysis, have been done to determine the number of Ca^{2+}-binding sites and the binding affinities. Upon immunoprecipitation, proteins of apparent of 100 kDa, 55 kDa and 42 kDa, coprecipitated with RCN (M. Ozawa, unpublished observation). These proteins could be the target molecules of RCN.

References

*Ozawa, M. (1995a) Cloning of human homologue of mouse reticulocalbin reveals conservation of structural domains in the novel endoplasmic reticulum-resident Ca^{2+}-binding protein with multiple EF-hand motifs. J. Biochem. **117**, 1113–1119.

*Ozawa, M. (1995b) Structure of the gene encoding mouse reticulocalbin, a novel endoplasmic reticulum resident Ca^{2+}-binding protein with multiple EF-hand motifs. J. Biochem. **118**, 154–160.

*Ozawa, M. and Muramatsu, T. (1993) Reticulocalbin, a novel endoplasmic reticulum resident Ca^{2+}-binding protein with multiple EF-hand motifs and a carboxyl-terminal HDEL sequence. J. Biol. Chem. **268**, 699–705.

Weis, K., Griffiths, G., and Lamond, A.I. (1994) The endoplasmic reticulum calcium-binding protein of 55 kDa is a novel

EF-hand protein retained in the endoplasmic reticulum by a carboxyl-terminal His-Asp-Glu-Leu motif. J. Biol. Chem. **269**, 19142–9150.

■ *Masayuki Ozawa:*
Department of Biochemistry,

Faculty of Medicine,
Kagoshima University,
Kagoshima 890,
Japan
Tel.: 81 992 75 5246
Fax: 81 992 64 5618

S100 proteins

Members of the S100 Ca²⁺-binding protein family are typically small, acidic proteins containing two Ca²⁺-binding sites. It has been suggested, that they are associated with cell cycle progression, differentiation, metabolism, and the generation of neoplastic cells. Each member of the S100 protein family shows a unique spatial and temporal expression pattern.

■ Members of this subfamily

At present 13 different S100 molecules have been identified from human sources (see Table 1). For all of these, cDNA sequences are available and the chromosomal location is known. In most cases, the genomic structure is also known (see below). In addition, one vertebrate S100 protein, which has not been purified or cloned from human, has been reported from porcine, rabbit, and chicken tissues (S100C or calgizzarin (Todoroki *et al.* 1991)). Two S100 proteins have been identified from fish species, one seems to be the fish homolog of S100A2 (Bettini *et al.* 1994), the other one called ictacalcin was reported to be a novel member of the S100

Table 1. Human S100 proteins

Name	Gene symbol	Synonyms	Chromosome
S100 calcium-binding protein A1	S100A1	S100, S100α	1q21
S100 calcium-binding protein A2	S100A2	S100L, CaN19	1q21
S100 calcium-binding protein A3	S100A3	S100E	1q21
S100 calcium-binding protein A4	S100A4	CAPL, p9Ka, 42A, pEL98, mts1, calvasculin, 18A2	1q21
S100 calcium-binding protein A5	S100A5	S100D	1q21
S100 calcium-binding protein A6	S100A6	calcyclin, 2A9, PRA, CaBP, 5B10	1q21
S100 calcium-binding protein A7	S100A7	psoriasin	1q21
S100 calcium-binding protein A8	S100A8	calgranulin A, CFAg, MRP8, p8, MAC387. 60B8Ag, L1Ag, CP-10, MIF, NIF	1q21
S100 calcium-binding protein A9	S100A9	calgranulin B, CFAg, MRP14, p14, MAC387, 60B8Ag, L1Ag, MIF, NIF	1q21
S100 calcium-binding protein A10	S100A10	calpactin light chain, p11, CLP11, p10, 42C, Ca[1]	1q21
S100 calcium-binding protein β	S100B	S100β, NEF, S100	21q22
Calbindin-D9k	CALB3	CaBP9K, calbindin 3, ICaBP	Xp22
S100 calcium-binding protein P	S100P		4p16
Profilaggrin	FLG		1q21
Trichohyalin	THH		1q21
S100C	S100C	calgizzarin	porcine, rabbit, chicken
Ictacalcin			catfish

The nomenclature given for the S100 protein family is taken from Schäfer *et al.* (1995) and corresponds to the approved and official entries in the Genome Database (GDB) for human genes or proteins. Human S100C, calgranulin C, and ictacalcin are not know and therefore they are listed in the lower part of the table, together with the species from which they have been isolated. Also shown in the lower part are profilaggrin and trichohyalin, which are found late in the terminally differentiating granular cells of the epidermis. They contain an S100-like domain at the amino terminus.

protein family (Ivanenkov et al. 1993). In contrast, no S100 protein has so far been isolated or cloned from invertebrates.

Interestingly, it was recently reported that two high molecular weight proteins, which are expressed late in terminally differentiating cells of the granular layer in the epidermis, contain in their precursor state an N-terminal S100 domain (Presland et al. 1992; Lee et al. 1993), which has also been recognized at the genomic level. In these two proteins (trichohyalin and profilaggrin) the N-terminal S100 domain is cleaved off during maturation. The fate of this processed S100 domain is not known at present.

Protein structure

Most S100 proteins have a molecular mass of 9–12 kDa. The degree of identity at the amino acid level ranges from 25% to 60%. S100A2 and S100A4 have the highest level of identity and S100A7 is the most distantly related S100 family member. In general, they can bind two Ca^{2+} ions in two distinct binding regions. Whereas the first Ca^{2+}-binding loop is typical for S100 proteins and binds Ca^{2+} only with low affinity (200–500 μM), the second loop is a canonical EF-hand with high affinity (20–50 μM) Ca^{2+} binding (Fig. 1). In addition to Ca^{2+}, several S100 proteins are able to bind zinc, although the zinc binding regions are less well-defined (Baudier et al. 1986). The two Ca^{2+}-binding loops are interrupted by a central hinge region, which is less conserved among different members of this subfamily and might therefore define functional specificity of S100 proteins. Upon binding of Ca^{2+}, S100 proteins display a change in conformation, thus exposing the more hydrophobic regions on the surface of the proteins. This allows for interactions with different target molecules, but seems also to be required for the observed oligomerization of some S100 proteins. Whereas S100A1 and S100β are known to both homo- and heterodimerize, for most other members of this family their state of oligomerization is not definitively known.

Gene structure and organization

The S100 family not only shows significant homologies at the level of the protein structure; their genes also are uni-

formly organized. In the human genome, 10 out of 13 known S100 genes are localized on chromosome 1q21 in a tight gene cluster. Within a stretch of about 300 kb in this chromosomal region, nine S100 genes could be localized (Schäfer et al. 1995). Hence, most of the S100 genes have been kept together during gene duplication events during evolution. Supporting this view, there is some evidence that the clustered organization of S100 genes has been conserved during evolution, since several mouse genes are located in a syntenic region on mouse chromosome 3 (Dorin et al. 1990). The clustered organization of S100 genes allowed the introduction of a logical nomenclature for these genes (and their corresponding proteins), thus eliminating the use of several different synonyms in the literature (see Table 1). The S100 genes are numbered according to their location within the cluster, S100A1 to S100A10. Genes not located on chromosome 1q21 are not affected. The names and symbols have been approved by the human nomenclature committee and are the official entries in the Genome Database (GDB), hence they are also used in this guidebook.

The similarities among S100 genes extends to the exon–intron organization. For almost all of the genes known, the coding region is interrupted by two introns, whereby the first intron is located in the 5' untranslated region of the mRNA and the second intron lies within the hinge region. Therefore, the two Ca^{2+}-binding loops are encoded by two separate exons. So far the only exception to this organization is the gene coding for S100A5, which contains an additional exon coding for 18 amino acids at the N-terminal end of the protein.

Typically, transcription of S100 genes is initiated at a TATA box; however, at the moment not much is known about the tissue-specific regulation of these genes. The question of gene regulation is especially interesting considering the clustered organization of S100 genes.

Biological activities

Is it possible to attribute a common function to all S100 proteins? At the moment, no such function (with the exception of Ca^{2+}-binding in most S100 members), has been described. Whereas there is a large body of literature describing the biochemical properties of S100 proteins, the functional aspects are only now beginning to emerge. A complication in the study of the general func-

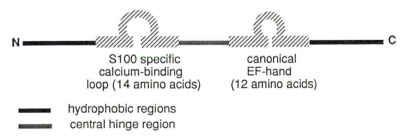

Figure 1. Basic structure of S100 proteins.

tion of S100 proteins is their distinct spatial and temporal pattern of expression. On top of that, there lies an additional level of complexity in the subcellular distribution. S100 proteins have been reported to be localized within the cytoplasm, to be associated with the cytoskeleton and the plasma membrane, and they can also be secreted from certain cells. Accordingly, a number of different functions have been attributed to S100 proteins, among them regulation of protein phosphorylation, of enzyme activity, of microtubule or microfilament polymerization, stimulation of neuronal differentiation, as well as chemotactic activity (reviewed in Donato 1991). Thereby it appears that at least some members of the S100 protein family can have dual or multiple functions, acting both intra- as well as extracellularly.

An interesting aspect of S100 proteins is their possible involvement in cell cycle control and tumorigenicity. Abnormalities in human chromosome region 1q21 (location of the S100 cluster) are found in a number of malignancies, including breast cancer, lymphomas, and leukemias. Furthermore, at least three *S100* genes located within the cluster (*S100A2, S100A4,* and *S100A6*) show deregulated expression in association with tumor progression. The S100 protein was reported to modulate the phosphorylation of the negative cell cycle regulator and tumor suppressor protein p53 (Baudier *et al.* 1992). Apart from these exemplary associations, direct evidence for a role of S100 proteins in tumor progression comes from transfection experiments. Overexpression of S100A4 in malignant rodent cells leads to an increase in their metastatic potential (Davies *et al.* 1993). However, these results have so far not been reproduced with human cells.

■ References

Baudier, J., Glasser, N., and Gérard, D. (1986) Ions binding to S100 proteins I. J. Biol. Chem. **261**, 8192–8203.

*Baudier, J., Delphin, C., Grunwald, D., Khochbin, S., and Lawrence, J.J. (1992) Characterization of the tumor suppressor protein p53 as a protein kinase C substrate and a S100b-binding protein. Proc. Natl. Acad. Sci. USA **89**, 11627–11631.

Bettini, E., Porta, A.R., Dahmen, N., Wang, H., and Margolis, F.L. (1994) Expressed sequence tags (EST) identify genes preferentially expressed in catfish chemosensory tissues. Mol. Brain Res. **23**, 285–291.

Davies, B.R., Davies, M., Gibbs, F., Barraclough, R., and Rudland, P.S. (1993) Induction of the metastatic phenotype by transfection of a benign rat mammary epithelial cell line with the gene for p9Ka, a rat calcium-binding protein, but not with the oncogene EJ-ras-1. Oncogene **8**, 999–1008.

*Donato, R. (1991) Perspectives in S-100 protein biology. Cell Calcium **12**, 713–726.

Dorin, J.R., Emslie, E., and Van Heiningen, V. (1990) Related calcium-binding proteins map to the same subregion of chromosome 1q and to an extended region of synteny on mouse chromosome 3. Genomics **8**, 420–426.

Ivanenkov, V.V., Gerke, V., Minin, A.A., Plessmann, U., and Weber, K. (1993) Transduction of Ca^{2+} signals upon fertilization of eggs; identification of an S-100 protein as a major Ca^{2+} binding protein. Mech. Dev. **42**, 151–158.

Lee, S.C., Kim, I.G., Marekov, L.N., Okeefe, E.J., Parry, D., and Steinert, P.M. (1993) The structure of human Trichohyalin–potential multiple roles as a functional EF-hand-like calcium-binding protein, a cornified cell envelope precursor, and an intermediate filament-associated (cross-linking) protein. J. Biol. Chem. **268**, 12164–12176.

Presland, R.B., Haydock, P.V., Fleckman, P., Nirunsuksiri, W., and Dale, B.A. (1992) Characterization of the human epidermal Profilaggrin gene–genomic organization and identification of an S-100-like calcium binding domain at the amino terminus. J. Biol. Chem. **267**, 23772–23781.

*Schäfer, B.W., Wicki, R., Engelkamp, D., Mattei, M.G., and Heizmann, C.W. (1995) Isolation of a YAC clone covering a cluster of nine S100 genes on human chromosome 1q21: Rationale for a new nomenclature of the S100 calcium-binding protein family. Genomics **25**, 638–643.

Todoroki, H., Kobayashi, R., Watanabe, M., Minami, H., and Hidaka, H. (1991) Purification, characterization and partial sequence analysis of a newly identified EF-hand type 13-kDa Ca-binding protein from smooth muscle and non-muscle tissues. J. Biol. Chem. **266**, 18668–18673.

■ *Beat W. Schäfer:*
University of Zürich,
Department of Pediatrics,
Division of Clinical Chemistry,
Steinwiesstrasse 75,
CH-8032 Zürich,Switzerland
Tel.: +41 1 266 7553
Fax: +41 1 266 7169
E-mail: schaefer@wavona.vmsmail.ethz.ch

S100A1

S100A1 is an intracellular Ca²⁺-binding protein expressed in a variety of tissues including the nervous system, skeletal muscle, heart, kidney, and fat. It is hypothesized to regulate a diverse group of cellular functions including cell–cell communication, cell growth, cell structure, energy metabolism, and intracellular signal transduction via interaction with and modulation of the activity of numerous target proteins.

■ Alternative names

Prior to the adaptation of a new nomenclature for the S100 family in 1995 (see Schäfer *et al.* 1995), S100A1 was called S100α. The dimeric forms of the protein have been referred to as S100a$_O$ (S100A1-S100A1 dimer) and S100a (S100A1-S100β dimer).

■ Identification/isolation

S100A1 was originally isolated as a component of a highly acidic, water soluble, nervous-tissue-specific fraction (Moore 1965). Early purification procedures utilized physical properties including acidity, heat stability, precipitation in saturated ammonium sulfate, and Ca²⁺-dependent interaction with hydrophobic resins such as phenyl- and phenothiazine-Sepharoses to isolate S100A1 from bovine brain (Isobe *et al.* 1981). The recent identification of tissues which express S100A1 and not S100β (heart and skeletal muscle) at levels equivalent or greater than that found in brain has eliminated the need for chromatographic steps to remove the S100A1-S100β and S100β-S100β dimers (Kato *et al.* 1986; Haimoto and Kato 1988; Donato *et al.* 1989). Functional S100A1 can be isolated from bacteria carrying an S100A1 expression plasmid by a two-step procedure which takes one day (Landar and Zimmer, unpublished observation).

■ Gene and sequences

The S100A1 genes are single copy genes and produce one mRNA species in the rat (Zimmer *et al.* 1991; S68809) and two mRNAs in human (Engelkamp *et al.* 1992; X58079) which may result from the usage of alternate polyadenylation signals. The organization and sequence of the human (Morii *et al.* 1991; M65210) and rat (Song and Zimmer 1994) S100A1 genes are similar to that reported for other members of the S100 family, i.e. three exons interrupted by two introns (Fig. 1). In the rat gene, the first exon contains 58 bases of 5′ untranslated sequence, the second exon contains 13 bases of 5′ untranslated sequence and codons for the first 47 amino acids, and the third exon contains codons for the remaining 46 amino acids and 158 bases of 3′ untranslated sequence. The human and rat S100A1 gene exon sequences are almost identical. However, the 5′ flanking sequences of the two genes are very different. While the rat gene contains

several potential regulatory elements such as a nonclassical TATA box (AGTAAA), two AP-1 elements, two reverse AP-2 elements, and a 20 GCT trinucleotide repeat, none of these elements are present in the human gene. The rat gene has been shown to be functional (Song and Zimmer, unpublished observation) while the human gene has not. The human S100A1 gene has been assigned to human chromosome 1 (Morii *et al.* 1991; Schäfer *et al.* 1995).

■ Protein

S100A1 is a 93 amino acid protein which has two EF-hand Ca²⁺-binding domains (Fig. 1). The amino terminal EF-hand is noncanonical and contains 14 amino acids. The carboxy-terminal EF-hand is canonical and contains 12 amino acids (see Zimmer *et al.* 1995). The protein is highly conserved among species with only four conservative amino acid changes between bovine and rat (Zimmer *et al.* 1991). The molecular mechanisms involved in target protein interaction have not been elucidated, although the single cysteine residue at amino acid 85 may be involved (see Zimmer *et al.* 1995). This cysteine residue is not involved in S100A1 dimerization (Masure *et al.* 1984; Donato *et al.* 1989).

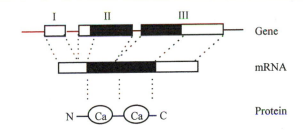

Figure 1. Diagrammatic representation of the S100A1 gene and protein. The boxes represent the exons and the lines introns. Open boxes denote the 5′ and 3′ untranslated regions and black boxes the coding regions. N- and C-represent the amino- and carboxy-termini of the protein, respectively. The two EF-hand calcium-binding domains are represented by the circles.

■ Antibodies

Antibodies specific for S100A1 have been prepared in a number of laboratories (Haimoto and Kato 1987; Zimmer and Van Eldik 1987; Donato *et al.* 1989; Zimmer and Landar 1995). Commercially available S100 antibodies from Sigma, Calbiochem, Chemicon, and Dako recognize S100A1 and S100B. Due to the high degree of homology among members of this family, it is not uncommon to observe crossreactivity of isoform specific antibodies with other members of the family.

Anatomical location

S100A1 exhibits a diverse pattern of tissue- and cell-type specific expression, with the highest levels found in brain, heart, slow-twitch muscle fibers, and kidney (see Zimmer *et al.* 1995). Although the data are limited, in skeletal muscle S100A1 colocalizes with the sarco-plasmic reticulum (Zimmer *et al.* 1991), in heart with the sarcolemma, sarcoplasmic reticulum, nuclei, and myofibrils (Haimoto and Kato 1988; Donato *et al.* 1989), in cultured neuroendocrine and skeletal muscle cells with the Golgi apparatus and secretory vesicles (Zimmer and Landar 1995), and in renal epithelial cells with the cytoplasm, nuclease, and plasma membrane (Kato *et al.* 1985).

Although S100A1 is undetectable in the serum of normal individuals, it is detectable in serum of patients with renal carcinoma where the levels directly parallel the clinical course of the disease (Kato *et al.* 1985). However, there is no evidence that S100A1 is actively secreted from cells and its presence in serum may be due to cell lysis. While Mariggio and coworkers (1994) have observed apoptosis in PC12 cells incubated in S100, this effect may be due to the S100β in the fraction and not S100A1.

Biological activities

S100A1 is thought to function as a Ca^{2+}-modulated protein and modulates the activity of other proteins, termed target proteins in a Ca^{2+}-dependent manner. Studies utilizing an S100 fraction containing both S100A1 and S100β have shown that the activity of p53, tubulin, the microtubule associated t protein and MAP2, GFAP, annexin 2, caldesmon, the myosin heavy chain, adenylate cyclase, neuromodulin, neurogranin, and p87 can be modulated by S100 (see Zimmer *et al.* 1995). For three target proteins (aldolase, the gap junction polypeptide, and glycogen phosphorylase a), the effects of S100A1 and S100β have been compared and only glycogen phospho-rylase a exhibits S100A1-specific regulation (see Zimmer *et al.* 1995)

Biological regulation

Although there are no data available regarding the molecular mechanisms which regulate S100A1 expression, studies have demonstrated that this gene product exhibits a unique pattern of tissue/cell-type specific expression which is regulated in a temporal and spatial

manner (see Zimmer *et al.* 1995). Furthermore, misregula-tion of S100A1 expression occurs in various cancers, and may occur in other disease states and in response to phar-macological and toxicological agents (see Zimmer *et al.* 1995).

References

Donato, R., Giambanco, I., Aisa, M.C., diGeronimo, G., Ceccarelli, P., Rambotti, M.G., and Spreca, A. (1989) Cardiac S-100a. protein: purification by a simple procedure and related immunocytochemical and immunochemical studies. Cell Calcium **10**, 81–92.

Engelkamp, D., Schafer, B.W., Erne, P., and Heizmann, C.W. (1992) S100a, CAPL, and CACY: molecular cloning and expression of three calcium-binding proteins from human heart. Biochem. **31**, 10258–10264.

Haimoto, H., and Kato, K. (1987) S100a. (αα) protein, a calcium-binding protein, is localized in the slow-twitch muscle fiber. J. Neurochem. **48**, 917–923.

Haimoto, H., and Kato, K. (1988) S100a. (αα) protein in cardiac muscle. Isolation from human cardiac muscle and ultrastructural localization. Eur. J. Biochem. **171**, 409–415.

Isobe, T., Ishioka, N., and Okuyama, T. (1981) Structural relation of the two S-100 proteins in bovine brain; subunit composition of S-100a protein. Eur. J. Biochem. **115**, 469–474.

Kato, K., Haimoto, H., Ariyoshi, Y., Horisawa, M., Washida, H., and Kimura S. (1985) High levels of S100a. (αα) protein in tumor tissues and in sera of patients with renal cell carcinoma. Jpn. J. Caۚer Res. (Gann) **76**, 856–862.

Kato, K., Kimura, S., Haimoto, H., and Suzuki, F. (1986) S100a. (αα) protein: distribution in muscle tissue of various animals and purification from human pectoral muscle. J. Neurochem. **46**, 1555–1560.

Mariggio, M.A., Fulle, S., Calissano, P., Nicoletti,I., and Fano, G. (1994) The brain protein S-100ab induces apoptosis in PC12 cells. Neuroscience **60**, 29–35.

Masure, H.R., Head, J.F., and Tice, H.M. (1984) Studies on the a-subunit of bovine brain S100 protein. Biochem. J. **218**, 691–696.

Moore, B.W. (1965) A soluble protein characteristic of the nervous system. Biochem. Biophys. Res. Comm. **19**, 739–744.

Morii, K., Tanaka, R., Takahashi, Y., Minoshima, S., Fukuyama, R., Shimizu, N., and Kuwano, R. (1991) Structure and chromosome assignment of human S100 a and b subunit genes. Biochem. Biophys. Res. Comm. **175**, 185–191.

Schäfer, B.W., Wicki, R., Engelkamp, D., Mattei, J.-G., and Heizmann, C.W. (1995) Isolation of a YAC clone covering a cluster of nine S100 genes on human chromosome 1q21: rationale for a new nomenclature for the S100 calcium-binding protein family. Genomics **25**, 18668–18673.

Song, W. and Zimmer, D.B. (1994) Isolation and characterization of a rat S100a gene. Soc. Neurosci. Abst. **20**, 50.

Zimmer, D.B. and Landar, A.H. (1995) Analysis of S100A1 expression during skeletal muscle and neuronal cell differentiation. J. Neurochem., **64**, 2727–2736.

Zimmer, D.B. and Van Eldik, L.J. (1987) Tissue distribution of rat S100a and S100b and S100-binding proteins. Am. J. Physiol. (Cell Physiol.) **252**, C285–C289.

Zimmer, D.B., Song, W., and Zimmer, W.E. (1991) Isolation of rat S100a cDNA and distribution of its mRNA in rat tissues. Brain Res. Bull. **27**, 157–162.

Zimmer, D.B., Cornwall, E.H., Landar, A., and Song, W. (1995) The S100 protein family: History, function and expression. Brain Res. Bull. **37**, 417–429.

■ Danna B. Zimmer:
Department of Pharmacology,
University of South Alabama,
Mobile, AL 36688, USA

Tel.: 334 460 7056
Fax: 334 460 6798
E-mail: dzimmer@jaguar1.usouthal.edu

S100A2

The S100A2 protein has originally been isolated from bovine lung and cDNAs have been cloned from bovine and human sources. S100A2 is preferentially expressed in normal human mammary epithelial cells and not in breast tumor cells, suggesting that it might play a role in suppressing tumor cell growth.

The human S100A2 protein has a calculated molecular mass of 11.1 kDa and a pI of 4.5. On the sequence level, it is most closely related to S100A4. The bovine S100A2 has been shown by antibody studies to be expressed at high levels in kidney, lung, heart, and skeletal muscle. In bovine kidney cells (MDBK), S100A2 was found to be localized both in the cytoplasm as well as in the nucleus (Glenney et al. 1989). It is not known whether S100A2 can be secreted from these cells as has been shown for other S100 proteins. Interestingly, the human S100A2 and S100A4 genes have an opposite expression pattern in mammary epithelial cells. While S100A2 expression seems to be restricted to normal epithelial cells, the expression of S100A4 increases in advanced metastatic breast tumors. This inverse regulation might be, at least in part, mediated by differential methylation (Lee et al. 1992; Pedrocchi et al. 1994).

Alternative names

S100L (Glenney et al. 1989), CaN19 (Lee et al. 1992).

Identification and isolation

S100A2 protein has so far only been purified from bovine lung tissue, while its cDNA has been cloned from both bovine and human. The human cDNA has been identified by subtractive hybridization involving normal and tumorigenic breast epithelial cells. It was one among about 30 sequences whose expression was down-regulated in tumor cells (Lee et al. 1992). Reexpression could be achieved in tumor cells by treatment with 5-azacytidine, a demethylating agent.

Gene and sequence

Human cDNA has been used to localize the S100A2 gene to the cluster of S100 genes on chromosome 1q21. The sequence is available from the GenBank under accession no. M87068. The genomic structure of S100A2 is at the moment not known.

■ Antibodies

Monoclonal antibodies against S100A2 are available from Chemicon, and from Affinity Research Products, but their specificity is not known.

■ References

Glenney, J.R., Kindy, M.S., and Zokas, L. (1989) Isolation of a new member of the S100 protein family: Amino acid sequence, tissue, and subcellular distribution. J. Cell Biol. **108**, 569–578.

Lee, S.W., Tomasetto, C., Swissheln, K., Keyomarsi, K., and Sager, R. (1992) Down-regulation of a member of the S100 gene family in mammary carcinoma cells and reexpression by azadeoxycytidine treatment. Proc. Natl. Acad. Sci. USA **89**, 2504–2508.

Pedrocchi, M., Schäfer, B.W., Mueller, H., Eppenberger, U., and Heizmann, C.W. (1994) Expression of Ca^{2+}-binding proteins of the S100 family in malignant human breast-cancer cell lines and biopsy samples. Int. J. Cancer **57**, 684–690.

■ Beat W. Schäfer:
University of Zürich,
Department of Pediatrics,
Division of Clinical Chemistry,
Steinwiesstrasse 75,
CH-8032 Zürich, Switzerland
Tel.: +41 1 266 7553
Fax: +41 1 266 7169
E-mail: schaefer@wawona.vmsmail.ethz.ch

S100A3

A cDNA has been cloned from human kidney and heart RNA which codes for an open reading frame of 101 amino acids. Sequence comparison revealed that the deduced protein product is a member of the S100 family. Its most prominent feature is the presence of 10 cysteine residues. The protein has so far not been isolated and characterized.

The deduced S100A3 protein has a calculated molecular mass of 11.7 kDa and a p*I* of 4.55. The highest sequence identities were found to S100A4, S100A5, and S100A6 (46%). S100A3 differs from all other S100 proteins by its high content of cysteine residues (Fig. 1). Among a total of 10 cysteines, five of them are located within the carboxy-terminal 21 amino acids. However, no sequence similarities were found to metallothioneins or zinc-finger proteins, which also have a high cysteine content (Engelkamp et al. 1993). Tissue distribution of S100A3 mRNA was examined in adult human tissues with a semi-quantitative PCR technique. Highest expression levels were found in lung and kidney, followed by heart, stomach, and skeletal muscle. No expression was seen in brain.

Alternative names

S100E (Engelkamp et. al.1993).

Identification

A genomic DNA clone from human chromosome 1q21 was isolated and partially sequenced. During the course of this work, one exon was discovered which could potentially code for a new S100 protein. Additional sequencing as well as cDNA amplification from human kidney and heart RNA led to the isolation of the gene and the complete cDNA coding for S100A3 (Fig. 1).

Gene and sequence

The gene coding for S100A3 contains three exons organized in a way typical of other *S100* genes. The first intron is located in the 5' nontranslated part of the RNA, whereas an additional intron is found between the two structural calcium-binding domains of S100A3. The gene is located in a cluster of S100 proteins on human chromosome 1q21. The sequence is available with the accession number Z18948 (cDNA) and Z18950 (genomic sequence) from the GenBank/EMBL databank.

Reference

Engelkamp, D., Schäfer, B.W., Mattei, G.M., Erne, P., and Heizmann, C.W. (1993) Six S100 genes are clustered on human chromosome 1q21: Identification of two genes coding for the

```
                                                                      ▼
AGTCTCAGATTGGTAAACACCCGAACTGGTCAACTCTCAAGAGACCATCTGGTTCAGGTTCCTGACTGGGCCAGCGAGTG    80

AGGATGGCCAGGCCTCTGGAGCAGGCGGTAGCTGCCATCGTGTGCACCTTCCAGGAATACGCAGGGCGCTGTGGGGACAA   160
   M   A   R   P   L   E   Q   A   V   A   A   I   V   C   T   F   Q   E   Y   A   G   R   C   G   D   K    26
                                                                              ___ ___ ___ ___ ___ ___
                                                          ▼
ATACAAGCTCTGTCCAGGCGGAGCTCAAGGAGCTGCTGCAGAAGGAGCTGGCCACCTGGACCCCCGACTGAGTTTCGGGAAT   240
 ___ Y   K   L   C   Q   A   E   L   K   E   L   L   Q   K   E   L   A   T   W   T   P   T   E   F   R   E    52

GTGACTACAACAAATTCATGAGTGTTCTGGACACCAACAAGGACTGCGAGGTGGACTTTGTGGAGTATGTGCGCTCACTT   320
C   D   Y   N   K   F   M   S   V   L   D   T   N   K   D   C   E   V   D   F   V   E   Y   V   R   S   L    79

GCCTGCCTCTGTCTCTACTGCCACGAGTACTTCAAGGACTGCCCCCTCAGAGCCCCCCTGCTCCCAGTAGCCTCTGCTCCA   400
A   L   C   L   Y   C   H   E   Y   F   K   D   C   P   S   E   P   P   C   S   Q   *              101

GGGGGTGCGCTGGCTGTCGGGGGCTGGGCATGTCTCCCACACCCCCTCCTACCCTCTCTCCTGTACCCCTTTCAATCTGG   480

ACTTGCCCAGGTCTTCTGCGATCAGTTAACCCATTTTACCTAGGAGGCCCAGAGATGTGAGGGCTCCTTCCTCAGGATGC   560

CCAGCGAATGAGGGGTAGAGCCACTCTGGGGCCCAGCCTGCCTGCCGCACCCCTGTGGCCTCCCTTGTGGATGGGAGGAG   640

GCGGGATCTGCTCTGAGGCCCTCGAGGCTCAGCAGAGCGTGCACCAATGAGACCACGATGGGAAAGGGCCTATTTAACTC   720

CTAATAAAAAACTGGCAT   738
```

Figure 1. Nucleotide and deduced amino acid sequence of the human S100A3 cDNA. Positions of the two introns in the genomic structure are marked by an arrowhead. The S100-specific motif is underlined by dashes whereas the canonical EF-hand is underlined continuously. The stop codon is marked by an asterisk. The polyA tail is not shown.

two previously unreported calcium-binding proteins S100D and S100E. Proc. Natl. Acad. Sci. USA **90**, 6547–6551.

■ *Beat W. Schäfer:*
University of Zürich,
Department of Pediatrics,

Division of Clinical Chemistry,
Steinwiesstrasse 75,
CH-8032 Zürich, Switzerland
Tel.: +41 1 266 7553
Fax: +41 1 266 7169
E-mail: schaefer@wawona.vmsmail.ethz.ch

S100A4

S100A4 has a widespread but specific distribution in normal cells; however, elevated levels in certain cultured tumour cells are associated with cell transformation and the ability of the cells to metastasize. S100A4 binds calcium with an affinity of 34–38 μM and appears to be associated with elements of the cytoskeleton.

S100A4 has a calculated molecular weight of approximately 11,600 and an isoelectric point of 5.5 (rat)–6.1 (human) under denaturing conditions. It consists of two EF-hand motifs which can bind calcium ions. S100A4 occurs widely in normal rat tissues (Gibbs *et al.* 1995) and has been isolated from rat cultured cells (Gibbs *et al.* 1994), bovine retina (Polans *et al.* 1993), aorta (Watanabe *et al.* 1992a), and human heart muscle (Pedrocchi *et al.* 1994).

In cultured cells, elevated levels of S100A4, or of its mRNA, accompany the differentiation of rat PC12 phaeochromocytoma cells induced by nerve growth factor (Masiakowski and Shooter 1988), an increase in growth rate of cultured murine fibroblasts induced by serum (Jackson-Grusby *et al.* 1987), the transformation of murine fibroblasts (Goto *et al.* 1988) or rat kidney cells (De Vouge and Mukherjee 1992) induced by oncogene or carcinogen, and the induced differentiation of human promyelocytic leukemia cells along the macrophagic or granulocytic lineages (Takenaga *et al.* 1994a). In cultured rodent mammary epithelial cells, elevated levels of S100A4 (Barraclough and Rudland 1994) or of its mRNA (Grigorian *et al.* 1993), correlate with the metastatic potential of the cells. Transfer of multiple expressed copies of the rat S100A4 gene into benign tumor-derived mammary epithelial cells induces the metastatic phenotype in some of the cells (Barraclough and Rudland 1994). Transfection of the mouse gene for S100A4 into non-metastatic murine melanoma cells has been reported to increase the ability of the cells to colonize the lungs when injected into the tail vein of recipient mice (Parker *et al.* 1994).

■ Alternative names

p9Ka (Barraclough *et al.* 1987), 18A2 (Jackson-Grusby *et al.* 1987), pEL98 (Goto *et al.* 1988), 42A (Masiakowski and Shooter 1988), *mts*1 (Grigorian *et al.* 1993), calvasculin (Watanabe *et al.* 1992a), CAPL (Pedrocchi *et al.* 1994).

■ Identification/isolation

Originally identified as a protein differentially expressed between related rat mammary cell lines (Barraclough and Rudland 1994), S100A4 has been purified from cultured cells using a combination of ion exchange and phenyl Sepharose chromatography (Gibbs *et al.* 1994). It was isolated from bovine retina using phenyl Sepharose and organomercurial chromatography (Polans *et al.* 1993) and from human heart by ammonium sulphate fractionation and phenyl Sepharose chromatography (Pedrocchi *et al.* 1994). S100A4 also binds to *N*-(2-aminoethyl)-*N*-[2-(4-chlorocinnamylamino)ethyl]-5-isoquinolinesulphonamide (W-66) (Watanabe *et al.* 1992a).

■ Genes and sequence

The nucleotide sequences of cDNAs for S100A4 from rat (Barraclough *et al.* 1987; Masiakowski and Shooter 1988; De Vouge and Mukherjee 1992: accession numbers X64022, X64023 and J03627), mouse (Goto *et al.* 1988: accession number D00208), and human (Engelkamp *et al.* 1992: accession numbers M77499 and M80563) are present in the GenBank database. Gene sequences for S100A4 from rat (Barraclough *et al.* 1987: accession number X06916), mouse (Grigorian *et al.* 1993: accession numbers M35147 and M36578), and human (Engelkamp *et al.* 1992: contained in accession number Z18950) are also in the GenBank database.

Derived or actual amino acid sequences of S100A4 for rat (Barraclough *et al.* 1987; Masiakowski and Shooter 1988; De Vouge and Mukherjee, 1992: accession number P05942), mouse (Jackson-Grusby *et al.* 1987; Goto *et al.* 1988; Grigorian *et al.* 1993: accession numbers P07091 and P20066), bovine (Polans *et al.* 1993: accession number P35466), and human (Engelkamp *et al.* 1993: accession number P26447) are present in the SWISS-PROT database.

The gene for S100A4 is located on mouse chromosome 3 and on human chromosome 1q21.

Protein

S100A4 contains two EF-hand domains which are typical of the S100 family. Amino acid sequences, either directly determined or derived from the nucleotide sequences of cloned genes, are available for four species: human, mouse, rat, and cow. There is 92% identity between rat and human, 94% identity between mouse and human, and 98% identity between cow and human. All amino acid substitutions are conservative replacements. S100A4 from rat or human source is N-terminally acetylated.

Anatomical localization

Immunocytochemical localization in the rat indicates that S100A4 is widely distributed amongst the tissues of the body, occurring in the gut, in the kidney, in the liver, in the skin, in smooth muscle, in the immune and peripheral nervous systems, but within most of these tissues it is highly localized to particular cell types (Gibbs et al. 1995). S100A4 is found in bovine retina, choroid (Polans et al. 1993), and aortic smooth muscle (Watanabe et al. 1992a). S100A4 is expressed in human monocytes, macrophages, and polymorphonuclear leukocytes (Takenaga et al. 1994a). There is some evidence for extracellular immunolocalization in the rat mammary gland (Gibbs et al. 1995), and secretion of S100A4 into the medium of cultures of smooth muscle cells has been reported (Watanabe et al. 1992b).

Biological activities

Using the method of flow dialysis, recombinant rat or human S100A4 binds calcium ions at two sites per molecule (Gibbs et al. 1994; Pedrocchi et al. 1994) with an overall K_d of 34–38 μM for the rat (Gibbs et al. 1994). The K_d is markedly raised in the presence of magnesium or potassium ions at physiological concentrations (Gibbs et al. 1994). The binding of calcium ions at two sites on a S100A4 dimer has also been reported (Watanabe et al. 1992a).

Biological regulation

In the mouse, the expression of S100A4 is thought to be modulated, at least in part, by regulatory regions in the first intron and by methylation of the DNA (Grigorian et al. 1993).

Interactions

Human, rat, and bovine S100A4 form homodimers, probably stabilized by cysteine bridges (Watanabe et al. 1992a; Pedrocchi et al. 1993; Gibbs et al. 1994).

In cultured cells, S100A4 localizes immunofluorescently to the actin and myosin microfilaments (Barraclough and Rudland 1994; Kriajevska et al. 1994). Using a range of techniques, S100A4 has been reported to interact in vitro with a number of different proteins, including a 36 kDa microfibril-associated glycoprotein (Watanabe et al. 1992b), with non-muscle tropomyosin (Takenaga et al. 1994b) both using affinity chromatography, with actin, using a co-precipitation assay (Watanabe et al. 1993), with non-muscle myosin using immunoprecipitation, sucrose gradient and gel overlay techniques (Kriajevska et al. 1994), all in a calcium-dependent manner.

References

*Barraclough, R. and Rudland, P. (1994) The S-100-related calcium-binding protein, p9Ka, and metastasis in rodent and human mammary cells. Eur. J. Cancer **30A**, 1570–1576.

*Barraclough, R., Savin, J., Dube, S.K., and Rudland, P.S. (1987) Molecular cloning and sequence of the gene for p9Ka, a cultured myoepithelial cell protein with strong homology to S-100, a calcium-binding protein. J. Mol. Biol. **198**, 13–20.

De Vouge, M.W. and Mukherjee, B.B. (1992) Transformation of normal rat kidney cells by v-K-ras enhances expression of transin 2 and an S-100-related calcium-binding protein. Oncogene **7**, 109–119.

Engelkamp, D., Schäfer, B.W., Erne, P., and Heizmann, C.W. (1992) S100a, CAPL, and CACY : Molecular cloning and expression analysis of three calcium-binding proteins from human heart. Biochemistry **31**, 10258–10264.

Engelkamp, D., Schäfer, B.W., Mattei, M.G., Erne, P., and Heizmann, C.W. (1993) Six S100 genes are clustered on human chromosome 1q21: Identification of two genes coding for the two previously unreported calcium-binding proteins S100D and S100E. Proc. Natl. Acad. Sci. USA **90**, 6547–6551.

Gibbs, F.E.M., Wilkinson, M.C., Rudland, P.S., and Barraclough, R. (1994) Interactions in vitro of p9Ka, the rat S-100-related, metastasis-inducing, calcium-binding protein. J. Biol. Chem. **269**, 18992–18999.

Gibbs, F.E.M., Barraclough, R., Platt-Higgins, A., Rudland, P., Wilkinson, M., and Parry, E. (1995) Immunocytochemical distribution of the calcium-binding protein p9Ka in normal rat tissues: Variation in the cellular location in different tissues. J. Histochem. Cytochem. **42, 43**, 169–180.

Goto, K., Endo, H., and Fujiyoshi, T. (1988) Cloning of the sequences expressed abundantly in established cell lines: identification of a cDNA clone highly homologous to S-I00, a calcium binding protein. J. Biochem. (Tokyo) **103**, 48–53.

*Grigorian, M., Tulchinsky, E., Zain, S., Ebralidze, A., Kramerov, D., Kriajevska, M., Georgiev, G., and Lukanidin, E. (1993) The mts1 gene and control of tumor metastasis. Gene **135**, 229–238.

Jackson-Grusby, L.L., Swiergiel, J., and Linzer, D.I.H. (1987) A growth-related mRNA in cultured mouse cells encodes a placental calcium binding protein. Nucl. Acids Res. **15**, 6677–6690.

Kriajevska, M., Cardenas, M., Grigorian, M., Ambartsumian, N., Georgiev, G., and Lukanidin, E. (1994) Non-muscle myosin heavy chain as a possible target for protein encoded by metastasis-related mts-1 gene. J. Biol. Chem. **269**, 19679–19682.

Masiakowski, P. and Shooter, E.M. (1988) Nerve growth factor induces the genes for two proteins related to a family of calcium-binding proteins in PC12 cells. Proc. Natl. Acad. Sci. USA **85**, 1277–1281.

Parker, C., Whittaker, P., Usmani, B., Lakshmi, M., and Sherbert, G. (1994) Induction of 18A2/*mts*1 gene expression and its effects on metastasis and cell cycle control. DNA and Cell Biol. **13**, 1021–1028.

Pedrocchi, M., Hauer, C., Schafer, B., Erne, P., and Heizmann, C. (1993) Analysis of Ca²⁺ binding S100 proteins in human heart by HPLC-electrospray mass spectrometry. Biochem. Biophys. Res. Commun. **197**, 529–535.

Pedrocchi, M., Schafer, B., Durussel, I., Cox, J., and Heizmann, C. (1994) Purification and characterisation of the recombinant human calcium-binding S100 proteins CAPL and CACY. Biochemistry. **33**, 6732–6738.

Polans, A., Palczewski, K., Asson-Batres, M.-A., Ohguro, H., Witkowska, D., Haley, T., Baizer, L., and Crabb, J. (1993) Purification and primary structure of Capl, an S-100-related calcium binding protein isolated from bovine retina. J. Biol. Chem. **269**, 6233–6240.

Takenaga, K., Nakamura, Y., and Sakiyama, S. (1994a) Expression of a calcium binding protein pEL98 (*mts*1) during differentiation of human promyelocytic leukaemia HL-60 cells. Biochem. Biophys. Res. Commun. **202**, 94–101.

Takenaga, K., Nakamura, Y., Sakiyama, S., Hasegawa, Y., Sato, K., and Endo, H. (1994b) Binding of pEL98 protein, an S100-related Calcium-binding protein, to non-muscle tropomyosin. J. Cell Biol. **124**, 757–768.

Watanabe, Y., Kobayashi, R., Ishikawa, T., and Hidaka, H. (1992a). Isolation and characterization of a calcium-binding protein derived from the mRNA termed p9Ka, pEL-98, 18A2, or 42A by the newly-synthesized vasorelaxant W-66 affinity chromatography. Arch. Biochem. Biophys. **292**, 563–569.

Watanabe, Y., Usuda, N., Tsugane, S., Kobayashi, R., and Hidaka, H. (1992b) Calvasculin, an encoded protein from mRNA termed pEL-98, 18A2, 42A or p9Ka, is secreted by smooth muscle cells in culture and exhibits Ca²⁺-dependent binding to 36-kDa microfibril-associated glycoprotein. J. Biol. Chem. **267**, 17136–17140.

Watanabe, Y., Usada, N., Minami, H., Morita, T., Tsugane, S.-I., Ishikawa, R., Kohama, K., Tomida, Y., and Hidaka, H. (1993) Calvasculin as a factor affecting the microfilament assemblies in rat fibroblasts transfected by *src* gene. FEBS Lett. **324**, 51–55.

■ Roger Barraclough:
Department of Biochemistry,
University of Liverpool,
PO Box 147,
Liverpool L69 3BX, UK
Tel.:+44 151 794 4327
Fax:+44 151 794 4349
E-mail: brb@liv.ac.uk

S100A5

A cDNA which codes for an open reading frame of 110 amino acids has been cloned from human kidney and heart. Sequence comparison revealed that the deduced protein product is a member of the S100 family. Its most prominent feature is the presence of 18 additional amino acid residues at the N terminus. The protein has so far not been isolated and characterized.

The deduced S100A5 protein has a calculated molecular mass of 12.8 kDa and a p*I* of 5.2. The highest sequence identities found were to S100A2, S100A4, and S100A6 (52–54%). S100A5 differs from all the other S100 proteins in having an additional 18 amino acids at the N-terminus (Fig. 1). This extension is highly hydrophobic and therefore might influence the cellular localization of the protein. However, no homology was found in the databank with other known proteins. Tissue distribution of S100A5 mRNA was examined in adult human tissues with a semi-quantitative PCR technique. Only low expression levels were found in the tissues examined, including skeletal muscle, heart, brain, kidney, stomach, lung, liver, and placenta.

■ Alternative names

S100D (Engelkamp *et al.* 1993).

■ Identification

During a search for novel S100 proteins, genomic DNA was amplified using degenerated oligonucleotides directed against conservative regions in the first, non-canonical calcium-binding loop of S100 proteins. This experiment led to the identification of a novel S100 sequence, whose cDNA was subsequently cloned by RACE (rapid amplification of cDNA ends). The expected protein product has not been purified from any source.

■ Gene and sequence

The gene coding for S100A5 is, in contrast to other genes coding for S100 proteins, interrupted not by two, but by three introns. The second exon codes for most of the N-terminal extension of the deduced protein and might have been inserted by exon shuffling during evolution. Also in contrast to other *S100* genes, transcription of the gene coding for S100A5 does not seem to start from a

```
TCCCACACTTCTGAGGTTTTCTTTCCAGGACAGCCTGGTTTCCCTTCTTCGGCTTATTGTTCCATCAGATTTCAGATTTT   80

GAGTTCTGATTTTTGGTCAGAAGAGTAAAGTTTCTGGGATTGGGGACGTGTGTGCTATGGGAACTCAGTGTGTCCCCAGC   160
                 ▼
CCTTGTTTGTAAACAAGGAAGGGACAGAGATCAGGGAAATAAAGGCAGAAGGCAGTGAGAGGGAGGCTATGCCTGCTGCT   240
                                                                        M  P  A  A    4
                                 ▼
TGGATTCTCTGGGCTCACTCCCACAGTGAGCTGCACACTGTGATGGAGACTCCTCTGGAGAAGGCCCTGACCACTATGGT   320
 W  I  L  W  A  H  S  H  S  E  L  H  T  V  M  E  T  P  L  E  K  A  L  T  T  M  V    31

GACCACGTTTCACAAATATTCGGGGAGAGAGGGTAGCAAACTGACCCTGAGTAGGAAGGAACTCAAGGAGCTGATCAAGA   400
  T  T  F  H  K  Y  S  G  R  E  G  S  K  L  T  L  S  R  K  E  L  K  E  L  I  K    57
                        ▼                       ●
AAGAGCTGTGTCTTGGGGAGATGAAGGAGAGCAGCATCGATGACTTGATGAAGAGCCTGGACAAGAACAGCGACCAGGAG   480
 K  E  L  C  L  G  E  M  K  E  S  S  I  D  D  L  M  K  S  L  D  K  N  S  D  Q  E   84

ATCGACTTCAAGGAGTACTCGGTGTTCCTGACCATGCTGTGCATGGCCTACAACGACTTCTTTCTAGAGGACAACAAGTG   560
 I  D  F  K  E  Y  S  V  F  L  T  M  L  C  M  A  Y  N  D  F  F  L  E  D  N  K  *   110

ACCAGGGCTGCCCTCCACCCTCACCCTCCACCCTTTGCTGCTGACCTCGGCTGCTCCTCTCACAGACCCTCTTTGGCCCC   640

CTGCCCTCCTCTCCCTCCCAGATGGACCCTTCCATGGGAGGAAATAAAGTTTCCATCGCAGGTGCTGGGA           710
```

Figure 1. Nucleotide and deduced amino acid sequence of the human S100A5 cDNA. Positions of the three introns in the genomic structure are marked by an arrowhead. The S100-specific motif is underlined by dashes whereas the canonical EF-hand is underlined continuously. The stop codon is marked by an asterisk. The polyA tail is not shown. The position of an allelic variant (A to G) is indicated by a filled dot.

promoter containing a conserved TATA-Box. The gene is located in a cluster of S100 proteins on human chromosome 1q21 (see introduction). An allelic variant was found at position 443 of the cDNA sequence, resulting in an amino acid change from Asp to Glu. This variant was found both on the cDNA as well as on the genomic level. It is not known if this amino acid exchange has any functional consequences. The sequence is available with the accession number Z18954 (cDNA) and Z18949/Z18950 (genomic sequence) from the GenBank/EMBL databank.

human chromosome 1q21: Identification of two genes coding for the two previously unreported calcium-binding proteins S100D and S100E. Proc. Natl. Acad. Sci. USA **90**, 6547–6551.

■ Beat W. Schäfer:
University of Zürich,
Department of Pediatrics,
Division of Clinical Chemistry,
Steinwiesstrasse 75,
CH-8032 Zürich, Switzerland
Tel.: +41 1 266 7553
Fax: +41 1 266 7169
E-mail: schaefer@wawona.vmsmail.ethz.ch

■ Reference

Engelkamp, D., Schäfer, B.W., Mattei, G.M., Erne, P., and Heizmann, C.W. (1993) Six S100 genes are clustered on

S100A6

S100A6 is an EF-hand cytosolic Ca²⁺-binding protein expressed in a tissue and cell-specific manner (it is abundant in fibroblasts and epithelial cells), and in cultured cells that are stimulated to proliferate by growth factors such as EGF and PDGF. S100A6 may play a role in secretion, but probably is not involved in cell-cycle progression, as originally suggested.

Alternative names

2A9, calcyclin (Baserga's group, 1–4[1]), CaBP (Kuznicki and Filipek 1987), PRA (Murphy *et al.* 1988), 5B10 (25), CACY (Engelkamp *et al.* 1992), caltropin/SMCaBP (43), S100A6 (Schäfer *et al.* 1995).

Isolation/identification

The S100A6 gene was identified as one of several cDNA clones isolated from quiescent cells which were stimulated to proliferate by different mitogens (1–4). The S100A6 protein was found in preparations of prolactin receptor (Murphy *et al.* 1988) and was purified to homogeneity from mouse Ehrlich ascites tumor cells (Kuznicki and Filipek 1987), various human tissues (17), rabbit lung (14), bovine heart (18), mouse decidua (30), human platelets (11), chicken smooth muscle (43), and mouse brain (Filipek *et al.* 1993). Purification of S100A6 is based on its Ca²⁺-dependent binding to matrices such as phenyl-Sepharose, W7- or W77-Sepharose, and fetuin-Sepharose. Recombinant S100A6 from rabbit (15) and human (Pedrocchi *et al.* 1994) have similar or identical properties to the native protein. S100A6 can be identified during urea-PAGE as a protein band with higher mobility in the absence of Ca²⁺ than in its presence (Kuznicki and Filipek 1987).

Gene and sequences

The sequences of rabbit (GenBank accession # D10885), human (J02763; M18981), and mouse S100A6 (X52278; X66449; M37761; and PIR Accession # S14090; A49738) are highly homologous. The S100A6 gene was found on mouse chromosome 3 and human chromosome 1q21 (Dorin *et al.* 1990) where it is clustered with several other S-100 proteins (Engelkamp *et al.* 1993; Schäfer *et al.* 1995). The 5' and 3' flanking sequences of human S100A6 are known (33). The 5' sequence contains a TATA box, GC boxes, a sequence with a high homology to the enhancer core of the SV40 promoter, and serum-responsive elements (Ghezzo *et al.* 1989). The S100A6 gene is composed of three exons and two introns, and the two EF-hand coding sequences are located on separate exons (II and III).

---

[1] The numbers in parentheses refer ro references in the review article about S100A6 (Filipek and Kuznick 1993).

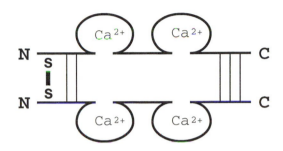

Figure 1. Hypothetical structure of mouse S100A6 dimer formed by S-S bridge and noncovalent forces (vertical lines).

Protein

Human recombinant S100A6 has a calculated molecular mass of 10,092 kDa, migrates on SDS gels with an apparent molecular mass of 10.5 kDa, and has an isoelectric point of 5.25 (Pedrocchi *et al.* 1994). S100A6 binds two Ca²⁺-ions with low affinity and positive cooperativity (Kuznicki and Filipek 1987; 10; Pedrocchi *et al.* 1994). S100A6 also binds Zn²⁺ (13), and sialic acid (18), but does not bind Mg²⁺ (Pedrocchi *et al.* 1994). S100A6 changes conformation upon Ca²⁺-binding and exposes hydrophobic regions (Kuznicki and Filipek 1987; 10; Pedrocchi *et al.* 1994), forms dimers by an S-S bridge (6; 10; 15; Pedrocchi *et al.* 1994), and noncovalent forces (Wojda and Kuznicki 1994) (Fig. 1). The N-terminal end of S100A6 is blocked by an acetyl group.

Antibodies

Rabbit antibodies against mouse S100A6 recognize mouse, rat, and human S100A6, but do not react with other S-100 proteins (9, Kuznicki *et al.* 1992). They are commercially available through Swant. Antibodies against S100A6 from rabbit (Okazaki *et al.* 1994) and human recombinant S100A6 (Pedrocchi *et al.* 1994) were also produced.

Anatomical localization

S100A6 immunoreactivity was found to be abundant in cytosol of human and rat fibroblasts and epithelial cells

(Kuznicki *et al.* 1992; Kordowska *et al.* 1994), and was detected in neurons, but not in glial cells (Filipek *et al.* 1993). S100A6 mRNA was found in mouse in the epithelia lining the gastrointestinal, respiratory, and urinary tracts, in the goblet cells in the small intestine (Timmons *et al.* 1993), and in tissues that support pregnancy such as chorioamnion and decidua (Waterhouse *et al.* 1992). The S100A6 transcripts were also detected in the corpus luteum, placenta, and nerves within the gut wall (Timmons *et al.* 1993). S100A6 mRNA was localized in the postmitotic keratogenous region of the murine hair follicle (31).

Biological activities

The physiological action of S100A6 protein is not known. It has been suggested that S100A6 is involved in cell cycle progression (4), interaction with cytoskeleton (8), neuroblastoma differentiation (Tonini *et al.* 1991), metastasis (25; Weterman *et al.* 1992), secretion of mouse placental lactogen II (30), exocytosis (Kuznicki *et al.* 1992), mucus secretion (Timmons *et al.* 1993), insulin secretion (Okazaki *et al.* 1994), and histamine release from mast cells (Fuji *et al.* 1994).

Biological regulation

S100A6 gene expression is activated upon stimulation of G_i-phase cells by serum or growth factors (1; 4), during differentiation of PC12 cells induced by nerve growth factor (23, 24), and during neuronal differentiation induced by retinoic acid (27). Serum-responsive elements were localized in the last 42 bp immediately upstream from the CAP site of the human S100A6 gene (Ghezzo *et al.* 1989).

Diseases/mutagenesis

S100A6 is overexpressed in some tumor cells (leukemia, melanoma, neuroblastoma, and colon). High levels of S100A6 mRNA were associated with the metastatic ability of ras-transformed cells (25), and S100A6 expression in human melanoma correlated with metastatic behavior in nude mice (Weterman *et al.* 1992). S100A6 immunoreactivity was used to detect changes in biliary epithelium in transplanted livers (44) and in experimentally induced biliary cirrhosis (Fig. 2) (Kordowska *et al.* 1994). Expression of S100A6 gene was enhanced during corneal wound healing (38). Different S100A6 mutants (15; Watanabe *et al.* 1993), and fragments of S100A6 (16) were described.

Interactions

The S100A6 protein interacts *in vitro* in a Ca^{2+}-dependent manner with annexin II, glyceraldehyde-3-phosphate dehydrogenase (8; Zeng *et al.* 1993), annexin VI (Zeng *et al.* 1993), annexin XI (14; 41; 42), sialic acid in fetuin (18), and caldesmon (Mani and Kay 1993).

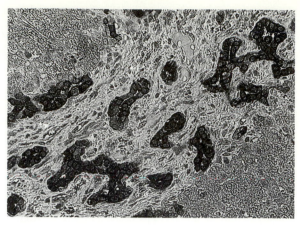

Figure 2. Section of rat liver with cirrhosis, stained with S100A6 antibodies.

References

Dorin, J.R., Emslie, E., and van Heyningen, V. (1990) Related calcium-binding proteins map to the same subregion of chromosome 1q and to an extended region of synteny on mouse chromosome 3. Genomics **8**, 420–426.

Engelkamp, D., Schafer, B.W., Erne, P., and Heizmann, C.W. (1992) S100 alpha, CAPL, and CACY: molecular cloning and expression analysis of three calcium-binding proteins from human heart. Biochemistry **31**, 10258–10264.

Engelkamp, D., Schaffer, B.W., Mattei, M.G., Erne, P., and Heizmann, C.W. (1993) Six S100 genes are clustered on human chromosome 1q21: Identification of two genes coding for the two previously unreported calcium-binding proteins S100D and S100E. Proc. Natl. Acad. Sci. USA **90**, 6547–6551.

*Filipek, A. and Kuznicki, J. (1993) Calcyclin – from basic research to clinical implications. Acta Biochim. Pol. **40**, 321–327.

Filipek, A., Puzianowska, M., Cieslak, B., and Kuznicki, J. (1993) Calcyclin-Ca^{2+}-binding protein homologous to glial S-100 beta is present in neurons. Neuroreport. **4**, 383–386.

Fujii, T., Kuzumaki, N., Ogoma, Y., and Kondo, Y. (1994) Effects of calcium-binding proteins on histamine release from permeabilized rat peritoneal mast cells. Biol. Pharm. Bull. **17**, 581–585.

Ghezzo, F., Valpreda, S., De Riel, J.K., and Baserga, R. (1989) Identification of serum-responsive elements in the promoter of human calcyclin, a growth-regulated gene. DNA **8**, 171–177.

Kordowska, J., Aple, A., Brand, I.A., and Kuznicki, J. (1994) Distribution and level of calcyclin in normal rat tissues and in experimentally induced liver cirrhosis biliaris. Acta Histochem. Cytochem. **27**, 205–218.

Kuznicki, J., and Filipek, A. (1987) Purification and properties of a novel Ca^{2+}-binding protein (10.5 kDa) from Ehrlich ascites tumor cells. Biochem. J. **247**, 663–667.

Kuznicki J., Kordowska, J., Puzianowska, M., and Worniewicz, B.M. (1992) Calcyclin as a marker of human epithelial cells and fibroblasts. Exp. Cell Res. **200**, 425–430.

Mani, R.S., and Kay, C.M. (1993) Calcium-dependent regulation of the caldesmon–heavy meromyosin interaction by caltropin. Biochemistry **32**, 11217–11223.

Murphy, L.C., Murphy, L.J., Tsuyuki, D., Duckworth, M.L., and Shiu, R.P. (1988) Cloning and characterization of a cDNA encoding a highly conserved, putative calcium binding protein, identified by an anti-prolactin receptor antiserum. J. Biol. Chem. **263**, 2397–2401.

*Okazaki, K., Niki, I., Iino, S., Kobayashi, S., and Hidaka, H. (1994) A role of calcyclin, a Ca²⁺-binding protein, on the Ca²⁺-dependent insulin release from the pancreatic beta cell. J. Biol. Chem. **269**, 6149–6152.

Pedrocchi, M., Schafer, B.W., Durussel, I., Cox, J.A., and Heizmann, C.W. (1994) Purification and characterization of the recombinant human calcium-binding S100 proteins CAPL and CACY. Biochemistry **33**, 6732–6738.

Schäfer, B.W., Wicki R., Engelkamp D., Mattei M.G., and Heizmann C.W. (1995) Isolation of a YAC clone covering a cluster of nine S100 genes on chromosome 1q21: rationale for a new nomenclature of the S100 calcium-binding protein family. Genomics **25**, 638–643.

*Timmons, P.M., Chan, C.T., Rigby, P.W., and Poirier, F. (1993) The gene encoding the calcium binding protein calcyclin is expressed at sites of exocytosis in the mouse. J. Cell Sci. **104**, 187–196.

Tonini, G.P., Casalaro, A., Cara, A., and Di Martino, D. (1991) Inducible expression of calcyclin, a gene with strong homology to S-100 protein, during neuroblastoma cell differentiation and its prevalent expression in Schwann-like cell lines. Cancer Res. **51**, 1733–1737.

Watanabe, M., Ando, Y., Tokumitsu, H., and Hidaka, H. (1993) Binding site of annexin XI on the calcyclin molecule. Biochem. Biophys. Res. Commun. **196**, 1376–1382.

Waterhouse, P., Parhar, R.S., Guo, X., Lala, P.K., and Denhardt, D.T. (1992) Regulated temporal and spatial expression of the calcium-binding proteins calcyclin and OPN (osteopontin) in mouse tissues during pregnancy. Mol. Reprod. Dev. **32**, 315–323.

Weterman, M.A., Stoopen, G.M., van Muijen, G.N., Kuznicki, J., Ruiter, D.J., and Bloemers, H.P. (1992) Expression of calcyclin in human melanoma cell lines correlates with metastatic behavior in nude mice. Cancer Res. **52**, 1291–1296.

Wojda, U. and Kuznicki, J. (1994) Calcyclin from mouse Ehrlich ascites tumor cells and rabbit lung form non-covalent dimers. Biochim. Biophys. Acta **1209**, 248–252.

Zeng, F.Y., Gerke, V., and Gabius, H.J. (1993) Identification of annexin II, annexin VI and glyceraldehyde–3-phosphate dehydrogenase as calcyclin-binding proteins in bovine heart. Int. J. Biochem. **25**, 1019–1027.

■ *Jacek Kuznicki:*
Nencki Institute of Experimental Biology,
3 Pasteur str., 02-093 Warsaw, Poland,
Tel.: 48 2 659 3123
Fax: 48 22 22 5342
E-mail: jacek@nencki.gov.pl

S100A7

S100A7 is a low molecular weight Ca²⁺-binding protein that is strongly upregulated in psoriatic keratinocytes as well as in abnormally differentiated cultured human keratinocytes. S100A7 is expressed mainly by stratified squamous epithelia and may play a role in skin inflammatory response.

S100A7, also known as psoriasin, which corresponds to IEF 3002 in the human keratinocyte protein database (Celis *et al.* 1994), has a calculated molecular mass of 11,457 Da and an isoelectric point (p*I*) of 6.77, values that are close to those observed in two-dimensional (2D) gels (apparent molecular mass = 11 kDa; p*I*, 6.2). It contains two EF-hand domains and binds Ca²⁺ as determined by the blot overlay assay (Hoffmann *et al.* 1994). S100A7 is partially external-ized to the medium by cultured keratinocytes in spite of the fact that it lacks a peptide signal sequence at its amino terminal end (Madsen *et al.* 1991). Several acidic variants of the protein have been found but the nature of the modification(s) is (are) at present unknown.

In the human fetus, S100A7 is expressed by tissues containing stratified epithelium. Keratinocytes from normal adult skin express low levels of S100A7 (Fig. 1A) but their

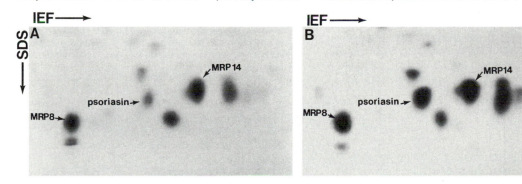

Figure 1. Localization of S100A7 in 2D gel autoradiograms [³⁵S]-methionine labelled proteins from (A) non-cultured, normal human keratinocytes and (B) psoriatic keratinocytes.

psoriatic counterparts show strong upregulation of this protein (Fig. 1B). Only transformed human keratinocyte cell lines that are able to differentiate (HaCat, UBJ) synthesize significant levels of S100A7, indicating that its expression is not compatible with a fully transformed phenotype. Lymphocytes, neutrophils, eosinophils, monocytes, fibroblasts, and endothelial cells do not synthesize detectable levels of S100A7. So far, only fetal calf serum (10% in the culture medium), Ca^{2+} (2 mM), and retinoic acid (4×10^{-7}M) have been shown to increase the levels of S100A7 in primary cultured human keratinocytes (Hoffmann et al. 1994).

Recently, it has been shown that S100A7 is also expressed in other skin diseases such as mycosis fungoides, atopic dermatitis, lichen sclerosus et atrophicus, and Darier's disease (Sitzmann et al. 1993), suggesting a general role in skin inflammatory response.

■ Alternative names

Psoriasin (Madsen et al. 1991).

■ Identification

S100A7 was originally identified by comparing 2D gel patterns of [^{35}S]-methionine labeled proteins from normal and psoriatic non-cultured human keratinocytes (Celis et al. 1990).

■ Gene and sequence

Oligodeoxynucleotide probes derived from part of a peptide sequence from S100A7 were used to screen a λgt11 cDNA library prepared from unfractionated epidermal keratinocytes obtained from psoriatic skin (Madsen et al. 1991). The open reading frame codes for a protein composed of 101 amino acids having a M_r of 11,457 and a calculated pI of 6.77 (GenBank accession number M86757). The gene for S100A7 has been mapped to chromosome 1q21 (Hoffmann et al. 1994).

As expected, the expression of the S100A7 specific transcript was found to be very high in psoriatic keratinocytes as compared to their normal counterparts. The transcript was not detected in SV40 transformed human keratinocytes (K14); A431 cells; AMA (transformed human amnion cells); MRC-5 V2 (SV40 transformed embryonal human lung fibroblasts), and MRC-5 (embryonal human lung fibroblasts) (Madsen et al. 1991).

■ Protein

S100A7 contains an N-terminal Ca^{2+}-binding signature (F_{17} to P_{41}) and a canonical EF-hand extending from L_{55} to I_{82}. Purified recombinant S100A7 produced in E. coli has been shown to bind Ca^{2+} in the same way as the native protein recovered from 2D gels (Hoffmann et al. 1994).

■ Antibodies

Rabbit polyclonal antibodies specific for S100A7–as determined by 2D gel Western blotting–have been prepared against the protein recovered from 2D gels (Celis et al. 1990). The antibodies are not suitable for immunofluorescence but work well in immunoblotting and immunoprecipitation. No commercial antibodies are available.

■ Biological regulation

So far only fetal calf serum (10% in the culture medium; Madsen et al. 1992), Ca^{2+} (2 mM) and retinoic acid (4×10^{-7}M) have been shown to increase the levels of S100A7 in primary cultured human keratinocytes (Hoffmann et al. 1994). No effect has been detected in cells treated with phorbol-12-myristate 13-acetate, INF-α or TNF-α.

■ References

Celis, J.E., Crüger, D., Kiil, J., Lauridsen, J.B., Ratz, G., Basse, B., Celis, and A. (1990) Identification of a group of proteins that are strongly up-regulated in total epidermal keratinocytes from psoriatic skin. FEBS Lett. **262**, 159–164.

Celis, J.E., Rasmussen, H.H., Olsen, E., Madsen, P., Leffers, H., Honoré, B., Dejgaard, K., Dejgaard, K., Gromov, P., Vorum, H., Vassilev, A., Baskin, Y., Liu, X., Celis. A., Basse, B., Lauridsen, J.B., Ratz, G.P., Andersen, A.H., Walbum, E., Kjærgaard, I., Andersen, I., Puype, M., Van Damme, J., and Vanderkerckhove, J. (1994) The human keratinocyte two-dimensional database (Update 1994): Towards an integrated approach to the study of cell proliferation, differentiation and skin diseases. Electrophoresis **15**, 1349–1458.

Hoffmann, H.H., Olsen, E., Etzerodt, M., Madsen, P., Thøgersen, H.C., Kruse, T., and Celis, J.E. (1994) Psoriasin binds calcium and is upregulated by calcium to levels that resemble those observed in normal skin. J. Invest Dermatol. **103**, 370–375.

Madsen, P., Rasmussen, H.H., Leffers, H., Honoré, B., Dejgaard, K., Olsen, E., Kiil, J., Walbum, E., Andersen, A.H., Basse, B., Lauridsen, J.B., Ratz, G.P., Celis, A., Vandekerckhove, J., and Celis, J.E. (1991) Molecular cloning, occurrence and expression of a novel secreted protein "psoriasin" that is highly up-regulated in psoriatic skin. J. Invest. Dermatol. **97**, 701–712.

Madsen, P., Rasmussen, H.H., Leffers, H., Honoré, B., and Celis J.E. (1992) Molecular cloning and expression of a novel keratinocyte protein [psoriasis-associated fatty acid binding protein (PA-FABP)] that is highly up-regulated in psoriatic skin and that shares similarity to fatty acid-binding proteins. J. Invest. Dermatol. **99**, 299–305.

Sitzmann, J., Algermissen, B., Czarnetski, B.M., and LeMotte, P. (1993) Expression of psoriasin mRNA in several human skin diseases. J. Invest. Dermatol. **100**, 220.

■ *Peder Madsen and Julio E. Celis:*
Department of Medical Biochemistry and
Danish Centre for Human Genome Research,
University of Aarhus,
Ole Worms Allé build. 170,
DK-8000 Aarhus C, Denmark
Tel.: +45 89 42 28 80
Fax:+45 86 13 11 60

S100A8 and S100A9

S100A8 and S100A9 are two Ca²⁺-binding proteins of the S100 familiy. They are expressed during myeloid differentiation by granulocytes and monocytes as well as by some epithelial cells, e.g. keratinocytes after inflammatory activation. S100A8 and S100A9 assemble to noncovalently associated complexes which are Ca²⁺-dependently translocated to membrane structures and intermediate filaments. Both proteins are supposed to play a role in intracellular signalling during activation of phagocytes.

S100A8 and S100A9 show molecular weights of about 10,800 and 13,200, respectively. Both proteins contain two Ca^{2+}-binding sites of the EF-type. S100A9 has been shown to be phosphorylated and to exist in two isotypes the smaller of which lacks the first four amino acids.

Expression of S100A8 and S100A9 is restricted to granulocytes and early stages of monocytic differentiation (Odink *et al.* 1987). Both are found in infiltrating myelomonocytic cells during various inflammatory disorders, whereas mature tissue macrophages do not express these proteins (Zwadlo *et al.* 1986; Roth *et al.* 1994). The abundance of S100A8 and S100A9 positive cells *in vivo* correlates with the activity of inflammatory processes (Hessian *et al.* 1993; Sunderkötter *et al.* 1993). S100A8 and S100A9 are released by a so far unknown mechanism and can be found at elevated concentrations in sera of patients suffering from various inflammatory diseases (Dorin *et al.* 1987; Roth *et al.* 1992; Hessian *et al.* 1993). Elevation of intracellular Ca^{2+} levels leads to the translocation of these proteins from the cytoplasma to the plasma membrane as well as to intermediate filaments (Roth *et al.* 1993). Translocation to membrane structures has been shown to correlate with activation of phagocytes, indicating a role of these proteins in intracellular signalling (Bhardwaj *et al.* 1992; Lemarchand *et al.* 1992).

■ Alternative names

Synonyms for S100A8 are MRP8, calgranulin A, p8, L1 complex light chain, and CP-10. S100A9 is referred to as MRP14, calgranulin B, p14, L1 complex heavy chain, and MAC387 antigen. In addition, the complex of these proteins has been called cystic fibrosis antigen, 60B8 antigen, and calprotectin (Hessian *et al.* 1993, Goebeler *et al.* 1994).

■ Identification/isolation

S100A8 and S100A9 were initially purified with a monoclonal antibody against the macrophage migration inhibitory factor (MIF) and cloned by screening of a human leukocyte cDNA libary (Odink *et al.* 1987). Approximately at the same time characterization of the so called cystic fibrosis antigen resulted in cloning of the S100A8 cDNA (Dorin *et al.* 1987). Both proteins can be purified from neutrophil cytosol using a fast-protein liquid chromatography technique (Edgeworth *et al.* 1991).

■ Gene and sequence

Human S100A8 and S100A9 are each encoded by single copy genes on chromosome 1. Both genes consist of three exons; exon two contains the translation initiation site. The S100A8 cDNA has an open reading frame of 279 nucleotides predicting a protein of 93 amino acids, S100A9 cDNA contains 342 nucleotides predicting 114 amino acids. The genomic DNA sequences of both genes have been cloned and several conserved regions and putative binding sites for transcriptional factors have been described (Lagasse and Clerc 1988; Kuwayama *et al.* 1993). Full length or at least partial sequences of S100A8 and S100A9 have been reported from mice, rat, rabbit, pork, and the bovine system.

■ Protein

S100A8 and S100A9 have molecular weights of 10,800 and 13,200, respectively. Both proteins contain two Ca^{2+}-binding sites of the EF-hand type. S100A9 has been shown to be posttranslationally modified by phosphorylation on threonine 113 and N-terminal acetylation. Phosphorylation seems to enhance its Ca^{2+} affinity. A S100A9 variant lacking the first four amino acids has been characterized. The functional relevance of these two isoforms is yet not clear (Odink *et al.* 1987; Edgeworth *et al.* 1989; Teigelkamp *et al.* 1991).

■ Antibodies

Various monoclonal antibodies against S100A8 and S100A9 are now commercially available (Dianova). The monoclonal antibody MAC387 which is widely used for phenotypical characterization of myelomonocytic cells, detects an epitope on S100A9 (Goebeler *et al.* 1994). Furthermore, employing the monoclonal antibody 27E10, which detects S100A8 and S100A9 heterodimers but not S100A8 or S100A9 monomers, it is possible to identify complex assembly of these proteins *in situ* (Bhardwaj *et al.* 1992).

Anatomical localization

S100A8 and S100A9 represent a major portion of the total cellular protein content in neutrophils and monocytes, whereas mature macrophages or lymphocytes do not contain these proteins at all. Expression of S100A8 and S100A9 in monocytes and neutrophils therefore reflects distinct cellular stages during myeloid differentiation which appear to be characterized by specific modes of reaction to Ca^{2+}-mediated stimuli. Expression of S100A8 and S100A9 by infiltrating neutrophils and monocytes has been shown to correlate with the activity of inflammatory processes during a variety of disorders in humans (Zwadlo et al. 1986, Hessian et al. 1993) as well as in models of experimental inflammation in mice (Sunderkötter et al. 1993). Furthermore, cells of epithelial origin, such as keratinocytes, express these proteins after inflammatory activation (Kelly et al. 1989).

S100A8 and S100A9 were initially described as cystic fibrosis antigen, which was found to be elevated in the sera of cystic fibrosis patients. However, elevated serum concentrations of these proteins are associated with various inflammatory processes. Their levels correlate significantly with local and systemic signs of disease activity. Little is known about the mechanism of their extracellular release (Dorin et al. 1987; Roth et al. 1992; Hessian et al. 1993).

Biological activities

S100A8 and S100A9 seem to play a role in Ca^{2+}-mediated intracellular signalling. Complexes of these proteins, but not their monomers, have been described as modulating the activity of protein kinases in vitro (Murao et al. 1989). Interestingly, complex formation is triggered by elevation of Ca^{2+}-levels. Ca^{2+}-dependent translocation of S100A8 and S100A9 to membrane structures and intermediate filaments (see below) refers to a modulatory role of S100A8 and S100A9 in the network of cytoskeletal/membrane interactions. Restriction of S100A8 and S100A9 expression to distinct stages of myelomonocytic differentiation suggests that these proteins are involved in highly specific pathways of intracellular signalling in phagocytes. Accordingly, Ca^{2+}-induced translocation of S100A8 and S100A9 to membrane structures has been shown to coincide with secretion of proinflammatory cytokines by monocytes (Bhardwaj et al. 1992), and enhanced superoxide release by neutrophils in vitro (Lemarchand et al. 1992).

In addition, S100A8 and S100A9 have been shown to exhibit antimicrobial actions in vitro. Antibacterial activity, however, was strongly influenced by the culture medium (Steinbakk et al. 1990; Murthy et al. 1993). A recent report on a chemotactic activity, of murine but not of human S100A8 on neutrophils has not been confirmed so far by other investigators (Lackmann et al. 1992)

Biological regulation

S100A8 and S100A9 expression is down-regulated by a Ca^{2+}-induced suppressor mechanism. De novo synthesis of repressor protein(s) seems to be responsible for Ca^{2+}-dependent regulation of these proteins (Roth et al. 1994). Interestingly, a recent study showed that nuclear factors not characterized yet bind to the 5' promotor region of S100A8 and S100A9 genes which has been shown to correlate with vitamin D_3-dependent induction of S100A8 and S100A9 transcription in HL-60 cells (Kuwayama et al. 1993).

Interactions

Elevation of intracellular Ca^{2+}-levels has been shown to lead to assembly of S100A8 and S100A9 to non-covalently linked complexes of 25, 36, and 48 kDa, which are supposed to represent the biologically active forms. The 25 kDa complex presents the S100A8 and S100A9 heterodimer, the 36 kDa band the $(S100A8)_2$ /S100A9 trimer, and the 48 kDa complex contains two S100A8 and two S100A9 chains (Teigelkamp et al. 1991). These protein complexes are Ca^{2+}-dependently translocated from the cytosol to membrane structures and intermediate filaments, and this has been shown to correlate with phagocytic activation (Bhardwaj et al. 1992; Lemarchand et al. 1992; Roth et al. 1993).

References

Bhardwaj, R.S., Zotz, C., Zwadlo-Klarwasser, G., Roth, J., Goebeler, M., Mahnke, K., Falk, M., Meinardus-Hager, G., and Sorg, C. (1992) The calcium-binding proteins MRP8 and MRP14 form a membrane associated heterodimer in a subset of monocytes/macrophages present in acute but absent in chronic inflammatory lesions. Eur. J. Immunol. **22**, 1891–1897.

Dorin, J.R., Novak, M., Hill, R.E., Brock, D.J.H., Secher, D.S., and van Heyningen, V. (1987) A clue to the basic defect in cystic fibrosis from cloning the CF antigen gene. Nature **326**, 614–617.

Edgeworth, J., Freemont, P., and Hogg, N. (1989) Ionomycin-regulated phosphorylation of the myeloid calcium-binding protein p14. Nature **342**, 189–192.

Edgeworth, J., Gorman, M., Bennett, R., Freemont, P., and Hogg, N. (1991) Identification of p8,14 as a highly abudant heterodimeric calcium binding protein complex of myeloid cells. J. Biol. Chem. **266**, 7706–7713.

Goebeler, M., Roth, J., Teigelkamp, S., and Sorg, C. (1994) The monoclonal antibody MAC387 detects an epitope on the calcium-binding protein MRP14. J. Leuko. Biol. **55**, 259–261.

Hessian, P.A., Edgeworth, J., and Hogg, N. (1993) MRP8 and MRP14, two abundant calcium-binding proteins of neutrophils and monocytes. J. Leuko. Biol. **53**, 197–204.

Kelly, S.E., Jones, D.B., and Fleming S. (1989) Calgranulin expression in inflammatory dermatoses. J. Pathol. **159**, 17–21.

Kuwayama, A., Kuruto, R., Horie, N., Takeishi, K., and Nozawa R. (1993) Appearance of nuclear factors that interact with genes for myeloid calcium binding proteins (MRP8 and MRP14) in differentiated HL-60 cells. Blood **81**, 3116–3121.

Lackmann, M., Cornich, C.J., Simpson, R.J., Moritz, R.L., and Geczy, C.L. (1992) Purification and structural analysis of a murine chemotactic cytokine (CP-10) with sequence homology to S100 proteins. J. Biol. Chem. **267**, 7499–7504.

Lagasse, E. and Clerc, R.G. (1988) Cloning and expression of two human genes encoding calcium-binding proteins that are regulated during myeloid differentiation. Mol. Cell. Biol. **8**, 2402–2410.

Lemarchand, P., Vaglio, M., Mauel, J., and Markert, M. (1992) Translocation of a small calcium-binding protein (MRP8) to plasma membrane correlates with human neutrophil activation. J. Biol. Chem. **267**, 19379–19382.

Murao, S., Collart, F.R., and Huberman, E. (1989) A protein containing the cystic fibrosis antigen is an inhibitor of protein kinases. J. Biol. Chem. **264**, 8356–8360.

Murthy, A.R.K., Lehrer, R.I., Harwig, S.S.L., and Miyasaki, K.T. (1993) In vitro candidastatic properties of the human neutrophil calprotectin complex. J. Immunol. **151**, 6291–6301.

Odink, K., Cerletti, N., Brüggen, J., Clerc, R.G., Tarcsay, L., Zwadlo, G., Gerhards, G., Schlegel, R., and Sorg, C. (1987) Two calcium-binding proteins in infiltrate macrophages of rheumatoid arthritis. Nature **330**, 80–82.

Roth, J., Teigelkamp, S., Wilke, M., Grün, L., Tümmler, B., and Sorg, C. (1992) Complex pattern of the myelo-monocytic differentiation antigens MRP8 and MRP14 during chronic airway inflammation. Immunobiol. **186**, 304–314.

Roth, J., Burwinkel, F., van den Bos, C., Goebeler, M., Vollmer, E., and Sorg, C. (1993) MRP8 and MRP14, S100-like proteins associated with myeloid differentiation, are translocated to plasma membrane and intermediate filaments in a calcium dependent manner. Blood **82**, 1875–1883.

Roth, J., Goebeler, M., Wrocklage, V., van den Bos, C., and Sorg, C. (1994) Expression of the calcium-binding proteins MRP8 and MRP14 in monocytes is regulated by a calcium-induced suppressor mechanism. Biochem. J. **301**, 655–660.

Steinbakk, M., Naess-Andresen, C.-F., Lingaas, E., Dale, I., Brandtzaeg, P., and Fagerhol, M.K. (1990) Antimicrobial actions of calcium binding leukocyte L1 protein, calprotectin. Lancet **336**, 763–765.

Sunderkötter, C., Kunz, M., Steinbrink, K., Meinardus-Hager, G., Goebeler, M., Bildau, H., and Sorg, C. (1993) Resistance of mice to experimental leishmaniasis is associated with more rapid appearance of mature macrophages in vitro and in vivo. J. Immunol. **151**, 4891–4901.

Teigelkamp, S., Bhardwaj, R. S., Roth, J., Meinardus-Hager, G., Karas, M., and Sorg, C. (1991) Calcium dependent complex assembly of the myeloic differentiation proteins MRP8 and MRP14. J. Biol. Chem. **266**, 13462–13467.

Zwadlo, G., Schlegel, R., and Sorg, C. (1986) A monoclonal antibody to a subset of human monocytes found only in the peripheral blood and inflammatory tissues. J. Immunol. **137**, 512–518.

■ *Johannes Roth and Clemens Sorg,*
Institute of Experimental Dermatology,
University of Münster,
von Esmarch Str. 56,
D-48149 Münster, Germany
Tel.: +49 251 89 77
Fax: +49 251 89 536

S100A10

S100A10 is a member of the S100 protein family found in a number of different tissues and cell lines. It is characterized by two mutated and thereby inactive EF-hand loops. S100A10 forms a heterotetrameric complex with the Ca^{2+}/lipid-binding protein annexin II. This binding is of regulatory importance and anchors the complex in the cell cortex where it is thought to play a role in membrane transport processes.

S100A10 is 96 amino acids in length and has an apparent molecular mass (M_r) of 11 kDa. Due to a three amino acid deletion in the first (N-terminal) EF-hand loop, and due to crucial amino acid substitutions in the second (C-teminal) EF-hand loop, the two putative Ca^{2+}-binding sites are inactive. S100A10 interacts with annexin II and thereby regulates the biochemical properties and the intracellular localization of this Ca^{2+}/lipid-binding protein. cDNAs encoding S100A10 have been cloned from human, cow, mouse, chicken, and *Xenopus laevis* (Saris *et al.* 1987; Kube *et al.* 1991). Identities in the determined or predicted amino acid sequences range from 60% (between *X. laevis* and human S100A10) to 100% (between pig and human S100A10) (Kube *et al.* 1991).

S100A10 is expressed in a number of different cell lines and tissues and most abundant in endothelial cells and certain epithelia (Zokas and Glenney 1987; Osborn *et al.* 1988). In its complex with annexin II it is found in the cortical region of the cell underlying the plasma membrane. Here the complex could be associated with the inner leaflet of the plasma membrane and/or the early endosomal membrane. S100A10 is thought to function as a key regulator of annexin II, with the annexin II–S100A10 complex most probably acting on membrane and/or cytoskeletal targets in the submembranous region (for reviews see Gerke 1989; Gruenberg and Emans 1993; Burgoyne and Clague 1994).

■ Alternative names

p11, Calpactin light chain (Glenney 1986), 42C (Masiakowski and Shooter 1988), CLP 11, p10, Ca[1].

■ Identification/isolation

S100A10 was first purified from intestinal epithelial cells and chicken embryo fibroblasts as a complex with annexin II (Erikson *et al.* 1984; Gerke and Weber 1984, 1985a). The purification protocol employed a Ca^{2+}-dependent protein fractionation and several conventional chromatographic steps. Dissociation of the annexin II–S100A10 complex was achieved by gel filtration in the presence of 9 M urea. Subsequently the separated subunits could be renatured individually by dialysis against urea-free buffer (Gerke and Weber 1985a). Direct protein sequencing of the S100A10 obtained using this protocol established the porcine S100A10 sequence (Gerke and Weber 1985b). Bovine and mouse S100A10 sequences were obtained by cDNA cloning (Saris *et al.* 1987). A rat S100A10 cDNA, called 42C, was isolated by subtractive hybridization from a phaeochromocytoma cell (PC12) cDNA library and S100A10 mRNA expression was shown to be induced in these cells by NGF (Masiakowski and Shooter 1988). Hybridization cloning led to the isolation of cDNAs for human, chicken, and *Xenopus laevis* S100A10 (Kube *et al.* 1991).

Gene and sequences

The GenBank/EMBL accession numbers for the S100A10 cDNAs are as follows: M16464 (bovine S100A10; Saris *et al.* 1987), M16465 (mouse S100A10; Saris *et al.* 1987), J03624 (Masiakowski and Shooter 1988), M38591 (human S100A10; Kube *et al.* 1991), M38592 (chicken S100A10; Kube *et al.* 1991), M38593 (*Xenopus laevis* S100A10; Kube *et al.* 1991). The gene encoding human S100A10 has been cloned and shown to contain two introns at positions conserved within the S100 family, i.e. in the 5′-untranslated region and in the protein coding region separating the two EF hands (Harder *et al.* 1992). The accession number for the 5′-nontranscribed region of the human S100A10 gene is M77483. The genes for mouse and human S100A10 have been mapped to chromosomes 3 and 1, respectively (Saris *et al.* 1987; Schäfer *et al.* 1995).

Protein

The amino acid of pig S100A10 is listed in the SwissProt database under the accession number P04163 (Gerke and Weber 1985b). Sequence identities between the different predicted protein sequences range from 60% (between *X. laevis* and human S100A10) to 100% (between pig and human S100A10). All S100A10 protein sequences predict the presence of two mutated EF-hand loops characterized by a three amino acid deletion in the N-terminal loop and by substitutions of consensus Ca^{2+} coordinating residues in the C-terminal loop. The second EF hand is followed by a unique C-terminal extension.

As predicted by the protein sequences, and as revealed by equilibrium dialysis experiments and spectroscopic studies, S100A10 does not bind Ca^{2+} (Gerke and Weber 1985b; Glenney 1986). Chemical cross-linking and hydrodynamic analysis revealed that S100A10 forms a homodimer (Gerke and Weber 1985a). Dimer formation requires the integrity of a conserved cysteine residue located in the C-terminal extension of the molecule (Cys82), as alkylation of this cysteine interferes with dimerization (Johnsson and Weber 1990).

Antibodies

Different monoclonal antibodies specific for S100A10 are commercially available through Swant, Zymed Laboratories Inc., Affinity Research Product Limited, and Glentech Inc. (addresses at the end of the book).

Localization

S100A10 has been identified in a number of tissues showing a distribution essentially identical to that of annexin II. Highest protein levels are found in intestine and lung, whereas moderate expression is observed in spleen, adrenal gland, kidney, and cardiac muscle (Zokas and Glenney 1987). Within the cell S100A10 is present in the peripheral region underlying the plasma membrane and seems to be associated with the cortical cytoskeleton (for review see Gerke 1989).

Biological activities

S100A10 is thought to function as a regulator of its intracellular protein ligand annexin II, as complex formation significantly alters the biochemical properties and the intracellular distribution of annexin II (Powell and Glenney 1987; Drust and Creutz 1988; Thiel *et al.* 1992). Biological activities discussed for the complex include the involvement in membrane transport processes during endo- and/or exocytosis as well as the establishment and regulation of membrane-cytoskeletal linkages (for reviews see Gerke 1989; Gruenberg and Emans 1993; Burgoyne and Claque 1994).

Biological regulation

Expression of the S100A10 mRNA is induced by NGF in PC12 cells (Masiakowski and Shooter 1988).

Mutagenesis studies

By employing site-directed mutagenesis and recombinant expression of human S100A10 in *E. coli* the unique C-terminal extension of S100A10 has been shown to be involved in annexin II binding. Tyrosine 85 and phenylalanine 86 located in this extension were found to participate in establishing the hydrophobic interaction with annexin II (Kube *et al.* 1992).

Interactions

S100A10 has been shown to bind to annexin II in a Ca^{2+}-independent manner. This interaction leads to the formation of a heterotetrameric annexin II_2 $S100A10_2$ complex. The protein–protein interaction between annexin II and S100A10 is driven by hydrophobic forces and occurs *in vitro* and *in vivo* (for review see Weber 1992).

References

Burgoyne, R.D. and Clague, M.J. (1994) Annexins in the endocytic pathway. Trends Biochem. Sci. **19**, 231–232.

Drust, D.S. and Creutz, C.E. (1988) Aggregation of chromaffin granules by calpactin at micomolar levels of calcium. Nature **331**, 88–91.

Erikson, E., Tomasiewicz, H.G., and Erikson, R.L. (1984) Biochemical characterization of a 34-kilodalton normal cellular substrate of pp60v-src and an associated 6-kilodalton protein. Mol. Cell. Biol. **4**, 77–85.

Gerke, V. (1989) Tyrosine protein kinase substrate p36: a member of the annexin family of Ca^{2+}/phospholipid-binding proteins. Cell Motil. Cytoskeleton **14**, 449–454.

Gerke, V. and Weber, K. (1984) Identity of p36K phosphorylated upon Rous sarcoma virus transformation with a protein purified from brush borders; calcium-dependent binding to non-erythroid spectrin and F-actin. EMBO J. **3**, 227–233.

Gerke, V. and Weber, K. (1985a) Calcium-dependent conformational changes in the 36-kDa subunit of intestinal protein I related to the cellular 36-kDa substrate of Rous sarcoma virus tyrosine kinase. J. Biol. Chem. **260**, 1688–1695.

Gerke, V. and Weber, K. (1985b) The regulatory chain in the p36-kd substrate complex of viral tyrosine-specific protein kinases is related in sequence to the S-100 protein of glial cells. EMBO J. **4**, 2917–2920.

Glenney, J.R. (1986) Phospholipid-dependent Ca^{2+}-binding by the 36-kDa tyrosine kinase substrate (calpactin) and its 33-kDa core. J. Biol. Chem. **261**, 7247–7252.

Gruenberg, J. and Emans, N. (1993) Annexins in membrane transport. Trends Cell Biol. **3**, 224–227.

Harder, T., Kube, E., and Gerke, V. (1992) Cloning and characterization of the human gene encoding p11; structural similarity to other members of the S-100 gene family. Gene **113**, 269–274.

Johnsson, N. and Weber, K. (1990) Alkylation of cysteine 82 of p11 abolishes the complex formation with the tyrosine-protein kinase substrate p36 (annexin 2, calpactin 1, lipocortin 2). J. Biol. Chem. **265**, 14464–14468.

Kube, E., Weber, K., and Gerke, V. (1991) Primary structure of human, chicken, and *Xenopus laevis* p11, a cellular ligand of the src kinase substrate, annexin II. Gene **102**, 255–259.

Kube, E., Becker, T., Weber, K., and Gerke, V. (1992) Protein–protein interaction studied by site-directed mutagenesis: characterization of the annexin II-binding site on p11, a member of the S-100 protein family. J. Biol. Chem. **267**, 14175–14182.

Masiakowski, P. and Shooter, E.M. (1988) Nerve growth factor induces the genes for two proteins related to a family of calcium binding proteins in PC12 cells. Proc. Natl. Acad. Sci. USA **85**, 1277–1281.

Osborn, M., Johnsson, N., Wehland, J. and Weber, K. (1988) The submembranous location of p11 and its interaction with the p36 substrate of pp60 src kinase *in situ*. Exp. Cell Res. **175**, 81–96.

Powell, M.A. and Glenney, J.R. (1987) Regulation of calpactin I phospholipid binding by calpactin I light-chain binding and phosphorylation by pp60v-src. Biochem. J. **247**, 321–328.

Saris, C.J.M., Kristensen, T., D'Eustachio, P., Hicks, L.J., Noonan, D.J., Hunter, T., and Tack, B.F. (1987) cDNA sequence and tissue distribution of the mRNA for bovine and murine p11, the S100-related light chain of the protein-tyrosine kinase substrate p36 (calpactin I). J. Biol. Chem. **262**, 10663–10671.

Schäfer, B.W., Wicki, R., Engelkamp, D., Mattei, M.G., and Heizmann, C.W. (1995) Isolation of a YAC clone covering a cluster of nine S100 genes on human chromosome 1q21: Rationale for a new nomenclature of the S100 calcium-binding protein family. Genomics **25**, 638–643.

Thiel, C., Osborn, M. and Gerke, V. (1992) The tight association of the tyrosine kinase substrate annexin II with the submembranous cytoskeleton depends on intact p11 and Ca^{2+} binding sites. J. Cell Sci. **103**, 733–742.

Weber, K. (1992) Annexin II: interaction with p11. In *The annexins* (ed. S.E. Moss), pp. 61–68. Portland Press, London.

Zokas, L. and Glenney, J.R. (1987) The calpactin light chain is tightly linked to the cytoskeletal form of calpactin I: studies using monoclonal antibodies to calpactin subunits. J. Cell Biol. **105**, 2111–2121.

■ *Volker Gerke:*
Clinical Research Group for Endothelial Cell Biology,
University of Münster,
Von-Esmarch-Str.56,
D-48149 Münster, Germany
Tel.: + 49 251 83 6722
Fax: + 49 251 83 6748
E-mail: gerke@wwupop.uni-muenster.de

S100β

S100β is an acidic Ca²⁺-binding protein synthesized and secreted by astroglial cells in the central nervous system. S100β interacts with a diverse range of intracellular target proteins and, as a disulfide-linked dimer, exhibits neurotrophic and mitogenic activities. Expression of S100β is abnormally regulated in certain neuropathological disorders.

S100β was originally isolated from bovine brain as a low molecular weight, acidic, protein fraction enriched in the nervous system, and called S100 to denote its partial solubility in 100% saturated ammonium sulfate (Moore 1965). A number of S100 proteins were subsequently identified and purified from the S100 fraction, and these proteins share extensive physicochemical and sequence similarities. S100β is the major form and the most extensively studied member of the S100 protein family, and is highly conserved in sequence and function among vertebrate species (for reviews, see Donato 1991; Hilt and Kligman 1991; Zimmer 1995). S100β has a molecular weight of 10,500, an isoelectric point of ~4.3, and two Ca²⁺-binding sites. The protein is most abundant in the nervous system, where it is localized primarily in glial cells. S100β levels are under tight and complex regulatory control, both at the transcriptional level and at the level of release from the cell. In addition, decreased or increased S100β production has been documented during development, in certain disease states, and in experimentally induced model systems. S100β has both intracellular and extracellular functions, as depicted schematically in Fig.1.

■ Alternative names

NEF: neurite extension factor (Kligman and Marshak 1985); S100b (ββ dimer).

■ Isolation/identification

S100β was first detected by starch gel electrophoresis of soluble extracts of bovine brain (Moore 1965). The protein was subsequently purified and characterized from the brains of several vertebrate species including bovine, porcine, rodent, and human, by a variety of purification methods that take advantage of S100β properties such as solubility, low molecular weight, acidic isoelectric point, heat stability, and Ca²⁺-binding activity. Production of recombinant S100β in *E. coli* provides a simple and rapid method to purify large amounts of

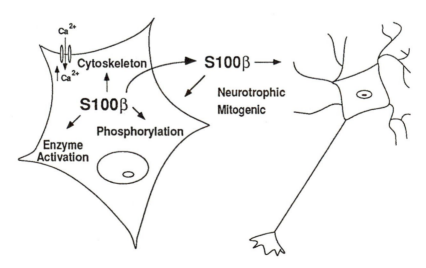

Figure 1. Potential biological roles of S100β. The Ca²⁺-binding protein S100β may transduce localized increases in cytoplasmic Ca²⁺ concentration into biological effects through its interaction with, and modulation of, intracellular binding proteins. S100β can also be released from the cell and, in a disulfide-linked dimeric form, exhibit neurotrophic or mitogenic activity on target cells.

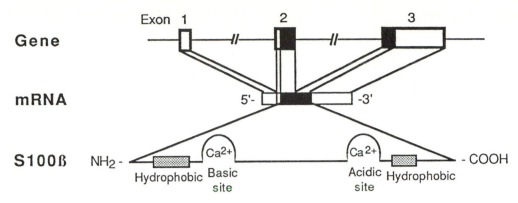

Figure 2. Schematic diagram of the organization of the S100β gene, mRNA, and protein. The S100β gene is composed of 3 exons (boxes), separated by introns (horizontal lines). Open boxes denote the 5'- and 3'-untranslated regions and black boxes denote the coding regions. The S100β amino acid sequence is encoded on exons 2 and 3. Exon 2 specifies amino acids 1–45 containing an N-terminal hydrophobic region and a helix-loop-helix Ca²⁺-binding domain rich in basic amino acids; exon 3 specifies amino acids 46–91 containing the acidic, canonical EF-hand Ca²⁺-binding domain and the C-terminal hydrophobic region.

biologically active S100β (Van Eldik *et al.* 1988; Barger *et al.* 1992).

Genes and sequences

The gene encoding human S100β is located on chromosome 21 in the Down syndrome region 21q22.2–22.3 (Duncan *et al.* 1989). The S100β gene has been isolated from human (Allore *et al.* 1990; GenBank accession numbers: M59486, M59487, M59488, J05600), rat (Maeda *et al.* 1991; S53517, S53522, S53527), and mouse (Jiang *et al.* 1993; L22144), and found to be conserved at both the nucleotide and amino acid sequence levels. For example, human and rodent S100β genes exhibit 85% identity in nucleic acid sequence in the protein-coding regions, and S100β proteins from human, cow, pig, rat, and mouse differ by only 1–4 amino acids. The exon/intron organization of the S100β genes is also similar, with exon 1 specifying the 5'-untranslated region, and exons 2 and 3 encoding the N- and C-terminal Ca²⁺-binding domains of the protein, respectively (Fig. 2).

Protein

S100β is soluble, acidic, and heat stable. No three-dimensional structure for S100β is available yet, but there are two Ca²⁺-binding domains characterized by an α-helix, loop, α-helix arrangement of the peptide chain. The C-terminal site resembles a canonical EF-hand similar to that found in calmodulin. The N-terminal site has a variant Ca²⁺-binding loop containing two extra amino acid residues, with a lower affinity for Ca²⁺. The Ca²⁺-binding properties of S100β can also be affected by the presence of Zn²⁺ or K⁺.

S100β can exist in several dimeric forms, including αβ heterodimers (termed S100a) and ββ homodimers (termed S100b). A disulfide-linked S100 ββ homodimer is required for neurotrophic activity, and dimerization of S100β can be enhanced by Ca²⁺ or lipid (Barger *et al.* 1992). Because S100β has two cysteine residues (amino acids 68 and 84), a number of dimeric forms are possible and the conformation of the biologically active dimer has not been defined yet.

Antibodies

Polyclonal and monoclonal antibodies against S100β are available commercially from a number of companies (e.g. Dako, Calbiochem, Chemicon, Sigma). Some antibodies generated against the bovine S100 fraction may show reactivity with multiple S100 proteins. Some antibodies made against purified S100β (e.g. East Acres Biologicals, Inc., Swant) are relatively selective for the S100β polypeptide (see addresses at the end of the book).

Anatomical localization

S100β is most abundant in the nervous system, but also present in other tissues, such as testis, adipose, skin, and cartilage. In the nervous system, S100β localizes primarily to glial cells and shows little or no expression in neurons. S100β is found throughout the cytoplasm, including the cell body and processes, and in association with some membranous structures (Zimmer 1995).

Biological activities

S100β has been implicated in regulation of cell growth, cell shape, energy metabolism, and modulation of signal transduction by targeting intracellular proteins. For example, S100β interacts with cytoskeletal elements including microtubule-associated proteins (tau, MAP2), actin-binding proteins (caldesmon, CAP-Z), and GFAP. S100β can activate enzymes in a Ca^{2+}-dependent manner and can inhibit phosphorylation of several protein kinase C substrates, including tumor suppressor protein p53, GAP43, p87, and neurogranin (Zimmer 1995).

S100β also acts extracellularly to promote neurite out-growth and/or neuronal survival of specific neuronal populations (e.g. cortical, dorsal root ganglia, serotoner-gic, and motor neurons) and to stimulate proliferation of glial cells (Barger et al. 1992). The mechanisms by which S100β exerts its trophic effects are unclear, although it has been found that S100β stimulates phosphoinositide hydrolysis, increases in cytoplasmic free Ca^{2+} concentration, and proto-oncogene expression (Barger and Van Eldik 1992; Barger et al. 1992). In vivo studies using various animal models have suggested that S100β may play a role in brain development, learning, and memory (Zimmer 1995).

Biological regulation

S100β expression is not constitutive, but can be regulated by a variety of factors, including cell cycle, cell density, differentiation state, cAMP, cytokines and growth factors, and in response to aging or injury (Hilt and Kligman 1991; Zimmer 1995). Analysis of the promoter region of S100β genes has suggested a complex transcrip-tional regulation, e.g. there is a potential cAMP response element in the human gene (Allore et al. 1990) and mul-tiple negative and cell type-specific regulatory elements in the murine gene (Jiang et al. 1993). S100β protein levels can also be regulated by changes in the ratio of intracellular to extracellular S100β. For example, S100β release can vary with cell growth parameters and can be stimulated by agonists such as isoproterenol or serotonin (Barger et al. 1992).

Mutagenesis studies

Transfected glial cell lines with altered S100β levels show changes in cell morphology, cytoskeletal organization and cell proliferation (Barger et al. 1992). A mouse strain with genetic polydactyly (multiple digits) and an abnor-mal development of cortex and hippocampus exhibits a marked reduction in brain S100β levels and serotonergic fiber density (Ueda et al. 1994). Overexpression of S100β in transgenic mice induces astrocytosis, axonal prolifera-tion, and behavioral abnormalities (Friend et al. 1992; Reeves et al. 1994). Increased S100β levels have also been documented in certain pathological states, such as cancer (Zimmer 1995), and in neuropathological disor-ders such as Down's syndrome and Alzheimer's disease

(Griffin et al. 1989). There is increasing evidence that S100β overexpression may be related to the degree of neuropathological involvement of different brain regions in Alzheimer's disease (Van Eldik and Griffin 1994).

References

Allore, R.J., Friend, W.C., O'Hanlon, D., Neilson, K.M., Baumal, R., Dunn, R.J., and Marks, A. (1990) Cloning and expression of the human S100β gene. J. Biol. Chem. **265**, 15537–15543.

Barger, S.W., and Van Eldik, L.J. (1992) S100β stimulates calcium fluxes in glial and neuronal cells. J. Biol Chem. **267**, 9689–9694.

*Barger, S.W., Wolchok, S.R., and Van Eldik, L.J. (1992) Disulfide-linked S100β dimers and signal transduction. Biochim. Biophys. Acta **1160**, 105–112.

Donato, R. (1991) Perspectives in S-100 protein biology. Cell Calcium **12**, 713–726.

Duncan, A.M.V., Higgins, J., Dunn, R.J., Allore, R., and Marks, A. (1989) Refined sublocalization of the human gene encoding the β subunit of S100 protein (S100β) and confirmation of a subtle t(9:21) translocation using in situ hybridization. Cytogenet. Cell Genet. **50**, 234–235.

Friend, W.C., Clapoff, S., Landry, C., Becker, L.E., O'Hanlon, D., Allore, R.J., Brown, I.R., Marks, A., Roder, J., and Dunn, R.J. (1992) Cell-specific expression of high levels of human S100β in transgenic mouse brain is dependent on gene dosage. J. Neurosci. **12**, 4337–4346.

Griffin, W.S.T., Stanley, L.C., Ling, C., White, L., MacLeod, V., Perrot, L.J. White, C.L., and Araoz, C. (1989) Brain interleukin 1 and S-100 immunoreactivity are elevated in Down syndrome and Alzheimer disease. Proc. Natl. Acad. Sci. USA **86**, 7611–7615.

Hilt, D.C. and Kligman, D. (1991) The S-100 protein family: a biochemical and functional overview. In Novel Calcium-Binding Proteins (ed. C.W. Heizmann), pp. 65–103. Springer-Verlag, Berlin.

Jiang, H., Shah, S., and Hilt, D.C. (1993) Organization, sequence, and expression of the murine S100β gene. J. Biol. Chem. **268**, 20502–20511.

*Kligman, D. and Marshak, D.R. (1985) Purification and characterization of a neurite extension factor from bovine brain. Proc. Natl. Acad. Sci. USA **82**, 7136–7139.

Maeda, T., Usui, H., Araki, K., Kuwano, R., Takahashi, Y., and Suzuki, Y. (1991) Structure and expression of rat S-100β subunit gene. Mol. Brain Res. **10**, 193–202.

Moore, B.W. (1965) A soluble protein characteristic of the nervous system. Biochem. Biophys. Res. Commun. **19**, 739–744.

Reeves, R.H., Yao, J., Crowley, M.R., Buck, S., Zhang, X., Yarowsky, P., Gearhart, J.D., and Hilt, D.C. (1994) Astrocytosis and axonal proliferation in the hippocampus of S100β transgenic mice. Proc. Natl. Acad. Sci. USA **91**, 5359–5363.

Ueda, S., Gu, X.F., Whitaker-Azmitia, P.M., Naruse, I., and Azmitia E.C. (1994) Neuro-glial neurotrophic interaction in the S-100β retarded mutant mouse (Polydactyly Nagoya). I. Immunocytochemical and neurochemical studies. Brain Res. **633**, 275–283.

*Van Eldik, L.J. and Griffin, W.S.T. (1994) S100β expression in Alzheimer's disease: relation to neuropathology in brain regions. Biochim. Biophys. Acta **1223**, 398–403.

Van Eldik, L.J., Staecker, J.L., and Winningham-Major, F. (1988) Synthesis and expression of a gene coding for the calcium-modulated protein S100β and designed for cassette-based, site-directed mutagenesis. J. Biol. Chem. **263**, 7830–7837.

Zimmer, D.B. *et al.* (1995) The S100 protein family: history, function, and expression. Brain Res. Bulletin, **37**, 417–429.

■ Linda J. Van Eldik and Jingru Hu:
   Dept. of Cell and Molecular Biology,

Northwestern University Medical School,
Chicago, IL 60611-3008, USA
Tel.: 1 312 503 0697
Fax: 1 312 503 0007
E-mail: vaneldik@nwu.ed

S100C

S100C is a novel member of the S100 family and abundant in porcine lung, kidney, and heart (Ohta et al. 1991). This protein binds to cytoskeletal components at physiological concentrations of Ca^{2+} and might act to regulate the cytoskeleton in a Ca^{2+} dependent manner (Naka et al., 1994).

The molecular mass of porcine heart S100C was about 11 kDa, as determined by SDS-PAGE. However, when subjected to analytical gel-filtration chromatography on a calibrated column of Sephacryl S-200, S100C eluted much earlier than would be expected for a 11 kDa monomer and its molecular mass appeared to be about 25 kDa. This result suggests that, under these conditions, the protein exists as a self-associated complex. Isoelectric focusing revealed that S100C had a slightly more basic isoelectric point (pI = 6.2) than S100a0 and S100b (Naka *et al.* 1994).

■ Alternative names

Calgizzarin (Todoroki *et al.* 1991; Watanabe *et al.* 1991).

■ Isolation/identification

S100C was purified to homogeneity from porcine cardiac muscle by Ca^{2+}-dependent hydrophobic and dye-affinity chromatography. Approximately 5 mg of S100C were purified from 2 kg of porcine heart. An immunoassay of the original 100 000 × ***g*** supernatant indicated that porcine cardiac muscle contained about 0.5 μg S100C/mg protein in the soluble fraction (Naka *et al.* 1994). Amino acid sequence determination of purified S100C from porcine heart revealed that it corresponded to that expected from the cloned cDNA. The cDNA gene coding for this protein was cloned from a porcine lung cDNA library (Ohta *et al.* 1991). The ability of the protein to bind Ca^{2+} was examined directly by the flow-dialysis or the dotblot assay.

■ Gene and sequences

The sequences of porcine heart S100C (Ohta *et al.* 1991; GenBank accession number D10705) and rabbit lung calgizzarin (Watanabe *et al.* 1991; GenBank accession number D10586) are homologous.

■ Protein

S100C may be a dimer, consisting of four EF-hand domains that bind Ca^{2+}. Amino acid sequence determination revealed that the subunit contained two Ca^{2+}-binding domains with the EF-hand motif. Sequence analysis of the cloned cDNA suggested that the protein is composed of 99 amino acid residues and its molecular weight was estimated to be 11.1 kDa (Ohta *et al.* 1991). A computer-assisted search of protein sequence libraries showed that the predicted amino acid sequence of S100C shared a significant homology with several other Ca^{2+}-binding proteins. Porcine S100C is homologous to rabbit S100C, chicken gizzard S100C, S100A10 (the calpactin light chain), bovine S100A1 and S100b subunits with homologies of 83%, 72.3%, 41.1%, 40.9%, and 37.5%, respectively. These homologies strongly suggest that S100C is structurally related to the S100 protein family. This conclusion was further supported by three additional observations. First, the best homology matching of the amino acid sequence was obtained without the introduction of gaps for any sequence compared. Second, many of the amino acid differences were conservative substitutions. Third, the homology between the S100C protein and the bovine S100A1 subunit was particularly striking (100%) in the regions where the highest conservation between the S100A1 and S100β was found. This analysis of homologies indicated that S100C is located in the earlier branch of the S100 subfamily lineage, between the S100A1 subunit and the S100A10.

■ Antibodies

Polyclonal antibodies against homogeneous preparations of S100 proteins have been raised in rabbits. The antibodies raised against S100C did not cross-react with S100A1, S100β, S100A2, and S100A10 (Naka *et al.* 1994).

▉ Localization

The presence of S100C was examined in several tissues by Northern and Western blotting analyses. S100C-specific mRNAs were most abundant in lung and kidney. Intermediate levels were found in heart and adrenal gland. In brain and liver, the levels were very low, since Northern blot analysis using 20 mg of total RNA from the tissue did not give rise to any detectable signals. These data were also confirmed by Western blotting analysis. It should be noted that the tissue distribution of S100C was different from that of other members of the S100 protein family.

▉ Biological activities

The Ca^{2+}-binding properties of S100C were characterized by the flow-dialysis technique with ^{45}Ca. Scatchard analysis of the data revealed that S100C bound 4 mol calcium/mol protein (dimer form) with apparent K_d-values of 16 and 8 mM, in the presence and absence of 100 mM KCl, respectively (Naka et al. 1994). The metachromatic carbocyanine dye Stains-All has been reported to bind to several Ca^{2+}-binding proteins, staining them blue or purple whereas other proteins stain red or pink. We investigated the staining properties of S100C and other S100 proteins with Stains-All. S100β stained blue, S100A1 stained blue or red, S100A2 stained red and S100C did not stain (Naka et al. 1994). These results suggest that the interaction of the dye with the anionic Ca^{2+}-binding sites within the S100C molecule is different from that of other S100 proteins.

▉ Interactions

For several members of the S100 family of proteins the functions are known. It is believed that, by analogy to the role of calmodulin and troponin C, the S100 proteins act to regulate the activities of their cellular target proteins via direct interactions. S100C does not activate cyclic nucleotide phosphodiesterase and myosin light chain kinase but is able to interact with cytoskeletal proteins in the presence of Ca^{2+}. In the presence of 100 mM KCl, the half maximal concentration of Ca^{2+} needed for binding was of about 3 μm. Analysis of the EGTA extract from porcine cardiac muscle by the gel-overlay procedure revealed the presence of several proteins that bound to 125I-S100C. Strong binding to S100C in a Ca^{2+}-dependent manner was observed for a protein of 36 kDa, annexinêl. The phosphorylation of annexin I by protein kinase C was markedly suppressed by S100C. Other S100 proteins had no effect. Under the same assay conditions, S100C did not inhibit the phosphorylation of histone IIIs by protein kinase C. Our results suggest that S100C may modulate the phosphorylation of annexin I by protein kinase C and that it has Ca^{2+}-dependent functions which differ from those of other members of the S100 family (Naka et al. 1994).

▉ References

*Naka, M., Zhao, Z.Q., Sasaki, T., Kise, H., Tawara, I., Hamaguchi, S., and Tanaka, T. (1994) Purification and characterization of a novel calcium-binding protein, S100C, from porcine heart. Biochim. Biophys. Act **1223**, 348–353.

*Ohta, H., Sasaki, T., Naka, M., Hiraoka, O., Miyamoto, C. Furuichi, Y., and Tanaka, T. (1991) Molecular cloning and expression of the cDNA coding for a new member of the S100 protein family from porcine cardiac muscle. Febs Lett. **295**, 93–96.

*Todoroki, H., Kobayashi, R., Watanabe, M., Minami, H., and Hidaka.H., (1991) Purification, characterization, and partial sequence analysis of a newly identified EF-hand type 13-kDa Ca^{2+}-binding protein from smooth muscle and non-muscle tissues. J. Biol.Chem. **266**, 18668–18673.

Watanabe, M., Ando, Y., Todoroki, H., Minami, H., and Hidaka.H., (1991) Molecular cloning and sequencing of a cDNA clone encoding a new calcium binding protein, named calgizzarin, from rabbit lung. Biochem. Biophys. Res. Commun. **181**, 644–649.

▉ Toshio Tanaka and Michiko Naka:
Department of Molecular and Cellular Pharmacology, Mie University School of Medicine, 2-174 Edobashi, Tsu, Mie 5l4, Japan
Tel.: +81 592 31 5006
Fax: +81 592 32 1765
E-mail: tanaka@doc.medic.mie-u.ac.jp

Calbindin-D9k

Calbindin-D9k is a cytosolic Ca²⁺-binding protein characteristic of mammals, abundant in the duodenum, placenta, uterus but also present in the yolk sac, fallopian tube, lung, kidney, cartilage, bone, and teeth. It may be involved in active transport of Ca²⁺ in the duodenum, kidney and placenta, contraction in the myometrium, and mineralization in bone and teeth. A protective role against Ca²⁺ toxicity has also been postulated. Expression of the calbindin-D9k gene is regulated in a tissue-specific manner at both transcriptional and post-transcriptional levels by 1,25-dihydroxyvitamin D₃ (calcitriol) in the duodenum and kidney, and by estrogens in the uterus.

Human calbindin-D9k (calbindin-D9k) is a 79-amino acid protein with a calculated molecular mass of 9,015 kDa. It is 89% homologous with the bovine and porcine calbindin-D9k sequences, 78% with rat, and 77% with mouse proteins. Calbindin-D9k migrates on SDS gels with an apparent molecular mass of 10 kDa and has an isoelectric point of 4.7. It consists of two EF-hand motifs (sites I and II) which each binds Ca^{2+} with high affinity (K_a 10^6 M^{-1}). Calbindin-D9k is more closely related to S100 protein than to calbindin-D28k. Antisera to calbindin-D9k do not cross-react with calbindin-D28k or S100 protein.

Calbindin-D9k was first found in rat intestine and its concentration in this tissue is correlated with active transcellular, vitamin D-dependent Ca^{2+} aborption. Calbindin-D9k is also associated with Ca^{2+} reabsorption in the kidney distal tubules and with Ca^{2+} transfer in the placenta. Calbindin-D9k has also been found in the uterus, yolk sac, lung, cartilage, bone, and teeth of mammals (for review Christakos et al. 1989), including human uterus (Miller et al. 1994).

■ Alternative names

Vitamin D-induced (-dependent) calcium-binding protein (CaBP9k) (Kallfelz et al. 1967), 9 kDa cholecalcin (Perret et al. 1985), 9 kDa calcium-binding protein (Gross and Kumar 1990).

■ Isolation/identification

Early studies using competitive ion exchange and equilibrium dialysis indicated that supplying vitamin D to vitamin D-deficient rats increased the Ca^{2+}-binding activity of crude extracts of intestinal mucosa (Kallfelz et al. 1967). Calbindin-D9k was purified by gel filtration and DEAE-cellulose column chromatography in the presence or absence of Ca^{2+} ions and used to raise specific rabbit antisera and produce a radioimmunoassay (Thomasset et al. 1982). A cDNA clone for rat intestinal calbindin-D9k was reported by Desplan et al. (1983) and by Darwish et al. (1987) , using a library constructed from size-selected mRNA from intestine of vitamin D-treated rats. The library was screened by differential *in situ* hybridization using enriched cDNAs (RNA from intestine of vitamin D replete rats) *v.* nonenriched probes (RNA from intestine

of vitamin D-deficient animals). cDNA encoding human calbindin-D9k has recently been reported (Howard et al. 1992; Jeung et al. 1992).

■ Gene and sequences

The structural organization of the entire rat calbindin-D9k gene was determined by analysis of overlapping genomic clones isolated from a rat genomic library using the rat intestinal calbindin-D9k cDNA (Perret et al. 1988a; GenBank accession number X16635). The gene is 2.5 kb long and contains three exons interrupted by two introns. The first exon contains the 5′ untranslated region; the second exon, the first EF-hand; and the third exon, the second EF-hand and the 3′ untranslated region. The two Ca^{2+}-binding sites are separated by a class o intron.

The sequence of the human calbindin-D9k gene (Jeung et al. 1994) is very similar. The human calbindin-D9k gene is on chromosome Xp 22.2 and is not linked to hypophosphatemic rickets (Howard et al. 1992; Oudet, personal communication). The promoter region contains the consensus TATAAA sequence and transcription is initiated at a single site (Perret et al. 1988a). The sequence contains elements which are very similar to consensus sequences for transcription factors: estrogen-responsive element (ERE), nuclear factor 1 (NF1) and Activator Protein 1 (AP-1) (Fig. 1).

■ Protein

Calbindin-D9k is a highly helical, heat stable, and acidic (p*I* ~ 4.7) protein, with two EF-hand regions which bind two Ca^{2+} with high affinity ($K_a = 10^6$ M^{-1}). Calbindin-D9k binds several other cations (Ca > Cd > Sr > Mn > Zn > Ba > Co > Mg), and Pb (Christakos et al. 1989 for review). The primary structures of bovine, porcine, and murine intestinal Ca^{2+}-binding proteins were obtained by amino acid sequencing (Gross and Kumar 1990, for review) and deduced from the sequence of appropriate rat (Desplan et al. 1983; Darwish et al. 1987), bovine (Gross and Kumar 1990) porcine (Jeung et al. 1992) and human (Howard et al. 1992; Jeung et al. 1992); cDNA clones. The bovine protein, which is a prototype for these proteins, is a 78-amino acid protein with a molecular weight of 8788. It is 87% and 81% homologous with the porcine and murine proteins. High-resolution X-ray crystallographic

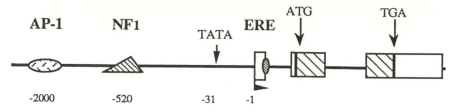

Figure 1. Organization of the calbindin-D9k gene. The 3 exons are represented by rectangles. The hatched rectangles indicate the sequence coding for calbindin-D9k. The position of transcription factors are noted.

structure of the bovine protein is in good agreement with the predicted secondary structure of the protein (Gross and Kumar 1990, for review). The protein contains two helix–loop–helix structures of 29 and 31 amino acids each that bind Ca^{2+}, consistent with the EF-hand concept defined by Kretsinger. Calbindin-D9k has a typical S100 EF-hand with a 14 amino acids loop. There is no evidence to indicate that calbindin-D9k has arisen from calbindin-D28k (Perret *et al.* 1988*b*).

■ Antibodies

Antisera to intestinal calbindin-D9k from one species do not cross-react with calbindin-D9k from other species in a radioimmunoassay, but there is weak cross-reactivity using immunostaining. Antisera to calbindin-D9k do not cross-react with calbindin-D28k or S100 protein. Commercial antibodies are available through Swant.

■ Anatomical localization

Calbindin-D9k is characteristic of mammals and present in several tissues (Thomasset *et al.* 1982). It represents 2%, 0.1%, 0.1%, and 0.01% of the soluble proteins of the duodenal mucosa, placenta, uterus, and lung (Dupret *et al.* 1992), respectively. Calbindin-D9k is present in absorptive epithelial cells of the rat duodenum. Its concentration increases from the crypt region to the villus tip. Calbindin-D9k gene expression decreases dramatically along the length of the small intestine, and calbindin-D9k is barely detectable in the distal ileum. The caecum contains significant amounts of calbindin-D9k (Thomasset *et al.* 1982; Perret *et al.* 1985). Calbindin-D9k is synthesized in the trophoblastic epithelium of the placenta. It is also expressed in the uterus, the myometrium and stroma of non-pregnant rats, and the epithelium of pregnant animals (Christakos *et al.* 1989 for review). This gene is also expressed at the basolateral membrane of the distal tubules cells of kidney (Bouhtiany *et al.* 1994), in the alveolar epithelial cells of the lung (Dupret *et al.* 1992), in the osteoblasts of bone, cartilage growth plate, and in the ameloblasts of teeth (Christakos *et al.* 1989, for review). The calbindin-D9k gene is not expressed in the liver.

■ Biological activities

Calbindin-D9k is thought to increase Ca^{2+} absorption by buffering cytoplasmic Ca^{2+}. It also increases ATP-

dependent Ca^{2+} transport in duodenal basolateral membrane vesicles and can bind to the regulatory calmodulin-binding domain of the plasma membrane Ca^{2+}-pump (Gross and Kumar 1990; Christakos *et al.* 1989 for review). Calbindin-D9k activates the Ca^{2+} pump in the basolateral membrane of both proximal and distal tubules (Bouhtiany *et al.* 1994). *In vivo*, vitamin D may enhance Ca^{2+} reabsorption in the distal segments through the synthesis of the two Ca^{2+}-binding proteins calbindin-D9k and calbindin D28k. The three-dimensional structure of calbindin-D9k in the presence and absence of Ca^{2+} suggests that calbindin-D9k responds to Ca^{2+} binding by small conformational changes compared to calmodulin and troponin C models (Skelton *et al.* 1994).

■ Biological regulation

The expression of the calbindin-D9k gene is regulated in a tissue-specific manner. Analysis of the chromatin structure of a 28 kb chromosome region containing the calbindin-D9k gene reveals several DNaseI-hypersensitive sites which define domains implicated in the tissue-specific control of calbindin-D9k gene expression (Perret *et al.* 1991).

Calbindin-D9k synthesis is under the control of the hormonal vitamin D_3 metabolite, $1,25(OH)_2D_3$, calcitriol, in the intestine of rats (Thomasset *et al.* 1982; Perret *et al.* 1985). $1,25(OH)_2D_3$ rapidly induces calbindin-D9k synthesis in rats fed a vitamin D-free diet for 5 weeks after weaning, and also *in vitro*. Run-on experiments (Dupret *et al.* 1987) suggest that calcitriol controls the expression of the calbindin-D9k gene at the transcriptional but also at the post-transcriptional levels. 1,25-dihydroxyvitamin-D_3 acts through its nuclear receptor (VDR), which is a DNA-binding protein belonging to the steroid receptor family. The VDR interacts with a specific DNA sequence, the VDRE (<u>v</u>itamin <u>D</u>-<u>r</u>esponsive <u>e</u>lement) which has been identified in the rat calbindin-D9k gene (Darwish and DeLuca 1992). Vitamin D may similarly regulate calbindin-D9k gene expression in kidney, placenta, bone, and teeth.

In the rat uterus, unlike the intestine, calbindin-D9k gene expression is under the control of estrogens and appears to be independent of the vitamin D status. Despite the presence of $1,25(OH)2D_3$ receptors, estradiol (17b-E2) is the major factor controlling calbindin-D9k gene expression in this tissue (L'Horset *et al.* 1990, 1993). Calbindin-D9k mRNAs are undetectable in the uterus of ovariectomized rats and a single injection of 17b-E2 rapidly induces the expression of the calbindin-D9k gene in this tissue. Estrogens control calbindin-D9k gene expression, at least in part, at the transcriptional level. Similarly, under physiological conditions, calbindin-D9k gene expression is maximal during the estrogen-dominated phase of the estrous cycle.

There is also *in vitro* evidence that the estradiol acts *via* an imperfect estrogen-responsive element ERE (Darwish *et al*. 1991) (Fig. 1). Progesterone has a late negative effect on this estradiol-induced expression of calbindin-D9k (L'Horset *et al*. 1993).

Calbindin-D9k gene expression in the lung is controlled by neither vitamin D nor estrogen (Dupret *et al*. 1992).

■ References

Bouhtiany, I., Lajeunesse, D., Christakos, S.,and Brunette, M.G. (1994) Two vitamin D3-dependent calcium binding proteins increase calcium reabsorption by different mechanisms II. Effect of CaBP9k. Kidney Intern. **45**, 469–474.

Christakos, S., Gabrielides, C.,and Rhoten, W.B. (1989) Vitamin D-dependent calcium binding proteins: chemistry, distribution, functional considerations, and molecular biology. Endocr. Rev. **10**, 3–25.

Darwish, H., Krisinger, J., Furlow, D., Smith, C., Murdoch, F.E.,and DeLuca, H.F. (1991) An estrogen-responsive element mediates the transcriptional regulation of calbindin-D9k gene in rat uterus. J. Biol. Chem., **266**, 551–558.

Darwish, H.M.and DeLuca, H.F. (1992) Identification of a 1, 25-dihydroxyvitamin-D3-response element in the 5'-flanking region of the rat calbindin-D9k gene. Proc. Natl. Acad. Sci. USA **89**, 603–607.

Darwish, H.M., Krisinger, J., Strom, M.,and DeLuca, H.F. (1987) Molecular cloning of the cDNA and chromosomal gene for vitamin D-dependent calcium-binding protein of rat intestine. Proc. Natl. Acad. Sci. USA **84**, 6108–6111.

Desplan, C., Heidmann, O., Lillie, J.W., Auffray, C.,and Thomasset, M. (1983) Sequence of rat intestinal vitamin D-dependent calcium-binding protein derived from a cDNA clone. Evolutionary implications. J. Biol. Chem. **258**, 13502–13505.

Dupret, J.M., Brun, P., Perret, C., Lomri, N., Thomasset, M.,and Cuisinier-Gleizes, P. (1987) Transcriptional and post-transcriptional regulation of vitamin D-dependent calcium-binding protein gene expression in the rat duodenum by 1,25-dihydroxycholecalciferol. J. Biol. Chem. **262**, 16553–16557.

Dupret, J.M., L'Horset, F., Perret, C., Bernaudin, J.F.,and Thomasset, M. (1992) Calbindin-D9k gene expression in the lung of the rat. Absence of regulation by 1,25-dihydroxy-vitamin D3 and estrogen. Endocrinology **131**, 2643–2648.

Gross, M. and Kumar, R. (1990) Physiology and biochemistry of vitamin D-dependent calcium binding protein. Am. J. Physiol. **259**, F195–F209.

Howard, A., Legon, S., Spurr, N.K.,and Walters, J.R.F. (1992) Molecular cloning and chromosomal assignment of human calbindin-D9k. Biochem. Biophys. Res. Commun., **185**, 663–669.

Jeung, E.B., Krisinger, J., Dann, J.L.,and Leung, P.C.K. (1992) Molecular cloning of the full-length cDNA encoding the human calbindin-D9k. FEBS Lett. **307**, 224–228.

Jeung, E.B., Leung, P.C.K.,and Krisinger, J. (1994) The human calbindin-D9k gene. Complete structure and implications on steroid hormone regulation. J. Mol. Biol. **235**, 1231–1238.

Kallfelz, F.A., Taylor, A.N.,and Wasserman, R.H. (1967) Vitamin D-induced calcium-binding factor in rat intestinal mucosa. Proc. Soc. Exp. Biol. Med. **125**, 54–58.

L'Horset, F., Perret, C., Brehier, A.,and Thomasset, M. (1990) 17-Estradiol stimulates the calbindin-D9k (CaBP9k) gene expression at the transcriptional and postranscriptional levels in the rat uterus. Endocrinology **127**, 2891–2897.

L'Horset, F., Blin, C., Brehier, A., Thomasset, M.,and Perret, C. (1993) Estrogen-induced calbindin-D9k gene expression in the rat uterus during the estrous cycle: late antagonistic effect of progesterone. Endocrinology **132**, 489–495.

Miller, E.K., Word, R.A., Goodall, C.A.,and Iacopino, A.M. (1994) Calbindin-D9k gene expression in human myometrium during pregnancy and labor. J. Clin. Endocrinol. Metabol. **79**, 609–615.

Perret, C., Desplan, C.,and Thomasset, M. (1985) Cholecalcin (a 9-kDa cholecalciferol-induced calcium-binding protein) messenger RNA. Distribution and induction by calcitriol in the rat digestive tract. Eur. J. Biochem. **150**, 211–217.

Perret, C., Lomri, N., Gouhier, N., Auffray, C.,and Thomasset, M. (1988*a*) The rat vitamin D-dependent calcium-binding protein (9-kDa CaBP) gene. Complete nucleotide sequence and structural organization. Eur. J. Biochem. **172**, 43–51.

Perret, C., Lomri, N.,and Thomasset, M. (1988*b*) Evolution of the EF-hand calcium-binding protein family: evidence for exon shuffling and intron insertion. J. Mol. Evol. **27**, 351–364.

Perret, C., L'Horset, F.,and Thomasset, M. (1991) DNase I-hypersensitive sites are associated, in a tissue-specific manner, with expression of the calbindin-D9k-encoding gene. Gene **108**, 227–235.

Skelton, H.J., Kördel, J., Akke, M., Forsén, S.,and Chazin, W.J. (1994) Signal transduction versus buffering activity in Ca^{2+}-binding proteins. Structural biology **1**, 239–244.

Thomasset, M., Parkes, C.O.,and Cuisinier-Gleizes, P. (1982) Rat calcium-binding proteins: distribution, development, and vitamin D dependence. Am. J. Physiol. **243**, E483–E488.

Wasserman, R.H. (1985) Nomenclature of the vitamin D induced calcium binding proteins. In (ed. A.W. Norman, K. Schaefer, H.G. Grigoleit and D.V. Herrath), p.321. Walter de Gruyter, Berlin.

■ *Monique Thomasset, Fabienne L'Horset, Claudine Blin, Mireille Lambert, Sabine Colnot, and Christine Perret:*
INSERM U.120,
Hôpital Robert Debré,
48 Bd Sérurier, 75019 Paris, France
Tel.: 331 40 03 19 15
Fax: 331 40 03 19 03
E-mail: perret@citi2.fr

S100P

S100P is a Ca^{2+}-binding protein of the S100 family purified from human placenta. It forms a homodimer, with each chain containing two functional EF-hands. Ca^{2+} binding to these sites leads to a conformational change involving the C-terminal extension of the molecule. Cellular protein ligands and the function of S100P are not known.

Human S100P is 95 amino acid residues in length. It has an apparent molecular mass of 10 kDa and a calculated isolectric point of 4.58. So far, the protein has only been identified in placenta, although a thorough analysis of its tissue distribution has not been carried out (Becker *et al.* 1992; Emoto *et al.* 1992). A biochemical and biophysical characterization of recombinantly expressed S100P revealed the presence of two Ca^{2+}-binding sites of different affinities. The low affinity site could be assigned to the N-terminal EF-hand whereas the high affinity site resides in the C-terminal EF-hand. Binding to both sites results in conformational changes (Becker *et al.* 1992).

■ Identification/isolation

S100P was purified from human placenta by exploiting its ability to interact with hydrophobic matrices in a Ca^{2+}-dependent manner (Becker *et al.* 1992; Emoto *et al.* 1992). The cDNA was cloned from a placenta cDNA library and used to express the protein recombinantly in *E. coli* (Becker *et al.* 1992). Both, authentic and bacterially expressed S100P, were shown to bind Ca^{2+} by a number of different assays (Becker *et al.* 1992; Emoto *et al.* 1992).

■ Gene and sequence

The cDNA sequence for human S100P is listed in the EMBL database under the accession number X65614. The predicted protein sequence shows the highest degree of similarity to S100A1 and S100β (approximately 50% identity). The gene encoding S100P has not been isolated. It has, however, been mapped to human chromosome 4 (B.W. Schäfer and C.W. Heizmann, personal communication).

■ Protein

S100P purified from human placenta was shown by UV difference spectroscopy, urea/alkaline gel electrophoresis, and ^{45}Ca overlay to bind Ca^{2+} (Emoto *et al.* 1992). Ca^{2+} binding to recombinantly expressed S100P was revealed by fluorescence spectroscopy recording either the internal tyrosine fluorescence or the fluorescence emission of a Prodan moiety linked to the sole cysteine residue of the molecule (Cys85). This analysis identified two Ca^{2+}-binding sites of low (K_d = 800 μM) and high affinity (K_d = 1.6 μM) located in the N- and C-terminal EF-hand, respectively (Becker *et al.* 1992). As revealed by chemical cross-linking, S100P forms a homodimer in aqueous solutions (Becker *et al.* 1992).

■ References

Becker, T., Gerke, V., Kube, E., and Weber, K. (1992) S100P, a novel Ca^{2+} binding protein from human placenta. cDNA cloning, recombinant protein expression and Ca^{2+} binding properties. Eur. J. Biochem. **207**, 541–547.

Emoto, Y., Kobayashi, R., Akatsuka, H., and Hidaka, H. (1992) Purification and characterization of a new member of the S100 protein from human placenta. Biochem. Biophys. Res. Commun. **182**, 1246–1253.

■ *Volker Gerke:*
Clinical Research Group for Endothelial Cell Biology, University of Münster,
Von-Esmarch-Strasse 56,
D-48149 Münster, Germany
Tel.: + 49 251 83 6722
Fax: + 49 251 83 6748
E-mail: gerke@wwupop.uni-muenster.de

Profilaggrin

Profilaggrin (PF) is a polymeric protein, consisting largely of multiple filaggrin repeats. It initially accumulates in keratohyalin granules in the granular layer of orthokeratinizing epithelia. Converted to multiple copies of filaggrin, it functions as an intermediate-filament associated protein. The amino-terminal region of PF has a pair of functional Ca^{2+}-binding domains of the S100 type, the role of which is as yet unknown.

Profilaggrin (PF) is a short-lived (6–48 hours), very large precursor protein (> 400 kDa for human, > 500 kDa for mouse, 1000 kDa for rat) expressed in the granular layer of all orthokeratinizing epithelia. It consists mainly of multiple, contiguous copies of filaggrin polypeptides which themselves show blocks of repeating sequences. These filaggrin units are joined by linker segments. PF is neutral to slightly acidic (pI 6.5 for mouse), this in contrast to the highly basic filaggrin monomers (pI 7.5–8.5 for human, > 11.5 for mouse [Dale *et al.* 1993; Mack *et al.* 1993]). The size, and some biochemical properties of PF and filaggrin vary in different mammalian species, but their major characteristics are common to all. The region of filaggrin repeats is flanked at its amino- and carboxyl-terminal ends by leader and tail peptide sequences. The amino-terminal leader sequence has two EF-hand domains with a significant homology to the S100 proteins (Presland *et al.* 1992; Markova *et al.* 1993).

PF is a highly phosphorylated polymeric protein. The conversion of PF to monomers of filaggrin, involves complete dephosphorylation and proteolytic removal of linker segments. Filaggrin acts as an intermediate filament-associated protein, whereas the function of the precursor protein PF and its Ca^{2+}-binding sites is as yet unknown. It is also unclear whether the amino-terminus cleaved from the filaggrin monomers still remains functional. The Ca^{2+}-binding domains may be involved in the regulation of PF processing in a Ca^{2+}-dependent manner, for example for its packing in keratohyalin granules, or in a tight control of its timely dephosphorylation, or for its proteolytic cleavage. Also, the Ca^{2+}-binding sites could participate in regulating calcium availability to Ca^{2+}-dependent enzymes. Lastly, by transduction of Ca^{2+} signals, these sites may play a role in the process of epidermal differentiation (Dale *et al.* 1993; Markova *et al.* 1993). Indeed, transfected keratinocytes which express an antisense PF-mRNA show perturbed differentiation beyond decreased PF synthesis (Haydock *et al.* 1993).

Alternative names

Filaggrin was named originally for its biochemical properties "stratum corneum basic protein" or "histidine-rich protein". It was renamed after identification of its function as keratin filament aggregating protein.

Isolation/identification

Various methods for isolation of PF from several species have been used successfully, such as extraction in high-salt buffers, urea, or thiocyanate solution, if proteolytic degradation was minimized (Ramsden *et al.* 1983). The large amount of phosphate allows purification by ion-exchange chromatography on DEAE-cellulose (Dale *et al.* 1990b). Pulse-chase experiments using radiolabelled histidine and phosphorus, peptide mapping, amino acid composition analysis, immunoassays, immuno-electron microscopy and immunohistochemistry identified PF as the precursor protein of filaggrin. The human PF gene was isolated from placenta-derived genomic libraries using cDNA probes coding for a filaggrin repeat (McKinley-Grant *et al.* 1989; Gan *et al.* 1990; Presland *et al.* 1992; Markova *et al.* 1993). So far, the complete PF genes of other species have not been isolated.

Gene and sequences

Human PF gene (23 kb) maps to chromosome 1q21, and mouse PF is located on chromosome 3. The sequence of human PF (EMBL/GenBank accession numbers L01088-L01090 and J02929) has been determined. Mouse and rat gene sequences are as yet only partially known. The organization of the human PF gene is similar to that of S100-like proteins. It has three exons and two introns (Fig. 1). The first intron interrupts the small 5′ non-coding region, the second is located in the middle of the linker region between the Ca^{2+}-binding domains, which have a high homology to those of other members of the S100 family of Ca^{2+}-binding proteins. Downstream of the second EF-hand domain in exon 3 are the filaggrin repeats which constitute the bulk of PF. Several potential regulatory elements have been identified in the human PF gene, such as AP1 sites, RARE-like sequences, and cytokeratin octamer sequences (Presland *et al.* 1992; Dale *et al.* 1993; Markova *et al.* 1993). The PF gene is clustered with genes encoding other structural proteins expressed in the epidermis and showing a similar gene organization (trichohyalin, PF, involucrin, the small proline-rich proteins, loricrin) and with Ca^{2+}-binding proteins of the S100 family (calcyclin, calpactin I light chain, calgranulin A and B) (Volz *et al.* 1993). This led to the hypothesis that PF (and trichohyalin) genes are the result of the fusion of an ancestral epidermal structural gene with a gene for a

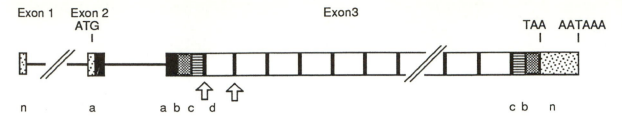

Figure 1. Schematic drawing of human PF gene organization (modified from Presland *et al.* 1992; Markova *et al.* 1993). Black boxes (a) represent EF hands, shaded boxes (b) represent N-terminal leader and C-terminal tail sequences, horizontal hatched boxes (c) represent truncated filaggrin repeats, dark columns (arrows) indicate sequences coding for linker segments between filaggrin repeats, white boxes (d) represent complete filaggrin repeats (number varies between species), and dotted boxes stand for noncoding 5′ and 3′ sequences (n).

Ca^{2+}-binding protein that resided in the same chromosomal locus (Markova *et al.* 1993).

■ Protein

Human profilaggrin codes for a large protein with various domains. The initiation codon is followed by a 292 amino acid (AA) leader peptide which shows two parts. The first part of 81 AA comprises the two EF-hands. The first (N-terminal) EF-hand contains a 14 amino acid loop, typical for the S100 protein family; the second (C-terminal) EF-hand is formed by a classical 12 residue loop. The overall homology of this domain of 81 AA and $S100\alpha$ is 38.3%, while comparison of the EF-hands themselves reveals a homology of > 60% with Ca^{2+}-binding proteins of the S100 protein family (Presland *et al.* 1992; Markova *et al.* 1993). Adjacent to the EF-hands is a hydrophilic domain of 212 AA. This leader peptide is followed by a truncated filaggrin repeat of 174 AA, prior to the first linker segement of 7 AA. What follows is a row of 10–12 filaggrin repeats of 316 AA, each joined by linker segments, and finally another truncated filaggrin repeat of 64 AA, followed by a tail peptide of 157 AA (Presland *et al.* 1992).

The functionality of both EF-hand domains of human PF was assessed on a recombinant 293-residue amino-terminal fragment expressed as a polyhistidine fusion protein in *E. coli*. Fluorescence emission spectroscopy reveals conformational changes of the recombinant protein upon Ca^{2+} binding, consistent with two functional binding sites. The K_d for the EF hands are estimated as $1.2\text{-}1.6 \times 10\text{-}4$ M and $1.1\text{-}1.4 \times 10\text{-}3$ M, respectively, indicating high- and low-affinity Ca^{2+}-binding. In quantitative Ca^{2+}-blots 1 mol of recombinant protein binds approximately 1.5 mol Ca^{2+} (Presland *et al.* 1995). Similarly, native mouse PF is a functional Ca^{2+}-binding protein (Markova *et al.* 1993).

PF shows considerable heterogeneity between species, although its general structure is presumably conserved. This is reflected in variation of number (10–12 in humans, number inherited in a Mendelian fashion, > 20 in mouse, depending on strain) and size of filaggrin units (37 kDa

for human, 26 kDa for mouse), and the species-specificity of most antibodies. PF is postranslationally phosphorylated by several kinases on multiple serine residues in each filaggrin repeat, linker domain, and in the amino- and carboxy-terminal ends. *In vitro* the phosphorylated precursor PF is unable to interact with intermediate filaments. Processing PF to functional filaggrin involves dephosphorylation followed by proteolytic cleavage. The proteolytic processing occurs in two distinct stages: first processing results in intermediates composed of several linked filaggrin domains. The second stage of PF proteolysis is Ca^{2+}-dependent and generates filaggrin monomers (Resing *et al.* 1993). After dephosphorylation and proteolysis, filaggrin aggregates keratin, vimentin, and desmin efficiently into tight macrofibril bundles. Thus, *in vivo* filaggrin is presumed to act as an intermediate filament-associated protein aggregating keratin filaments. This function is probably only a temporary scaffolding in the lower portion of the stratum corneum, until the keratin filaments are covalently linked. Then, filaggrin is degraded to be the main source of free amino acids in the upper layers of the stratum corneum, providing its high osmolarity for retention of water and thus its flexibility. Eventually, urocanic acid derived from histidine, serves as UV filter (Dale *et al.* 1994). Further, small amounts of filaggrin are found within the cornified cell envelope of corneocytes. Mouse and human filaggrins have almost no sequence homology, except in regions containing potential phosphorylation sites and, to some extent, at proteolytic processing sites, and the linker domains. In humans even the filaggrin repeats are heterogeneous at nearly 40% of the amino acid residues. Most of the amino acid sequence variations are conservative, few involve exchanges between hydrophilic and hydrophobic residues (McKinley-Grant *et al.* 1989; Gan *et al.* 1990a). Thus, the precise sequence of filaggrin may not be critical for its function, which may reside on the overall charge distribution. Human and mouse filaggrin have been shown to possess a conserved distribution of positive and negative charges and a secondary structure of tetrapeptide repeats that adopt a β-turn motif. It has been proposed that filaggrin binds intermediate filaments by ionic interaction, where positive and negative charges on the frequent β-turns of filaggrin interface with the negative and positive charges of the α-helical rod domains of intermediate filaments (Mack *et al.* 1993).

Similarities of PF with trichohyalin are discussed elsewhere (see chapter on trichohyalin).

■ Antibodies

The monoclonal antihuman PF/filaggrin antibody AKH1 (Dale *et al.* 1987) is commercially available through Biomedical Technologies Inc.

■ Anatomical localization

PF is expressed, together with or after the keratins K1 and K10, in orthokeratinizing epithelia, such as epidermis, hard palate, gingiva, interpapillary and papillary tongue epithelium, oesophagus and forestomach (rodents), exocervix, and at very low levels in non-keratinized buccal mucosa. In humans, PF is a major component of the keratohyalin granules, microscopically visible basophilic non-membrane bound aggregates in the granular layer of orthokeratinizing epithelia. Associated with polyribosomes, keratohyalin granules are sites of active protein synthesis; they increase in size progressively from the deeper granular layer towards the stratum corneum. Other proteins are deposited together with PF in the keratohyalin granules, for example the cell envelope proteins loricrin, cystatin A, and eventually the Ca^{2+}-binding protein trichohyalin (O'Guin and Manabe 1991; Dale *et al.* 1994). In rodents, PF accumulates in the phosphorous-rich type of keratohyalin granules (F-granules); in these animals loricrin is deposited separately in another type of granule, the sulfur-rich granules (L-granules) (Manabe *et al.* 1991; Dale *et al.* 1994). The redistribution of profilaggrin from keratohyalin granules to the cytoplasm of the corneocyte has been demonstrated by immunohistochemistry and ultrastructural immunolocalization. Filaggrin is the electron-dense matrix protein which embeds electron-lucent keratin filaments in the cornified cell to form a filament-matrix assembly described ultrastructurally as the "keratin pattern" (Dale *et al.* 1993, 1994).

■ Biological regulation

PF expression is regulated at the level of transcription. Modulators of its expression are extra- and intracellular Ca^{2+} levels, and retinoids. Keratinocytes cultured in medium with low Ca^{2+} levels (< 0.1mM) do not synthesize PF. BAPTA, a Ca^{2+} chelator, when injected intracellularly, blocks its expression (Dale *et al.* 1993; Dlugosz and Yuspa 1993). Within the epidermis an intra- and extracellular Ca^{2+}-gradient from the basal layer (low Ca^{2+}) to the granular layer (high Ca^{2+}) has been demonstrated and it is likely that also *in vivo* Ca^{2+} regulates the expression and processing of PF. Ca^{2+} is also required for posttranslational processing of filaggrin by trans-

glutaminases and peptidylarginine deiminase. PF expression and its processing to filaggrin is negatively regulated by retinoids. PF is not processed to filaggrin in cultured keratinocytes unless the cultures are lifted to the air–liquid interface (Dale *et al.* 1993). Filaggrin breakdown to free amino acids is regulated *in vivo* and *in vitro* by the environmental humidity (Scott and Harding 1986).

■ Diseases with altered PF expression

Reduced PF expression is observed in ichthyosis vulgaris, a common genodermatosis characterized by dry skin. The reduction of PF synthesis correlates with severity of the disease (Manabe *et al.* 1991). In some forms of harlequin ichthyosis PF seems to be blocked in the state of dephosphorylation, unable to convert to filaggrin (Dale *et al.* 1990a).

■ References

Dale, B.A., Gown, A.M., Fleckman, P., Kimball, J.R., and Resing, K.A. (1987) Characterization of two monoclonal antibodies to human epidermal keratohyalin: reactivity with filaggrin and related proteins. J. Invest. Derm. **88**, 306–313.

Dale, B.A., Holbrook, K.A., Fleckman, P., Kimball, J.R., Brumbaugh, S., and Sybert, V.P. (1990a) Heterogeneity in harlequin ichthyosis, an inborn error of epidermal keratinization: Variable morphology and structural protein expression and a defect in lamellar granules. J. Invest. Derm. **94**, 6–18.

Dale, B.A., Resing, K.A., and Haydock, P.V. (1990b) Filaggrins. In Cellular and *molecular biology of intermediate filaments*. (ed. R.D. Goldman and P.M. Steinert), pp. 393–412. Plenum Press, New York.

Dale, B.A., Presland, R.B., Fleckman, P., Kam, E., and Resing, K.A. (1993) Phenotypic expression and processing of filaggrin in epidermal differentiation. In *Molecular biology of the skin: the keratinocyte* (ed. M. Darmon and M. Blumenberg), pp. 79–106. Academic Press, New York.

Dale, B.A., Resing, K.A., and Presland, R.B. (1994) Keratohyalin granule proteins. In *The keratinocyte handbook* (ed. I.M. Leigh, E.B. Lane, and F.M. Watt), pp. 323–350. Cambridge University Press, New York.

Dlugosz, A.A. and Yuspa, S.H. (1993) Coordinate changes in gene expression which mark the spinous to granular cell transition in epidermis are regulated by protein kinase C. J. Cell. Biol. **120**, 217–225.

Gan, S.-Q., McBride, O.W., Idler, W.W., Markova, N., and Steinert, P.M. (1990a) Organization, structure, and polymorphisms of the human profilaggrin gene. Biochemistry **29**, 9432–9440.

Gan, S.-Q., McBride, O.W., Idler, W.W., Markova, N., and Steinert, P.M. (1990b) Correction. Biochemistry **30**, 5814.

Haydock, P.V., Blomquist, C., Brumbaugh, S., Dale, B.A., Holbrook, K.A., and Fleckman, P. (1993) Antisense profilaggrin RNA delays and decreases profilaggrin expression and alters *in vitro* differentiation of rat epidermal keratinocytes. J. Invest. Derm. **101**, 118–126.

Mack, J.W., Steven, A.C., and Steinert, P.M. (1993). The mechanism of interaction of filaggrin with intermediate filaments. The ionic zipper hypothesis. J. Mol. Biol. **232**, 50–66.

McKinley-Grant, L.J., Idler, W.W., Bernstein, I.A., Parry, D.A.D., Cannizzaro, L., Croce, C.M., Huebner, K., Lessin, S.R., and Steinert, P.M. (1989) Characterization of a cDNA clone encoding human filaggrin and localization of the gene to chromosome region 1q21. Proc. Natl. Acad. Sci. USA **86**, 4848–4852.

Manabe, M., Sanchez, M., Sun, T.-T., and Dale, B.A. (1991) Interaction of filaggrin wit keratin filaments during advanced stages of normal human epidermal differentiation and in ichthyosis vulgaris. Differentiation **48**, 43–50.

*Markova, N.G., Marekov, L.N., Chipev, C.C., Gan, S.-Q., Idler, W.W., and Steinert, P.M. (1993) Profilaggrin is a major epidermal calcium-binding protein. Mol. Cell. Biol. **13**, 613–625.

O'Guin, W.M. and Manabe, M. (1991) The role of trichohyalin in hair follicle differentiation and its expression in nonfollicular epithelia. Ann. NY Acad. Sci. **642**, 51–63.

*Presland, R.B., Haydock, P.V., Fleckman, P., Nirunsuksiri, W., and Dale, B.A. (1992) Characterzation of the human epidermal profilaggrin gene. Genomic organization and identification of an S-100-like calcium binding domain at the amino terminus. J. Biol. Chem. **267**, 23772–23781.

*Presland, R.B., Bassuk, J.A., Kimball, J.R., and Dale, B.A. (1995) Characterization of two distinct calcium-binding sites in the amino-terminus of human profilaggrin. J. Invest. Derm. **104**, 218–223.

Ramsden, M., Loehren, D., and Balmain, A. (1983) Identification of a rapidly labelled 350k histidine-rich protein in neonatal mouse epidermis. Differentiation **23**, 243–249.

Resing, K.A., Al-Alawi, N., Blomquist, C., Fleckman, P., and Dale, B.A. (1993) Independent regulation of two cytoplasmic processing stages of the intermediate filament-associated protein filaggrin and role of Ca^{2+} in the second stage. J. Biol. Chem. **268**, 25139–25145.

Scott, I.R. and Harding, C.R. (1986) Filaggrin breakdown to water binding compounds during development of the rat stratum corneum is controlled by the water activity of the environement. Dev. Biol. **115**, 84–92.

Volz, A., Korge, B.P., Compton, J.G., Ziegler, A., Steinert, P., and Mischke, D. (1993) Physical mapping of a functional cluster of epidermal differentiation genes on chromosome 1q21. Genomics **18**, 92–99.

■ *Pierre A. de Viragh:*
Depts of Dermatology and Cell Biology,
Baylor College of Medicine,
Houston, TX 77030, USA
Tel.: +713 798 6350
Fax: +713 790 0545

Trichohyalin

Trichohyalin (TH) is a putative intermediate filament-associated protein expressed in the inner root sheath and the medulla of the hair follicle, and in various other tissues. It consists mainly of tandem peptide repeats that form an elongated α-helical rod presumed to interact with keratin intermediate filaments. The amino terminus of TH has two Ca^{2+}-binding domains of the S100 type, the role of which is as yet unknown.

Trichohyalin (TH) is a highly charged protein that consists mainly of a series of peptide repeats adopting an α-helical configuration. TH differs in molecular mass in different species from 190 (sheep, calculated 201 kDa) to 220 kDa (human, calculated 248 kDa) , with a p*I* of 5.4 (human) to 5.6 (sheep, pig) (Rothnagel and Rogers, 1986; O'Guin et al. 1992; Fietz et al. 1993; Lee et al. 1993). In pig, dog, sheep, and mouse, unlike in cow and human, TH forms protein doublets varying by approx. 10 kDa, indicating allelic differences in the numbers of repeats. The amino terminus of TH has two EF-hand domains which are very similar to those of the S100 proteins (Rogers et al. 1991; Fietz et al. 1993; Lee et al. 1993).

Most of the protein is presumed to act as a structural protein by interaction of its α-helical tandem repeats with keratin intermediate filaments. The function of the two Ca^{2+}-binding domains of TH is as yet unknown. Presumably, they may play a role in the regulation of the proteins own post-translational processing. TH is a sub-strate for Ca^{2+}-dependent enzymes, peptidylarginine deiminase and transglutaminases (Rogers et al. 1991; Fietz et al. 1993; Lee et al. 1993). Eventually the EF-hand domains are involved in the regulation of the intracellular Ca^{2+} level which regulates differentiation in skin (Fairley 1991).

TH is similar to profilaggrin and in some instances these proteins are coexpressed in the same tissue. They accumulate first in granules before being dispersed into the cytoplasm. Both are modified by peptidylarginine deiminase and transglutaminases upon their release from the granules, share a putative function as intermediate filament-associated proteins, and are characterized by repetitive sequences preceded by two EF-hand domains. Their genes co-localize on the same chromosome, and share a similar exon/intron organization. In contrast to profilaggrin, however, TH is a non-phosphorylated protein which functions as a large protein without decay into smaller functional units.

Isolation/identification

Denatured TH protein was extracted from follicles in guanidine-HCl buffer and was purified by gel-filtration chromatography (Fietz et al. 1986; Rothnagel and Rogers, 1986). Undenatured TH was extracted from tongue epithelium using a citric acid/sodium citrate insoluble pellet as starting material (Hamilton et al. 1992; O'Keefe et al. 1993). Ca^{2+}-binding by TH was demonstrated by Ca^{2+} blots using purified TH from pig tongue and was estimated, after correction for the number of Ca^{2+}-binding sites, to be as efficient as calmodulin (Lee et al. 1993). The human TH gene was isolated from a placental genomic library screened with a cDNA probe prepared from foreskin (Lee et al. 1993). The sheep TH gene was isolated from a genomic library using a cDNA probe prepared from wool follicles (Fietz et al. 1986). The sheep cDNA probe also served to isolate most of the rabbit gene (Rogers et al. 1991). Recently, the isolation of the mouse gene has been reported (O'Guin et al. 1994).

Gene and sequence

The human TH gene maps to chromosome 1q21, and the mouse TH gene is located on chromosome 3. The organization of all TH genes (EBML/GenBank accession numbers: human, L09190; sheep, Z18361; rabbit, Z18361) is similar to that of other members of the S100 family. They have three exons and two introns (Fig. 1). The first intron interrupts a small 5'-noncoding region, the second is located in the middle of the linker region between the Ca^{2+}-binding domains. Downstream of the second EF-hand domain in exon 3 are the repetitive sequences which constitute the bulk of the protein. The TH gene is clustered with genes encoding other structural proteins expressed in the skin and showing a similar gene organization, and with Ca^{2+}-binding proteins of the S100 family. It originated possibly as a fusion of an ancestral epidermal structural gene with a gene for a Ca^{2+}-binding protein (see entry on profilaggrin) (Volz et al. 1993).

Protein

TH is a rod-like protein that consists mainly of highly conserved tandem repeats forming segments with an α-helical conformation interrupted by occasional β-turn sequences (Rothnagel and Rogers 1986; Fietz et al. 1993; Lee et al. 1993). Between species, TH shows a relatively high degree of sequence homology (58% between human and sheep) and antibodies cross-react (O'Keefe et al. 1993). It is synthesized as a hydrophilic protein and only becomes insoluble upon release from the granules. This insolubilization is accomplished by the modification of some arginine residues by peptidylarginine deiminase to become citrulline and by the crosslinking by trans-glutaminase of glutamine and lysine residues to form ε-(γ-glutamyl)lysine crosslinks. The EF-hand domains have a high homology to those of other S100-like proteins, with a typical 14 amino acids (N-terminal) Ca^{2+}-binding loop of the first EF-hand loop (Rogers et al. 1991; Fietz et al. 1993; Lee et al. 1993). The second (C-terminal) EF-hand loop is formed by a classical 12 residue loop.

The biological function of TH probably is manifold. Morphologic data raised by means of three monoclonal antibodies recognizing different epitopes suggest that TH is an intermediate filament-associated protein and binds covalently to keratin filaments in a periodic manner, thus contributing to structural stability. Confirmation of this presumed function by in vitro studies has as yet not been possible, but this presumption is corroborated by information derived from the amino acid sequence (O'Guin et al. 1992). The large α-helical rod-like structure consisting of tandem repeats is similar to that of involucrin, a cell envelope protein which is abundant in the epidermis and the hair follicle, suggesting that it could also function as a cell envelope protein. The Ca^{2+}-binding properties suggest a role in the regulation of Ca^{2+}-dependent enzymes (Fietz et al. 1993; Lee et al. 1993).

Anatomical localization

TH is a major component of the inner root sheath and of the medulla of the hair follicle, where it accumulates in microscopically visible eosinophilic non-membrane bound aggregates (TH granules) that become larger in size as the cells grow further from the hair matrix. In the inner root sheath dispersion of TH granules occurs with the appearance of intermediate filaments. Finally the granules abruptly disappear and the intermediate filaments are embedded in an amorphous matrix. In the medulla TH is not associated with intermediate filaments

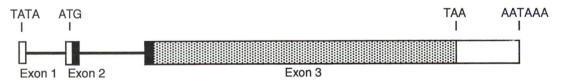

Figure 1. Schematic drawing of TH gene organization (modified from Fietz et al. 1993; Lee et al. 1993). Black boxes represent EF hands, dotted box represents remaining coding region, open boxes represent non-coding sequences.

but forms amorphous deposits (O'Guin *et al.* 1992). TH has also been found in small amounts in human neonatal foreskin epithelium, a few scattered cells of human inter-follicular epidermis (Hamilton *et al.* 1991; O'Guin and Manabe 1991; Lee *et al.* 1993; O'Keefe *et al.* 1993), in the ventral matrix of human nail (agranular) (O'Keefe *et al.* 1993), fetal sheep hoof (Fietz *et al.* 1993), and in a specific region (E' region) of the filiform papillae of the tongue of human, mouse, cow, sheep, and dog (O'Guin and Manabe 1991; O'Keefe *et al.* 1993). The cells that express TH in the epidermis and the tongue are a subset of the cells that express profilaggrin. TH eventually forms hybrid granules with profilaggrin. Thymic epithelium of Hassall's corpuscles also expresses TH (O'Guin and Manabe 1991), as does sheep rumen epithelium (Fietz *et al.* 1993).

◼ Diseases with altered TH expression

In some epidermal diseases characterized by hyperplasia, such as psoriasis, TH expression is induced in the granular layer (O'Guin and Manabe 1991). However, no hair or skin disease has so far been identified to be caused by an abnormal TH or by its abnormal regulation.

◼ References

Fairley, J.A. (1991) Calcium: a second messenger. In *Physiology, biochemistry, and molecular biology of the skin.* (ed. L.A. Goldsmith), pp. 314–328. Oxford University Press, New York

Fietz, M.J., Presland, R.B., and Rogers, G.E. (1986) The cDNA-deduced amino acid sequence for trichohyalin, a differentiation marker in the hair follicle, contains a 23 amino acid repeat. J. Cell. Biol. **102**, 1419–1429.

*Fietz, M.J., McLaughlan, C.J., Campbell, M.T., and Rogers, G.E. (1993) Analysis of the sheep trichohyalin gene: potential structural and calcium-binding roles of trichohyalin in the hair follicle. J. Cell. Biol. **121**, 855–864.

Hamilton, E.H., Payne, R.E., and O'Keefe, E.J. (1991) Trichohyalin: presence in the granular layer and stratum corneum of normal human epidermis. J. Invest. Derm. **96**, 666–672.

Hamilton, E.H., Sealock, R., Wallace, N.R., and O'Keefe, E.J. (1992) Trichohyalin: purification from porcine tongue epithelium and characterization of the native protein. J. Invest. Derm. **98**, 881–889.

*Lee, S.-C., Kim, I.-G., Marekov, L.N., O'Keefe, E.J., Parry, D.A.D., and Steinert, P. (1993) The structure of human trichohyalin. Potential multiple roles as a functional EF-hand-like calcium-binding protein, a cornified cell envelope precursor, and an intermediate filament-associated (cross-linking) protein. J. Cell Biol. **268**, 12164–12176.

O'Guin, W.M. and Manabe, M. (1991) The role of trichohyalin in hair follicle differentiation and its expression in nonfollicular epithelia. Ann. NY Acad. Sci. **642**, 51–63.

O'Guin, W.M., Sun, T.-T., and Manabe, M. (1992) Interaction of trichohyalin with intermediate filaments: three immuno-logically defined stages of trichohyalin maturation. J. Invest. Derm. **98**, 24–32.

O'Guin, W.M., Sun, T.-T., and Loomis, C.A. (1994) The cloning and characterization of the gene encoding murine trichohyalin. J. Invest. Derm. **102**, 607 (abstract).

O'Keefe, E.J., Hamilton, E.H., Lee, S.-C., and Steinert, P. (1993) Trichohyalin: a structural protein of hair, tongue, nail, and epidermis. J. Invest. Derm. **101**, 65S–71S.

*Rogers, G.E., Fietz, M.J., and Fratini, A. (1991) Trichohyalin and matrix proteins. Ann. NY Acad. Sci. **642**, 64–81.

Rothnagel, J.A. and Rogers, G.E. (1986) Trichohyalin, an intermediate filament-associated protein of the hair follicle. J. Cell Biol. **102**, 1419–1429.

Volz, A., Korge, B.P., Compton, J.G., Ziegler, A., Steinert, P., and Mischke, D. (1993) Physical mapping of a functional cluster of epidermal differentiation genes on chromosome 1q21. Genomics **18**, 92–99.

◼ *Pierre A. de Viragh:*
Depts of Dermatology and Cell Biology,
Baylor College of Medicine,
Houston, TX 77030, USA
Tel. +713 798 6350
Fax: +713 790 0545

Sorcin

Sorcin is a Ca²⁺-binding protein initially identified as an abundant protein in cells selected for resistance to natural product cancer drugs, such as vincristine and adriamycin. Among normal tissues, it is abundant in heart, skeletal, and smooth muscle, as well as in other tissues, including brain and kidney. The major form of sorcin in resistant cells has a molecular weight of 22,000, whereas normal tissues may express a family of sorcin-related proteins. Transfection of sorcin into fibroblasts produces cells manifesting a muscle-like, caffeine-stimulated release of Ca²⁺ from intracellular stores.

The molecular weight of sorcin, calculated from amino acid sequences deduced from cloned cDNAs, is 22,000 and the protein has a pI of 5.7 by isoelectric focusing. *In vitro*, sorcin is phosphorylated in the presence of protein kinase A catalytic subunit and the protein is phosphorylated in intact cells. The major molecular weight form of sorcin in multidrug-resistant cells is 22 kDa; however, sorcin may have several isoforms and may be a family of proteins in normal tissues. Sorcin is abundant in striated and smooth muscle cells, including cardiomyocytes; sarco(endo)plasmic reticulum (SR/ER) of heart cells have been shown, by electron microscopy, to be intensely stained by sorcin antibodies. Sorcin is associated with cardiac ryanodine receptor. Transfection of sorcin cDNA into hamster fibroblasts yielded cells which manifested a caffeine-sensitive Ca²⁺-release property usually reserved for "excitable" cells, such as heart and muscle. The intra-cellular localization of sorcin and Ca²⁺-release properties of the transfectants suggest a role for sorcin in intra-cellular Ca²⁺ release (Meyers and Biedler 1981; Van der Bliek *et al*. 1986a; Meyers 1988, 1990; Meyers *et al*. 1993; Meyers *et al*. 1995b)

■ Alternative names

Sorcin has been referred to as V19 (vincristine (V)-resistant cells overproduced a 19 kDa protein) or as CP$_{22}$. Sorcin (soluble resistance-related calcium-binding protein) is the accepted name for the 22 kDa Ca²⁺-binding protein overproduced by some multidrug-resistant cells (Meyers and Biedler 1981; Koch *et al*. 1986; Meyers *et al*. 1987; Meyers 1991).

■ Identification/isolation

Sorcin was first detected on two-dimensional gels display-ing soluble proteins from multidrug-resistant Chinese hamster (DC-3F/VCRd-5L) and mouse (MAZ/VCR and QUA/ADj) cells. These cells contained chromosomes bearing cytogenetic manifestations of gene amplification (homogeneously staining regions and double minute chromosomes) and cloning of amplified sequences showed that sorcin was one of six amplifiable genes (or gene classes) in those cells. The other identified gene in that tandemly arranged group encodes the P-glycoprotein, a membrane-bound drug transporter. Cells selected for resistance to a wide variety of natural product cancer drugs may amplify and overexpress genes encoding P-glycoprotein (considered to be the basis of a major mechanism for drug resistance); only a subset of those cell lines overproduce sorcin. Sorcin genes may be fortuitously amplified and overexpressed in multidrug-resistant cells because of their proximity to P-gly-coprotein. Sorcin's function, if any, in development or maintenance of the multidrug resistance phenotype is unknown (Meyers and Biedler 1981; Meyers *et al*. 1985; de Bruijn *et al*. 1986; Van der Bliek *et al*. 1986a, b; Endicott and Ling 1989).

Sucrose density fractionation of RNA from vincristine-resistant Chinese hamster lung cells (DC-3F/VCRd-5L) and *in vitro* translation showed that a 1.0 kb transcript encodes the 22 kDa sorcin. Cloned sorcin cDNAs hybridize to 1.0 and 2.5 kb transcripts in cultured cells and normal tissues; the role of the larger transcript is not known (de Bruijn *et al*. 1986; Van der Bliek *et al*. 1986a; Meyers and Biedler 1991).

The protein was purified from actinomycin D-resistant mouse cells by preparative gel electrophoresis. Sequences of tryptic peptides obtained from those samples were identical to those deduced from cloned sorcin cDNAs (Van der Bliek *et al*. 1986a). Sorcin has been purified from multidrug-resistant cells, normal tissues, and recombinant bacteria by ion exchange chromatography (Meyers 1991; Meyers *et al*. 1995). Two proteins in normal tissues, a 26 and a 47 kDa species, cross-react with sorcin antibodies. They are seen on Western blots and have been isolated by ion exchange chromatography of soluble heart pro-teins (Meyers 1988). The relationship of these species to the 22 kDa sorcin is under investigation.

The 22 kDa form of sorcin is found in soluble fractions of DC-3F/VCRd-5L cells or rabbit heart tissue lysed in the absence of Ca²⁺ and subjected to differential centrifuga-tion, whereas, when cells were lysed in the presence of Ca²⁺, sorcin was absent from supernatant fractions and present, instead, in pelleted fractions. Sorcin may, therefore, have soluble (Ca²⁺-free) and membrane (Ca²⁺-bound) biochemical or conformational forms and may undergo Ca²⁺-mediated translocation in the living cell (Meyers *et al*. 1995).

Gene and sequence

Sorcin's deduced amino acid sequence shows homology to calpain and grancalcin. Specific features of the sequence are: a 30–35 amino acid hydrophobic, glycine- and proline-rich N-terminus region, two "EF-hand" Ca^{2+}-binding domains with good homology to those in calmodulin, two atypical Ca^{2+}-binding domains with protein kinase A recognition sites at the beginning of those domains, and a Ca^{2+}-calmodulin kinase site. Hamster, mouse, and human sorcin show a high degree of homology (Van der Bliek *et al.* 1986a; Van der Bliek *et al.* 1988; Meyers *et al.* 1995).

The six-gene amplicon containing sorcin, P-glycoprotein, and four unidentified genes linked in tandem, is conserved in hamster, mouse, and human. The amplicon maps to chromosomes 1, 5, and 7 in hamster, mouse, and human, respectively (Jongsma *et al.* 1987; Van der Bliek, *et al.* 1988; Stahl, *et al.* 1992). To date, only one sorcin gene has been mapped; somatic cell hybrid studies suggest the possibility of another sorcin gene on human chromosome 4 (Van der Bliek *et al.* 1988).

Protein

Sorcin has been shown to bind Ca^{2+} by $^{45}Ca^{2+}$-overlay assay, by gel filtration Ca^{2+}-affinity procedures, and by intrinsic fluorescence measurements. The protein has at least one high affinity Ca^{2+} binding site ($K_d \sim 1$ μM), presumably an 'EF-hand' domain. Ca^{2+}-mediated conformational changes have been measured by circular dichroism and fluorescence spectroscopic procedures. Unlike calmodulin and other Ca^{2+}-binding proteins, sorcin is more fluorescent in the absence of Ca^{2+} than in the presence (Meyers *et al.*, in press).

Phosphorylation of sorcin purified from multidrug-resistant cells, heart tissue, and recombinant bacteria is catalyzed by protein kinase A catalytic subunit, and 1–2% of 22 kDa sorcin in multidrug-resistant cells is metabolically labeled with $^{32}P_i$ (Meyers 1990; Meyers *et al.* 1995a).

Biological activities

Sorcin's biological role is not known, although intracellular localization of sorcin to cardiac SR and the above-mentioned caffeine-sensitive Ca^{2+} release property of sorcin transfectants suggest that sorcin may participate in trans-sarcolemmal Ca^{2+} transport (Meyers *et al.* 1993).

References

de Bruijn, M.H.L., Van der Bliek, A.M., Biedler, J.L., and Borst, P. (1986) Differential amplification and disproportionate expression of five genes in three multidrug-resistant Chinese hamster lung cell lines. Mol. Cell. Biol. **6**, 4717–4722.

Endicott, J.A. and Ling, V. (1989) The biochemistry of P-glycoprotein-mediated multidrug resistance. Annu. Rev. Biochem. **58**, 137–171.

Jongsma, A.P.M., Spengler, B.A., Van der Bliek, A.M., Borst, P., and Biedler, J.L. (1987) Chromosomal localization of three genes coamplified in the multidrug-resistant CH^{R}C5 Chinese hamster ovary line. Cancer Res. **47**, 2875–2878.

Koch, G., Smith, M., Twentyman, P., and Wright, K. (1986) Identification of a novel calcium-binding protein (CP22) in multidrug-resistant murine and hamster cells. FEBS Lett. **195**, 275–279.

Meyers, M.B. (1988) Sorcin is a cardiac calcium-binding protein. Proc. Am. Assoc. Cancer Res. **30**, 505.

Meyers, M.B. (1990) Sorcin, a calcium-binding protein overproduced in many multidrug-resistant cells. In *Stimulus response coupling: the role of intracellular calcium-binding proteins,* (ed. V.L. Smith and J.R. Dedman), pp. 159–171. CRC Press, Boca Raton, Florida.

Meyers, M.B. (1991) A 22 kDa calcium-binding protein, sorcin, is encoded by amplified genes in multidrug-resistant cells. In *Novel calcium-binding proteins. fundamentals and clinical implications,* (ed. C.W. Heizman), pp. 385–399. Springer-Verlag, Heidelberg.

Meyers, M.B. and Biedler, J.L. (1981) Increased synthesis of a low molecular weight protein in vincristine-resistant cells. Biochem. Biophys. Res. Commun. **99**, 228-235.

Meyers, M.B. and Biedler, J.L. (1991) Protein changes in multidrug-resistant cells. In *Molecular and cellular biology of multidrug resistance in tumor cells,* (ed. I.B. Roninson), pp. 243–261. Plenum Publishing Corporation, New York.

Meyers, M.B., Spengler, B.A., Chang, T.-D., Melera, P.W., and Biedler, J.L. (1985) Gene amplification-associated cytogenetic aberrations and protein changes in vincristine-resistant Chinese hamster, mouse, and human cells. J. Cell Biol. **100**, 588–597.

* Meyers, M.B., Schneider, K.A., Spengler, B.A., Chang, T.-D., and Biedler, J.L. (1987) Sorcin (V19), a soluble acidic calcium-binding protein overproduced in multidrug-resistant cells. Identification of the protein by anti-sorcin antibodies. Biochem. Pharmacol. **36**, 2373–2380.

Meyers, M.B., Song, C.H., Scotto, K.W., Kerr, A.H., and Sheu, S–S. (1993) Analysis of Chinese hamster lung cells transfected with the calcium-binding protein, sorcin. Proc. Am. Assoc. Cancer Res. **34**, 432.

* Meyers, M.B., Zamparelli, C., Verzili, D., Dicker, A.P., Blanck, T.J.J., and Chiancone, E. (1995a) Calcium-dependent translocation of sorcin to membranes: functional relevance in contractile tissue. FEBS Lett. **357**, 230.

Meyers, M.B., Pickel, V.M., Sheu, S.S., Sharma, V.K., Scotto, K.W., and Fishman, G.I. (1995b) Association of sorcin with the cardiac ryanodine receptor. J. Biol. Chem. **270**, 26411–26418.

Stahl, F., Wettergren, Y., and Levan, G. (1992) Amplicon structure in multidrug-resistant murine cells: a nonrearranged region of genomic DNA. Mol. Cell. Biol. **12**, 1179–1187.

* Van der Bliek, A.M., Meyers, M.B., Biedler, J.L., Hes, E., and Borst, P. (1986a) A 22-kd protein (sorcin/V19) encoded by an amplified gene in multidrug-resistant cells, is homologous to the calcium-binding light chain of calpain. EMBO J. **5**, 3201–3208.

Van der Bliek A.M., Van der Velde-Koerts, T., Ling, V., and Borst, P. (1986b) Overexpression and amplification of five genes in a multidrug-resistant Chinese hamster ovary cell line. Mol. Cell. Biol. **6**, 1671–1678.

Van der Bliek, A.M., Baas, F., Van der Velde-Koerts, T., Biedler, J.L., Meyers, M.B., Ozols, R.F., Hamilton, T.C., Joenje, H., and Borst, P. (1988) Genes amplified and overexpressed in human multidrug-resistant cell lines. Cancer Res. **48**, 5927–5932.

■ *Marian B. Meyers:*
   Albert Einstein College of Medicine,
   Department of Medicine/Division of Cardiology,
   1300 Morris Park Avenue,
   Bronx, New York 10461, USA
   Tel.: (718) 430 2619
   Fax: (718) 430 8989

SPARC

SPARC is an extracellular multidomain glycoprotein with domains also found in other modular proteins. Two Ca²⁺-binding sites have been demonstrated: a low affinity site presumably binding several Ca^{2+} ions and a single high affinity site similar to the EF-hand Ca^{2+}-binding motif which binds one Ca^{2+} ion. SPARC is expressed in a variety of tissues in nematodes and vertebrates. Its physiological role is still unclear, but localization studies and in vitro data suggest multiple functions in cell-matrix interactions.

SPARC, BM-40, and osteonectin are synonyms for identical proteins initially identified from different sources, such as bone (Termine *et al.* 1981), endothelial cells (Sage *et al.* 1984; Mason *et al.* 1986), platelets (Stenner *et al.* 1986), and basement membranes (Dziadek *et al.* 1986). Comparison of cDNA sequences have shown that all these proteins are identical molecules or interspecies homologs and that they are the product of a single gene. The acronym SPARC (secreted protein acidic and rich in cysteine) is perhaps the most appropriate name for this protein, because both other names refer to only part of its widespread extracellular tissue localization.

SPARC is a member of a new modular protein family which has several domains in common (Fig. 1): the family includes SC1, a rat brain protein associated with synaptic junctions (Guermah *et al.* 1991), a quail retinal protein, QR1, which is exclusively expressed in the neuroretina (Johnston *et al.* 1990), a human testicular proteoglycan, testican (Alliel *et al.* 1993), and TGF-β induced protein

tsc36 (Shibanuma *et al.* 1993). The functions of all of the homologs of SPARC have not been established so far.

■ Alternative names

SPARC (Mason *et al.* 1986), BM-40 (Dziadek *et al.* 1986), and osteonectin (Termine *et al.* 1981)

■ Isolation

1) From bone under demineralizing conditions (Romberg *et al.* 1985).
2) From platelets by immunoaffinity chromatography (Kelm and Mann 1990).
3) From mouse Engelbreth–Holm–Swarm tumor under nondenaturing conditions (Dziadek *et al.* 1986).
4) From conditioned media of PYS cells under denaturing conditions (Sage *et al.* 1984).

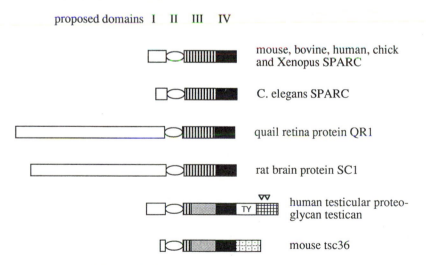

Figure 1. Domain organization of SPARC and related proteins. Domain organization as predicted by secondary structure analyses is indicated by roman number I–IV (Engel *et al.* 1987). Domains II, III, and IV are conserved within this protein family. Domains I are not homologous to each other, but have an acidic character in common. Domain II is a ten cysteine-containing follistatin-like module. Domain III is a novel domain. Hatched areas indicate low similarity. Domain IV contains a single Ca^{2+}-binding site analogous to the EF-hand superfamily. TY denotes a thyroglobulin-like domain; triangles, glycosaminoglycan attachment sites.

5) From conditioned media of stably transfected embryonic kidney cell lines under nondenaturing conditions (Pottgiesser et al. 1994).

Gene and sequences

Accession numbers of SPARC in EMBL and GenBank databases are L21758 (*C. elegans*), X62483 (*Xenopus*), L24906 (chick), X12697 (mouse), J03233 (bovine), and J03040 (human). The gene is located on chromosome 5 of humans, on 11 of mouse, and chromosome 4 of nematodes. Vertebrate SPARCs are encoded on 10 exons while the nematode gene contains six exons. No alternative splice variants have been detected. In the 5′ UTR positive and negative regulatory elements, GGA boxes and elements responsive to retinoic acid, cAMP, steroids, and heat shock are located. *In vitro* models show that SPARC is indeed inducible with morphogens, cytokines, and hormones (Lane and Sage 1994).

Protein

Figure 2A shows an illustrative model of SPARC as deduced from secondary structure predictions in accordance with the exon structure of the gene (Engel et al. 1987; McVey et al. 1988). Domain I, comprising the first 52 amino acids of the protein, features primarily two segments of 15 residues each of which contains 7–8 glutamic acids in short clusters that impart a negative charge at physiological pH. Domain II is homologous to the follistatin-like module as found in follistatin and agrin. It contains 10 cysteines, two clusters of positive charges and Asn-linked glycosylation sites. Glycosylation accounts for about 10–20% of the molecular mass (40 kDa) of SPARC and is tissue specific (Kelm, *et al*. 1992; Pottgiesser et al. 1994). Domain III was predicted to be predominantly α-helical. It is linked to domain IV by a proline-rich stretch of about 30 residues. Domain IV contains an EF-hand analog Ca^{2+}-binding motif with a predicted helix–loop–helix secondary structure (Fig. 2B) and the short C-terminus with 10 residues. However, experimental data indicate that postulated domains III and IV presumably form together one independently folded protein unit (Pottgiesser *et al*. 1994). Domains II, III, and IV are conserved within the family of SPARC-related proteins (Fig. 1).

Two different Ca^{2+}-binding sites have been detected in SPARC. A low affinity site presumably binding several Ca^{2+} ions with a K_d larger than 5 mM was localized in domain I (Maurer et al. 1992). This domain is implicated in hydroxyapatite binding; however, direct experimental data are missing so far. Furthermore, SPARC contains a single high affinity Ca^{2+}-binding site. Its K_d ranges between 80 and 300 nM dependent on the species (Romberg et al. 1985; Pottgiesser et al. 1994). Ca^{2+} binding to this site induces a large conformational change resulting in a 30% increase of α-helical content. Point mutations demonstrated that the EF-hand analog motif in domain IV is the high affinity Ca^{2+}-binding site of SPARC (Fig. 2B; Pottgiesser et al. 1994). The conformational change upon Ca^{2+} binding is not restricted to the EF-hand analog motif itself but is transmitted to domain III via strong interactions. The high affinity Ca^{2+}-binding site will always be saturated at millimolar Ca^{2+} concentrations in the extracellular space and thus cannot be involved in regulation. However, this site may be important for folding and secretion of SPARC (Pottgiesser et al. 1994).

Anatomical localization

During development SPARC expression is regulated spatially and temporally. In adult organisms four types of SPARC-producing tissues can be distinguished in principle (Lane and Sage 1994):

1. All matrix-producing tissues such as ligaments, endometrium and decidua, expressing cell types are osteoblasts, odontoblasts, chrondrocytes, and endothelial cells of blood vessels.
2. Corticosteroid-secreting tissues such as the adrenal cortex (type I astrocytes), ovaries, and testes (Leydig cells).
3. Highly proliferative epithelia as found in gut, skin, salivary gland, lactating mammary gland, in the renal tubule of the kidney, and in testicular Sertoli cells.
4. Platelets (megakaryocytes).

Activities

SPARC was shown to bind to hydroxyapatite and to inhibit hydroxyapatite crystal growth. Furthermore, binding affinities to a variety of extracellular proteins have been demonstrated *in vitro*: to collagens, to plasminogen, to plasminogen activator, to albumin, and to platelet-derived growth factor (PDGF). SPARC inhibits binding of PDGF isoforms to their receptor. SPARC also binds to thrombospondin and is secreted as a complex upon platelet stimulation (for references see Lane and Sage 1994).

Cellular effects of SPARC *in vitro* include inhibition of cell migration and spreading, induction of cell rounding, and modulation of cell cycle progression. However, these effects have only been demonstrated for aortic endothelial cells and a general physiological function is unclear so far. Developmental anomalies observed in *Xenopus* following microinjection of SPARC antibodies and in *C. elegans* upon overexpression of SPARC agree with a function of SPARC in the modulation of cell-matrix interactions (for references see Lane and Sage 1994).

References

Alliel, P.M., Perin, J.-P., Jolles, P., and Bonnet, F.J. (1993) Testican, a multidomain testicular proteoglycan resembling modulators of cell social behaviour. Eur. J. Biochem. **214**, 347–350.

Dziadek, M., Paulsson, M., Aumailley, M., and Timpl, R. (1986) Purification and tissue distribution of a small protein (BM-40) extracted from basement membrane tumor. Eur. J. Biochem. **161**, 455–464.

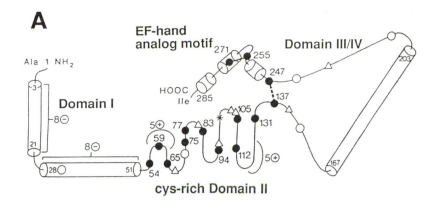

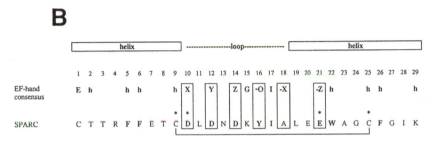

Figure 2. Domain model and EF-hand analog motif of SPARC. (A) Domain model of murine SPARC based on secondary structure predictions (Engel *et al.* 1987). Regions of the protein predicted to be α-helical are represented by cylinders, cysteines are indicated by filled circles. The glycosylation site is indicated by a star. (B) The EF-hand analog motif in murine SPARC is compared to the consensus sequence of the EF-hand superfamily. Conserved amino acids are shown in bold, Ca²⁺-coordinating ligands are boxed. h denotes hydrophobic amino acids. The bracket indicates the disulfide bridge in the motif of SPARC. Stars mark the amino acids which affect Ca²⁺ affinity when replaced by site-directed mutagenesis (Pottgiesser *et al.* 1994).

Engel, J., Taylor, M., Paulsson, M., Sage, H., and Hogan, B.L.M. (1987) Calcium-binding domains and calcium-induced conformational transition of SPARC/BM-40/osteonectin, an extracellular glycoprotein expressed in mineralized and non-mineralized tissues. Biochemistry **26**, 6958–6965.

Guermah, M., Crisanti, P., Langier, D., Dezelee, P., Bidou, L., Pessac, B., and Calothy, G. (1991) Transcription of a quail gene expressed in embryonic retinal cells is shut off sharply at hatching. Proc. Natl. Acad. Sci. USA **88**, 4503–4507.

Hohenester, E., Maurer, P., Hohenadi, C., Timpl, R., Jansonius, J.N., and Engel, J. (1996) Structure of a novel extracellular Ca(2+)-binding module in BM-40. Nat. Struct. Biol. 3, 67–73.

Johnston, I.G., Paladino, T., Gurd, J.W., and Brown, I.R. (1990) Molecular cloning of SC1: a putative brain extracellular matrix glycoprotein showing partial similarity to osteonectin/BM-40/SPARC. Neuron **2**, 165–176.

Kelm, R.J. and Mann, K.G. (1990) Human platelet osteonectin: release, surface expression and partial characterization. Blood **75**, 1105–1113.

Kelm, R.J., Hair, G.A., Mann, K.G., and Grant, B.W. (1992) Characterization of human osteoblast and megakaryocyte-derived osteonectin (SPARC). Blood **80**, 3112–3119.

Lane T.F. and Sage, H. (1994) The biology of SPARC, a protein that modulates cell-matrix interactions. FASEB J. **8**, 163–173.

McVey, J.H., Nomura, S., Kelly, P., Mason, I.J., and Hogan, B.L.M. (1988) Characterisation of the mouse SPARC/osteonectin gene: intron/exon organization and an unusual promoter region. J. Biol. Chem. **263**, 11111–11116.

Mason, I.J., Taylor, A., Williams, J.G., Sage, H., and Hogan, B.L.M. (1986) Evidence from molecular cloning that SPARC, a major product of mouse embryo parietal endoderm, is related to an endothelial cell "culture shock" glycoprotein. EMBO J. **5**, 1465–1472.

Maurer, P., Mayer, U., Bruch, M., Jenö, P., Mann, K., Landwehr, R., Engel, J., and Timpl, R. (1992) High and low affinity calcium binding and stability of the multidomain extracellular glyco-protein BM-40/SPARC/osteonectin. Eur. J. Biochem. **205**, 233–240.

Pottgieser, J., Maurer, P., Mayer, U., Nischt, R., Mann· K., Timpl, R., Krieg, T., and Engel, J. (1994) Changes in calcium and collagen IV binding caused by mutations in the EF hand and other domains of extracellular matrix protein BM-40/SPARC/osteonectin. J. Mol. Biol. **238**, 563–574.

Romberg, R.W., Werness, P.G., Lollar, P., Riggs, B.L., and Mann, K.G. (1985) Isolation and characterization of native adult osteonectin. J. Biol. Chem. **260**, 2728–2736.

Sage, H., Johnson, C., and Bornstein, P. (1984) Characterization of a novel serum albumin-binding glycoprotein secreted by endothelial cells in culture. J. Biol. Chem. **259**, 3993–4007.

Shibanuma, M., Mashimo, J., Mita, A., Kuroki, T., and Nose, K. (1993) Cloning from a mouse osteoblastic cell line of a set of transforming-growth-factor 1-regulated genes, one of which seems to encode a follistatin-related polypeptide. Eur. J. Biochem. **217**, 13–19.

Stenner, D.D., Tracy, R.P., Riggs, B.L., and Mann, K.G. (1986) Human platelets contain and secrete osteonectin, a major protein of mineralized bone. Proc. Natl. Acad. Sci. (USA), **83**, 6892–6896.

Termine, J.D., Kleinman, H.K., Whitson, S.W., Conn, K.M., McGarvey, M.L., and Martin, G.R. (1981) Osteonectin, a bone-specific protein linking mineral to collagen. Cell **26**, 99–105.

Note added in proof:

The crystal structure of the C-terminal portion of SPARC has been solved (Hohenester *et al.* 1996). Surprisingly this demonstrated two paired, Ca²⁺-binding EF-hands with a novel variation of the EF-hand loop structure.

■ *Patrick Maurer:*
Institute for Biochemistry,
Medical Faculty,
University of Köln,
Joseph-Stelzmann-Str.52
D-50931 Köln, Germany.
Tel.: 49 251 478 6997
Fax: 49 251 478 6977

Spectrin (Brain)

Spectrin belongs to the family of actin-binding proteins. It is a structural protein associated with the cytoplasmic surface of the plasma membrane. It is composed of an α- and β-subunit and was first defined in red blood cells. It has been found in most metazoans including vertebrates and higher plants. Non-erythroid forms exist in a variety of tissues and are most abundant in nervous tissue. The α-subunit of brain spectrin contains two EF-hands and binds calmodulin and Ca²⁺(for review, see, 1989; Goodman et al. 1988; Coleman et al., Michaud et al. 1991; Bennet and Gilligan 1993; Winkelman and Forget 1993).

■ Isolation/identification

Brain spectrin comprises 2–3% of the total brain proteins. It is isolated via a synaptosomal membrane preparation, followed by extraction at low ionic strength, by a zonal sedimentation through a sucrose gradient, then spectrin tetramers are obtained by gel filtration chromatography (Riederer *et al.* 1986). Some procedures isolate spectrin from membranes using either high ionic strength buffers or a preparative electrophoresis. The later isolation usually yields a mixture of brain spectrin isoforms. The preparation of recombinant spectrin is another way to obtain individual spectrin subunits (Dubreuil *et al.* 1991), e.g. for the study of the calmodulin-binding and EF-hand Ca²⁺-binding properties of *Drosophila* α-spectrin polypeptides.

■ Alternative names

In early studies a variety of names were given to brain spectrin: *calmodulin binding proteins-I* binding f-actin (Davis and Klee 1981); *calspectin*, a calmodulin-binding protein (Kakiuchi *et al.* 1982); *fodrin*, an axonally trans-ported protein doublet found at the internal periphery of neurons (Levine and Willard 1981); or *brain actin-binding protein*, BABP, binding to actin and stimulating actomyosin Mg²⁺-ATPase (Shimo-oka *et al.* 1983). Erythrocyte and brain forms of spectrin obtained from chicken cerebellum were named *α-, β-, β′- and γ-subunits* (Lazarides and Nelson 1983). In mammalian CNS, *brain spectrin240/235*, *brain spectrin240/235E* (E standing for erythrocyte-related) were found segregated in the axonal and somatodendritic parts of neurons, respectively (Riederer *et al.* 1986), while *brain spectrin240/235A* (A standing for astroglia-related) was found in astrocytes (Goodman *et al.* 1989). Due to the confusing nomencla-ture, and the extreme genetic heterogeneity, Zimmer *et al.* (1992) and Winkelmann and Forget (1993) have proposed that the spectrins be classified as αSp and βSp followed by roman numerals, i.e. I for erythroid and II for non-erythroid gene products. The symbol Σ would designate "subtypes", followed by an arabic numeral to designate known isoforms, or by an asterix * to desig-nate suspected isoforms. Erythroid α- and β-spectrins are thus termed αSpIΣ1 and βSpIΣ1. α- and β-brain spectrin, fodrin, calspectin or 240/235 become αSpIIΣ1 and βSpIIΣ1. Brain spectrin 235E or β′-spectrin is termed βSpIΣ2. The presence of αSpIΣ2 in brain tissue is suspected, but until its molecular characterization is defined it is termed αSpIΣ* (Riederer *et al.* 1988; Clark *et al.* 1994).

■ Genes and sequences

The αSp II gene has been mapped to chromosome 9 in humans. The βSp II gene has been mapped to chromo-some 11 in the mouse and chromosome 2 in humans, and the β-spectrin I gene has been mapped to chromosome 14 in humans (reviewed by Winkelman and Forget, 1993; Goodman *et al.* 1995). α-spectrin is a 2429 amino acid polypeptide and β-spectrin II contains 2363 residues. Their amino acid sequences can be obtained e.g. from SwissProt under SPCA, SPCB, SPCN, FODA and FODB, accession numbers P02549, P13395, P19546, P07751, Q00963 and P11277; or GenBank accession number S59200 for mouse βSpIIΣ1.

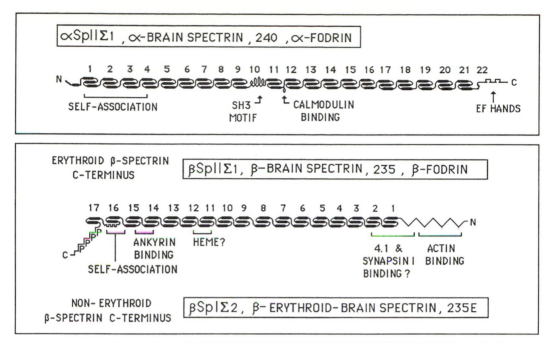

Figure 1. The structures of the brain spectrin forms are summarized schematically. For details see text.

Proteins

Brain spectrin is a filamentous, flexible, rod-shaped structure of 200 nm length and 10^6 kDa molecular mass. It is composed of two $\alpha\beta$ heterodimers which, by head-to-head interaction, form a heterotetramer. The actin-binding sites are located at both ends of the tetrameric complex. The α-subunit has a calculated molecular mass of 280 kDa and migrates on SDS gels with an apparent M_r of 240 kDa, while the molecular mass of the β-subunit, based on the amino acid sequence is 275 kDa and it shows on SDS gels an apparent M_r of 235 kDa. The β-subunit has an isoelectric point of pH 5.78. Differences in brain spectrin isoforms, i.e. erythroid-related or non-erythroid related forms, arise by the alternate splicing of pre-mRNAs that originate from two α-spectrin or two β-spectrin genes, respectively. All spectrin subunits exhibit an internal 106 amino acid repeating motif, with 22 repeats for α- and 17 repeats for β-spectrin. These repeated segments are typical for other members of the family of actin-binding proteins, including dystrophin and α-actinin and consist of three helix bundles. In α-brain spectrin the self-association site is located at the N-terminal end. Segment 10 has a high homology to the modulatory *src*-tyrosine kinase (SH3) domain. A high-affinity calmodulin binding site is located between repeats 11 and 12 and is typical for non-erythroid α-spectrin. The C-terminal domain 22 includes two EF-hand motifs, which bind Ca^{2+} with high affinity (Fig. 1). Brain βSpII contains an f-actin, a protein 4.1/synapsin I, an ankyrin binding site, a self-association

region, and a sequence with a high homology to globins, possibly a heme-binding domain which may relate to oxygen binding and electron transfer (Ma *et al.* 1993).

Antibodies

A variety of poly- and monoclonal antibodies, directed against erythroid and non-erythroid spectrin of a variety of species are commercially available. Companies to contact are: Biodesign Int., Calbiochem Corp., Chemicon International Inc., East-Acres Biologicals, ICN Immunochemicals, Serotec, Sigma.

Localization

A variety of brain spectrin isoforms were found in mammalian and avian brains. One neuronal form is localized throughout neurons (chicken), or in axons (mouse), a second form is present in perikarya and dendrites (Lazarides and Nelson 1983; Riederer *et al.* 1986), while a third form is exclusive to astroglia (Goodman *et al.* 1989). The variety of non-erythroid spectrin in different tissues is due mainly to the presence of variable β-spectrin forms (Coleman *et al.* 1989; Bennett and Gilligan 1993). At the subcellular level, brain spectrin isoforms were found not to associate exclusively with the neuronal plasma membrane, but to form a structural connection with the membranes of mitochondria, endoplas-

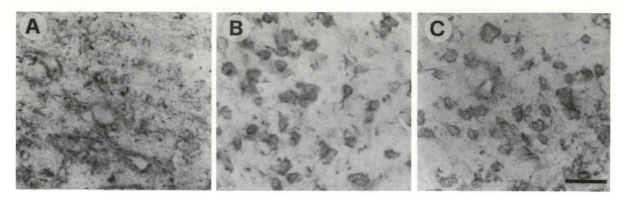

Figure 2. The immunocytochemical distribution of brain spectrin isoforms in the vestibular nucleus of adult mouse brain, with antisera: (A) anti-human αSpIIΣ1, (B) anti-human αSpIΣ*, and (C) anti-mouse βSpIΣ2; the bar represents 50 μm (for methods see Riederer *et al.* 1988). Note the axonal and synaptic distribution of αSpIIΣ1, and the somato-dendritic location of αSpIΣ* and βSpIS2.

mic reticulum, and vesicles, as well as with cytoskeletal structures (Zagon *et al.* 1986).

■ Biological activities

Brain spectrin associates with high affinity (K_d = 5–10 nM) with proteins in brain synaptosomal membranes. Calmodulin in the presence of submicromolar concentrations of Ca^{2+} inhibits spectrin association with synaptosomal membranes (Steiner *et al.* 1989). Brain spectrin associates with a variety of structural and regulatory proteins: actin, microtubules, intermediate filaments (NF-L), calpactin 1, Ca^{2+}- and phospholipid-binding proteins, N-CAM, protein 4.1, synapsin I, and Na^+/K^+-ATPase. Four high affinity sites for Ca^{2+} binding with a K_d = 20–300 nM and 1–3 μM, and with a low affinity binding component (K_d = 100–200 μM) have been found. In αSpIIΣ1, two sites are at the EF-hand structures and one is located at the hypersensitive cleavage site in the region of repeats 11 and 12. The fourth Ca^{2+}-binding site is found in the N-terminal domain of β-spectrin, βSpIIΣ1, near the acting-binding site. Magnesium inhibits Ca^{2+} binding to the low affinity site with a K_i = 1.21 mM (Wallis *et al.* 1992). Ca^{2+} binds to spectrin with higher affinity than to many other Ca^{2+}-binding proteins. The location of Ca^{2+}-binding sites is consistent with a direct modulation of the spectrin-actin-protein 4.1, synapsin I interaction, Ca^{2+}-regulated release of neurotransmitters and exocytosis (Goodman *et al.* 1995). Brain spectrin is a good substrate for calpain I, which is activated by Ca^{2+} in the μM range. The cleavage site in α-brain spectrin is close to the calmodulin-binding site, and higher Ca^{2+} content results in cleavage of both subunits, with a loss in actin binding and subunit dimerization (Harris and Morrow 1990). The presence of calmodulin increases the extent of calpain-induced hydrolysis of αSpIIΣ1, and α and βSpIIΣ1 are more sensitive to calpain-induced degradation than the erythroid

counterparts αSpIΣ* and βSpIΣ2 (Johnson *et al.* 1991). Interestingly, *erythrocyte spectrin* has 25 times more Ca^{2+} binding sites per dimer than non-erythroid spectrin. This Ca^{2+} possibly binds to the repetitive sequences and stabilizes their folded conformation (Wallis *et al.* 1993).

■ References

Bennet, V. and Gilligan, D.M. (1993) The spectrin-based membrane skeleton and micron-scale organization of the plasma membrane. Annu. Rev. Cell Biol. **9**, 27–66.

Clark, M.B., Ma, Y., Bloom., M.L., Barker, J.E., Zagon, I.S., Zimmer, W.E., and Goodman, S.R. (1994) Brain α-erythroid spectrin: identification, compartmentalization and β-spectrin association. Brain Res. **663**, 223–236.

Coleman, T.R., Fishkind, D.J., Mooseker, M.S., and Morrow, J.S. (1989) Functional diversity among spectrin isoforms. Cell Motil. **12**, 225–247

Davis, P.J.A., and Klee, C.B. (1981) Calmodulin-binding proteins: A high molecular weight calmodulin-binding protein from bovine brain. Biochem. Int. **3**, 203–212.

Dubreuil, R.R., Brandin, E., Reisberg, J.H.S., Goldstein, L.S.B., and Branton, D. (1991) Structure, calmodulin-binding, and calcium-binding properties of recombinant α-spectrin polypeptides. J. Biol. Chem. **266**, 7189–7193.

Goodman, S.R., Krebs, K.E., Whitfield, C.F., Riederer, B.M., and Zagon, I.S. (1988) Spectrin and related molecules. CRC Crit. Rev. Biochem. **23**, 171–274.

Goodman, S.R., Lopresti, L.I. Riederer, B.M., Sikorski, A., and Zagon, I.S. (1989) Brain spectrin (240/235A): a novel astrocyte specific spectrin isoform. Brain Res. Bull. **23**, 311–316.

Goodman, S.R., Zimmer, W.E., Clark, M.B., Zagon, I.S., Barker, J.E. and Bloom, M.L. (1995) Brain spectrin: of mice and men. Brain Res. Bull. **36**, 593–606.

Harris, A.S. and Morrow, J.S. (1990) Calmodulin and calcium-dependent protease I coordinately regulate the interaction of fodrin with actin. Proc. Natl. Acad. Sci. USA **87**, 3009–3013.

Hohenester, E., Maurer, P., Hohenadl, C., Timpl, R., Jansonius, J.N., and Engel, J. (1996) Structure of a novel Ca^{2+}-binding module in BM-40. Nature Structural Biology **3**, 67–73.

Johnson, G.V., Litersky, J.M., and Jope, R.S. (1991) Degradation of microtubule-associated protein 2 and brain spectrin by calpain: a comparative study. J. Neurochem. **56**, 1630–1638.

Kakiuchi, S., Sobue, K., Morimoto, K., and Kanda, K. (1982) A spectrin-like calmodulin-binding protein (calspectin) of brain. Biochem. Int. **5**, 755–762.

Lazarides, E. and Nelson, W.J. (1983) Erythrocyte form of spectrin in cerebellum: appearance at a specific stage in the terminal differentiation of neurons. Science **222**, 931–933.

Levine, J. and Willard, M. (1981) Fodrin: axonally transported protein associated with the internal periphery of many cells. J. Cell Biol. **90**, 631–643.

Ma, Y., Zimmer, W.E., Riederer, B.M., Bloom, M.L., Barker, J.E., and Goodman, S.R. (1993) The complete amino acid sequence for brain β spectrin (β fodrin): relationship to globin sequence. Mol. Brain Res. **18**, 87–99.

Michaud, D., Guillet, G., Rogers, P.A., and Charest, P.M. (1991) Identification of a 220 kDa membrane-associated plant cell protein immunologically related to human β spectrin. FEBS Lett. **294**, 77–80.

Riederer, B.M., Zagon, I.S., and Goodman, S.R. (1986) Brain spectrin(240/235) and brain spectrin(240/235E): two distinct spectrin subtypes with different locations within mammalian neural cells. J. Cell Biol. **102**, 2088–2096.

Riederer, B.M., Lopresti, L.L., Krebs, K.E., Zagon, I.S., and Goodman, S.R. (1988) Brain spectrin(240/235) and brain spectrin(240/235E): Conservation of structure and location within mammalian neural tissue. Brain Res. Bull. **21**, 607–616.

Shimo-oka, T., Ohnisji, K., and Watanabe, Y. (1983) Further characterization of a brain high molecular weight actin-binding protein (BABP): interaction with brain actin and ultrastructural studies. J. Biochem. **93**, 977–987.

Steiner, J.P., Walke, H.T., and Bennett, V. (1989) Calcium/calmodulin inhibits direct binding of spectrin to synaptosomal membranes. J. Biol. Chem. **264**, 2783–2791.

Wallis, C.J., Wenegieme, E.F., and Babitch, J.A. (1992) Characterization of calcium binding to brain spectrin. J. Biol. Chem. **267**, 4333–4337.

Wallis, C.J., Babitch, J.A., and Wenegieme, E.F. (1993) Divalent cation binding to erythrocyte spectrin. Biochem. **32**, 5045–5450.

Winkelmann, J.C. and Forget, B.G. (1993) Erythroid and nonerythroid spectrins. Blood **81**, 3173–3185.

Zagon, I.S., Higbee, R., Riederer, B.M., and Goodman, S.R. (1986) Spectrin subtypes in mammalian brain: an immunoelectron microscopic study. J. Neurosci. **6**, 2977–2986.

Zimmer, W.E., Ma, Y., Zagon, I.S., and Goodman, S.R. (1992) Developmental expression of brain β-spectrin isoform messenger RNAs. Brain Res. **594**, 75–83.

■ *Beat M. Riederer:*
Institute of Anatomy,
University of Lausanne,
Rue du Bugnon 9,
1005 Lausanne,
Switzerland
Tel.: +41 21 692 5100
Fax: +41 21 692 5105
E-mail: briedere@eliot.unil.ch

Troponin C

Troponin C (TnC) is an EF-hand Ca^{2+}-binding protein that is a constitutive subunit of the troponin complex on the thin filament of striated muscle. Cyclic binding and release of Ca^{2+} from the N-terminal Ca^{2+}-binding sites of TnC regulates muscle contraction.

There are two isoforms of TnC (see Fig. 1); one is expressed in fast skeletal muscle (sTnC), while another is expressed in cardiac and slow skeletal muscle (cTnC) (for reviews see Leavis and Gergely 1984; Collins 1991; Gergely *et al.* 1993). The molecular weights of human sTnC and cTnC are 18,102 and 18,382, respectively, with isoelectric points between 4.1 and 4.6. Troponin C, together with troponin I (TnI) and troponin T (TnT), form the heterotrimer troponin complex which is bound to the thin filament of striated muscle near the overlap region between adjacent tropomyosin dimers.

TnC has four Ca^{2+}-binding sites (I, II, III, and IV; see Fig. 1). Site I in cTnC is inactive. The C-terminal, high-affinity metal-binding sites III and IV are probably saturated with Ca^{2+} or Mg^{2+} during relaxation and contraction and function to allow constitutive association of TnC with the troponin complex (K_d $Ca^{2+} \approx 6 \times 10^{-8}$ M; K_d $Mg^{2+} \approx 3 \times 10^{-4}$ M). Sites I and II in sTnC and site II in cTnC have a lower affinity for Ca^{2+} ($K_d \approx 3 \times 10^{-6}$ M), but are Ca^{2+}-specific. Cyclic binding and release of Ca^{2+} from the low-affinity N-terminal Ca^{2+}-binding sites of TnC regulates muscle contraction.

■ Identification/isolation

The troponin complex was first identified in 1965 as a factor that promoted the aggregation of tropomyosin (Ebashi and Kodama 1965), and TnC (initially called troponin A) was identified in 1968 (Hartshorne and Mueller 1968).

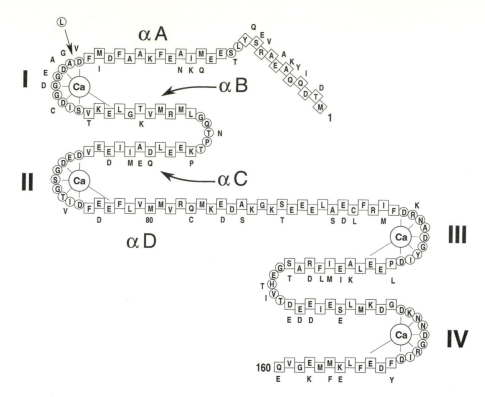

Figure 1. The primary sequence of mammalian sTnC. Ca²⁺-binding sites I–IV, α-helices αA–αD, and residues that differ between cTnC and sTnC are indicated, including an insertion in site I. Helical and nonhelical regions are indicated by boxes and circles, respectively.

High-level expression of sTnC requires a basal promoter located in the 5′-flanking region of the gene and an enhancer located in the first intron (Parmacek *et al.* 1990). Minimally, expression of the cTnC gene in cardiac myocytes requires basal promoter/enhancer elements in the immediate 5′-flanking region ($\approx$ −100 to +30), while expression in skeletal myotubes requires additional enhancer elements in the first intron and sequences upstream of the basal promoter/enhancer (Christensen *et al.* 1993; Parmacek *et al.* 1994).

Purification of TnC, as well as the other troponin subunits, can be performed by variations of the method of Potter (1982). A crude troponin fraction is first prepared from muscle ether powder by sequential salt extraction, isoelectric precipitation, and two ammonium sulfate cuts. The troponin subunits are then dissociated by dialysis against 6 M urea and EDTA, and TnC is isolated by anion exchange chromatography under conditions in which TnI will not bind and TnT binds poorly. Variations of this procedure are adequate for the isolation of cTnC if protease inhibitors are included. Smaller amounts of sTnC and cTnC can be isolated by selective extraction of TnC from isolated myofibrils by low ionic strength and EDTA followed by anion exchange chromatography (Cox *et al.* 1981).

Gene sequences and regulation

Genomic and cDNA clones for TnC have been isolated from a variety of species. Introns in the genes for sTnC and cTnC do not partition the amino acid coding sequence into discrete Ca²⁺-binding domains. However, the intron-exon boundaries are nearly identical for cTnC, sTnC, calmodulin, and parvalbumin. Sequences for full-length clones of vertebrate TnC isoforms, which are available in the GenBank, are listed below.

TnC	Species	Clone	GenBank
sTnC	human	cDNA	HSTC2
sTnC	rabbit	cDNA	RABTNC
sTnC	chicken	cDNA	CHKTNC
sTnC	human	gene	HUMTNC1 and 2
sTnC	mouse	gene	MUSFSTC6
cTnC	human	cDNA	HSTNS
cTnC	mouse	cDNA	MUSCTNCA
cTnC	chicken	cDNA	CHKCAMA
cTnC	human	gene	HUMTROC
cTnC	mouse	gene	MUSCTNC

Protein characterization

The crystal structure for sTnC revealed an elongated protein in which the paired Ca^{2+}-binding sites I/II, and III/IV form two globular domains that are separated by a long central helix (for review see Strynadka and James 1989). A model has been proposed for Ca^{2+}-dependent transitions in the N-terminal domain of sTnC in which a lobe composed of helices B/C moves as a unit away from helix D (Herzberg et al. 1986; see Fig. 2). The basic features of this model are consistent with a variety of experimental data.

Protein/protein interactions

In addition to TnC, the troponin complex consists of troponin I and troponin T (for review see Zot and Potter 1987). Troponin I is the inhibitory subunit of the troponin complex, since it can inhibit actomyosin ATPase activity. Peptide studies have shown that a region near the middle of TnI encodes its inhibitory activity and is called the inhibitory region or inhibitory peptide.

TnC interacts with TnI at multiple Ca^{2+}-dependent and Ca^{2+}-independent interfaces. The association of TnC with either TnI or the inhibitory peptide neutralizes the inhibition of actomyosin ATPase activity by TnI. Based on these observations, it is thought that in the absence of Ca^{2+} a domain of TnI, which includes the inhibitory region, binds to actin and inhibits ATPase activity. Binding Ca^{2+} to TnC causes this domain to shift from actin to TnC, thus relieving inhibition of ATPase activity by subsequent positional changes of tropomyosin on the thin filament.

Recent studies have shown that TnC and TnI associate in an anti-parallel fashion in which the C-terminal domain of TnC associates with the N-terminal domain of TnI, and vice versa (Farah et al. 1994; Kobayashi et al. 1994). Both TnI and TnC are in an extended conformation in a binary complex (Olah et al. 1994). A model has been proposed in which TnI wraps around TnC with the inhibitory peptide of TnI near the central helix of TnC (Olah and Trewhella 1994).

References

Christensen, T.H., Prentice, H., Gahlmann, R., and Kedes, L. (1993) Regulation of the human cardiac/slow-twitch troponin C gene by multiple, cooperative, cell-type-specific, and MyoD-responsive elements. Mol. Cell. Biol. **13**, 6752–6765.

Collins, J.H. (1991) Myosin light chains and troponin C: Structural and evolutionary relationships revealed by amino acid sequence comparisons. J. Muscle Res. Cell Motil. **12**, 3–25.

Cox, J.A., Comte, M., and Stein, E.A. (1981) Calmodulin-free skeletal-muscle troponin-C prepared in the absence of urea. Biochem. J. **195**, 205–211.

Ebashi, S. and Kodama, A. (1965) A new protein factor promoting aggregation of tropomyosin. J. Biochem. **58**, 107–108.

Farah, C.S., Miyamoto, C.A., Ramos, C.H.I., da Silva, A.C., Quaggio, R.B., Fujimori, K., Smillie, L.B., and Reinach, F.C., (1994) Structrual and regulatory functions of the NH$_2$- and COOH-terminal regions of skeletal muscle troponin I. J. Biol. Chem. **269**, 5230–5240.

Gergely, J., Grabarek, Z. and Tao, T. (1993) The molecular switch in troponin C. Adv. Exp. Med. Biol. **332**, 117–123.

Hartshorne, D.J. and Mueller, H. (1968) Fractionation of troponin into two distinct proteins. Biochem. Biophys. Res. Commun. **31**, 647–653.

Herzberg, O., Moult, J. and James, M.N. (1986) A model for the Ca^{2+}-induced conformational transition of troponin C. A trigger for muscle contraction. J. Biol. Chem. **261**, 2638–2644.

Kobayashi, T., Tao, T., Gergely, J. and Collins, J.H. (1994) Structure of the troponin complex: implications of photocross-linking of troponin C thiol mutants. J. Biol. Chem. **269**, 5725–5729.

Leavis, P.C. and Gergely, J. (1984) Thin filament proteins and thin filament-linked regulation of vertebrate muscle contraction. CRC. Crit. Rev. Biochem. **16**, 235–305.

Olah, G.A. and Trewhella, J. (1994) A model structure of the muscle protein complex 4Ca^{2+}-troponin C-troponin I derived from small-angle scattering data: Implications for regulation. Biochemistry **33**, 12800–12806.

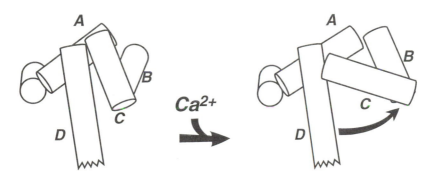

Figure 2. Calcium-dependent movement of α-helices in the N-terminal domain of sTnC.

Olah, G.A., Rokop, S.E., Wang, C.-L.A., Blechner, S.L., and Trewhella, J. (1994) Troponin I encompasses an extended troponin C in the Ca^{2+}-bound complex: A small-angle X-ray and neutron scattering study. Biochemistry **33**, 8233–8239.

Parmacek, M.S., Bengur, A.R., Vora, A.J., and Leiden, J.M. (1990) The structure and regulation of expression of the murine fast skeletal troponin C gene. Identification of a developmentally regulated, muscle-specific transcriptional enhancer. J. Biol. Chem. **265**, 15970–15976.

Parmacek, M.S., Ip, H.S., Jung, F., Shen, T., Martin, J.F., Vora, A.J., Olson, E.N., and Leiden, J.M. (1994) A novel myogenic regulatory circuit controls slow/cardiac troponin C gene transcription in skeletal muscle. Mol. Cell. Biol. **14**, 1870–1885.

Potter, J.D. (1982) Preparation of troponin and its subunits. Methods in Enzymology **85**, 241–263.

Strynadka, N.C.J. and James, M.N.G. (1989) Crystal structures of the helix-loop-helix calcium-binding proteins. Annu. Rev. Biochem. **58**, 951–998.

Zot, A.S. and Potter, J.D. (1987) Structural aspects of troponin-tropomyosin regulation of skeletal muscle contraction. Annu. Rev. Biophys. Biophys. Chem. **16**, 535–559.

■ *John A. Putkey:*
Department of Biochemistry and Molecular Biology,
University of Texas Medical School,
Houston, Texas 77030, USA
Tel.: (713) 792 5600
Fax: (713) 794 4150
E-mail: jputkey@utmmg.med.uth.tmc.edu

Annexins

Annexins

The annexins are a family of widely distributed Ca²⁺- and phospholipid-binding proteins all of which possess a conserved repeated domain. These proteins are found in both intracellular and extracellular locations and, despite being associated with many distinct cellular processes, their exact functions are not known for certain.

At present ten mammalian annexins are known and fully sequenced (I, II, III, IV, V, VI, VII, VIII, XI, and XIII). With the exception of erythrocytes, every mammalian cell type examined expresses one or more annexins. The sequences of two *Drosophila* (annexin IX and X) and one *Hydra* (XII) annexin have also been described. In addition, annexins have been identified and partially characterized from plants, *Dictyostelium*, sponges, sea urchin and fish (loach and torpedo). Two protozoan proteins, $\alpha 1$ and $\alpha 2$ giardin, from the protist *Giardia lamblia* have been found to have sequence homology with mammalian annexins (Fiedler and Simons, 1995) and may represent primordial members of the annexin family. The common feature of all of the annexins is a conserved domain that is repeated four times, or eight times in the case of annexin VI, to form the core of the annexin (Fig. 1). The annexins are distinguished from each other by variable N-terminal domains that may confer specific functions on the Ca²⁺- and phospholipid-binding core. The Ca²⁺-binding affinities of the annexin in the presence of phospholipids varies widely between members of the family, over the low to high micromolar range.

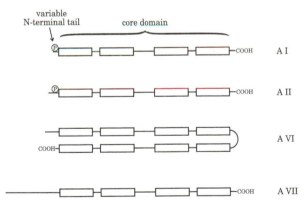

Figure 1. Structure of the annexins. The domain structure of selected mammalian annexins are shown to illustrate the general features of the annexins. They all possess the core conserved domains. Annexin VI has eight repeats, all other annexins have four. Each annexin has a unique N-terminal tail of variable length.

■ Discovery of the annexins

Proteins that are now known to be members of the annexin family were originally discovered in many different contexts and related to a variety of cellular functions. The first annexin to be purified was annexin VII (synexin), following a search for proteins from the adrenal medulla involved in exocytosis, based on the ability of synexin to bind to and aggregate chromaffin granules in the presence of Ca²⁺ (Creutz et al., 1978). Additional chromaffin granule-binding proteins, including several other annexins (I, II, IV, V and VI), were later identified in adrenal medullary cytosol in Ca²⁺-dependent binding assays (Creutz 1981; Geisow and Burgoyne 1982; Creutz et al. 1983). The pattern of polypeptides isolated in these studies was very similar to that of a series of proteins isolated by fluphenazine affinity chromatography (Moore and Dedman 1982) which were also shown subsequently to be annexins. Annexin VI was identified in studies on proteins showing Ca²⁺-dependent binding to the cytoskeleton of lymphocyte plasma membranes (Owens and Crumpton 1984). These studies were all based on searches for Ca²⁺-dependent proteins, but mammalian annexins were also discovered independently by quite different approaches. Annexin II was first identified as a major cellular substrate for tyrosine phosphorylation in cells transformed by Rous sarcoma virus (Radke and Martin 1979) and subsequently purified in bulk from intestinal epithelium (Gerke and Weber 1984). Annexin I (lipocortin) was discovered in the search for proteins released from cells in response to glucocorticoids and which could control inflammation by inhibition of phospholipase A₂ (Flower and Blackwell 1979).

A Ca²⁺- and phospholipid-binding protein was isolated from the electric organs of *Torpedo marmorata* in 1982 based on a similar approach to that used for adrenal medullary chromaffin granule-binding proteins, i.e. Ca²⁺-dependent membrane binding (Walker 1982). Antiserum against the *Torpedo* protein provided the first clear evidence of a relationship between the various proteins isolated in different laboratories since it was found to cross-react with mammalian membrane binding proteins of 68 kDa (annexin VI) and 32 kDa (annexin IV) and with the tyrosine kinase substrate p36 (annexin II) (Geisow et al. 1984; Sudhof et al. 1984). The first sequence data available to support the relatedness of the proteins came from protein sequencing of tryptic peptides from

Torpedo and from mammalian p36 and p32 (Geisow et al. 1986). This study revealed the presence of a conserved common domain, referred to as the endonexin fold, and that this was present in multiple copies in the proteins. In addition, it was quickly realized that this repeated domain was also present in lipocortin (annexin I) for which the full sequence had been published from cDNA sequencing shortly before (Wallner et al. 1986). Within the same year publication of the full sequence of annexin II from cDNA cloning revealed the close similarity between annexins I and II (Saris et al. 1986).

In the next few years the relationships of the various mammalian annexins were resolved as their sequences were determined. Several other proteins were found to be annexins when sequenced and two additional annexins (XI and XIII) were identified by cDNA cloning. Other mammalian annexins, as yet unidentified, may exist. A new terminology (Table 1) based on the common name annexin, was proposed and accepted by the majority of workers in this field (Crumpton and Dedman 1990). The first crystal structure of an annexin, that of annexin V, was described in 1990 (Huber et al. 1990). The structures of the other annexins have been predicted to be closely similar to that of annexin V but in most cases this remains to be established. It is clear that the Ca^{2+}-binding motifs in the annexins differs from the classic EF-hand domain.

It is now clear that the designation of members of this family in studies on mammalian tissues must be based on sequence analysis or the use of proven mono-specific antibodies. Due to the sequence similarities between the annexins, care is required to establish the specificity of antisera and lack of cross-reactivity with other annexins. Many of the non-mammalian and plant annexins are still only known from recognition by antisera, Ca^{2+}-dependent phospholipid binding and, in some cases, partial protein sequencing.

■ Cellular functions of the annexins

The major unanswered, and most controversial, question about the annexins is their exact cellular function. As they were identified from several independent approaches they have been associated with many biological functions (Raynal and Pollard 1994). It may well be that they do not have single sites of actions but act in multiple cellular processes and these could vary between cell types. The idea that they function extracellularly in the control of inflammation seems unlikely to be a major explanation since this could not explain their expression in plants and protozoa. This particular aspect has generated considerable controversy. The original observation was that annexin I was released from cells in response to glucocorticoids and then acted to prevent eicosonoid generation by inhibition of phospholipase A2 (PLA$_2$). The annexins do not have signal sequences and the ability of cells to secrete these proteins has been disputed. There is, however, now clear evidence that several of the annexins including annexin I (Flower and Rothwell 1994) and annexin II (Ma et al. 1994), for example, can be found in

Table 1. The annexin family

Annexin	Previous names
I	Lipocortin I Calpactin II p35 Chromobindin 9
II	Calpactin I heavy chain Lipocortin II p36 Chromobindin 8 Protein I Placental anticoagulant protein IV
III	Lipocortin III Placental anticoagulant protein III 35-α calcimedin
IV	Endonexin I Protein II 32.5 kDa calelectrin Lipocortin IV Chromobindin 4 Placental anticoagulant protein II Placental protein 4-X 35-β Calcimedin
V	Placental anticoagulant protein I Inhibitor of blood coagulation Lipocortin V 35 kDa calelectrin Endonexin II Placental protein 4 Vascular anticoagulant (VAC)-α 35-γ Calcimedin Calphobindin I Anchorin CII
VI	p68, p70, 73k 67 kDa Calelectrin Lipocortin VI Protein III Chromobindin 20 67 kDa Calcimedin Calphobindin II
VII	Synexin
VIII	Vascular anticoagulant (VAC)-β
IX and X	*Drosophila melanogaster* annexins
XI	Calcyclin-associated annexin (CAP-50)
XII	*Hydra vulgaris* annexin
XIII	Intestine-specific annexin (ISA)

extracellular fluids and on the external surface of the plasma membrane. However, the ability of glucocorticoids to induce annexin I expression and secretion has been questioned (reviewed in Raynal and Polland 1994) and the inhibition of PLA$_2$ by the annexins may be due to substrate depletion by phospholipid binding rather than a direct inhibition of the enzyme (Haigler et al. 1987).

The annexins have been suggested to function in intra-cellular vesicular traffic (Burgoyne and Geisow 1989; Creutz 1992; Burgoyne and Clague 1994; Wilton *et al.* 1994) and direct evidence suggests that annexin II acts in exocytosis (Drust and Creutz 1988; Ali *et al.* 1989) and in endosome–endosome fusion (Emans *et al.* 1993; Harder and Gerke 1993; Mayorga *et al.* 1994). Several studies have shown that various annexins translocate from cytosol to plasma or organelle (including secretory granule) membranes on cell activation and elevation of intracellular Ca^{2+}. The ability of annexin II to associate with cytoskeletal proteins has suggested that annexins may regulate cytoskeletal interactions with membranes (Gerke and Weber 1984). Other studies have, in contrast, suggested that annexin II functions in DNA replication (Vishwanatha and Kumble 1993) or as an extracellular membrane receptor for plasminogen activator (Hajjar *et al.* 1994), tenascin C (Chung and Erickson 1994), and cytomegalovirus (Wright *et al.* 1994). Many attempts have been made to determine whether annexins have enzymatic functions. It was claimed that annexin III has inositol 1,2-cyclic phosphate 2-phosphohydrolase activity (Ross *et al.* 1990) but this has not been substantiated or confirmed. Recently, it has been suggested that a plant 68 kDa annexin has ATPase activity (McClung *et al.* 1994).

Clearly, determination of the exact intracellular and extracellular functions of the annexins remains a major challenge for future studies on this protein family and it is likely that resolution of this issue will require extensive analysis of gene knock-out and/or mutations in cells and transgenic animals. In the only study of this type so far, the single known annexin gene in *Dictyostelium discoideum* encoding an annexin VII homolog was disrupted. No major effect on development or survival was detected (Doring *et al.* 1991) but further work using such approaches will be essential in the future.

■ References

Ali, S.M., Geisow, M.J., and Burgoyne, R.D. (1989) A role for calpactin in calcium-dependent exocytosis in adrenal chromaffin cells. Nature **340**, 313–315.

Burgoyne, R.D. and Clague, M.J. (1994) Annexins in the endocytic pathway. Trends Biochem. Sci. **19**, 231–232.

Burgoyne, R.D. and Geisow, M.J. (1989) The annexin family of calcium-binding proteins. Cell Calcium, **10**, 1–10.

Chung, C.Y. and Erickson, H.P. (1994) Cell surface annexin II is a high affinity receptor for the alternatively spliced segment of tenascin-C. J. Cell Biol. **126**, 539–548.

Creutz, C.E. (1981) Secretory vesicle cytosol interactions in exocytosis: isolation by Ca^{2+}-dependent affinity chromatography of proteins that bind to the chromaffin granule membranes. Biochem. Biophys. Res. Comm. **103**, 1345–1400.

Creutz, C.E. (1992) The annexins and exocytosis. Science **258**, 924–931.

Creutz, C.E., Pazoles, C.J., and Pollard, H.B. (1978) Identification and purification of an adrenal medullary protein (synexin) that causes calcium dependent aggregation of isolated chromaffin granules. J. Biol. Chem. **253**, 2858–2866.

Creutz, C.E., Dowling, L.G., Sando, J.J., Villar-Palasi, C., Whipple, J.H., and Zaks, W.J. (1983) Characterisation of the chromobindins. Soluble proteins that bind to the chromaffin granules in the presence of Ca^{2+}. J. Biol. Chem. **258**, 14664–14674.

Crumpton, M.J. and Dedman, J.R. (1990) Protein terminology tangle. Nature **345**, 212.

Doring, V., Schleicher, M., and Noegel, A.A. (1991) Dictyostelium annexin VII (synexin)-cDNA sequence and isolation of a gene disruption mutant. J. Biol. Chem. **266**, 17509–17515.

Drust, D.S. and Creutz, C.E. (1988) Aggregation of chromaffin granules by calpactin at micromolar levels of calcium. Nature **331**, 88–91.

Emans, N., Gorvel, J.P., Walter, C., Gerke, V., Kellner, R., Griffiths, G., and Gruenberg, J. (1993) Annexin II is a component of fusogenic endosomal vesicles. J. Cell Biol. **120**, 1357–1370.

Fiedler, K. and Simons, K. (1995) Annexin homologues in Giardia lamblia. Trends Biochem. Sci. **20**, 177–178.

Flower, R.J. and Blackwell, G.J. (1979) Anti-inflammatory steroids induce biosynthesis of a phospholipase A2-inhibitor which prevents prostaglandin generation. Nature **278**, 456–459.

Flower, R.J. and Rothwell, N.J. (1994) Lipocortin-1: Cellular mechanisms and clinical relevance. Trends Pharmacol. Sci. **15**, 71–76.

Geisow, M.J. and Burgoyne, R.D. (1982) Calcium-dependent binding of cytosolic proteins by chromaffin granules from adrenal medulla. J. Neurochem. **38**, 1735–1741.

Geisow, M.J., Childs, J., Dash, B., Harris, A., Panayotou, G., Sudhof, T., and Walker, J.H. (1984) Cellular distribution of three mammalian Ca^{2+}-binding proteins related to Torpedo calelectrin. EMBO J. **3**, 2969–2974.

Geisow, M.J., Fritsche, U., Hexham, J.M., Dash, B., and Johnson, T. (1986) A consensus amino-acid sequence repeat in *Torpedo* and mammalian Ca^{2+}-dependent membrane-binding proteins. Nature **320**, 636–638.

Gerke, V. and Weber, K. (1984) Identity of p36k phosphorylated upon Rous sarcoma virus transformation with a protein from brush borders: calcium-dependent binding to nonerythroid spectrin and F-actin. EMBOJ. **3**, 227–233.

Haigler, H.T., Schlaepfer, R.D., and Burgess, W.H. (1987) Characterisation of lipocortin I and an immunologically unrelated 33-kDa protein as epidermal growth factor/kinase substrates and phospholipase A2 inhibitors. J. Biol. Chem. **262**, 6921–6930.

Hajjar, K.A., Jacovina, A.T., and Chacko, J. (1994) A endothelial cell receptor for plasminogen/tissue plasminogen activator I. Identity with annexin II. J. Biol. Chem. **269**, 21191–21197.

Harder, T. and Gerke, V. (1993) The subcellular distribution of early endosomes is affected by the annexin IIp112 complex. J. Cell Biol. **123**, 1119–1132.

Huber, R., Romish, J., and Paques, E. (1990) The crystal and molecular structure of human annexin V, an anticoagulant protein that binds to calcium and membranes. EMBOJ. **9**, 3867–3874.

Ma, A.S.P., Bell, D.J., Mittal, A.A., and Harrison, H.H. (1994) Immunocytochemical detection of extracellular annexin II in cultured human skin keratinocytes and isolation of annexin II isoforms enriched in the extracellular pool. J. Cell Sci. **107**, 1973–1984.

McClung, A.D., Carroll, A.D., and Battey, N.H. (1994) Identification and characteristics of ATPase activity associated with maize (*Zea mays*) annexins. Biochem. J. **303**, 709–712.

Mayorga, L.S., Beron, W., Sarrout, M.N., Colombo, M.I., Creutz, C.E., and Stahl, P.D. (1994) Calcium-dependent fusion among endosomes. J. Biol. Chem. **269**, 30927–30934.

Moore, P.B. and Dedman, J.R. (1982) Calcium-dependent protein binding to phenothiazine columns. J. Biol. Chem. **257**, 9663–9667.

Owens, R.J. and Crumpton, M.J. (1984) Isolation and characterisation of a novel 68,000-M, Ca²⁺-binding protein of lymphocyte plasma membrane. Biochem. J. **219**, 309–316.

Radke, K. and Martin, G.S. (1979) Transformation by Rous sarcoma virus: effects of *src* gene expression on the synthesis and phosphorylation of cellular polypeptides. Proc. Natl. Acad. Sci. USA **76**, 5212–5216.

Raynal, P. and Pollard, H.B. (1994) Annexins: the problem of assessing the biological role of a gene family of multifunctional calcium- and phospholipid-binding proteins. Biochim. Biophys. Acta. **1197**, 63–93.

Ross, T.S., Tait, J.F., and Majerus, P.W. (1990) Identity of 1,2-cyclic phosphate 2-phosphohydrolase with lipocortin III. Science **248**, 605–607.

Saris, C.J.M., Tack, B.F., Kristensen, T., Glenney, J.R., and Hunter, T. (1986) The cDNA sequence for the protein-tyrosine kinase substrate p36 (calpactin I heavy chain) reveal a multi domain protein with internal repeats. Cell **46**, 201–212.

Sudhof, T.C., Ebbecke, M., Walker, J.H., Fritsche, U., and Boustead, C. (1984) Isolation of mammalian calelectrins: a new class of ubiquitous Ca²⁺-regulated proteins. Biochem. **23**, 1103–1109.

Vishwanatha, J.K. and Kumble, S. (1993) Involvement of annexin II in DNA replication: evidence from cell-free extracts of *Xenopus* eggs. J. Cell Sci. **105**, 533–540.

Walker, J.H. (1982) Isolation from cholinergic synapses of a protein that binds to membranes in a calcium-dependent manner. J. Neurochem. **39**, 815–823.

Wallner, B.P., Mattaliano, R.J., Hessian, C., Cate, R.L., Tizard, R., Sinclair, L.K., Foeller, C., Chow, E.P., Browning, J.L., Ramachandran, K.L., and Repinsky, R.B. (1986) Cloning and expression of human lipocortin, a phospholipase A2 inhibitor with potential anti-inflammatory activity. Nature **320**, 77–81.

Wilton, J.C., Matthews, G.M., Burgoyne, R.D., Mills, C.D., Chipman, J.K., and Coleman, R. (1994) Fluorescent choleretic and cholestatic bile salts take different paths across the hepatocyte: transcytosis of glycolithocholate leads to an extensive redistribution of annexin II. J. Cell Biol. **127**, 401–410.

Wright, J.F., Kurosky, A., and West, S. (1994) An endothelial cell surface form of annexin II binds human cytomegalavirus. Biochem. Biophys. Res. Comm. **198**, 983–989.

■ *Robert D. Burgoyne:*
The Physiological Laboratory,
University of Liverpool,
Crown Street,
Liverpool,
L69 3BX,
UK
Tel.: +44-151-794-5305
Fax: +44-151-794-5337
E-mail: burgoyne@liverpool.ac.uk

Annexin I

Annexin I is a primarily cytosolic protein capable of binding phospholipids and Ca²⁺. This protein is present in many differentiated cell types and can associate with the cell membrane. Annexin I is thought to function in cell signaling, growth and differentiation.

Annexin I is a member of the superfamily of annexin Ca²⁺-binding proteins and exhibits a relative molecular mass of ~ 37,000. All contain four or eight putative Ca²⁺- and phospholipid-binding domains, each exhibiting ~ê50% identity to each other at the amino acid level (Horseman 1992). Ca²⁺/phospholipid-binding in the first domain has been mapped to amino acid positions 42–99 (Ernst 1993). Although annexin I is a cytosolic protein, it can be secreted by the prostate gland into seminal plasma of mammals (Christmas et al. 1991). Annexin I has also been observed to be in rat peritoneal exudates, bronchoalveolar lavage fluid, serum, and amniotic fluid (as reviewed by Haigler and Schlaepfer 1992). Pigeons express two annexin I proteins, specified as cp35 (Horseman 1989), and cp37 (Haigler et al. 1992). Cp35 is regulated by prolactin, yet cp37 is expressed constituitively.

■ Alternative names

Lipocortin I (Di Rosa et al. 1984; Wallner et al. 1986), calpactin II (Saris et al. 1986), p35 (Fava and Cohen 1984).

■ Isolation/identification

Annexin I can inhibit phospholipase A₂ activity (as reviewed by Flower 1990). Annexin I was purified from rat peritoneal lavage fluid (Wallner et al. 1986). Purification schemes for annexin I involved size exclusion, ion-exchange and phospholipase affinity chromatography (as reviewed by Flower 1990).

Gene and sequence

Human annexin I was purified, sequenced, and the cDNA isolated by Wallner *et al.* (1986). The pigeon annexin I cDNA, cp35, was identified independently by using differential screening of a prolactin-stimulated cDNA library (Pukac and Horseman 1987). Other annexin I cDNAs were isolated subsequently by routine cDNA screening techniques. All members of the annexin I gene family contain 13 exons and 12 introns, as shown in Fig. 1 (Horseman 1992). Exons 1 and 13 are non-coding 5′ and 3′ regions, respectively. The translational start codon is located close to the 5′ border of exon 2. Exons 2 and 3 encode the amino terminal region of the protein. Exons 4 through 12 encode the Ca^{2+}- and phospholipid-binding domains. Each domain is 70 amino acids in length. Exon 8 is not within one of the four binding domains, but codes for amino acids acting as a linker region between domains II and III. Mammalian annexin I genes are 17–19 kb in length, while the pigeon annexin I genes are somewhat smaller, being 15 kb in length.

Genomic and cDNA accession numbers: human (X05908), mouse (M69249 to M69260, X07486, X07484, M24554), rat (Y00446, M19967), pigeon cp35 (M22635, M36969 to M36977), pigeon cp37 (M91008, L02504), cow (X56649), sponge (X16980).

Protein

Mammalian annexin I contains phosphorylation sites for the epidermal growth factor (EGF) receptor tyrosine kinase and protein kinase C in the N2 region (Horseman 1992). Cp35 lacks both of these sites, cp37 possesses both, and chicken annexin I has only the protein kinase C

target sequence (Horseman 1992; Sidis and Horseman 1993). Annexin I has been shown to be associated with cellular vesiculation (Meers *et al.* 1992). By using 3T3 cells, it was demonstrated that phosphorylation of annexin I occurs in multivesicular bodies (Futter *et al.* 1993). It has been postulated that EGF receptor kinase activity stimulates vesiculation by the phosphorylation of annexin I.

Antibodies

Antibodies specific for annexin I, which do not cross-react with other known annexins, are commercially available from Santa Cruz Biotechnology, Transduction Laboratories and Zymed Laboratory, Inc.

Localization

Annexin I is expressed widely in many tissue types. The protein is primarily located in differentiated cell types (Fava and Piltch 1987; Fava *et al.* 1989), but has also been observed to increase in abundance in actively dividing cells, *in vitro* (Haigler and Schlaepfer 1990). Most annexins are associated with the cellular membranes.

Biological regulation

Mammalian annexin I appears to be either directly or indirectly regulated by glucocorticoids (Blackwell *et al.* 1982; Flower 1990). No effect on gene activity was observed in several human cell types when exposed to glucocorticoids (Bronnegard *et al.* 1988). Mammalian annexin I genes have putative glucocorticoid response elements (GRE) either in the 5′ non-coding region or in

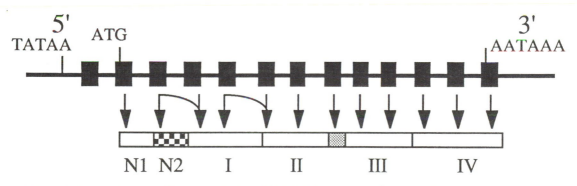

Figure 1. Annexin I gene structure. Exons are indicated by black boxes (top). The gene 5′ and 3′ borders are indicated and gene size ranges from 15 to 19 kb. Introns are not drawn to scale. TATAA, ATG start site and AATAAA polyadenylation signals are mapped to their relative positions on the gene. Arrows indicate portions of the protein (bottom) encoded by specific exons. The Ca^{2+}-binding domains are numbered I through IV. These repeat domains are 70 amino acids in length and exhibit ~50% amino acid identity. Amino terminal subdomains N1 and N2 regulate the protein's function. Phosphorylation sites are in the domain, N2. The black bar is a linker between regions II and III.

the first intron (as reviewed by Horseman 1992). Other sequences, termed slow GRE, have been reported in mammalian annexin I genes. These slow GRE sites, occur in similar locations, 5' to the transcriptional start site, and are possibly involved in gene regulation (Horseman 1992).

Cp35 is induced by prolactin. The cp35 gene contains two γ-interferon-like response sequences (Sidis and Horseman 1994) and these sequences bind proteins termed signaling transducers and activators of transcription (STAT). STAT proteins are phosphorylated after prolactin binds to its receptor.

■ References

Blackwell, G.J., Curnurcio, R., Di Rosa, M., Flower, R.J., Langham, C.S.J., Parente, L., Persico, P., Russell-Smith, N.C., and Stone, D. (1982) Glucocorticoids induce the formation and release of anti-inflammatory and anti-phospholipase proteins into the peritoneal cavity of the rat. Br. J. Pharmacol. **76**, 185–194.

Bronnegard, M., Andersson, O., Edwall, D., Lund, J., Norstedt, G., and Caristedt-Duke, J. (1988) Human calpactin II (lipocortin I) messenger ribonucleic acid is not induced by glucocorticoids. Mol. Endocrinol. **2**, 732–739.

Christmas, P., Callaway, J., Fallon, J., Jones, J., and Haigler, H.T. (1991) Selective secretion of annexin I, a protein without a signal sequence, by the human prostate gland. J. Biol. Chem. **266**, 2499–2507.

Di Rosa, M., Flower, R.J., Hirata, F., Parente, L., and Russo-Marie, F. (1984) Nomenclature announcement. Anti-phospholipase proteins. Prostaglandins **28**, 441–442.

Ernst, J.D. (1993) Epitope mapping of annexin I: antibodies that compete with phospholipids and calcium recognize amino acids 42–99. Biochem. J. **289**, 539–542.

Fava, R.A. and Cohen, J. (1984) Isolation of a calcium-dependent 35-kilodalton substrate of the epidermal growth factor receptor/kinase from A-431 cells. J. Biol. Chem. **259**, 2636–2645.

Fava, R.A. and Piltch, A.S. (1987) Histological distribution of the 35-kd protein substrate of the epidermal growth factor receptor/kinase in thymus. J. Histochem. Cytochem. **35**, 1309–1315.

Fava, R.A., Mikanna, J., and Cohen, S. (1989) Lipocortin I (p35) is abundant in a restricted number of differentiated cell types in adult organs. J. Cell. Physiol. **141**, 284–293.

Flower, R. J. (1990) Cytokines and lipocortins in inflammation and differentiation. Lipocortin, pp. 11–25. Wiley-Liss Inc.

Flower, R. J., Wood, J.N., and Parente, L. (1984) Macrocortin and the mechanism of action of the glucocorticoids. Adv. Inflammation Res. **7**, 61–69.

Futter, C.E., Felder, S., Schlessinger, J., Ullrich, A., and Hopkins, C. (1993) Annexin I is phosphorylated in the multivesicular body during the processing of the epidermal growth factor receptor. J. Cell. Biol. **120**, 77–83.

Haigler, H.T. and Schlaepfer, D.D. (1990) Expression of lipocortin I and endonexin II as a function of cellular growth state. Prog. Clin. Biol. Res. **349**, 91–108.

Haigler, H.T. and Schlaepfer, D.D. (1992) Annexin I phosphorylation and secretion. In The annexins (ed. S.E. Moss), pp. 11–22. Portland Press, London.

Haigler, H.T., Mangili, J.A., Gao, Y., Jones, J., and Horseman, N.D. (1992) Identification and characterization of columbid annexin I-cp37: Insights into the evolution of annexin I phosphorylation sites. J. Biol. Chem. **267**, 19123–19129.

Horseman, N.D. (1989) Aprolactin-inducible gene product which is a member of the calpactin/lipocortin family. Mol. Endocrinol. **3**, 773–779.

Horseman, N.D. (1992) Annexin I genes: diversity and regulation. In The annexins (ed. S. E. Moss), pp. 23–34. Portland Press, London.

Meers, P., Mealy, T., Pavlotsky, N., and Tauber, A.I. (1992) Annexin I-mediated vesicular aggregation: mechanism and role in human neutrophils. Am. Chem. Soc. **31**, 6373–6382.

Pukac, L. and Horseman, N.D. (1987) Regulation of cloned prolactin-inducible genes in pigeon crop. Mol. Endocrinol. **1**, 188–194.

Saris, C.J.M., Tack, B.F., Kristensen, T., Glenney, J.R., Jr., and Hunter, T. (1986) The cDNA sequence for the protein-tyrosine kinase substrate p36 (Calpactin I heavy chain) reveal a multidomain protein with internal repeats. Cell **46**, 201–212.

Sidis, Y. and Horseman, N.D. (1993) The hinge region of chicken annexin I contains no site for tyrosine phosphorylation. FEBS Lett. **329**, 296–300.

Sidis, Y. and Horseman, N.D. (1994) Prolactin induces rapid p95/p70 tyrosine phosphorylation, and protein binding to GAS-like sites in the anx I cp35 and cFos genes. Endocrinol **134**,1979–1985.

Wallner, B.P., Mattalian, R.J., Hession, C., Cate, R.L., Tizard, R., Sinclair, L.K., Foeller, C., Chow, E.P., Browning, J.L., Pamachanchan, K.L., and Pepinsky, R.B. (1986) Cloning and expression of human lipocortin, a phospholipase A2 inhibitor with potential anti-imflammatory activity. Nature. **320**, 77–81.

■ Scott L. Pratt and Nelson D. Horseman:
Department of Molecular and Cellular Physiology,
University of Cincinnati,
College of Medicine,
P.O. Box 670576,
Cincinnati, OH 45267-0576, USA
Tel.: (513) 558-3019
Fax: (513) 558-5738

Annexin II

Annexin II is a Ca^{2+}/lipid-binding protein expressed in various tissues and cell lines. The so-called type II Ca^{2+}-binding sites of this annexin are present in the annexin homology segments (annexin repeats) 2, 3, and 4, respectively, and are required for phospholipid binding and the proper intracellular localization of the protein. Annexin II forms a heterotetrameric complex with the S100 protein p11. This complex is located in the submembranous region of the cell and has been implicated in membrane fusion processes and membrane - cytoskeleton linkage.

Annexin II is 338 amino acids in length and has an apparent molecular mass of 36 kDa. The protease-resistant protein core of the molecule (amino acids 30–338 if generated by limited chymotrypsin treatment) is built of four so-called annexin repeats, segments which are 70–75 amino acids in length and share sequence homologies with one another and with the repeats in other annexins. The core harbours the binding sites for Ca^{2+}, phospholipid, and F-actin (for review see Gerke 1992). The N-terminal head region contains phosphorylation sites for serine- and tyrosine-specific protein kinases and the binding site for the intracellular protein ligand p11 (S100A10), a member of the S100 protein family. This p11 binding site is contained within the 14 N-terminal residues (including the *N*-acetyl group of the N-terminal serine) which form an amphiphatic α-helix (for review see Weber 1992). Binding of the p11 dimer leads to the formation of a heterotetrameric annexin II_2p11_2 complex which has altered Ca^{2+}- and/or phospholipid-binding properties as compared to the monomer (for review see Gerke 1992).

Within the cell the heterotetrameric annexin II_2p11_2 complex is found in the periphery on, or close to, the cytoplasmic face of the plasma membrane and on early endosomal membranes, whereas monomeric annexin II seems to be a cytosolic protein (Zokas and Glenney, 1987; Thiel *et al.* 1992; Emans *et al.* 1993). Extracellular locations of annexin II, e.g. on the surface of endothelial cells, have also been reported (Chung and Erickson 1994; Hajjar *et al.* 1994).

Alternative names

36K phosphoprotein, calpactin I heavy chain, chromobindin 8, lipocortin II, p36, protein I, anticoagulant protein IV (for review see Moss 1992).

Identification/isolation

Annexin II was initially described as a major substrate for the tyrosine kinase encoded by the *src* oncogene (Radke and Martin 1979; Erikson and Erikson 1980). The first large-scale purification was carried out using intestinal epithelial cells as starting material and exploited the ability of the protein to interact Ca^{2+}-dependently with membranes and/or cytoskeletal elements (Gerke and Weber 1984). Following this protocol membrane/cytoskeleton-associated annexin II was obtained by cell fractionation in the presence of Ca^{2+}, separated from soluble components by centrifugation and specifically released by adding a Ca^{2+}-chelating agent. Subsequent conventional chromatographic procedures yielded a highly pure annexin II_2p11_2 complex which could be dissociated by gel filtration in the presence of 9 M urea. The separated subunits could be renatured individually by dialysis against urea-free buffer (Gerke and Weber 1985).

Genes and sequences

The following annexin II cDNA sequences have been reported and are listed in the GenBank/EMBL databases: human (accession number M14043), mouse (M14044), rat (X66871), bovine (M14056), chicken (X53334), *Xenopus laevis* type-1 (M60768), *X. laevis* type-2 (M60769), *X. laevis* A3 (M58575), *X. laevis* C4 (M58576), *X. laevis* E4/F4 (M58577). Moreover, a partial protein sequence for pig annexin II is listed in the SwissProt database under the accession number P19620.

The genes encoding human and mouse annexin II have been cloned and mapped to chromosomes 15 and 9, respectively. Both show an identical organization characterized by 13 exons. Three human annexin II pseudogenes have also been identified and mapped to chromosomes 4, 9, and 10, respectively. Human genomic sequences are listed under the GenBank accession numbers M33162, M33163, M33164 and M33165. All original references are cited with the individual database entries.

Protein

Annexin II interacts Ca^{2+}-dependently with negatively charged liposomes with half-maximal phospholipid binding occurring at Ca^{2+} concentrations ranging between 0.2 and 20 μM. p11-induced formation of the heterotetrameric annexin II_2p11_2 complex increases this affinity significantly (for review see Gerke 1992). The complex is also able to aggregate chromaffin granules at micromolar Ca^{2+} concentrations (Drust and Creutz 1988). Phospholipid binding and lipid vesicle aggregation are subject to regulation by phosphorylation. Tyrosine phosphorylation by the src kinase decreases the affinity for phosphatidylserine liposomes, and serine phosphorylation by protein kinase C markedly reduces the rate and extent of vesicle aggregation (Powell and Glenney 1987; Johnstone *et al*. 1992). Annexin II also interacts with the cytoskeletal elements F-actin and non-erythroid spectrin (Gerke and Weber 1984). Binding of the annexin II_2p11_2 complex to F-actin occurs in the presence of micromolar Ca^{2+} concentrations with high affinity and in a cooperative manner (Ikebuchi and Waisman 1990). Extracellular high-affinity ligands reported for annexin II include plasminogen and the tissue plasminogen activator as well as tenascin-C (Chung and Erickson 1994; Hajjar *et al*. 1994).

A schematic model of the structural organization of the annexin II molecule is given in Fig. 1. Limited proteolysis identified two principal protein domains, a protease-sensitive N-terminal region harbouring the p11 binding site as well as the major phosphorylation sites and a protease-resistant protein core consisting of the four annexin repeats and containing the binding sites

for Ca^{2+}, phospholipid and F-actin (for review see Gerke 1992).

■ Antibodies

Monoclonal antibodies directed against annexin II are commercially available through Zymed Laboratories Inc., and Affinity Research Product Limited.

■ Localization

Annexin II is most abundant in intestinal epithelium, lung, and placenta; moderately expressed in spleen, adrenal gland, kidney, and cardiac muscle; and seems absent from, or present at only low levels, in brain and red blood cells (Zokas and Glenney 1987). Within the cell annexin II seems to exist in two forms: the monomeric protein, which seems not, or only loosely, associated with the cortical cytoskeleton, and the annexin II_2p11_2 complex, which is anchored in the submembranous cytoskeleton and is also found on early endosomal membranes (Zokas and Glenney 1987; Osborn *et al*. 1988; Emans *et al*. 1993; Harder and Gerke 1993). Extracellular annexin II has been reported, e.g. on the surface of endothelial cells (Chung and Erickson 1994; Hajjar *et al*. 1994, and references therein).

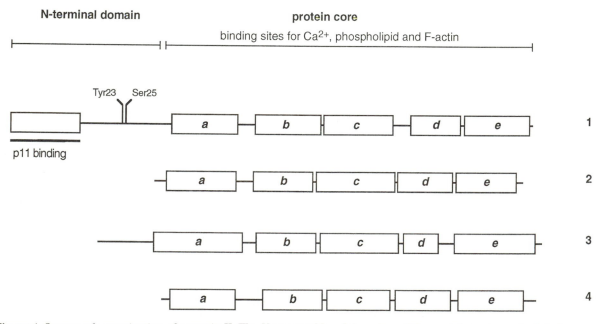

Figure 1. Structural organization of annexin II. The N-terminal head domain and the protein core are depicted separately to illustrate the domain structure of the molecule. Sites for p11 binding and phosphorylation by protein kinase C (Ser25) and the src tyrosine kinase (Tyr23) are present in the N-terminal region (residues 1 - 29). The protein core (residues 30–338) is defined by its resistance against limited proteolysis. It is composed of four annexin repeats (1–4) and contains Ca^{2+}-, phospholipid- and F-actin binding sites. Boxes indicate predicted α-helices: the N-terminal helix harbouring the p11 binding site and the five helices (*a–e*) present in each repeat which have been identified in the crystal structure of the related annexin V (Huber *et al*. 1990).

Biological activities

The annexin II_2p11_2 complex has been shown to stimulate Ca^{2+}-activated secretion in permeabilized chromaffin cells after soluble protein leakage and progressive loss of the secretory response, and thus has been implicated in Ca^{2+}-regulated exocytosis (Ali *et al.* 1989; Sarafian *et al.* 1991). Annexin II has also been linked to endocytotic processes as it is found on early endosomal membranes and is transferred from a donor to an acceptor endosomal membrane in an *in vitro* fusion assay (Emans *et al.* 1993). Moreover, a trans-dominant mutant for the annexin II_2p11_2 complex specifically affects the intracellular distribution of early endosomes in polarized epithelial cells, indicating that the complex is involved in positioning early endosomes in the periphery of such cells (Harder and Gerke 1993). An involvement in transcytosis across hepatocytes has also been suggested since the transcytosis of glycolithocholate leads to an extensive redistribution of annexin II (Wilton *et al.* 1994). Furthermore, extracellular activities as a cell surface receptor for tissue plasminogen activator and tenascin-C have been reported (Chung and Erickson 1994; Hajjar *et al.* 1994).

Biological regulation

The expression of annexin II is subject to regulation in a variety of different cells and an increased expression is usually observed during differentiation, e.g. in cells of the differentiating chicken lens, in mouse fibroblasts after serum stimulation, in human U937 cells after phorbol ester induced differentiation into macrophage-like cells, and in rat phaeochromocytoma PC12 cells after NGF treatment (for review see Gerke 1992).

Mutagenesis studies

Mutagenesis studies carried out with human annexin II led to the identification of acidic residues which are involved in the formation of Ca^{2+}-binding sites. Three so-called type II Ca^{2+}-binding sites are located in repeats 2, 3, and 4, and have been shown to involve the acidic residues Asp161, Glu246, and Asp321, respectively. Two so-called type III sites are present in the first repeat, with residues Glu52 and Glu95 participating in the formation of these sites (Jost *et al.* 1994).

Interactions

Annexin II has been shown to interact with p11 in a Ca^{2+}-independent manner. The protein–protein interaction is driven by hydrophobic forces and occurs *in vitro* and *in vivo* (for review see Weber 1992).

References

*Ali, S.M., Geisow, M.J., and Burgoyne, R.D. (1989) A role for calpactin in calcium dependent exocytosis in adrenal chromaffin cells. Nature **340**, 313–315.

Chung, C.Y. and Erickson, H.P. (1994) Cell surface annexin II is a high affinity receptor for the alternatively spliced segment of tenascin-C. J. Cell Biol. **126**, 539–548.

*Drust, D.S. and Creutz, C.E. (1988) Aggregation of chromaffin granules by calpactin at micromolar levels of calcium. Nature **331**, 88–91.

*Emans, N., Gorvel, J.P., Walter, C., Gerke, V., Kellner, R., Griffiths, G., and Gruenberg, J. (1993) Annexin II is a major component of fusogenic endosomal vesicles. J. Cell Biol. **120**, 1357–1369.

Erikson, E. and Erikson, R.L. (1980) Identification of a cellular protein substrate phosphorylated by the avian sarcoma virus-transforming gene product. Cell **21**, 829–836.

Gerke, V. (1992) Evolutionary conservation and three-dimensional folding of annexin II. In *The annexins* (ed. S.E. Moss), pp. 47–59. Portland Press, London.

Gerke, V. and Weber, K. (1984) Identity of p36K phosphorylated upon Rous sarcoma virus transformation with a protein from brush borders; calcium-dependent binding to nonerythroid spectrin and F-actin. EMBO J. **3**, 227–233.

Gerke, V. and Weber, K. (1985) Calcium dependent conformational changes in the 36-kDa subunit of intestinal protein I related to the cellular 36 kDa target of Rous sarcoma virus tyrosine kinase. J. Biol. Chem. **260**, 1688–1695.

Hajjar K.A., Jacovina A.T., and Chacko, J. (1994) An endothelial cell receptor for plasminogen/tissue plasminogen activator. J. Biol. Chem. **269**, 21191–21197.

*Harder, T. and Gerke, V. (1993) The subcellular distribution of early endosomes is affected by the annexin II_2p11_2 complex. J. Cell Biol. **123**, 1119–1132.

Huber, R., Römisch, J., and Paques, E.P. (1990) The crystal and molecular structure of human annexin V, an anticoagulant calcium, membrane binding protein. EMBO J. **9**, 3867–3874.

Ikebuchi, N.W. and Waisman D.M. (1990) Calcium-dependent regulation of actin filament bundling by Lipocortin-85. J. Biol. Chem. **265**, 3392–3400.

Johnstone, S.A., Hubaishy I., and Waisman D.M. (1992) Phosphorylation of Annexin II tetramer by protein kinase C inhibits aggregation of lipid vesicles by the protein. J. Biol. Chem. **267**, 25976–25981.

Jost, M., Weber, K., and Gerke, V. (1994) Annexin II contains two types of Ca^{2+}-binding sites. Biochem. J. **3**, 553–559.

Moss, S.E. (1992) The annexins. In *The annexins* (ed. S.E. Moss), pp. 1–9. Portland Press, London.

Osborn, M., Johnsson, N., Wehland, J., and Weber, K. (1988) The submembraneous location of p11 and its interaction with the p36 substrate of pp60 src kinase *in situ*. Exp. Cell Res. **175**, 81–96.

Powell, M.A. and Glenney, J.R., Jr., (1987) Regulation of calpactin I phospholipid binding by calpactin I light-chain binding and phosphorylation by p60[v-src]. Biochem. J. **247**, 321–328.

*Radke, K. and Martin, G.S. (1979) Transformation by Rous sarcoma virus: effects of *src* gene expression on the synthesis and phosphorylation of cellular polypeptides. Proc. Natl. Acad. Sci. USA **76**, 5212–5216.

Sarafian, T., Pradel, L.-A., Henry, J.-P., Aunis, D., and Bader, M.-F. (1991) The participation of annexin II (calpactin I) in calcium-evoked exocytosis requires protein kinase C. J. Cell Biol. **114**, 1135–1147.

Thiel, C., Osborn, M., and Gerke, V. (1992) The tight association of the tyrosine kinase substrate annexin II with the submembranous cytoskeleton depends on intact p11- and Ca^{2+}-binding sites. J. Cell Sci. **103**, 733–742.

Weber, K. (1992) Annexin II: interaction with p11. In *The annexins* (ed. S.E. Moss), pp. 61–68. Portland Press, London.

Wilton, J.C., Matthews, G.M., Burgoyne R.D., Mills C.O., Chipman, J.K., and Coleman, R. (1994) Fluorescent choleretic and cholestatic bile salts take different paths across the hepatocyte: transcytosis of glycolithocholate leads to an extensive redistribution of annexin II. J. Cell Biol. **127**, 401–410.

Zokas, L. and Glenney, J.R. (1987) The calpactin light chain is tightly linked to the cytoskeletal form of calpactin I: studies using monoclonal antibodies to calpactin subunits. J. Cell Biol. **105**, 2111–2121.

■ Matthias Jost and Volker Gerke:
Clinical Research Group for Endothelial Cell Biology, University of Münster,
Von-Esmarch Str. 56,
D-48149 Münster, Germany
Tel.:+49 251 83 6722
Fax: +49 251 83 6748
E-mail: jost@uni-muenster.de
gerke@wwupop.uni-muenster.de

Annexin III

Annexin III is one of the less ubiquitous annexins since it is expressed almost exclusively in differentiated cells of the monophagocytic cell lineage. It is also a unique annexin in having an identified enzymatic activity, namely inositol 1,2-cyclic phosphate 2-phosphohydrolase.

Annexin III, a member of the annexin family, has an apparent molecular mass of 33 kDa, it contains 322 amino acids and its isoelectric point is 6.2. This family of proteins that bind to phospholipids in a Ca^{2+}-dependent manner now consists of 13 members that have been identified in a number of different tissues and cell types in higher and lower eukaryotes (Moss 1992; Raynal and Pollard 1994; Swairjo and Seaton 1994). Annexin III is composed of four highly conserved 70 amino acid repeats. The amino termini of annexins are diverse in sequence and length and confer specific functions on each protein. In the case of annexin III, the 16 amino-acid long N-terminus carries a protein kinase C phosphorylation site. Like other members of the family, annexin III possesses anti-coagulant and anti-phospholipase A_2 properties. Unlike some members of the family, annexin III does not bind to actin.

■ Alternative names

Lipocortin III (Pepinsky *et al.* 1988; Coméra *et al.* 1990); 35 α calcimedin (Kaetzel *et al.* 1989); placental anticoagulant protein III or PAP III (Tait *et al.* 1988).

■ Identification/isolation

Annexin III has always been isolated from different tissues using classical biochemical purification procedures. Pepinsky *et al.* (1988) purified it from rat peritoneal lavage fluid using DEAE-cellulose chromatography and analysed its sequence; Coméra *et al.* (1989, 1990) purified it from human peripheral mononuclear cells using a Ca^{2+}-EGTA precipitation procedure followed by anion exchange column chromatography before sequencing it; Kaetzel *et al.* (1989) purified it from rat liver using

various chromatographic steps before sequencing it. Tait *et al.* (1988) identified it in human placenta and Ernst *et al.* (1990) from human neutrophils, also using various chromatographic steps and further sequencing the protein.

cDNA cloning was performed either after constructing antisense oligonucleotide hybridization probes derived from the amino acid sequences (Pepinsky *et al.* 1988), or using standard methods of immunoscreening of a λgt11 cDNA library (Tait *et al.* 1988).

Annexin III is available as a recombinant fusion protein linked to glutathione-S-transferase (GST) and is produced in *E. coli* (Favier *et al.*, unpublished results).

■ Gene and sequence

The cDNA sequence of human annexin III is available in the GenBank under the name "HUMLC3"; the rat sequence is also available under the name "RATLC3" (Pepinsky *et al.* 1988). The genomic DNA of human annexin III has been analysed (Tait *et al.* 1991, 1993). The GenBank accession number is M63310. Annexin III gene is localized to human chromosome 4q21. The transcribed region spans 58 kb and contains 12 introns and 13 exons. There are two first exons: exons 1A and 1B but only the shortest exon, 1A, gave rise to a transcript. Northern blots showed one single mRNA of 1.7 kb in all tissues examined. Three intragenic polymorphisms were identified: a microsatellite polymorphism with at least six alleles and two restriction site polymorphisms. The 5′ region of the gene has no recognizable TATA box; however, there are two perfect GGGCG sequences and one imperfect CCAAT sequence within exon 1A. As a whole, the annexin III gene organization is similar to that of all other annexins.

Protein

The annexin III primary structure is similar to all annexins (40–60% identity), consisting of four 70 amino acid domains. The structure contains Ca^{2+}-binding sites similar to annexin V in domains I, II and IV. In domain III, it has a tryptophan at the same position as annexin V. Good-quality crystals have been obtained and the X-ray structure has been refined to 1.8 Å resolution (Favier-Perron et al. 1996). The N-terminal end of annexin III is unique, in that it carries a putative phosphorylation site for protein kinase C. Annexin III is a substrate for protein kinase C both in vitro (Coméra et al. 1989) and in permeabilized neutrophils (Stoehr et al. 1990).

Antibodies

Antibodies specific for annexin III (polyclonal and monoclonal) are not commercially available. Nevertheless all laboratories working with annexin III have raised their own antibodies.

Localization

Northern blots and immunoblots have permitted localization of annexin III in different tissues and cells (Kaetzel et al. 1989; Tait et al. 1993). Annexin III has a specific distribution, its mRNA levels differing from tissue to tissue, with highest levels in lung and heart, lower levels in skeletal muscle, kidney, and pancreas, and undetectable levels in brain and liver. This pattern generally agrees with levels of annexin III protein in rat tissues as determined by immunoblot. It seems that neutrophils do contain the highest amount of annexin III among cells, followed by monocytes–macrophages (Coméra et al. 1989, 1990; Ernst et al. 1990). In general, the presence of annexin III is correlated with differentiation (Kaetzel et al. 1989; LeCabec et al. 1992). In cells, annexin III is mostly found associated with cytosolic granules, but it translocates to the membrane upon cell activation and most specifically to the periphagosomal membrane in neutrophils during phagocytosis (Ernst 1991).

Biological activities

Annexin III shares the same biological activities as other annexins, i.e. it has anti-coagulant properties (Tait et al. 1988) and anti-phospholipase A_2 properties (Coméra et al. 1989, 1990). Both of these properties are known to be related to the annexin propensity to bind negatively charged phospholipids in the presence of Ca^{2+}. Although its participation in intracellular traffic has not been clearly demonstrated, the fact that it is found associated to neutrophil-specific granules and that it translocates to the periphagosomal membrane upon induction of phagocytosis indicates that it may play a role in the organelle traffic in neutrophils. Annexin III is also unique in having an identified enzymatic activity, namely inositol 1,2-cyclic phosphate 2-phosphohydrolase, an enzyme that converts inositol 1,2-cyclic phosphate to inositol 1-phosphate, which is implicated in the control of cell proliferation (Ross et al. 1990, 1991; Ross and Majerus 1991).

References

Coméra, C., Rothhut, B., Cavadore, J.C., Vilgrain, I., Cochet, C., Chambaz, E., and Russo-Marie, F. (1989) Further characterization of four lipocortins from human peripheral blood mononuclear cells. J. Cell Biochem. **40**, 361–370.

*Coméra, C., Rothhut, B., and Russo-Marie, F. (1990) Identification and characterization of phospholipase A2 inhibitory proteins in human mononuclear cells. Eur. J. Biochem. **188**, 139–146.

Ernst, J.D. (1991) Annexin III translocates to the periphagosomal region when neutrophils ingest opsonized yeast. J. Immunol. **146**, 3110–3114.

Ernst J.D., Hoye, E., Blackwood, R.A., and Jaye, D. (1990) Purification and characterization of an abundant cytosolic protein from human neutrophils that promote Ca^{2+}-dependent aggregation of isolated specific granules. J. Clin. Invest. **85**, 1065–1075.

Favier-Perron A., Lewit-Bentley A., and F. Russo-Marie (1996) The high resolution crystal structure of human annexin III shows subtle differences with annexin V. Biochem. **35**, 1740–1744.

Kaetzel, M.A., Harazika, P., and Dedman, J.R. (1989) Differential tissue expression of three 35-kDa annexin calcium-dependent phospholipid-binding proteins. J. Biol. Chem. **264**, 14463–14470.

LeCabec, V., Russo-Marie, F., and Maridonneau-Parini, I. (1992) Differential expression of two forms of annexin III in human neutrophils and monocytes and along their differentiation. Biochem. Biophys. Res. Commun. **189**, 1471–1476.

Moss, S.E. (1992) The annexins, (ed.), Portland Press, London.

*Pepinsky, R.B., Tizard, R., Mattaliano, R.J., Sinclair, L.K., Miller, G.T., Browning, J.L., Chow, E.P., Burne, C., Huang, K.S., Pratt, D., Watcher, L., Hession, C., Frey, A.Z., and Wallner, B.P. (1988) Five distinct calcium and phospholipid binding proteins share homology with lipocortin I. J. Biol. Chem. **263**, 10799–10811.

Raynal, P. and Pollard, H.B. (1994) Annexins: the problem of assessing the biological role for a gene family of multifunctional calcium- and phospholipid-binding proteins. Biochim. Biophys. Acta **1197**, 63–93.

Ross, T.S. and Majerus, P.W. (1991) Inositol-1, 2-cyclic-phosphate-inositolphosphohydrolase. Substrate specificity and regulation of activity by phospholipids, metal ion chelators, and inositol 2-phosphate. J. Biol. Chem. **266**, 851–856.

*Ross, T.S., Tait, J.F., and Majerus, P.W. (1990) Identity of inositol 1,2-cyclic phosphate 2-phosphohydrolase with lipocortin III. Science **248**, 605–607.

Ross, T.S., Whiteley, B., Graham, R.A., and Majerus, P.W. (1991) Cyclic hydrolase-transfected 3T3 cells have low levels of inositol 1,2-cyclic phosphate and reach confluence at low density. J. Biol. Chem. **266**, 9086–9092.

Stoehr, S.J., Smolen, J., and Suchard, S.J. (1990) Lipocortins are major substrates for protein kinase C in extracts of human neutrophils. J. Immunol. **144**, 3936–3945.

Swairjo, M.A., and Seaton, B.A. (1994) Annexin structure and membrane interactions: a molecular perspective. Ann. Rev. Biophys. Biomol. Struct. **23**, 193–213.

Tait, J.F., Sakata, M., McMullen, B.A., Miao, C.H., Funakoshi, T., Hendrickson, L.E., and Fujikawa, K. (1988) Placental anticoagulant proteins: isolation and comparative characterization of four members of the lipocortin family. Biochemistry **27**, 6268–6276.

Tait, J.F., Frankenberry, D.A., Miao, C.H., Killary, A.M., Adler, D.A., and Disteche, C.M. (1991) Chromosomal localization of the human annexin III gene. Genomics, **10**, 441–448.

Tait, J.F., Smith, C., Lei Xu, and Cookson, B.T. (1993) Structure and polymorphisms of the human annexin III gene. Genomics **18**, 79–86.

Weng, X., Luecke, H. , Song, I.S., Kang, D.S., Kim, S-H., and Huber, R. (1993) Crystal structure of human annexin I. Protein Science **2**, 448–458.

■ *Beatrice Perron:LURE-Centre Universitaire Paris Sud,*
F-91405 Orsay Cedex
and INSERM U332 et ICGM,
22 rue Méchain 75014-Paris, France
E-mail: favier@lure.u-psud.fr

■ *Anita Lewit-Bentley:LURE-Centre Universitaire Paris Sud,*
F-91405 Orsay Cedex, France
Tel.: 33 1 64 46 80 50
Fax: 33 1 64 46 41 48
E-mail: anita@lure.u-psud.fr

■ *Françoise Russo-Marie:INSERM U332 et ICGM,*
22 rue Méchain,
F-75014-Paris, France
Tel.: 33 1 40 51 64 42
Fax: 33 1 40 51 77 49
E-mail: russo@citi2.fr

Annexin IV

Annexin IV is a ubiquitous member of the annexin family of Ca^{2+}-dependent, phospholipid-binding proteins. It is composed of four canonical 70 amino acid imperfect repeats characteristic of the annexin family and a short N-terminal tail unique to annexin IV.

On two-dimensional SDS gels annexin IV exhibits a molecular mass of 32 kDa and a p*I* of 5.9 (Creutz *et al*. 1987). The human protein has a calculated molecular mass of 35,959 Da (Grundmann *et al*. 1988). The porcine and bovine proteins are 96.5% and 94.7% identical in sequence to the human protein (Weber *et al*. 1987; Hamman *et al*. 1988).

The relative Ca^{2+}-dependence of the binding of annexin IV to membranes varies according to the concentration and type of negatively charged phospholipids in the membrane (Junker and Creutz 1994). With membranes composed of phosphatidylcholine and a single negatively charged or zwitterionic lipid present at 30 mole %, the sensitivity to calcium varies in the following order: cardiolipin (half maximal binding at 17 μM Ca^{2+}), phosphatidylserine (48 μM), phosphatidic acid (48 μM), phosphatidylglycerol (55 μM), phosphatidylinositol-bis-phosphate (65 μM), phosphatidylinositol (114 μM) and phosphatidylethanolamine (2 mM).

Annexin IV promotes the aggregation of secretory vesicles (chromaffin granules) in a Ca^{2+}-dependent manner (half maximal effect at 140 to 160 μM Ca^{2+}; Zaks and Creutz 1990; Nelson and Creutz 1995*a*, *b*).

Annexin IV can be phosphorylated *in vitro* on a threonine residue in the N-terminus by protein kinase C, although it is a poorer substrate than annexins I or II (Wang and Creutz 1992). The phosphorylation does not appear to influence significantly the membrane-binding properties of annexin IV, although it has not been determined if the membrane aggregating activity of the protein is altered by phosphorylating as it is in the case of annexin I.

The functions of annexin IV are unknown but may include modulation of lipid metabolism and membrane organization (Fauvel *et al*. 1987; Junker and Creutz 1993), regulation of ion transport (Kaetzel *et al*. 1994), and membrane–membrane interactions in exocytosis or membrane trafficking (Creutz 1992).

■ Alternative names

Endonexin I, protein II, chromobindin 4, 32.5 calelectrin, lipocortin IV, placental anticoagulant protein II, placental protein 4-x, 35βcalcimedin.

■ Identification/isolation

Annexin IV has been identified as a Ca^{2+}-dependent lipid-binding (Weber *et al*. 1987) or membrane-binding (Creutz *et al*. 1987) protein and as an anticoagulant protein (Grundmann *et al*. 1988). It may be purified by Ca^{2+}-dependent binding to lipids or hydrophobic matrices. Typical sources are bovine liver (Creutz *et al*. 1987) or lung (Khanna *et al*. 1990), human placenta (Tait *et al*. 1988) and recombinant proteins produced in bacteria (Romisch *et al*. 1990; Nelson and Creutz 1995*a*) or yeast (Creutz *et al*. 1992).

Gene and sequences

Sequences for annexin IV currently in GenBank include human (M82809) and bovine (M22248), and in the NBRF Protein Database, porcine (LUPG4). The human annexin IV gene (ANX4) has been partially characterized and mapped to a single locus on chromosome 2 at band 2p13 (Tait *et al.* 1992).

Protein

Similar to other annexins, annexin IV has a protease-resistant core composed predominantly of four 70 amino acid repeats, each of which may bind one or two Ca^{2+} ions in a phospholipid-dependent manner. The N-terminal domain is particularly short, 14 residues long, and contains the single site for phosphorylation by protein kinase C (Thr8).

Antibodies

Monoclonal antibodies cross-reactive with mammalian annexins IV are available from Zymed Laboratories.

Anatomical localization

Annexin IV is generally found intracellularly, diffusely distributed in the cytoplasm, in the nucleus, or near the apical surface of epithelial cells (Walker *et al.* 1990; Kaetzel *et al.* 1994; Kojima *et al.* 1994). Although present in many tissues, differential distributions among cell types have been observed in the brain (Eberhard *et al.* 1994).

Mutagenesis studies

Mutagenesis of the Ca^{2+}-binding sites has been found to influence the Ca^{2+}-sensitivity of the interactions of the protein with chromaffin granule membranes (Nelson and Creutz 1995b). The first and fourth repeats appear most important in promoting the binding to membranes at low concentrations of Ca^{2+}; the second repeat is particularly important for promoting membrane aggregation.

Interactions

Annexin IV undergoes Ca^{2+}-dependent self-association both in solution and on surfaces of natural and artificial membrane surfaces. This has been detected by the measurement of energy transfer between labelled annexin IV molecules in solution or on the surfaces of isolated chromaffin granules or synthetic lipid vesicles containing acidic phospholipids (Zaks and Creutz 1991). This self-association may be important for promoting cooperative binding of annexin IV to membranes and membrane–membrane aggregation.

References

*Creutz, C.E. (1992) The annexins and exocytosis. Science **258**, 924–931.

Creutz, C.E., Zaks, W.J., Hamman, H.C., Crane, S., Martin, W.H., Gould, K.L., Oddie K.M., and Parsons, S.J. (1987) Identification of Chromaffin granule binding proteins: Relationship of the chromobindins to calelectrin, synhibin, and the tyrosine kinase substrates p35 and p36. J. Biol. Chem. **262**, 1860–1868.

Creutz, C.E., Kambouris, N.G., Snyder, S.L., Hamman, H.C., Nelson, M.R., Liu, W., and Rock, P. (1992) Effects of the expression of mammalian annexins in yeast secretory mutants. J. Cell Sci. **103**, 1177–1192.

Eberhard, D.A., Brown, M.D., and VandenBerg, S.R. (1994) Alterations of annexin expression in pathological neuronal and glial reactions: Immunohistochemical localization of annexin I, annexin II (p36 and p11 subunits), annexin IV, and annexin VI in the human hippocampus. Amer. J. Pathol. **145**, 640–649.

Fauvel, J., Salles, J.-P., Roques, V., Chap, H., Rochat, H., and Douste-Blazy, L. (1987) Lipocortin-like anti-phospholipase A2 activity of endonexin. FEBS Lett. **216**, 45–50.

Grundmann, U., Abel, K.-J., Bohn, H., Lobermann, H., Lottspeich, F., and Kupper, H. (1988) Characterization of cDNA encoding human placental anticoagulant protein (PP4): Homology with the lipocortin family. Proc. Natl. Acad. Sci. USA **85**, 3708–3712.

Hamman, H.C., Gaffey, L.C., Lynch, K.R., and Creutz, C.E. (1988) Cloning and characterization of a cDNA encoding bovine endonexin (chromobindin 4). Biochem. Biophys. Res. Commun. **156**, 660–667.

Junker, M. and Creutz, C.E. (1993) Endonexin (annexin IV)-mediated lateral segregation of phosphatidylglycerol in phosphatidylglycerol/phosphatidylcholine membranes. Biochemistry **32**, 9968–9974.

Junker, M. and Creutz, C.E. (1994) Ca^{2+}-Dependent binding of endonexin (annexin IV) to membranes: Analysis of the effects of membrane lipid composition and development of a predictive model for the binding interaction. Biochemistry **33**, 8930–8940.

Kaetzel, M.A., Chan, H.C., Dubinsky, W.P., Dedman, J.R., and Nelson, D.J. (1994) A role for annexin IV in epithelial cell function: Inhibition of calcium-activated chloride conductance. J. Biol. Chem. **269**, 5297–5302.

Khanna, N.C., Helwig, E.D., Ikebuchi, N.W., Fitzpatrick, S., Bajwa, R., and Waisman, D.M. (1990) Purification and characterization of annexin proteins from bovine lung. Biochemistry **29**, 4852–4862.

Kojima, K., Utsumi, H., Ogawa, H., and Matsumoto, I. (1994) Highly polarized expression of carbohydrate-binding protein p33/41 (annexin IV) on the apical plasma membrane of epithelial cells in renal proximal tubules. FEBS Lett. **342**, 313–318.

Nelson, M.R. and Creutz, C.E. (1995a) Comparison of the expression of native and mutant bovine annexin IV in *E. coli* using four different expression systems. Protein Expression and Purification **6**, 132–140.

*Nelson, M.R. and Creutz, C.E. (1995b) Combinatorial mutagenesis of the four domains of annexin IV: Effects on chromaffin granule binding and aggregating activities. Biochemistry **34**, 3121–3132.

Romisch, J., Grote, M., Withmann, K.U., Heimburger, N., and Amann, E. (1990) Annexin proteins PP4 and PP4-X. Biochem. J. **272**, 223–229.

Tait, J.F., Sakata, M., McMullen, B.A., Miao, C.H., Funakoshi, T., Hendrickson, L.E., and Fujikawa, K. (1988) Placental anticoagulant proteins: Isolation and comparative characterization of four members of the lipocortin family. Biochemistry **27**, 6268–6276.

Tait, J.F., Smith, C., Frankenberry, D.A., Miao, C.H., Adler, D.A. and Disteche, C.M. (1992) Chromosomal mapping of the human annexin IV (ANX4) gene. Genomics **12**, 313–318.

Walker, J.H., Boustead, C.M., Brown, R., Koster, J.J., and Middleton, C.A. (1990) Tissue and subcellular distribution of endonexin, a calcium-dependent phospholipid-binding protein. Biochem. Soc. Trans. **18**, 1235–1236.

Wang, W. and Creutz, C.E. (1992) Regulation of the chromaffin granule aggregating activity of annexin I by phosphorylation. Biochemistry **31**, 9934–9939.

*Weber, K., Johnsson, N., Plessmann, U., Van, P.N., Soling, H.-D., Ampe, C., and Vandekerckhove, J. (1987) The amino acid sequence of protein II and its phosphorylation site for protein kinase C; the domain structure of Ca^{2+}-modulated lipid-binding proteins. EMBO J. **6**, 1599–1604.

Zaks, W.H. and Creutz, C.E. (1990) Annexin-chromaffin granule membrane interactions: A comparative study of synexin, p32 and p67. Biochem. Biophys. Acta **1029**, 149–160.

Zaks, W.H. and Creutz, C.E. (1991) Ca^{2+}-dependent annexin self-association on membrane surfaces. Biochemistry **30**, 9607–9615.

■ *Carl E. Creutz:*
Department of Pharmacology,
University of Virginia,
Charlottesville, VA 22908, USA
Tel.: 804 924 5029
Fax: 804 982 3878

Annexin V

Annexin V is one of the proteins of the annexin family which has been most thoroughly studied by biophysical methods. Its physiological role is not clear yet. The sequence shows four repeats which fold into four domains, each one built up by five α-helices. The Ca^{2+}-binding sites are different to those of the proteins of the EF-hand family.

Annexin V binds in a Ca^{2+}-dependent manner to phospholipids. It is a typical member of this protein family, although there are minor differences, e.g. annexin V is not phosphorylated. The proposed biological roles are mostly the same as for the other annexins (reviewed in Raynal and Pollard 1994; the references for all facts presented in this text and not explicitly cited can be found in this publication).

The protein consists of 320 amino acids (including the first methionine) with a calculated molecular mass of 35,935 Da which is more than the observed migration behavior in denaturing polyacrylamide gels. Annexin V isoforms have been found. These differ presumably in their N-termini. Annexin V has a p*I* of 4.8 and the absorption of a solution of 1 mg/ml of pure protein is 6.0 at a wavelength of 280 nm (Funakoshi *et al*. 1987). The dissociation constant is 500 μM for Ca^{2+} without phospholipid and 100 μM for Ca^{2+} in the presence of phosphatidylserine. This value is strongly influenced by the nature of the phospholipid. Annexin V can be found in a variety of eucaryotic cells.

■ Alternative names

Placental anticoagulant protein I (PAP), inhibitor of blood coagulation, lipocortin V, 35 kDa calelectrin, endonexin II, placental protein 4, vascular anticoagulant protein-α (VAC α), 35-g-calcimedin, calphobindin I, anchorin CII (Crumpton and Dedman 1990).

■ Isolation/identification

Annexin V was discovered in the mid 1980s by groups who investigated extracts from human placenta which had anticoagulating activities. Partial amino acid sequence determination helped to develop gene probes which led to the isolation of the cDNA sequence from human cDNA libraries (see e.g. Funakoshi *et al*. 1987). Annexin V can be very easily expressed in *E. coli* (see e.g. Amann *et al*. 1988) in a soluble form without fusing it to any other protein. Protocols for the purification of the recombinant protein (see e.g. Burger *et al*. 1993) or the natural protein from human placenta are available (Römisch and Heimburger, 1990). Recombinant and natural protein seem to be very similar. Most of the purification procedures make use of the reversible Ca^{2+}-mediated binding to phospholipid vesicles.

■ Gene and sequences

cDNA sequences have been found for the human (Genbank code: HUMENN; accession number M19348), rat (RATLC5) and chicken protein (CHKANCC2A; A35381), see

Barton *et al.* (1991) for references. The sequence contains four repeats, which are highly homologous to one another as well as to other annexins. The N-terminal sequence is relatively short, namely 15 amino acids (including the starting methionine), similar to annexin IV (16 residues) rather than to other annexins. Sequence alignments can be found in Barton *et al.* (1991) or in Huber *et al.* (1992), especially with regard to the 3D-structure. The genomic sequence is known for the chicken (Pfannmüller *et al.* 1993) and the human annexin V gene (Cookson *et al.* 1994). The human gene maps to the chromosomal locus 4q26–q28. The chicken gene is about 25 kb long and contains 13 short exons (as the human gene) very similar to other known annexin genes. In the first two domains the exon boundaries correspond to one or more α-helices whereas this is not the case in the domains three and four.

■ The protein and its three-dimensional structure

Human annexin V was the first annexin to be structurally characterized (Huber *et al.* 1992). The four repeats fold into four domains of similar structure which consist of five α-helices wound into a right-handed super-helix (Fig. 1). The four domains are arranged in a planar, cyclic array which surrounds a very hydrophilic pore which is an ion conduction pathway (Berendes *et al.* 1993*a*; Burger *et al.* 1994). This arrangement exhibits a concave and a convex surface which becomes more planar when the protein is membrane bound (Voges *et al.* 1994). The N-terminus is located at the concave side and adopts an extended conformation. All calcium-binding sites are on the convex side. The main Ca^{2+}-binding sites in annexin V are formed by the sequence motif -G-X-G-T-X_{39}-(D,E)-. Ca^{2+} is hepta-coordinated by three carbonyl oxygens, the two oxygens of an acidic amino acid and two water molecules. These Ca^{2+}-binding sites are similar to the active site of phospholipase A_2 (Thunissen *et al.* 1990). Three of the four domains possess these Ca^{2+}-binding sites. Recent crystallographic and spectroscopic studies (Berendes *et al.* 1993*a*; Concha *et al.* 1993; Burger *et al.* 1994; see also Sopkova *et al.* (1994) for more references) showed the presence of another Ca^{2+}-binding site which is formed after a conformational change in domain III so that the arrangement of the Ca^{2+}-binding sites reflects the symmetry of the whole molecule. The structures of rat (Concha *et al.* 1993) and chicken (Bewley *et al.* 1993) annexin V are also known.

The membrane-bound form of annexin V has been studied by electron microscopy (Voges *et al.* 1994). It forms two-dimensional crystals on phospholipid monolayers allowing the investigation of the membrane-bound structure at a resolution of 15 Å. Annexin V becomes more flat upon membrane binding, although the overall structure remains unchanged. Studies using circular dichroism, UV absorption, fluorescence and neutron dif-

fraction have also been carried out, especially in regard to Ca^{2+} and/or phospholipid binding (see Sopkova *et al.* (1994) for references).

■ Antibodies

No antibodies specific for annexin V are commercially available.

■ Localization

Annexin V is found in multicellular organisms in various cell types in high amounts (up to 2% of the total protein). Each cell type exhibits a special annexin expression pattern. Annexin V is found primarily to be cytosolic, although there are reports that annexin V can be found in the nucleus and outside the cell. The annexin V cDNA misses a signal sequence so that the mechanism for the export is not clear.

■ Biological activities

A lot of different activities have been found for annexin V (reviewed in Raynal and Pollard 1994). In contrast to the other annexins, annexin V does not aggregate membranes and is only a poor substrate for protein kinases, whereas it has been proposed that it is an inhibitor of protein kinase C. Annexin V inhibits phospholipase A_2 *in vitro* and was therefore proposed to have anti-inflammatory activities. It has also anticoagulant activities *in vitro*. Both functions might be explained by substrate depletion as annexin V covers phospholipid membranes (Voges *et al.* 1994) thereby preventing the contact of the membrane with other proteins. Annexin V expression is enhanced in differentiating cells. When PC12 cells are stimulated to differentiate by the addition of nerve growth factor the amount of annexin V (as well as annexin II) is increased. Annexin V has therefore been proposed to be involved in cell proliferation and differentiation processes. Annexin V also binds to different cytoskeletal proteins. A possible involvement in membrane trafficking processes is under discussion. It has also been found that annexin V binds to hepatitis virus B surface antigen.

In vitro annexin V possesses ion channel activity with moderate selectivity for Ca^{2+} versus other monovalent cations, and a clear voltage dependence. This has been demonstrated by patch clamp experiments (Rojas *et al.* 1990) and by an assay which is sensitive for the protein-mediated accumulation of Ca^{2+} in fura-2 loaded vesicles (Berendes *et al.* 1993*b*). Annexin V does not penetrate the membrane (Voges *et al.* 1994) and therefore it has been proposed that the protein makes the membrane locally permeable by the disturbance of the bilayer caused by binding of phospholipids and by "microscopic" electroporation (for a review see Demange *et al.* 1994).

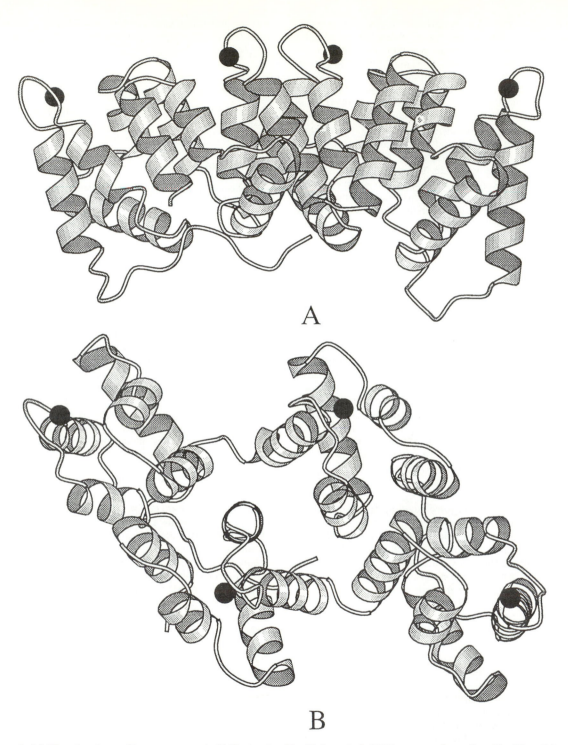

Figure 1. (a) The structure of human annexin V (first solved by Huber *et al.* 1992) as seen from the side. The ribbons represent α-helices. The concave side (on the bottom) bears the N-terminus, whereas the Ca^{2+}-binding sites (Ca^{2+} ions are depicted as black spheres) are located on the convex side. (b) Structure as seen from the concave side. The four domains built up by five α-helices are visible. The ion conductance pathway is in the middle. The location of the major Ca^{2+}-binding reflects the symmetry of the molecule. Figures kindly provided by Dr F. Russo-Marie, Paris.

Amino acids which are responsible for the ion selectivity, voltage dependence, and regulation of ion conductance (Berendes *et al.* 1993a; Burger *et al.* 1994; Demange *et al.* 1994) have been determined. Therefore annexin V seems to be a valuable model system for ion channels as it has a known 3D-structure. The significance of the ion channel activity for the physiological role is not clear.

■ References

Amann, E., Ochs, B., and Abel, K.-J. (1988) Tightly regulated tac promotor vectors useful for the expression of unfused and fused proteins in *E. coli*. Gene **69**, 301–315.

Barton, G.J., Newman, R.H., Freemont, P.S., and Crumpton, M.J. (1991) Amino acid sequence analysis of the annexin supergene family of proteins. Eur. J. Biochem. **198**, 749–760.

*Berendes, R., Voges, D., Demange, P., Huber, R., and Burger, A. (1993a) Structure-function analysis of the ion channel selectivity filter in human annexin V. Science **262**, 427–430.

Berendes, R., Burger, A., Voges, D., Demange, P., and Huber, R. (1993b) Calcium influx through annexin V ion channels into large unilamellar vesicles measured with fura-2. FEBS Lett. **317**, 131–134.

Bewley, M.C., Boustead, C.M., Walker, J.H., Waller, D.A., and Huber, R. (1993) Structure of chicken annexin V at 2.25 Å resolution. Biochemistry **32**, 3923–3929.

Burger, A., Berendes, R., Voges, D., Huber, R., and Demange, P. (1993) A rapid and efficient method of purification of recombinant annexin V. FEBS Lett. **329**, 25–28.

Burger, A., Voges, D., Demange, P., Peréz, C. R., Huber, R., and Berendes, R. (1994) Structural and electrophysiological analysis of annexin V mutants. J. Mol. Biol. **237**, 479–499.

Concha, N.O., Head, J.F., Kaetzel, M.A., Dedman, J.R., and Seaton, B.A. (1993) Rat annexin V crystal structure–Ca^{2+} induced conformational changes. Science **261**, 1321–1324.

Cookson, B.T., Engelhardt, S., Smith, C., Bamford, H.A., Prochazka, M., and Tait, J.F. (1994) Organization of the human annexin V (Anx5) gene. Genomics **20**, 463–467.

Crumpton, M. J., and Dedman, J. R. (1990) Protein terminology tangle. Nature (London) **345**, 212.

Demange, P., Voges, D., Benz, J., Liemann, S., Goettig, P., Berendes, R., Burger, A., and Huber, R. (1994) Annexin V: The key to understanding ion selectivity and voltage regulation. Trends. Biochem. Sci. **19**, 272–276.

Funakoshi, T., Heimark, R. L., Hendrickson, L. E. McMullen, B. A., and Fujikawa, K. (1987) Human placental anticoagulant protein: isolation and characterization. Biochemistry **26**, 5572–5578.

*Huber, R., Berendes, R., Burger, A., Schneider, M., Karshikov, A., Luecke, H., Römisch, J., and Paques, E. (1992) Crystal and molecular structure of human annexin V after refinement. J. Mol. Biol. **223**, 683–704.

Pfannmüller, E., Turnay, J., Bertling, W., and von der Mark, K. (1993) Organisation of the chicken annexin V gene and its correlation with the tertiary structure of the protein. FEBS Lett. **336**, 467–471.

Raynal, P., and Pollard, H.B. (1994) Annexins: the problem of assessing the biological role for a gene family of multifunctional calcium and phospholipid-binding proteins. Biochim. Biophys. Acta **1197**, 63–93.

Rojas, E., Pollard, H.B., Haigler, H.T., Parra, C., and Burns, A.L. (1990) Calcium-activated endonexin II forms calcium channels across acidic phospholipid bilayer membranes. J. Biol. Chem. **265**, 21207–21215.

Römisch, J., and Heimburger, N. (1990) Purification and characterization of 6 annexins from human placenta. Biol. Chem. Hoppe-Seyler **371**, 383–388.

Sopkova, J., Gallay, J., Vincent, M., Pancoska, P., and Lewit-Bentley, A. (1994) The dynamic behavior of annexin V as a function of calcium ion binding: a circular dichroism, UV absorption, and steady-state and time resolved fluorescence study. Biochemistry **33**, 4490–4499.

Thunissen, M. M. G., Eiso, A. B., Kalk, K. H., Drenth, J., Dijkstra, B. W., Kuipers, O. P., Dijkman, R., de Haas, G. H., and Verhej, H. M. (1990) X-ray structure of phospholipase A2 complexed with a substrate derived inhibitor. Nature (London) **347**, 689–691.

Voges, D., Berendes, R., Burger, A., Demange, P., Baumeister, W., and Huber, R. (1994) Three dimensional structure of membrane bound annexin V: a correlative electron-microscopy X-ray-crystallography study. J. Mol. Biol. **238**, 199–213.

■ *Alexander Burger:*
MediGene GmbH,
Lochhamerstr 11,
Tel.: +49 8956 320
Fax: +49 8956 3220
D-82152 Martinsried, Germany.
E-mail: watzmann@mips.embnet.org

Annexin VI

Annexin VI is an abundant intracellular protein which binds Ca^{2+} dependently to phospholipids. It is the largest member of the annexin family of Ca^{2+}-binding proteins uniquely comprising two sets of the four conserved repetitive domains that characterise all annexins. It is often found closely associated with the plasma membrane and other membraneous organelles. Although its function remains unclear, it has been linked with membrane trafficking events such as endo- and exocytosis, membrane–microfilament attachment, PLA2-inhibition and blood anti-coagulation, regulation of the sarcoplasmic reticulum Ca^{2+}-channel and Ca^{2+} release from chromaffin granules.

Annexin VI is a 68–70 kDa protein with a p*I* of 5.8 that migrates on SDS gels as a closely spaced doublet. It is reported to have a single binding site for Ca^{2+} in the absence of phospholipid with a K_d in the micromolar range, and in the presence of phospholipid the number of sites is increased to eight (Yoshizaki *et al.* 1989). Unlike annexins I and II which have been reported to be good substrates for *in vitro* phosphorylation by many kinases, annexin VI is not phosphorylated by tyrosine kinases and is only poorly phosphorylated by PKC. However, *in vivo,* serine and threonine phosphorylation of annexin VI does occur in a growth dependent manner in Swiss 3T3 cells and human lymphocytes, and the protein is also subject to a post-translational modification, incorporating phosphate, the chemical nature of which remains unclear (Moss *et al.* 1992).

As with other annexins, annexin VI is characterized by its ability to bind Ca^{2+} dependently to phospholipids, largely by ionic interactions between the protein and the phospholipid headgroup via bound Ca^{2+}, rather than an increase in hydrophobicity as seen with proteins such as calmodulin. There is some evidence that a hierarchy for binding to phospholipids/membranes exists between various members of the annexin family, many of which are often present in the same cell type (Edwards and Booth 1987) and also in the type of phospholipid bound (Edwards and Crumpton 1991; Moss *et al.* 1991). Some reports suggest there may be membrane-bound populations of annexin VI which cannot be released by the removal of Ca^{2+}, but purified annexin VI is invariably hydrophilic in nature. Although generally considered to be an intracellular protein, annexin VI has been identified at the surface of several metastatic tumour cell lines (Yeatman *et al.* 1993).

Alternative names

p68, p70, 73K, 67 kDa-calelectrin, 67 kDa-calcimedin, lipocortin VI, chromobindin 20, calphobindin II (Crumpton and Dedman 1990).

Identification and isolation

Annexin VI is defined by its ability to bind Ca^{2+} dependently to phospholipids, its molecular weight, 68 kDa and its structure, i.e. the presence of eight repeats of the conserved 70 amino acid domains. Specific antibodies are essential for the identification of annexin VI if sequences are not available; the high degree of relatedness within the annexin family and the existence of the covalently linked homodimer of annexin I (Hayashi *et al.* 1989) may lead to incorrect assignment. Isolation of annexin VI can be achieved by the EGTA extraction of detergent-solubilised plasma membranes which have been prepared in the presence of Ca^{2+}, followed by ion exchange chromatography on a Mono S FPLC column. Annexin VI is then eluted using a salt gradient (0–0.5 M). Placenta provides an excellent source of plasma membranes (Edwards and Crumpton 1991).

Antibodies

Antibodies are commercially available from Chemicon, ICN, Zymed.

Gene and sequence

Genbank accession numbers for:

Human	67 kDa-calelectrin	J03578
	Calphobindin	IID00510
	p68	Y00097
	Annexin VI gene; exon I	X77673
Chicken	Annexin VI	S67466
Mouse	p68	X13460

The human annexin VI gene is located on chromosome 5q and the murine gene on the syntenic chromosome II (Davies *et al.* 1989). The human gene is about 60 kb, comprising 26 exons with a similar structure to that of other annexins. Exon 21 contains the alternative splice site that gives rise to the two forms of annexin VI present in many cell types. There is a region of Z DNA in the midpoint of the gene which suggests that annexin VI arose from gene duplication (Smith and Moss 1994). The putative annexin VI gene promoter has now been cloned (Smith *et al.* 1994).

Protein

Annexin VI consists of eight repetitions of the conserved 70 amino acid domains common to all annexins, linked by variable regions of 7–40 amino acids. The N-terminal is the region of greatest diversity in the annexin family and in annexin VI this is relatively short. Each half of the core domains shares about 50% sequence identity with the other, such that domain 1 is closest to domain 5, 2 to 6, 3 to 7 and 4 to 8. (Crompton *et al.* 1988; Moss *et al.* 1988). Analysis of the crystal structure and amino acid sequence of annexin V suggests there are six potential binding sites for Ca^{2+} in annexin VI in domains 1, 2, 4, 5, 6 and 8 (Huber *et al.* 1990).

Localization

In humans, annexin VI is present in most tissues studied, but is restricted to specific cell types. It is absent from platelets and non-secretory epithelia, but present in the secretory epithelia. Annexin VI expression correlated well with endocrine cells (Clark *et al.* 1991). Within the cell the protein is most commonly located to the plasma membrane, but is also associated with many intracellular organelles especially those associated with the sequestering or release of Ca^{2+} (e.g. Drust and Creutz 1991).

Biological functions

Annexin VI has been reported to be required for the budding of coated pits from the plasma membrane during receptor-mediated endocytosis (Lin *et al.*,1992), however in another report (Smythe *et al.* 1994) its presence or absence was found to have no effect on the internalization or recycling of transferrin receptors.

Annexin VI has also been linked with membrane microfilament attachment, it has been shown to bind Ca^{2+} dependently to detergent extracted plasma membrane cytoskeletons (Edwards and Booth 1987), and to bind actin as a component of slow axonal transport (Sekimoto *et al.* 1991). This and its ability to bind to phospholipid make it a candidate for membrane–microfilament attachment.

Several reports have shown that annexin VI can act as a voltage-gated Ca^{2+}-channel in artificial membranes (Demange *et al.* 1994) and it is reported to alter radically the gating properties of the ryanodine-sensitive Ca^{2+}-channel isolated from the sarcoplasmic reticulum of skeletal muscle, by increasing both the mean open time and number of channels open (Dedman and

Kaetzel,1992). It has also been shown to release specifically sequestered Ca^{2+} from chromaffin granules in a dose-dependent manner (Jones *et al.* 1994).

When annexin VI is expressed in A431 squamous carcinoma cells it has been shown to have an anti-proliferative effect, significantly reducing the growth rate in a serum-dependent manner, such that cell growth is arrested in G1 (Theobald *et al.* 1994).

Other functions with which annexin VI is commonly associated include those of phospholipase-A2 inhibition and anti-blood coagulation, both of which can be attributed to its ability to bind Ca^{2+} dependently to phospholipids. (For a recent review on the functional analysis of annexin VI, see Edwards and Moss 1995.)

References

Clark, D.M., Moss, S.E., Wright, N.A., and Crumpton, M.J. (1991) Expression of annexin VI (p68, 67kDa-calelectrin) in normal human tissues: evidence for developmental regulation in B- and T-lymphocytes. Histochem. **96**, 405–412.

Crompton, M.R., Owens, R.J., Totty, N.F., Moss, S.E., Waterfield, M.D., and Crumpton, M.J. (1988) Primary structure of the human, membrane-associated calcium-binding protein p68: a novel member of a protein family. EMBO J. **7**, 21–27.

Crumpton, M.J. and Dedman, J.R. (1990) Protein terminology tangle. Nature (Lond) **345**, 212.

Davies, A.A., Moss, S.E., Crompton, M.R., Jones, T.A., Spurr, N.K., Sheer, D., Kozak, C., and Crumpton, M.J. (1989) The gene coding for the p68 calcium-binding protein is localised to bands q32-q34 of human chromosome 5, and to mouse chromosome 11. Hum. Genet. **82**, 234–238.

Dedman, J.R. and Kaetzel, M.A. (1992) Annexin VI. In (ed. S.E. Moss). *The annexins*. Portland Press, London.

Demange, P., Voges, D., Benz, J., Leimann, S., Göttig, P., Berrendes, R., Burger, A., and Hüber, R. (1994) Annexin V: the key to understanding ion selectivity and voltage regulation? Trends Biochem. Sci. **19**, 272–276.

Drust, D.S. and Creutz, C.E. (1991) Differential subcellular distribution of p36 (the heavy chain of calpactin I) and other annexins in the adrenal medulla. J. Neurochem. **56**, 469–478.

Edwards, H.C. and Booth, A.G. (1987) Calcium sensitive, lipid binding cytoskeletal proteins of the human placental microvillar region. J. Cell Biol. **105**, 303–311.

Edwards, H.C. and Crumpton, M.J. (1991) Calcium-dependent phospholipid and arachidonic acid binding by the placental annexins VI and IV. Eur. J. Biochem. **198**, 121–129.

Edwards, H.C. and Moss, S.E. (1995) Functional and genetic analysis of annexin VI. Mol. Cell. Biochem. **149–150**, 293–299.

Hayashi, H., Owada, M.K., Sonobe, S., and Kakunaga, T. (1989) Characterisation of two distinct Ca^{2+}-dependent phospholipid-binding proteins of 68 kDa isolated from human placenta. J. Biol. Chem. **264**, 17222–17230.

Huber, R., Römisch, J., and Paques, E-P. (1990) The crystal and molecular structure of human annexin V, an anticoagulant protein that binds to calcium and membranes. EMBO J. **9**, 3867–3874.

*Jones, P.G., Fitzpatrick, S., and Waisman, D.M. (1994) Chromaffin granules release calcium on contact with annexin VI: Implications for exocytosis. Biochemistry **33**, 8180–8187.

Lin, H.C., Sudhof, T.C., and Anderson, R.G.W. (1992) Annexin VI is required for the budding of clathrin-coated pits. Cell **70**, 283–291.

Moss, S.E., Crompton, M.R., and Crumpton, M.J. (1988) Molecular cloning of murine p68, a calcium-binding protein of the lipocortin family. Eur. J. Biochem. **177**, 21–27.

Moss, S.E., Edwards, H.C., and Crumpton, M.J. (1991) Diversity in the annexin family. In Novel calcium-binding proteins (ed. C.W. Heizmann), . Springer-Verlag, Berlin.

Moss, S.E., Jacob, S.M., Davies, A.A., and Crumpton, M.J. (1992) A growth-dependent post-translational modification of annexin VI. Biochim. Biophys. Acta **1160**, 120–126.

Sekimoto, S., Tashiro, T., and Komiya, Y. (1991) Two 68-kDa proteins in slow axonal transport belong to the 70-kDa heat shock protein family and the annexin family. J. Neurochem. **56**, 1774–1782.

Smith, P.D. and Moss, S.E. (1994) Z-DNA-forming sequences at a putative duplication site in the human annexin VI-encoding gene. Gene **138**, 239–242.

Smith, P.D., Davies, A., Crumpton, M.J., and Moss, S.E. (1994) Structure of the human annexin VI-encoding gene. Proc. Natl. Acad. Sci. USA **91**, 2713–2717.

*Smythe, E., Smith, P.D., Jacob, S.M., Theobald, J., and Moss, S.E. (1994) Endocytosis occurs independently of annexin VI in human A431 cells. J. Cell Biol. **124**, 301–306.

Theobald, J., Smith, P.D., Jacob, S., and Moss, S.E. (1994) Expression of annexin VI in A431 carcinoma cells suppresses proliferation: a possible role for annexin VI in cell growth regulation. Biochim. Biophys. Acta **1131**, 383–390.

Yeatman, T.J., Updyke, T.V., Kaetzel, M.A., Dedman, J.R. and Nicolson, G.L. (1993) Expression of annexins on the surfaces of non-metastatic and metastatic human and rodent tumor cells. Clin. Exp. Metastasis **11**, 37–44.

Yoshizaki, H., Arai, K., Mizoguchi, T., Shiratsuchi, M., Hattori, Y., Nagoya, T., Shidara, Y., and Maki, M. (1989) Isolation and characterisation of an anticoagulant protein from human placenta. J. Biochem. **105**, 178–183.

■ *Helena Edwards and Stephen E. Moss:*
Department of Physiology,
University College London,
Gower Street,
London WC1E 6BT, UK
Tel.: 0171 380 7744
Fax: 0171 413 8395
E-mail: ucgbsem@ucl.ac.uk

Annexin VII

Annexin VII is a Ca^{2+}-dependent phospholipid-binding and membrane fusion protein which occurs predominantly in an intracellular vesicle and plasma membrane-bound state and is expressed in small amounts in virtually every cell. In vitro, annexin VII binds GTP in a Ca^{2+}-conditional manner, and GTP potentiates the Ca^{2+}-dependent processes of granule aggregation and membrane fusion. Annexin VII also forms voltage-dependent Ca^{2+} channels in natural and artificial membranes. Annexin VII has thus been implicated in the mechanism of Ca^{2+}- and GTP-dependent exocytosis.

Human annexin VII has a calculated molecular weight (M_r) of 50,200 and migrates on SDS gels with an apparent M_r of 51,000 (Burns *et al.* 1989). Although the bovine protein has an apparent pI between 6 and 7 (Scott *et al.* 1985), the human protein has a calculated isoelectric point of 5.8. Annexin VII contains the highly conserved 16 amino acid endonexin fold in the C-terminal tetrad repeat core domain of the annexin family and the unique N-terminal is distinguished from other family members by its large and hydrophobic character (Raynal and Pollard 1994). Annexin VII is distributed throughout the body; however, in heart, skeletal muscle, and brain a higher molecular mass form of 53 kDa arises by alternative splicing of a cassette exon (Magendzo *et al.* 1991). While a soluble form of annexin VII can be extracted from tissue under low Ca^{2+} conditions (Creutz *et al.* 1978), immuno-electron microscopy in intact chromaffin cells, indicates that annexin VII is mostly membrane-associated (Kuijpers *et al.* 1992). In addition, approximately 70% of total annexin VII in chromaffin cells is resistant to detergent extraction (Cardenas *et al.* 1995). Upon stimulation of cells by cholinergic agonists, annexin VII antigen remains on the membranes. However, as defined by interaction with the monoclonal antibody 10E7, rapid and specific changes in local conformation occur. These data suggest a dynamic link between annexin VII and exocytosis. The potential role for annexin VII in the exocytotic secretion process may be to serve both as a calcium and GTP sensor, and as a driver for membrane fusion.

■ Alternative names

Synexin (Creutz *et al.* 1978).

Identification/isolation

During the search for proteins involved in membrane fusion during exocytotic secretion, annexin VII was discovered in chromaffin cells and purified by a series of steps including ammonium sulfate fractionation and AcA34 gel filtration followed by chromatofocusing (Scott *et al.* 1985, Brocklehurst and Pollard 1990). The human cDNA was isolated from a lambda gt11 expression library from liver (Burns *et al.* 1989) using an oligonucleotide derived from amino acid sequences of peptides from a tryptic digest of the purified human lung synexin. Purified recombinant human annexin VII possesses both Ca²⁺-dependent granule aggregation and liposome fusion activity as well as Ca²⁺-channel activity, identical to activities of the purified native protein (Burns *et al.* 1990).

Gene and sequence

Mammalian annexin VII occurs as single copy genes of *ca.* 34 kb with 14 exons, including an alternatively spliced cassette exon (#6) of 66 bp (Shirvan *et al.* 1994; Zhang-Keck *et al.* 1994). The sequences of human (Burns *et al.* 1989: Genbank accession number J04543), mouse (Zhang-Keck *et al.* 1993: GenBank accession number L13129), *Xenopus* (Srivastava *et al.* 1996: GenBank accession number U16365) and *Dictyostelium* (Doring *et al.* 1991; Gerke 1991: GenBank accession number M69022) show that Annexin VII molecules are highly homologous in the conserved C-terminal tetrad repeat region. However, the deduced amino acid sequences in the N-terminal domain of mouse, *Xenopus* and *Dictyostelium* are 88%, 45%, and 34% identical to those of human annexin VII. In heart, muscle, and brain, human and mouse annexin VII express a highly conserved, alternatively spliced cassette exon containing 66 bp (22 amino acids) in the unique N-terminal regulatory region (Magendzo *et al.* 1991). By contrast, in *Xenopus*, this domain is replaced in different adult tissues and embryonic stages by different numbers of tandem PGQM repeats. In addition, the PGQM repeat region appears to have distinct, tissue specific protein targets (Srivastava *et al.* 1996, and unpublished). However, *Dictyostelium* is not reported to contain any isoforms. In addition, in the case of human annexin VII, the polymorphisms have been traced to multiple polyadenylation sites from a single annexin VII gene (Magendzo *et al.* 1991; Shirvan *et al.* 1994). However, the mRNA variants in mouse may reflect an entirely different polymorphism mechanism due to the occurrence of 800 bp in the 3' untranslated region associated with two nucleotide changes in one of the forms and not the other (Zhang-Keck *et al.* 1993). The introns of the human and mouse annexin VII genes are in the same positions (Shirvan *et al.* 1994; Zhang-Keck *et al.* 1994) and do not coincide with the coding regions of the four tetrad repeats. In addition, they are located somewhat differently from the splice junctions of annexin I, II, and III. Human and mouse C-terminal tetrad repeats and the location of splice junctions of annexin I, II, and VII, and mammalian sequence variants are shown in extended form in Fig. 1, in which alphahelical domains are based on the crystal structure of the homologous annexin V. In the 5' untranslated regions, the human and mouse annexin VII differ in that the mouse promotor has a TATA and CCATT box while the human promotor lacks these elements. In addition, many putative but different transcription factor sites are evident on both systems. The human gene is

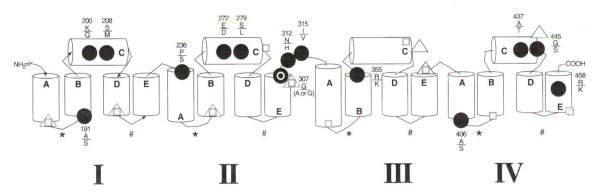

Figure 1. Expanded molecular form of conserved C-terminal tetrad repeat to show the locations of splice sites on human and mouse annexin VII relative to helical domains, and allowed mutations in human/mouse annexin VII. The four individual repeats in the C-terminal domain are indicated by roman numerals. Each repeat contains sets of anti-parallel alpha-helices (A,B and D,E) arranged perpendicular to helix C in the crystal structure. The (*) and (#) symbols represents S1 ("endonexin fold") and S2 regions in the nomenclature of Guy *et al.* (1991). Each solid circle (●) locates a difference between human and mouse residues (human amino acid/mouse amino acid), numbered according to the human sequence. The target symbol locates a possible allelic site in mouse. The positions of the intron–exon are shown for annexin I (□), II (▒), and VII (△) (after Zhang-Keck *et al.* 1993).

located on chromosome 10q21 while the mouse gene is located on the homologous chromosome 14.

Protein

Annexin VII contains the highly conserved C-terminal tetrad repeat common to other members of the annexin gene family, as well as a lengthy, unique hydrophobic N-terminal domain. The C-terminal core domain harbors the binding sites for Ca^{2+} and phospholipid, and, based on studies of gating currents (Rojas and Pollard 1988) and Ca^{2+} ion conductance (Fig. 2; Pollard and Rojas 1987), the molecule appears to penetrate the target membrane and form ion channels (Pollard and Rojas 1988; Burns *et al.* 1989; Pollard *et al.* 1991). Once the penetration has occurred, the unique N-terminal domain seems to be important for completion of the membrane fusion process. The N-terminal region and the conserved first C-terminal repeat contain sequences which somewhat resemble the five ras-consensus domains identified with phosphate and guanine binding, and with the GTP effector domain. These consensus sequences G-1 through G-5 are found in most members of the GTPase superfamily (Bourne *et al.* 1991). Indeed, annexin VII can bind GTP in a Ca^{2+}-dependent manner, and GTP hydrolysis is dependent upon Ca^{2+} and other divalent cations (Caohuy *et al.* 1996).

Antibodies

No commercially available antibodies are known for annexin VII.

Anatomical localization

The immunogold labeling of synexin using mono-clonal antibody 10E7 or goat polyclonal antibody ("Ramon","Ramon II"), identifies annexin VII in close proximity to the chromaffin granule membranes, plasma membrane, and nucleoplasm. Upon stimulation with nicotine over a 90 -sec. time period, and using the mono-clonal antibody, a decrease of annexin VII immuno-reactivity is detected in all compartments, especially in the granule membrane (Kuijpers *et al.* 1992). In contrast, no change in the polyclonal label occurs. Thus, annexin VII is localized to membranes, and upon stimulation, changes occur in the orientation of the 10E7 epitope to the aqueous phase. A polyclonal antibody to the peptide defined by the cassette exon clearly shows that in skeletal muscle, annexin VII is specifically localized to myosin-rich regions of the sarcomere (see Fig. 3). Similarly an anti-PGQM antibody localizes *Xenopus* skeletal muscle annexin VII in the identical myosin-rich regions.

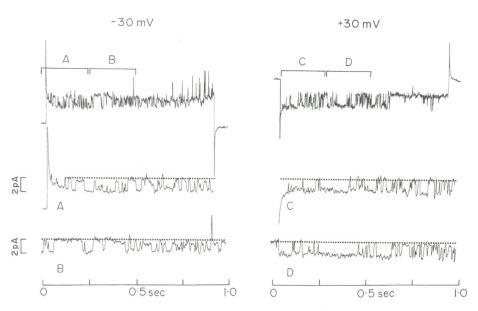

Figure 2. Voltage-dependent Ca^{2+} channels formed by annexin VII in a phosphatidyl serine bilayer in a patch pipette. The pipette contains 50 mM Ca^{2+}, while the bath contains *ca.* 50 nM Ca^{2+}. Current flow, from pipette to bath, is driven by the electrochemical potential. At V_n = -30 mV, the channel has a low open time probability, while at V_n = +30 mV, the channel has a high time probability. (From Pollard and Rojas 1988.)

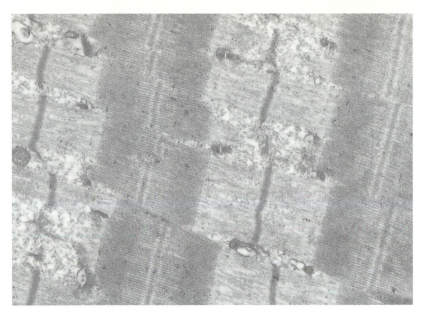

Figure 3. Specific localization of annexin VII to myosin-rich regions in human skeletal muscle by the immunogold method. The polyclonal antibody is directed against the cassette exon defined by the 22-residue peptide specific to brain, skeletal, and cardiac muscle (contributed by G.A.J. Kuijpers and G. Goping, LCBG, NIH).

■ Biological activity

Purified synexin binds Ca^{2+} and drives chromaffin granule aggregation in a Ca^{2+}-dependent manner. For both events the K_d for Ca^{2+} is approximately 200 μM (Creutz et al. 1978, 1979). This affinity for Ca^{2+} is in the physiological range for exocytosis, as defined by numerous caged Ca^{2+} studies in chromaffin and other cells. Annexin VII also forms 175pS voltage-dependent Ca^{2+} channels in natural and artificial membranes (Pollard and Rojas 1988). The cation selectivity for annexin channels in the patch pipette studies parallel annexin VII's cation dependence for both chromaffin granule aggregation and PS liposome aggregation and fusion (Pollard and Rojas 1988). Annexin VII fuses chromaffin granule ghosts (Stutzin 1985; Nir et al. 1987) and acidic phospholipid liposomes (Hong et al. 1981). The mechanism of membrane fusion appears to involve the formation of a "hydrophobic bridge" between fusion membrane partners, and individual fusion occurs in approximately 4 μs (Pollard et al. 1987; Pollard et al. 1990, Pollard et al. 1991; Fig. 4). The mechanism of the activation of membrane fusion by GTP has been viewed in terms of a cycle of Ca^{2+}-conditional activation of annexin VII to a GTP-bound state, and subsequent inactivation by GTP hydrolysis (Fig. 5; Caohuy et al. 1995). The GTP-bound state of Ca^{2+}-activated annexin VII appears to be a strong driver of membrane aggregation, fusion, and ion channel activity, suggesting that annexin VII provides a common site for both Ca^{2+} and GTP action in the exocytotic process.

■ References

Bourne, H.R., Sanders, D.A., and McCormick, F. (1991) The GTPase superfamily: conserved structure and molecular mechanism. Nature **349**, 117–127.

Brocklehurst. K.W. and Pollard, H.B. (1990) Cell Biology of Secretion. In *Peptide hormone secretion. A practical approach* (ed. J.C. Hutton and K. Siddle) pp. 233–255. IRL Press, Oxford.

Burns, A.L., Magendzo, K., Shirvan, A., Srivastava, M., Rojas, E., Alijani, M. and Pollard, H.B. (1989) Calcium channel activity of purified human synexin and structure of the human synexin gene. Proc. Natl. Acad. Sci. USA **86**, 3798–3802.

Burns, A.L., Magendzo, K., Rojas, E., Parra, C., Fuente, M., Cultraro, C., Shirvan, A., Vogel, T., Heldman, J., Caohuy, H., Tombaccini, D., and Pollard, H.B. (1990) Human synexin (annexin VII) polymorphisms: Tissue specificity and expression in *Escherichia coli*. Biochem. Soc. Trans. **18**, 1118–1121.

Caohuy, H., Srivastava, M., and Pollard, H.B. (1996) Membrane fusion protein synexin (annexin VII) as a Ca^{2+}/GTP sensor in exocytotic secretion. (submitted).

Cardenas, A.M., Kuijpers, G.A.J., and Pollard, H.B. (1995) Effect of protein inhibitors on synexin levels and secretory response in bovine adrenal medullary chromaffin cells. Biochim. Biophys. Acta. **1234**, 255–260.

Creutz, C.E., Pazoles, C.J., and Pollard, H.B. (1978) Identification and purification of an adrenal medullary protein (synexin) that causes calcium-dependent aggregation of chromaffin granules. J. Biol. Chem. **253**, 2858–2866.

Creutz, C.E., Pazoles, C.J., and Pollard H.B. (1979) Self-association of synexin in the presence of calcium: Correlation with synexin-induced membrane fusion and examination of the structure of synexin aggregates. J. Biol. Chem. **254**, 553–558.

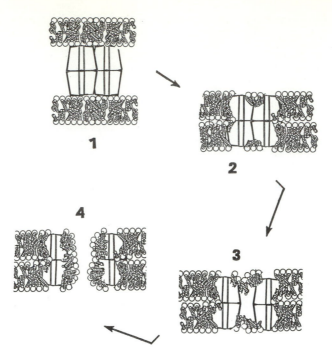

Figure 4. Hydrophobic bridge hypothesis for membrane fusion. 1. When exposed to Ca^{2+}, annexin VII forms polymers and binds to phospholipid head groups on two adjoining membranes. 2. Phospholipids cross over the hydrophobic bridge provided by the annexin VII polymer. 3. Annexin VII polymer dissociates in the low dielectric medium. 4. Phospholipids migrate over the newly exposed annexin VII surfaces to complete the fusion process. (From Pollard *et al.* 1991.)

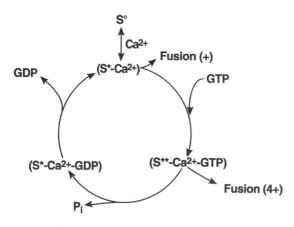

Figure 5. Cyclic model for synexin-driven membrane fusion regulated by GTP-binding and hydrolysis. Upon binding Ca^{2+}, annexin VII (S^o) becomes activated to S^*-Ca^{2+} and capable of modest fusion activity. Optimal fusion activity ensues when GTP binds to the complex to form S^{**}-Ca^{2+}-GTP. When annexin VII hydrolyzes bound GTP to form S^*-Ca^{2+}-GDP, the activity drops to baseline levels. Upon dissociation of GDP, S^*-Ca^{2+} is reformed and the cycle starts once again. (From Caohuy *et al.* 1996.)

Doring, V., Schleicher, M., and Noegel, A.A. (1991) *Dictyostelium* annexin VII (synexin): cDNA sequence and Isolation of a gene disruption mutant. J. Biol. Chem. **266**, 17509–17515.

Gerke, V. (1991) Identification of a homologue for annexin VII (synexin) in *Dictyostelium discoideum*. J. Biol. Chem. **266**, 1697–1700.

Guy, H.R., Rojas, E.M., Burns, A.L., Rojas, E., and Pollard, H.B. (1991) A TIM-barrel model of synexin channels. Biophys. J. **59**, 372a.

Hong, K., Düzgunes, N., and Papahadjopoulos, D. (1981) Role of synexin in membrane fusion. Enhancement of calcium-dependent fusion of phospholipid vesicles. J. Biol. Chem. **256**, 3641–3644.

Kuijpers, G.A.J., Lee, G., and Pollard, H.B. (1992) Immunolocalization of synexin (annexin vii) in adrenal chromaffin granules and chromaffin cells: Evidence for a dynamic role in the secretory process. Cell Tissue Res. **269**, 323–330.

Magendzo, K., Shirvan, A., Cultraro, C., Srivastava, M., Pollard, H.B., and Burns, A.L. (1991) Alternative splicing of human synexin mRNA in brain, cardiac, and skeletal muscle alters the unique N-terminal domain. J. Biol. Chem. **266**, 3228–3232.

Nir, S., Stutzin, A., and Pollard, H.B. (1987) Effect of synexin on aggregation and fusion of chromaffin granule ghosts at pH 6. Biochim. Biophys. Acta **903**, 309–318.

Pollard, H.B. and Rojas, E. (1988) Calcium activated synexin forms highly selective, voltage-gated channels in phosphatidylserine bilayer membranes. Proc. Natl. Acad. Sci. USA **85**, 2974–2978.

Pollard, H.B., Rojas, E., and Burns, A.L. (1987) Synexin and chromaffin granule membrane fusion. A novel "hydrophobic bridge" hypothesis for the driving and directing of the fusion process. Ann. NY Acad. Sci. **493**, 524–551.

Pollard, H.B., Rojas, E., and Burns, A.L. (1990) Synexin (annexin VII): a cytosolic calcium-binding protein which promotes membrane fusion and forms calcium channels on artificial bilayer and natural membranes. J. Membr. Biol. **117**, 101–112.

Pollard, H.B., Rojas, E., Pastor, R.W., Rojas, E.M., Guy, H.R., and Burns, A.L. (1991) Synexin: Molecular mechanism of calcium-dependent membrane fusion and voltage-dependent calcium channel activity. Evidence in support of the "hydrophobic bridge hypothesis" for exocytotic membrane fusion. Ann. NY Acad. Sci. **635**, 328–351.

Raynal, P. and Pollard, H.B. (1994) Annexins: The problem of assessing the biological role for a gene family of multi-functional calcium and phospholipid-binding proteins. Biochim. Biophys. Acta **1197**, 63–93.

Rojas, E. and Pollard, H.B. (1987) Membrane capacity measurements suggest a calcium-dependent insertion of synexin into phosphatidylserine bilayers. FEBS Lett. **217**, 25–31.

Scott, J.M., Kelner, K.L., and Pollard, H.B. (1985) Purification of synexin by pH step elution from chromatofocusing media in the absence of ampholytes. Anal. Biochem. **149**, 163–165.

Shirvan, A., Srivastava, M., Wong, M.G., Cultraro, C., Magendzo, K., McBride, O.W., Pollard, H.B., and Burns, A.L. (1994) Divergent structure of the human synexin (annexin VII) gene and assignment to chromosome 10. Biochemistry **33**, 6888–6901.

Srivastava, M., Zhang-Keck, Z.-Y., Caohuy, H., McPhie, P., and Pollard, H.B. (1996) Novel isoforms of synexin in *Xenopus laevis*: multiple tandem PGQM repeats distinguish mRNA's in specific adult tissues and embryonic stages. Biochem. J. (in press).

Stutzin, A. (1985) A fluorescence assay for monitoring and analyzing fusion of biological membranes *in vitro*. FEBS Letts. **197**, 274–280.

Zhang-keck, Z.-Y., Burns, A.L., and Pollard, H.B. (1993) Mouse synexin (annexin VII) polymorphisms and a phylogenetic comparison with other annexins. Biochem. J. **289**, 735–741.

Zhang-Keck, Z.-Y., Srivastava, M., Kozak, C.A., Caohuy, H., Shirvan, A., Burns, A.L., and Pollard, H.B. (1994) Genomic organization and chromosomal localization of the mouse synexin gene. Biochem. J. **301**, 835–845.

■ *M. Srivastava, E., Rojas, H. Caohuy, and Harvey B. Pollard: LCBG, NIDDK, National Institutes of Health, Bethesda, MD 20892, USA*
Tel.: 301 496 3435
Fax: 301 402 3298
E-mail: hpollard@helix.nih.gov

Annexin XI

Annexin XI is a protein in the annexin family that is expressed at moderate levels in a wide variety of tissues and isolated cells in culture. Annexin XI interacts with S100A6 and localizes to nuclei in certain rapidly growing cells, prompting speculation that it functions in cell cycling. However, nuclear localization is not strictly tied to proliferation, so roles in differentiated cell function or development have been postulated.

Bovine annexin XI is a 503 amino acid protein with a calculated molecular mass of 54,018 Da and an isoelectric point of 7.66 as predicted from the cDNA sequence. The protein consists of a core domain of four imperfect annexin repeats and a long amino terminal domain rich in glycine, proline, and tyrosine (Towle and Treadwell 1992).

■ Alternative names

CAP-50 (Tokumitsu *et al*. 1992*b*).

■ Isolation/identification

Two annexin XI cDNA clones, corresponding to mRNAs generated by alternative splicing of identical primary transcripts, were identified in a bovine chondrocyte cDNA library (Towle and Treadwell 1992; Towle *et al*. 1992). Rabbit and bovine lung annexin XI proteins were purified by ion exchange and calcyclin-affinity chromatography using calcyclin binding as an assay (Mizutani *et al*. 1992; Tokumitsu *et al*. 1992*a*).

■ Gene and sequences

Two distinct bovine annexin XI mRNA species encoding protein isoforms differing at the amino terminus are predicted from separate cDNA clones (accession numbers M82802 and Z11742). These mRNAs are generated by an unusual, mutually exclusive pattern of alternative splicing: the primary transcript of a single annexin XI gene is processed into either of two different mRNAs each having one of two specific exons. The predominant annexin XI isoform lacks a signal peptide, consistent with its intracellular localization. The second protein isoform is predicted to have a signal peptide-like amino terminus, but this variant has been identified only at the mRNA level (Towle et al. 1992). The rabbit cDNA homologue was cloned as CAP-50, a 50 kDa, S100A6 binding protein (accession number D10883). Rabbit annexin XI cDNA was reported to be 94% identical to the bovine cDNA sequence (Tokumitsu et al. 1992b). Human annexin XI amino acid sequence is ~92% identical with the bovine protein (Misaki et al. 1994; accession number L19605).

Protein

The ~55 kDa annexin XI protein consists of four tandem annexin domains and a non-conserved amino terminal domain rich in glycine, proline, and tyrosine. This extended hydrophobic domain accounts for nearly half the protein and contains the site predicted to differ in the proteins encoded by alternative annexin XI transcripts.

Biological regulation

Annexin XI is a ubiquitously expressed gene, suggesting that the encoded protein plays a role in basic cellular function (Towle and Treadwell 1992). The subcellular localization of annexin XI is regulated in a developmental and tissue-specific fashion. Using immunochemical techniques, the protein was localized to nuclei in rat fibroblast 3Y1 cells (Mizutani et al. 1992) and in undifferentiated mesenchymal cells of 14-day rat embryos, but it was cytosolic in day-18 fetal connective tissues (Mamiya et al. 1994). There was no evidence of an obligatory relationship between nuclear localization and proliferation. Rather, the presence of annexin XI in the nucleus was thought to be related to differentiation or developmental processes (Mamiya et al. 1994). Annexin XI is phosphorylated (serine and threonine) in v-src-transformed rat fibroblast 3Y1 cells, and the modification appears to alter nuclear localization and phospholipid binding (Mizutani et al. 1993). Only a small fraction of the total cellular annexin XI is phosphorylated, and the significance of the phosphorylation is unclear.

Interactions/biological activities

Like other family members, annexin XI binds to phospholipids in a Ca^{2+}-dependent manner. This probably accounts for the inhibition of phospholipase A_2 reported for this and other annexins (Tokumitsu et al. 1992a). It also exhibits specific, Ca^{2+}-dependent, and stoichiometric binding with S100A6 (Minami et al. 1992; Mizutani et al. 1992; Tokumitsu et al. 1992a). Experiments using proteolysis and deletion mutagenesis localized binding to the amino terminal region of annexin XI, probably in the vicinity of Tyr27 to Leu52 of the rabbit protein (Tokumitsu et al. 1993).

Pathology

Human cDNA clones were identified by immunoscreening using anti-56K autoantibodies present in the sera of patients with various autoimmune diseases. Reactivity was with the extended amino terminal hydrophobic domain. Thus, annexin XI may be an important target in auto immune diseases (Misaki et al. 1994).

References

Mamiya, N., Iino, S., Mizutani, A., Kobayashi, S., and Hidaka, H. (1994) Development-related and cell-type specific nuclear localization of annexin XI: Immunolocalization analysis in rat tissues. Biochem. Biophys. Res. Comm. **202**, 403–409.

Minami, H., Tokumitsu, H., Mizutani, A., Watanabe, Y., Watanabe, M., and Hidaka, H. (1992) Specific binding of CAP-50 to calcyclin. FEBS Lett. **305**, 217–219.

Misaki, Y., Pruijn, G.J.M., van der Kemp, A.W.C.M., and van Venrooij, W.J. (1994) The 56K autoantigen is identical to human annexin XI. J. Biol. Chem. **269**, 4240–4246.

Mizutani, A, Usuda, N., Tokumitsu, H., Minami, H., Yasui, K., Kobayashi, R., and Hiroyoshi, H. (1992) CAP-50, a newly identified annexin, localizes in nuclei of cultured fibroblast 3Y1 cells. J. Biol. Chem. **267**, 13498–13504.

Mizutani, A., Tokumitsu, H., Kobayashi, R., and Hidaka, H. (1993) Phosphorylation of annexin XI (CAP-50) in SR-3Y1 cells. J. Biol. Chem. **268**, 15517–15522.

Tokumitsu, H., Mizutani, A., Minami, H., Kobayashi, R., and Hidaka, H. (1992a) A calcyclin-associated protein is a newly identified member of the Ca^{2+}/phospholipid binding proteins, annexin family. J. Biol. Chem. **267**, 8919–8924.

*Tokumitsu, H., Mizutani, A., Muramatsu, M., Yokota, T., Arai, K., and Hidaka, H. (1992b) Molecular cloning of rabbit CAP-50, a calcyclin-associated annexin protein. Biochem. Biophys. Res. Comm. **186**, 1227–1235.

Tokumitsu, H., Mizutani, A., and Hidaka, H. (1993) Calcyclin-binding site located on the NH2-terminal domain of rabbit CAP-50 (Annexin XI): functional expression of CAP-50 in Escherichia coli. Arch. Biochem. Biophys. **303**, 302–306.

*Towle, C.A. and Treadwell, B.V. (1992) Identification of a novel mammalian annexin. J. Biol. Chem. **267**, 5416–5423.

*Towle, C.A., Weissbach, L., and Treadwell, B.V. (1992) Alternatively spliced annexin XI transcripts encode proteins that differ near the amino terminus. Biochim. Biophys. Acta **1131** 223–226.

■ Christine A. Towle:
Orthopedic Research Laboratories,
Massachusetts General Hospital and Harvard Medical School,
Boston, MA 02114, USA
Tel.: (617) 724 3744
Fax: (617) 724 7396

3

Other Proteins

Bacterial calcium-binding proteins

Bacterial proteins concerned with Ca^{2+} regulation include primary and secondary transporters responsible for efflux, voltage-gated calcium channels responsible for influx, and calmodulin-like proteins. These proteins implicate calcium in the control of functions that may include heat shock, pathogenicity, chemotaxis, differentiation, and the progression of the cell cycle.

The importance of Ca^{2+} in bacterial physiology is at last being confirmed (for references see Lynn and Rosen 1987; Norris *et al*. 1991a; Onek and Smith 1992). Almost 20 years after Ca^{2+} was first implicated in bacterial chemotaxis, manipulations of putative Ca^{2+} channels and intracellular Ca^{2+} levels in *Escherichia coli* have been clearly shown to affect chemotaxis (Tisa *et al*. 1993). Examples of bacterial differentiation that reveal a connection with Ca^{2+} now include sporulation, fruiting body formation, gliding and heterocyst formation. Ca^{2+} is also implicated in the cell cycle, with intracellular Ca^{2+} apparently increasing during cell division in *E. coli*. Such division entails formation of non-bilayer structures which may depend on Ca^{2+} (Rietveld *et al*. 1993). Clarification of the role of Ca^{2+} in the heat shock response awaits discovery of a role for Ca^{2+} in phosphorylation of DnaK *in vivo* (see below). The role of Ca^{2+} in bacterial disease now extends from the expression of virulence-related genes in strains of *Yersinia pestis* and dental plaque formation *in Streptococcus mutans* to nodulation in the "parasitic" relationship between *Rhizobium* spp. and plants. Such roles indicate that the diverse Ca^{2+}-binding proteins described below are likely to be involved in more than a simple buffering of intracellular Ca^{2+}. Indeed, these proteins may have the same activites as their eukaryotic homologues.

◼ Efflux

There has been evidence for the presence of primary pumps in bacteria for over a decade (Lynn and Rosen 1987; Norris *et al*. 1991a). Recently, a Ca^{2+} pump has been cloned from the cyanobacterium *Synechococcus* sp. PCC7942, sequenced and characterized as a P-type ATPase (Kanamaru *et al*. 1993; Berkelman *et al*. 1994). Another Ca^{2+} pump, purified from the soil and water bacterium *Flavobacterium odoratum*, fulfils all the criteria expected of a P-type ATPase and shows a remarkable similarity to the eukaryotic calcium-ATPase from sarcoplasmic reticulum (Gambel *et al*. 1992). Evidence for primary exchangers, based on ATP-dependence and orthovanadate inhibition, has also been reported for various species of *streptococci* including *S. sanguis* and *S. lactis* (Lynn and Rosen 1987) and the cyanobacterium, *Anabaena variabilis* (Lockau and Pfeffer 1983).

A number of secondary Ca^{2+} exchangers have also been identified in bacteria (Lynn and Rosen 1987). A Ca^{2+}/proton antiporter that exchanges one divalent Ca^{2+} ion for three protons and is, therefore, electrogenic has been identified in *E. coli*. This exchanger is not specific and will transport other ions with relative affinities Ca>Mn>Sr>Ba (for references see Lynn and Rosen 1987). The relationship between this exchanger and the recently discovered ChaA Ca^{2+}/proton exchanger from *E. coli* remains to be determined (Ivey *et al*. 1993). ChaA, which appears to be involved in Ca^{2+} ion circulation at alkaline pH (Ohyama *et al*. 1994), possesses an aspartic acid/glutamic acid sequence with an intriguing similarity to sequences found in eukaryotic Ca^{2+}-binding proteins such as calsequestrin (Ivey *et al*. 1993).

In addition to Ca^{2+}/proton exchangers, there is evidence for other secondary exchanger systems for Ca^{2+} in prokaryotes. In *E. coli*, a secondary exchanger has been identified in which Ca^{2+} and phosphate are co-exported in a 1:1 ratio in exchange for protons (Ambudkar *et al*. 1984). This exchanger also differs from the Ca^{2+}/proton antiporter in its lack of sensitivity to proteases and aminoacyl-modifying reagents and in its response to the presence of the *calC* and *calD* mutations which confer sensitivity to Ca^{2+} (Ambudkar *et al*. 1984). In *Bacillus* sp. A-007 and *Halobacterium salinarium*, which live in a high salt environment, a strategy of sodium/Ca^{2+} exchange has been adopted (Lynn and Rosen 1987). Finally, a Ca^{2+}/sodium exchanger involved in Ca^{2+} efflux and influx, lysis and competence for genetic transformation has been identified in *Streptococcus pneumoniae* on the basis of inhibition studies with the amiloride derivative 2′,4′-dimethylbenzamil (Trombe *et al*. 1994).

◼ Influx

In *Bacillus subtilis*, Ca^{2+} uptake into right-side-out vesicles mediated by a protein displaying 'L-type' Ca^{2+} channel properties has been reported (Kusaka and Matsushita 1987; Matsushita *et al*. 1989). In this case, ^{45}Ca^{2+} uptake was dependent on membrane depolarization, was inhibited in the presence of dihydropridine and phenylalkylamine antagonists and lanthanum, and activated by BAY K 8644. Significantly, Ca^{2+} channel blockers inhibit chemotaxis in both *B. subtilis* and *E. coli* (Matsushita *et al.* 1988; Tisa *et al.* 1993).

A very different mechanism also leads to divalent ion entry into bacteria. The uptake of inorganic phosphate depends on divalent ions such as calcium, magnesium, manganese, and cobalt in both the Pit system of *E. coli* and in similar systems of *Acinetobacter johnsonii* 210A and probably of other bacteria (van Veen *et al.* 1994). In these systems, the metal phosphate is transported in symport with a proton. Finally, in *E. coli* a non-proteinaceous Ca^{2+} channel composed of a complex of the lipidic polymer, poly-3-hydroxybutyrate, and Ca^{2+} polyphosphate has been described (Bramble and Reusch 1995).

■ Calmodulin-like proteins

One of the first bacterial proteins resembling calmodulin to be described was protein S which is involved in fruiting body formation in the Gram-negative, differentiating bacterium, *Myxococcus xanthus*. Protein S is an acidic and heat stable protein with a primary structure that contains amino acid sequences resembling EF-hands (Inouye *et al.* 1983). These properties are shared by calerythrin, a calmodulin-like protein present in an antibiotic-producing bacterium, *Saccharopolyspora erythraea*. This protein also shows the expected gel shift but is not an activator of cyclic nucleotide phosphodiesterase, PDE (Swan *et al.* 1987). In the Gram-positive, sporulating bacterium, *B. subtilis*, a calmodulin-like protein(s) has also been described. This is heat stable, acidic, cross-reacts with anti-calmodulin antibodies, activates PDE and NAD kinase in a Ca^{2+}-dependent way and is inhibited by trifluoperazine, a compound that inhibits eukaryotic calmodulin (Fry *et al.* 1991), although its specificity can be questioned. In *Bacillus cereus*, where a calmodulin-like protein has been identified on the basis of antibody cross-reactivity, heat stability and Ca^{2+}-binding (Shyu and Foegeding 1989), Ca^{2+} is required for formation of spores (Greene and Slepecky 1972; but see Youatt 1993). Calmodulin-like proteins were reported in 1981 in *E. coli* on the basis of Ca^{2+}-dependent activation and inhibition of PDE (Iwasa *et al.* 1981) as well as heat stability and Ca^{2+} binding (Harmon *et al.* 1985). More recently, calmodulin-like proteins have been described in *E. coli* that are heat stable, acidic, bind Ca^{2+}, are induced by EGTA and cross-react with anti-calmodulin antibodies (Laoudj *et al.* 1994). However, a mutant strategy to clone a calmodulin gene from *E. coli* on the basis of sensitivity to the calmodulin antagonist 48/80 resulted, curiously, in the cloning of the gene encoding leu3 tRNA (Chen *et al.* 1991).

Calmodulin-like proteins have been discovered in several cyanobacteria (for a review see Onek and Smith 1992). These include *Anabaena* spp. where heat stable proteins activate NAD kinase in a Ca^{2+}-dependent manner and cross-react with anti-calmodulin antibodies (Pettersson and Bergman 1989), and *Nostoc* PCC 6720 where acidic proteins bind Ca^{2+}, activate PDE and NAD kinase in a Ca^{2+}-dependent manner and cross-react with

anti-calmodulin antibodies (Onek and Smith 1992). The first evidence for a calmodulin-like protein in an archaeon, *Halobacterium salinarium*, has recently been obtained on the basis of p*I*, Ca^{2+}-binding and activation of PDE (Rothärmel and Wagner 1995).

■ Protein kinases

In response to changes in osmolarity, EnvZ, the osmotic sensor in the inner membrane of *E. coli*, phosphorylates OmpR, a DNA-binding protein that determines the differential transcription of two outer membrane porins, OmpF and OmpC. Using an EnvZ fusion protein, addition of 60 μM Ca^{2+} to an *in vitro* assay stimulated both autophosphorylation of the fusion protein and phosphorylation of OmpR (Rampersaud *et al.* 1991). Intriguingly, manganese at similar concentrations had similar effects. However, the Ca^{2+} chelator EGTA is a better chelator of manganese, zinc, and iron than Ca^{2+} and reversal of EGTA inhibition of phosphorylation by addition of Ca^{2+} does not necessarily imply that the kinase is dependent on Ca^{2+}. For example, in pursuit of Ca^{2+}-stimulated kinases in *E. coli* (Norris *et al.* 1991*b*), we have observed that EGTA inhibition of protein phosphorylation is reversed more frequently by manganese than by Ca^{2+} (Freestone *et al.* 1995).

DnaK, the *E. coli* equivalent of eukaryotic Heat Shock Protein 70, is induced by stress and has an autophosphorylation activity stimulated tenfold by Ca^{2+} *in vitro*. *In vivo*, phosphorylation of DnaK, albeit on a different residue, increases with temperature and determines binding to denatured substrates (Sherman and Goldberg 1993). The Ca^{2+}-dependence of this phosphorylation is not known. However, in view of the evidence for calmodulin-like proteins in bacteria, it may be significant that DnaK has a sequence with 60% identity to the classic 21 residue calmodulin-binding site (Stevenson and Calderwood 1990). One speculation is that Ca^{2+} levels serve as part of an intracellular thermometer and, in line with this, optimal growth of L-forms of *E. coli* occurs at 32°C and at 37°C in media containing 0.1 mM and 1 mM Ca^{2+}, respectively (Onoda and Oshima 1988).

Histone phosphorylation is commonly used to characterise eukaryotic kinases. Phosphorylation of eukaryotic histones by a purified, endogenous kinase from *Legionella micdadei* was stimulated threefold by Ca^{2+} (Saha *et al.* 1988). Other evidence for eukaryotic-style kinases in a variety of bacteria includes the presence of Ca^{2+}-, phosphatidylserine-, and TPA-stimulated kinases reminiscent of eukaryotic protein kinase C in *E. coli* (Norris *et al.* 1991*b*) and *B. subtilis* (Sandler *et al.* 1989), Ca^{2+}- and manganese-stimulation and PKC-like inhibition of phosphorylation in *Streptomyces griseus* (Hong *et al.* 1993), involvement of calmodulin-like proteins in protein phosphorylation in *Clostridium thermohydrosulfuricum* (Londesborough 1986) and in the cyanobacterium, *Anabaena* spp. (Mann *et al.* 1991), and about 25 protein serine/threonine kinases in *Myxococcus xanthus* (Munoz-Dorada *et al.* 1993).

Other calcium-binding proteins

The periplasmic D-galactose-binding protein involved in transport and chemotaxis in *E. coli* is predicted by X-ray crystallography to contain the classical Ca^{2+}-binding structure, the EF-hand (Vyas *et al.* 1987). Data-base searches for EF-hands identified four bacterial candidates: the elongation factor EF-Ts, the transcription factor, Rho and the replication initiation factor for the plasmid R6K (all from *E. coli*) and the secreted protein, haemolysin from *E. coli* (Kretsinger 1991). A haemolysin-like protein, NodO, exported from *Rhizobium leguminosarum*, binds Ca^{2+} and is proposed to have a Ca^{2+}-dependent interaction with plant root cells (Economou *et al.* 1990).

The future

Although the study of prokaryotic Ca^{2+} has not benefited from the same investments and activity as that of eukaryotic Ca^{2+}, a critical state has now been reached. The genes encoding bacterial Ca^{2+}-binding proteins can be mutagenized and phenotypes studied and related to measurements of intracellular Ca^{2+} by techniques that have recently become available. The results should lead to an exciting advance in our understanding of calcium's varied roles in both prokaryotic and eukaryotic cells.

References

Ambudkar, S. V., Zlotnick, G. W., and Rosen, B. P. (1984) Calcium efflux from *Escherichia coli*. J. Biol. Chem. **259**, 6142–6146.

Berkelman, T., Garret-Engele, P., and Hoffman, N. E. (1994) The *pacL* gene of *Synechococcus* sp strain PCC 7942 encodes a Ca^{2+}-transporting ATPase. J. Bacteriol. **176**, 4430–4436.

Bramble, L. L. and Reusch, R. N. (1995) Poly-3-hydroxybutyrate/polyphosphate complexes form voltage-gated calcium channels in *Escherichia coli* plasma membranes. Biophys. J. **68**, A148.

Chen, M. X., Bouquin, N., Norris, V., Casaregola, S., Seror, S. J., and Holland, I. B. (1991) A single base change in the acceptor stem of tRNA₃Leu confers resistance upon *Escherichia coli* to the calmodulin inhibitor, 48/80. EMBO J. **10**, 3113–3122.

Economou, A., Hamilton, W. D. O., Johnston, A. W. B., and Downie, J. A. (1990) The *Rhizobium* nodulation genes *nodO* encodes a Ca^{2+}-binding protein that is exported without N-terminal cleavage and is homologous to haemolysin and related proteins. EMBO J. **9**, 349–354.

Freestone, P., Grant, S., Toth, I., and Norris, V. (1995) Identification of phosphoproteins in *Escherichia coli*. Mol. Microbiol. **15**, 573–580.

Fry, I. J., Becker-Hapak, M., and Hageman, J. H. (1991) Purification and properties of an intracellular calmodulin-like protein from *Bacillus subtilis* cells. J. Bacteriol. **173**, 2506–2513.

Gambel, A. M., Desrosiers, M. G., and Menick, D. R. (1992) Characterization of a P-type Ca^{2+}-ATPase from *Flavobacterium odoratum*. J. Biol. Chem. **267**, 15923–15931.

Greene R. A. and Slepecky, R. A. (1972) Minimal requirements for commitment to sporulation in *Bacillus megaterium*. J. Bacteriol. **111**, 557–565.

Harmon, A. C., Prasher, D., and Cormier, M. J. (1985) High-affinity calcium-binding proteins in *Escherichia coli*. Biochem. Biophys. Res. Comm. **127**, 31–36.

Hong, S-K., Matsumoto, A., Horinouchi, S., and Beppu, T. (1993) Effect of protein kinase inhibitors on *in vitro* protein phosphorylation and cellular differentiation of *Streptomyces griseus*. Mol. Gen. Genet. **236**, 347–354.

Inouye, S., Franceshini, T., and Inouye, M. (1983) Structural similarities between the developmental-specific protein S from a Gram-negative bacterium, *Myxococcus xanthus*, and calmodulin. Proc. Natl. Acad. Sci. USA **80**, 6828–6833.

Ivey, D. M., Guffanti, A. A., Zemsky, J., Pinner, E., Karpel, R., Padan, E., Schuldiner, S., and Krulwich, T. A. (1993) Cloning and characterization of a putative $Ca^{2+}/H+$ antiporter gene from *Escherichia coli* upon functional complementation of Na+/H+ antiporter-deficient strains by the overexpressed gene. J. Biol. Chem. **268**, 11296–11303.

Iwasa, Y., Yonemitsu, K., Matsui, K., Fukunaga, K., and Miyamoto, E. (1981) A heat-stable inhibitor protein for bovine brain cyclic nucleotide phosphodiesterase from *Escherichia coli*. FEBS Lett. **128**, 311–314.

Kanamaru, K., Kashiwagi, S., and Mizuno, T. (1993) The cyanobacterium, *Synechococcus* sp pcc7942, possesses 2 distinct genes encoding cation-transporting P-type ATPases *FEBS Lett.* **330**, 99–104.

Kretsinger, R. H. (1991) in *Novel calcium-binding proteins* (ed. C. Heizman), Springer-Verlag, Berlin.

Kusaka, I. and Matsushita, T. (1987) Characterization of a Ca^{2+} uniporter from *Bacillus subtilis* by partial purification and reconstitution into phospholipid vesicles. J. Gen. Microbiol. **133**, 1337–1342.

Laoudj, D., Andersen, C. L., Bras, A., Goldberg, M., Jacq, A., and Holland, I. B. (1994) EGTA induces the synthesis in *Escherichia coli* of 3 proteins that cross-react with calmodulin antibodies. Mol. Microbiol. **13**, 445–457.

Lockau, W. and Pfeffer, S. (1983) ATP-dependent calcium transport in membrane vesicles of the cyanobacterium, *Anabaena variabilis*. Biochem. Biophys. Acta. **733**, 124–132.

Londesborough, J. (1986) Phosphorylation of proteins in *Clostridium thermohydrosulfuricum*. J. Bacteriol. **165**, 595–601.

Lynn, A. R. and Rosen, B. P. (1987) Calcium transport in prokaryotes. in *Ion transport in prokaryotes* (ed. B.P. Rosen and S. Silver), pp. 181–201., Academic Press, New York.

Mann, N. H., Rippka, R., and Herdman, M. (1991) Regulation of protein phosphorylation in the cyanobacterium *Anabaena* PCC 7120. J. Gen. Microbiol. **137**, 331–339.

Matsushita, T., Hirata, H., and Kusaka, I. (1988) Calcium channel blockers inhibit bacterial chemotaxis. FEBS Lett **236**, 437–440.

Matsushita, T., Hirata, H., and Kusaka, I. (1989) Calcium channels in bacteria: Purification and characterization. New York Acad. Sci. **560**, 426–429.

Munoz-Dorada, J., Inouye, S., and Inouye, M. (1993) Eukaryotic-like protein serine/threonine kinases in *Myxococcus xanthus*, a developmental bacterium exhibiting social behaviour. J. Cell. Biochem. **51**, 29–33.

Norris, V., Chen, M., Goldberg, M., Voskuil, J., McGurk, M., and Holland, I. B. (1991*a*) Calcium in bacteria: a solution to which problem? Mol. Microbiol. **5**, 775–778.

Norris, V., Baldwin, T. J., Sweeney, S. T., Williams, P. H., and Leach, K. L. (1991*b*) A protein kinase C-like activity in *Escherichia coli*. Mol. Microbiol. **5**, 2977–2981.

Ohyama, T., Igarashi, K., and Kobayashi (1994) Physiological role of the *chaA* gene in sodium and calcium circulations at a high pH in *Escherichia coli*. J. Bacteriol. **176**, 4311–4315.

Onek, L. A. and Smith, R. J. (1992) Calmodulin and calcium mediated regulation in prokaryotes. J. Gen. Micro. **138**, 1039–1049.

Onoda, T. and Oshima, A. (1988) Effects of Ca²⁺ and a protonophore on growth of an *Escherichia coli* L-form. J. Gen. Micro. **134**, 3071–3077.

Pettersson, A. and Bergman, B. (1989) Calmodulin in heterocystous cyanobacteria: biochemical and immunological evidence. FEMS Microbiol. Lett. **60**, 95–100.

Rampersaud, A., Utsumi, R., Delgaso, J., Forst, S.A., and Inouye, M. (1991) Ca²⁺-enhanced phosphorylation of a chimeric protein kinase involved with bacterial signal transduction. J.Biol. Chem. **266**, 7633–7637.

Rietveld, A.G., Killian, J.A., Dowhan W., and de Kruijff, B. (1993) Polymorphic regulation of membrane phospholipid composition in *Escherichia coli*. J. Biol. Chem. **268**, 12427–12433.

Rothärmel, T. and Wagner, G. (1995) Isolation and characterization of a calmodulin-like protein from *Halobacterium salinarium*. J. Bacteriol. **177**, 864–866.

Saha, A. K., Dowling, J. N., Mukhopadhyay, N. K., and Glew, R. H. (1988) Demonstration of two protein kinases in extracts of *Legionella micdadei*. J. Gen. Microbiol. **134**, 1275–1281.

Sandler, N., Dvir, A., Simon, A., Keynan, A., and Milner, Y. (1989) *7th International Conference on Cyclic Nucleotides, Calcium and Protein Phosphorylation*, Kobe, Japan.

Sherman, M. Y. and Goldberg, A. L. (1993) Heat shock of *Escherichia coli* increases binding of dnaK (the hsp70 homolog) to polypeptides by promoting its phosphorylation. Proc. Natl. Acad. Sci. USA. **90**, 8648–8652.

Shyu, Y. and Foegeding, P. M. (1989) Presence of calmodulin-like calcium-binding protein in *Bacillus cereus* T spores. FEMS Microbiol. Lett. **59**, 235–240.

Stevenson, M. A. and Calderwood, S. K. (1990) Members of the 70-kilodalton heat shock protein family contain a highly conserved calmodulin-binding domain. Molec. Cell Biol. **10**, 1234–1238.

Swan, D. G., Hale, R. S., Dhillon, N., and Leadlay, P. F. (1987) A bacterial calcium-binding protein homologous to calmodulin. Nature, **329**, 84–85.

Tisa, L. S., Olivera, B. M., and Adler, J. (1993) Inhibition of *Escherichia coli* chemotaxis by w-conotoxin, a calcium ion channel blocker. J. Bacteriol. **175**, 1235–1238.

Trombe, M.-C., Rieux, V., and Baille, F. (1994) Mutations which alter the kinetics of calcium-transport alter the regulation of competence in *Streptococcus pneumoniae*. J. Bacteriol. **176**, 1992–1996

van Veen, H. W., Abee, T., Kortstee, G. J. J., Konings, W. N., and Zehner, A. J. B. (1994) Translocation of metal phosphate via the phosphate inorganic transport system of *Escherichia coli*. Biochemistry **33**, 1766–1770.

Vyas, N. K., Vyas, M. N., and Quiocho, F. A. (1987) A novel calcium binding site in the galatose-binding protein of bacterial transport and chemotaxis. Nature **327**, 635–638.

Youatt, J. (1993) Calcium and Micro-organisms. Crit. Rev. Microbiol. **19**, 83–97.

■ *V., Norris*, M. Trinei, S. Atkinson, and D.J. Raine†:*
Department of Microbiology and Immunology, PO Box 138, University of Leicester, Leicester LE1 9HN, UK
†Department of Physics and Astronomy, University of Leicester, Leicester LE1 7RH, UK
Tel.: 44 116 2525094
Fax: 44 116 2525030
*E-mail: vjn@leicester.ac.uk

Ca²⁺-ATPase (Plasma membrane)

The plasma membrane Ca²⁺ ATPase (PMCA) or Ca²⁺ pump is an integral membrane protein which is present in all mammalian cells. It belongs to the family of the P-type ATPases. The pump transports Ca²⁺ ions out of the cells, by using the energy stored in ATP and is essential in the control of the Ca²⁺ concentration in the cytosol.

Indications for the existence of an ATP driven Ca²⁺ pump came from experiments with red blood cells (Schatzmann 1966). The observation that the pump was directly activated by calmodulin allowed its purification (Niggli *et al*. 1979) which was essential for its biochemical characterization. A large amount of experimental data has now been obtained on its functional domains (Carafoli 1994). The pump is a single polypeptide of 135–140 000 Da (approximately 1200 amino acids), anchored to the membrane by ten transmembrane domains (Fig. 1). The C-terminal portion of the pump contains the binding site for calmodulin (James *et al*. 1988) and other regulatory sites. Like other calmodulin-modulated proteins, the activity of

the pump is repressed in the absence of calmodulin and is stimulated by the binding of this protein.

As in other members of the P-type ATPase family, the PMCA protein forms a phosphoenzyme intermediate by transferring the γ-phosphate of ATP to an aspartic acid residue (D475, Fig. 1) in the catalytic site (Carafoli and Guerini 1993). The enzyme cycle is reversible, in fact, under certain conditions, the PMCA pump can form ATP from phosphate (Chiesi *et al*. 1984).

Amino acid sequences of the pump purified from red blood cell membranes, revealed the presence of two PMCA proteins (PMCA1 and PMCA4). These two isoforms can be considered the housekeeping pumps, whereby the

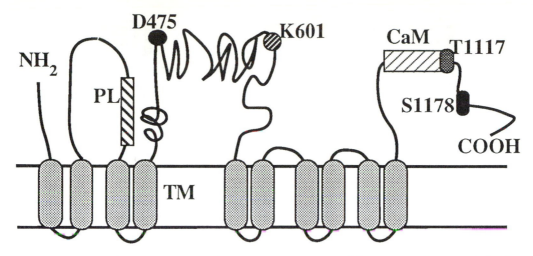

Figure 1. Schematic structure of the PMCA pump. Transmembrane domains (TM) are grey; PL: phospholipid binding domain; CaM: calmodulin-binding domain; D475: the aspartic acid involved in the catalytic cycle of the enzyme, to which the γ-P of the ATP is transiently transferred; K601: component of the ATP binding site; T1117: phosphorylation site by protein kinase C, S1178: phosphorylation site by protein kinase A.

products of the two other PMCA genes (PMCA2 and PMCA3) have a very restricted tissue distribution (Keeton *et al.* 1993; Stauffer *et al.* 1993). Overexpression of the PMCA4 and PMCA2 pump in the baculovirus system has revealed differences in the activation by calmodulin and in the formation of the enzyme intermediate (Hilfiker *et al.* 1994).

■ Alternative names

Plasma membrane Ca^{2+} ATPase (PMCA), plasma membrane Ca^{2+}-pump, calmodulin-dependent Ca^{2+}-pump, calmodulin-dependent Ca^{2+} ATPase (Carafoli 1994).

■ Identification and isolation

The PMCA pump protein was isolated from membranes of red blood cells (ghosts) (Niggli *et al.* 1979). The PMCA protein represents about 0.1% of the total protein of the ghosts. After solubilization of the membranes in Triton X-100 and stabilisation of the pump by the addition of phospholipids, the latter is purified by affinity chromatography on calmodulin-Sepharose. The Ca^{2+} pump can be specifically eluted by complexing the Ca^{2+} in the buffer. The protein isolated by this method is highly active and can be reconstituted as an active Ca^{2+}-transporting system in liposomes (Niggli *et al.* 1981).

■ Gene and sequences

Four different genes for the PMCA pump have been identified in the rat and in humans (Carafoli and Guerini

1993). In addition, a very complex pattern of alternative splicing at two different sites has been identified (Keeton *et al.* 1993; Stauffer *et al.* 1993; see Fig. 2). Complete cDNA sequences have been obtained for rat PMCA1, 2, 3; human PMCA1, 2, 4; pig PMCA1 (accession numbers: J03753, J03754, J05097, J04027, L20977, M25974, X53546). In addition, partial sequences for rat PMCA4, human PMCA3, and cow PMCA4 are available. The four human genes have been mapped to chromosomes 12 (q12–q23) (PMCA1), 1 (q25–q32) (PMCA4), 3 (3p26–p25) (PMCA2), and X (q28) (PMCA3) (Olson *et al.* 1991; Wang *et al.* 1994). The genes for rat PMCA3 (Burk and Shull 1992) and that for human PMCA1 (Hilfiker *et al.* 1993) have been characterized. The two genes contain particularly large introns at the 5' region. The promoter region of the human PMCA1 gene does not contain a TATA box, but elements typical for the housekeeping gene sequences are present. The gene structures of rat PMCA3 and human PMCA1 are very similar and most of the 22-(23) exons containing the coding sequence are identical in length. The only difference was observed in the exons which were involved in the alternative splicing and at the 5 ' end.

■ Protein

The PMCA protein consists of a single polypeptide of approximately 1200 amino acids. The variation in length arises mostly from alternative splicing processes (Carafoli and Guerini 1993; Carafoli 1994). The pump is composed of 10 putative transmembrane domains (Fig. 1), which are likely to form the putative Ca^{2+} channel (Carafoli and Guerini 1993), where the high affinity Ca^{2+}-binding sites

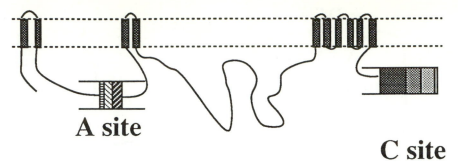

A site

C site

Figure 2. Alternative splicing. Two major sites of alternative splicing have been found, one located N-terminally (A site) and one C-terminally (C-site). The striped and shadowed boxes are sequences which can be inserted or omitted in the mature protein (additional combinations are possible). For a more detailed picture, see Carafoli and Guerini (1993).

must be located. It has been proposed that negatively charged amino acids in the transmembrane helices are involved in the Ca^{2+}-binding, but no known Ca^{2+}-binding motif has been found. The N-terminus and the C-terminus of the pump are in the cytosol (Carafoli 1994). The transmembrane domains are connected on the outside of the cells by very short loops, so that less than 5% of the protein sequence is exposed to the extracellular medium. 80% of the amino acids are located in the cytosol (Fig. 1): of these, about 100 precede the first transmembrane domain and about 160 follow the last. The two large cytosolic loops are located between transmembrane domains 2 and 3 (130 amino acids) and 3 and 4 (360 amino acids). Although the first loop is essential for the activity of the pump and contains a phospholipid-binding domain (Fig. 1), its role is not well defined. By contrast, the second loop contains the amino acids which are involved in the catalytic cycle of the pump (Fig. 1) (Carafoli 1994).

■ Antibodies

A monoclonal antibody (5F-10) against the human PMCA pump is now commercially available from Chemicon. This antibody recognizes the central region of the protein, (the epitope is located at the end of the second large cytosolic loop (Adamo et al. 1992)). Since this region is highly conserved in all isoforms and in the different organisms, this antibody recognizes the PMCA equally well in all mammalian tissues and species tested so far.

■ Biological function

The PMCA pump transports one Ca^{2+} ion per hydrolysed ATP (Carafoli 1994). The activity of the purified enzyme varies between 3000 and 5000 nmoles hydrolysed ÅTP/min . mg. The apparent K_m for Ca^{2+} is around 10 μM in the absence, and 0.4–0.5 μM in the presence, of calmodulin. Calmodulin also increases by 4 to 10 times

the V_{max} of the pump (Carafoli 1991). Alternatively, activation can be induced by the addition of acidic phospholipids (Niggli et al. 1981), by phosphorylation by protein kinase A and protein kinase C (James et al. 1989; Wang et al. 1991) or by proteolysis (Carafoli 1991). Since the neutral Ca^{2+}-dependent protease calpain can specifically remove the calmodulin binding site it was suggested that irreversible activation of the pump could occur *in vivo* (Carafoli 1991).

■ References

Adamo, H.P., Caride, A.J., and Penniston, J.T. (1992) Use of expression mutants and monoclonal antibodies to map the erythrocytes Ca^{2+} pump. J. Biol. Chem. **267**, 14244–14249.

Burk, S.E. and Shull, G.E. (1992) Structure of the rat membrane Ca^{2+}-ATPase isoform 3 gene and characterisation of alternative splicing and transcription products. J. Biol. Chem. **267**, 19683–19690.

Carafoli, E. (1991) Calcium pump of the plasma membrane. Physiol. Rev. **71**, 129–153.

*Carafoli E. (1994) Biogenesis: plasma membrane calcium ATPase: 15 years of work on the purified enzyme. FASEB J. **8**, 993–1002.

*Carafoli, E. and Guerini, D. (1993) Molecular and cellular biology of plasma membrane calcium ATPase. Trends in Cardivasc. Med. **3**, 177–184.

Chiesi, M., Zurini. M., and Carafoli, E. (1984) ATP synthesis catalysed by the purified erythrocyte Ca^{2+}-ATPase in the absence of calcium gradient. Biochemistry **23**, 2595–2600.

Hilfiker, E., Strehler, M.-A., Carafoli, E., and Strehler, E.E. (1993)Structure of the Gene encoding the human plasma membrane calcium isoform 1. J. Biol. Chem. **268**, 19717–19725.

Hilfiker, E., Guerini, D., and Carafoli, E. (1994) Cloning and expression of Isoform 2 of the human plasma membrane Ca^{2+}-ATPase. J. Biol. Chem. **269**, 26178–26183.

Keeton, T.P., Burk, S.E., and Shull, G.E. (1993) Alternative splicing of exons encoding the calmodulin-binding domains and C termini of plasma membrane Ca^{2+}-ATPase isoforms 1, 2, 3 and 4. J. Biol. Chem. **268**, 2740–2748.

James, P.H., Maeda, M., Fisher, R., Verma, A.K., Krebs, J., Penniston, J.T., and Carafoli, E. (1988) Identification and primary structure of a calmodulin binding domain of the Ca^{2+} pump of human erythrocytes. J. Biol. Chem. **263**, 2905–2910.

James, R.H., Pruschy, M., Vorherr, T., Penniston, J.T., and Carafoli, E. (1989) Primary structure of the cAMP-dependent phosphorylation site of the plasma membrane calcium pump. Biochemistry **28**, 4253–4258.

Niggli, V., Penniston, J.T., and Carafoli, E. (1979) Purification of the (Ca^{2+}-Mg^{2+})-ATPase from human erythrocyte membranes using a calmodulin affinity column. J. Biol. Chem. **254**, 9955–9958.

Niggli, V., Adunyah, E.S., Penniston, J.T., and Carafoli, E. (1981) Purified (Ca^{2+}-Mg^{2+}) ATPase of the erythrocyte membranes: reconstitution and effect of calmodulin and phospholipids. J. Biol. Chem. **256**, 8588–8592.

Olson, S., Wang, M.G., Carafoli, E., Strehler, E.E., and McBride, O.W. (1991) Localisation of two genes encoding plasma membrane Ca^{2+}-transporting ATPases to human chromosomes 1q25–32 and 12q21–23. Genomics **9**, 629–641.

Schatzmann, H.J. (1996) ATP-dependent Ca^{2+} extrusion from human red cells. Experientia Basel **22**, 363-368.

Stauffer, T.P., Hilfiker, H., Carafoli, E., and Strehler, E.E. (1993) Quantitative analysis of alternative splicing options of human plasma membrane calcium pump genes. J. Biol. Chem. **268**, 25993–26003.

Wang, K., Wright, L.C., Madian, C.L., Allen, B.G., Conigrave, A.D., and Roufogalis, B.D. (1991) Protein kinaseC phosphorylates the carboxyl terminus of the plasma membrane Ca^{2+}-ATPase from human erythrocytes. J.Biol.Chem **266**, 9078–9085.

Wang, M.G., Yi, H.-F., Hilfiker, H., Carafoli, E., Strehler, E.E., and McBride, O.W. (1994) Localisation of two genes encoding plasma membrane Ca^{2+}-ATPases isoforms 2 (ATP2B2) and 3 (ATP2B3) to human chromosomes 3p26 and Xq28, respectively. Cytogenet. Cell Genet. **67**, 41–45.

■ *Danilo Guerini and Ernesto Carafoli:*
Laboratory of Biochemistry III,
Federal Institute of Technology (ETH),
CH-8092 Zürich, Switzerland
Tel.: +41 1 632 31 42
Fax: +41 1 632 12 13

Calmegin

Calmegin is a cytosolic Ca^{2+}-binding protein abundant in specific stages of the development of male germ cells. Hypothetical functions in germ cells include Ca^{2+} storage and molecular chaperoning.

Mouse calmegin has a calculated molecular mass of 69 kDa, migrates on SDS-gels with an apparent molecular mass of 93 kDa and has an isoelectric point of 5.2. Calmegin has two sets of highly conserved repetitive amino acid sequences. One of them consists of four repeats of IPDPSAVKPEDWDD, and the other consists of four repeats of GEWXPPMIPNPXYQ. These repetitive sequences are also conserved in calnexin and calreticulin. Calmegin does not have domains containing EF-hand motifs.

■ Isolation/identification

A calmegin cDNA clone was isolated from a λgt 11 expression library using the monoclonal antibody TRA 369. This monoclonal antibody reacts specifically with mouse testicular germ cells in pachytene spermatocyte to spermatid stage (Watanabe *et al.* 1992). Purified recombinant calmegin produced in *E. coli* was tested in ^{45}Ca-overlay techniques and Western blots.

■ Gene and sequences

The whole sequence of the calmegin gene has not yet been published. The calmegin promoter region contains GC-rich sequences and potential binding sites for AP-2 and SP-1, but lacks the TATA sequence. The control locus of the specific expression of the calmegin gene in specific stages of germ cell differentiation is encoded in 152 base pairs at the 5′ flanking region. This has been deduced from studying tissue-specific expression in transgenic mice (Watanabe *et al.*, submitted for publication).

■ Protein

The deduced amino acid sequence of calmegin has two hydrophilic regions, one at the center and one at the COOH terminus of the amino acid sequence. The first contains two sets of highly conserved repetitive amino acid sequences. One of them consists of four repeats of IPDPSAVKPEDWDD, and the other consists of four repeats of GEWXPPMIPNPXYQ. This repetitive region contains a number of proline and highly charged amino acid residues (D,E,K). The second COOH-terminal hydrophilic region also contains a number of charged amino acid residues (D,E,K,R).

The computer-based analysis of the published nucleotides and amino acid sequences reveals significant homology (58% in amino acid) with dog calnexin (Wada *et al.* 1991), as well as partial homologies with calreticulin (Fliegel *et al.* 1989; Smith and Koch 1989) and with human Ro/SS-A autoantigen (McCauliffe *et al*. 1990). The hydrophilic internal repetitive amino acid sequences are located in this region. These common characteristic amino acid sequences are highly conserved in these proteins.

■ Antibody

A monoclonal antibody (TRA 369) was derived from hybridomas of rats immunized with mouse testicular germ cells by the histological selection method, using sections of testicles (Watanabe *et al*. 1992). The same antibody was used for the isolation of the calmegin cDNA.

■ Localization

TRA 369 has been used in studies on testicular germ cell differentiation. It is an excellent marker for germ cell differentiation since it reacts specifically with germ cells at pachytene spermatocyte to spermatid stage. It doesn't recognize any other somatic cells. In germ cells, calmegin occurs in the microsomal fraction.

■ Biological activities

The only known function of calmegin is its binding of Ca^{2+}. We postulate a role for this molecule as a molecular chaperone in the regulation of Ca^{2+}-dependent retention mechanisms for luminal proteins of the endoplasmic reticulum. It may also play a role in gene activation (Wada *et al*. 1991; Burns *et al*. 1994; Dedhar *et al*. 1994).

■ References

Burns, K., Duggan, B., Atkinson, E.A., Famulski, K.S., Nemer, M., Bleackley, R.C., and Michalak, M. (1994) Modulation of gene expression by calreticulin binding to the glucocorticoid receptor. Nature **367**, 476–480.

Dedhar, S., Rennie, P.S., Shago, M., Hagesteijn, C.-Y.L., Yang, H., Filmus, J., Hawley, R.G., Bruchovsky, N., Cheng, H., Matusik, R.J., and Giguere, V. (1994) Inhibition of nuclear hormone receptor activity by calreticulin. Nature **367**, 480–483.

Fliegel, L., Burns, K., MacLennan, D.H., Reithmeier, R.A.F., and Michalak, M. (1989) Molecular cloning of the high affinity calcium-binding protein (calreticulin) of skeletal muscle sarcoplasmic reticulum. J. Biol. Chem. **264**, 21522–21528.

McCauliffe, D.P., Zappi, E., Lieu, T.-S., Michalak, M., Sontheimer, R.D., and Capra, J.D. (1990) A human Ro/SS-A autoantigen is the homologue of calreticulin and is highly homologous with Onchocercal RAL-1 antigen and an Aplysia "memory molecule". J. Clin. Invest. **86**, 332–335.

Smith, M.J. and Koch, G.L.E. (1989) Multiple zones in the sequence of calreticulin (CRP55, calregulin, HACBP), a major calcium binding ER/SR protein. EMBO J. **8**, 3581–3586.

Wada, I., Rindress, D., Cameron, P.H., Ou, W., Doherty II, J.J., Louvard, D., Bell, A.W., Dignar, D.D., Thomas, D.Y., and Bergeron, J.J.M. (1991) SSRα and associated calnexin are major calcium binding proteins of the endoplasmic reticulum membrane. J. Biol. Chem. **266**, 19599–19610.

Watanabe, D., Sawada, K., Koshimizu, U., Kagawa, T., and Nishimune, Y. (1992) Characterization of male meiotic germ cell-specific antigen (Meg 1) by monoclonal antibody TRA 369 in mice. Mol. Reprod. Dev. **33**, 307–312.

Watanabe, D., Yamada, K., Nishina, Y., Tajima, Y., Koshimizu, U., Nagata, A., and Nishimune, Y. (1994) Molecular cloning of a novel Ca^{2+}-binding protein (Calmegin) specifically expressed during male meiotic germ cell development. J. Biol. Chem. **269**, 7744–7749.

■ *Yoshitake Nishimune:*
Research Institute for Microbial Diseases,
Osaka University,
Yamadaoka Suita, Osaka 565, Japan
Tel.: +81 6 879 8338
Fax: +81 6 879 8339
E-mail: nishimun@biken.osaka-u.ac.jp

Calnexin

Calnexin is one of the major Ca^{2+}-binding proteins of the endoplasmic reticulum (ER) membrane and has been demonstrated to interact transiently with nascent proteins. This membrane-bound chaperone is proposed to be directly involved in the quality-control mechanism of the ER.

Canine calnexin is a type I membrane protein with no oligosaccharide chain (Wada *et al*. 1991). Although the primary transcript of calnexin cDNA encodes for a 56,403 Da polypeptide, this acidic phosphoprotein migrates abnormally on SDS-PAGE and gives an apparent molecular mass of *ca*. 90 kDa.

Calnexin is found in the ER of virtually all eukaryotic cells including yeast (de Virgilio *et al*. 1993; Jannatipour and Rokeach 1995), plants (Huang *et al*. 1993), parasites (Hawn *et al*. 1993; Schue *et al*. 1994), and mammals (Wada *et al*. 1991; Galvin *et al*. 1992; David *et al*. 1993; Tjoelker *et al*. 1994). Calnexin binds transiently to newly synthesized membrane and soluble proteins that are destined for the secretory pathway (see Bergeron et al. 1994 for references). Most of the ligands are N-linked glycoproteins (Ou et al. 1993). Stable, if not permanent, complex formation has been reported with unassembled multi-subunits (Jackson et al. 1994; Rajagopalan et al. 1994) and misfolded proteins (Hammond et al. 1994; Loo and Clarke, 1994; Pind et al. 1994).

■ Alternative names

p88 (Degen and Williams 1991; Ahluwalia et al. 1992), IP90 (Hochstenbach et al. 1992; David et al. 1993), p93 (Gilchrist and Pierce 1993). Testicular specific calnexin-like proteins; calmegin (Watanabe et al. 1994), calnexin-t (Ohsako et al. 1994).

■ Identification/isolation

Calnexin was originally identified as one of the major phosphorylated proteins in the detergent phase of Triton X-114 extracted microsomes of dog pancreas and purified by a series of conventional column chromatographies

(Wada et al. 1991). $^{45}Ca^{2+}$ overlay blotting demonstrated that calnexin represented one of the major Ca^{2+}-binding proteins of microsomal membranes. Calnexin has also been identified by means of "Stains-All" and/or Ruthenium red staining of hepatic nuclear membranes (Gilchrist and Pierce 1993) and cardiac sarcoplasmic reticulum (Cala et al. 1993; Gilchrist and Pierce 1993). Functional identification of calnexin as a molecular chaperone has been made by crosslinking proteins in the extracts of cells which have been metabolically labeled with ^{35}S-methionine (Degen and Williams 1991).

■ Gene and sequence

Human calnexin is located on the distal end of the long arm of chromosome 5, at 5q35 (Tjoelker et al. 1994).

GenBank accession numbers of calnexin cDNA sequences are: for dog, X53616 (Wada et al. 1991); for human, L10284 (David et al. 1993) and M98452 (Galvin et al. 1992); for mouse, L18888 (Tjoelker et al. 1994); for rat, L18889 (Tjoelker et al. 1994); for Schistosoma mansoni, L08641 (Hawn et al. 1993); for Arabidopsis thaliana, Z18242 (Huang et al. 1993); for Saccharomyces cerevisiae,

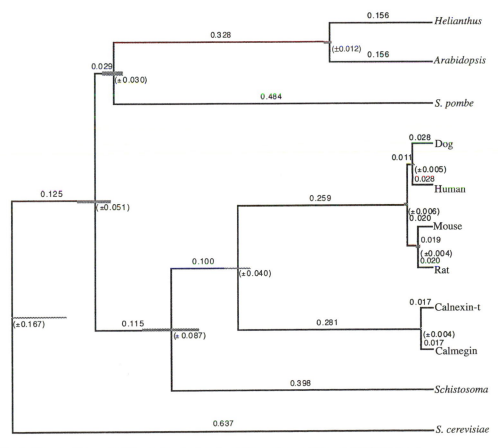

Figure 1. Evolutionary distance of the calnexin family at the amino acid level (UPGMA tree).

X66470 (de Virgilio *et al.* 1993); for *Schizosaccharomyces pombe,* U13389 (Jannatipour and Rokeach, 1995); and for mouse testis, U08373(calnexin-t) (Ohsako *et al.* 1994) and D14117(calmegin) (Watanabe *et al.* 1994) (Fig. 1).

Protein

Calnexin consists of a short cytoplasmic tail, a membrane-spanning domain and a large luminal domain containing two sets of four consecutive repeats (Fig. 2) (Wada *et al.* 1991; Tjoelker *et al.* 1994). When expressed as fusion proteins in *E. coli*, the first subdomain containing PXXIPDPXAXKPEDWDE repeats (Fig. 2, repeat 1) showed the highest binding to $^{45}Ca^{2+}$, whereas the second one containing GXWXPPXIXNPXYX (Fig. 2, repeat 2) did not bind $^{45}Ca^{2+}$ (Tjoelker *et al.* 1994). These two subdomains are also conserved in calreticulin, a major Ca^{2+}-binding protein of the ER lumen. The COOH-terminal six residues RKPRRE (human) are essential for ER retention (Rajagopalan *et al.* 1994; Tjoelker *et al.* 1994).

In vitro phosphorylation sites have been identified as Thr-[74] in the luminal domain and Ser-[535] or/and Ser-[545] in the cytoplasmic tail (Cala *et al.* 1993). Casein kinase II has been shown to be responsible for the phosphorylation *in vitro* (Ou *et al.* 1992).

Antibodies

Antibodies are commercially available through Stressgen.

Localization

In NRK (normal rat kidney) cells as well as in all cultured cells tested so far, calnexin has been immunolocalized to regions of reticular network concentrated around the nuclear periphery (Wada *et al.* 1991). Calnexin may be used as a marker for the ER.

While calnexin is thought to exist ubiquitously in all types of eukaryotic cells, two isoforms expressed specifically in testis have been identified (Ohsako *et al.* 1994; Watanabe *et al.* 1994).

Biological activity

Calnexin retains the unassembled multi-subunit complex in the ER (Jackson *et al.* 1994; Rajagopalan *et al.* 1994). Misfolded proteins, including the naturally occurring mutants, delta F[508] CFTR (Pind *et al.* 1994) or null_{Hong Kong} variant of a α1-antitrypsin (Le *et al.* 1994; Pind *et al.* 1994), form stable complexes with calnexin, thereby indicating a putative role for calnexin in their pre-Golgi retention. Although dissociation of nascent polypeptides from calnexin correlates with the progress of folding (Ou *et al.* 1993; Hammond *et al.* 1994; Hammond and Helenius 1994; Wada *et al.* 1994), the precise role of calnexin in the folding process is not known.

Interactions

The first observation of calnexin chaperone function was made during studies of the assembly of the major histocompatibility complex class I molecule (Degen and Williams 1991). Transient association has been reported with a wide array of soluble (Ou *et al.* 1993; Le *et al.* 1994; Wada *et al.* 1994) and membrane proteins (see Bergeron *et al.* 1994 for references) during the early stage of their maturation. While the dissociation process correlates with the event of proper folding (Ou *et al.* 1993; Hammond *et al.* 1994; Hammond and Helenius 1994; Wada *et al.* 1994), the association was abolished when glucosidases were blocked (Hammond *et al.* 1994). The latter finding, as well as an observation that calnexin (up to 60 min) associated stably with misfolded G protein tsO45[1] which possesses mostly monoglucosylated

---

[1] A temperature-sensitive mutant of VSV. Due to a single point mutation in the G protein, the newly synthesized mutant G protein remains in the ER at nonpermissive temperature.

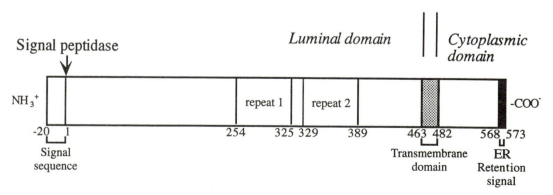

Figure 2. Schematic diagram of calnexin (canine).

oligosaccharides, led to the hypothesis that calnexin is a lectin with a specificity for monoglucosylated oligosaccharides (Hammond *et al.* 1994). This particular intermediate is continuously regenerated by the action of UDP:glucose glycoprotein glucosyltransferase until completion of folding of nascent chains (Sousa *et al.* 1992). When this hypothesis was directly tested, a weak but specific interaction with the $Glc_1Man_9GlcNAc_2$ oligosaccharides was found. However, endoglycosidase H treatment did not abolish the association (Ware *et al.* 1995). Therefore, calnexin has been proposed to be a polypeptide binding protein, the association being triggered by recognizing $Glc_1Man_9GlcNAc_2$.

■ References

Ahluwalia, N., Bergeron, J.J., Wada, I., Degen, E., and Williams, D.B. (1992) The p88 molecular chaperone is identical to the endoplasmic reticulum membrane protein, calnexin. J. Biol. Chem. **267**, 10914–10918.

Bergeron, J.J., Brenner, M.B., Thomas, D.Y., and Williams, D.B. (1994) Calnexin: a membrane-bound chaperone of the endoplasmic reticulum. Trends Biochem. Sci. **19**, 124–128.

Cala, S.E., Ulbright, C., Kelley, J.S., and Jones, L.R. (1993) Purification of a 90-kDa protein (Band VII) from cardiac sarcoplasmic reticulum. Identification as calnexin and localization of casein kinase II phosphorylation sites. J. Biol. Chem. **268**, 2969–2975.

David, V., Hochstenbach, F., Rajagopalan, S., and Brenner, M.B. (1993) Interaction with newly synthesized and retained proteins in the endoplasmic reticulum suggests a chaperone function for human integral membrane protein IP90 (calnexin). J. Biol. Chem. **268**, 9585–9592.

*Degen, E. and Williams, D.B. (1991) Participation of a novel 88-kD protein in the biogenesis of murine class I histocompatibility molecules. J. Cell Biol. **112**, 1099–1115.

de Virgilio, C., Burckert, N., Neuhaus, J.M., Boller, T., and Wiemken, A. (1993) CNE1, a *Saccharomyces cerevisiae* homologue of the genes encoding mammalian calnexin and calreticulin. Yeast **9**, 185–188.

Galvin, K., Krishna , S., Ponchel, F., Frohlich, M., Cummings, D. E., Carlson, R., Wands, J. R., Isselbacher, K. J., Pillai, S., and Ozturk, M. (1992) The major histocompatibility complex class I antigen-binding protein p88 is the product of the calnexin gene. Proc. Natl. Acad. Sci. USA **89**, 8452–8456.

Gilchrist, J. S. and Pierce, G. N. (1993) Identification and purification of a calcium-binding protein in hepatic nuclear membranes. J. Biol. Chem. **268**, 4291–4299.

Hammond, C. and Helenius, A. (1994) Folding of VSV G protein: sequential interaction with BiP and calnexin. Science **266**, 456–458.

*Hammond, C., Braakman, I., and Helenius, A. (1994) Role of N-linked oligosaccharide recognition, glucose trimming, and calnexin in glycoprotein folding and quality control. Proc. Natl. Acad. Sci. USA **91**, 913–917.

Hawn, T. R., Tom, T. D., and Strand, M. (1993) Molecular cloning and expression of SmIrV1, a *Schistosoma mansoni* antigen with similarity to calnexin, calreticulin, and OvRal1. J. Biol. Chem. **268**, 7692–7698.

Hochstenbach, F., David, V., Watkins, S., and Brenner, M. B. (1992) Endoplasmic reticulum resident protein of 90 kilodaltons associates with the T- and B-cell receptors and major histocompatibility complex antigens during their assembly. Proc. Natl. Acad. Sci. USA **89**, 4734–4738.

Huang, L., Franklin, A. E., and Hoffman, N. E. (1993) Primary structure and characterization of an *Arabidopsis thaliana* calnexin-like protein. J. Biol. Chem. **268**, 6560–6566.

Jackson, M. R., Cohen, D. M., Peterson, P. A., and Williams, D. B. (1994) Regulation of MHC class I transport by the molecular chaperone, calnexin (p88, IP90). Science **263**, 384–387.

Jannatipour, M. and Rokeach, L. A. (1995) The *Schizosaccharomyces pombe* homologue of the chaperone calnexin is essential for viability. J. Biol. Chem. **270**, 4845–4853.

Le, A., Steiner, J. L., Ferrell, G. A., Shaker, J. C., and Sifers, R. N. (1994) Association between calnexin and a secretion-incompetent variant of human alpha 1-antitrypsin. J. Biol. Chem. **269**, 7514–7519.

Loo, T. W. and Clarke, D. M. (1994) Prolonged association of temperature-sensitive mutants of human P-glycoprotein with calnexin during biogenesis. J. Biol. Chem. **269**, 28683–28689.

Ohsako, S., Hayashi, Y., and Bunick, D. (1994) Molecular cloning and sequencing of calnexin-t. An abundant male germ cell-specific calcium-binding protein of the endoplasmic reticulum. J. Biol. Chem. **269**, 14140–14148.

Ou, W. J., Thomas, D. Y., Bell, A. W., and Bergeron, J. J. (1992) Casein kinase II phosphorylation of signal sequence receptor alpha and the associated membrane chaperone calnexin. J. Biol. Chem. **267**, 23789–23796.

*Ou, W. J., Cameron, P. H., Thomas, D. Y., and Bergeron, J. J. (1993) Association of folding intermediates of glycoproteins with calnexin during protein maturation. Nature **364**, 771–776.

Pind, S., Riordan, J. R., and Williams, D. B. (1994) Participation of the endoplasmic reticulum chaperone calnexin (p88, IP90) in the biogenesis of the cystic fibrosis transmembrane conductance regulator. J. Biol. Chem. **269**, 12784–12788.

Rajagopalan, S., Xu, Y., and Brenner, M. B. (1994) Retention of unassembled components of integral membrane proteins by calnexin. Science **263**, 387–390.

Schue, V., Green, G. A., Girardot, R., and Monteil, H. (1994) Hyperphosphorylation of calnexin, a chaperone protein, induced by *Clostridium difficile* cytotoxin. Biochem. Biophys. Res. Commun. **203**, 22–28.

Sousa, M. C., Ferrero, G. M., and Parodi, A. J. (1992) Recognition of the oligosaccharide and protein moieties of glycoproteins by the UDP-Glc:glycoprotein glucosyltransferase. Biochemistry **31**, 97–105.

Tjoelker, L. W., Seyfried, C. E., Eddy, R. J., Byers, M. G., Shows, T. B., Calderon, J., Schreiber, R. B., and Gray, P. W. (1994) Human, mouse, and rat calnexin cDNA cloning: identification of potential calcium binding motifs and gene localization to human chromosome 5. Biochemistry **33**, 3229–3236.

Wada, I., Rindress, D., Cameron, P. H., Ou, W.-J., Doherty, J. J., Jr, Louvard, D., Bell, A. W., Dignard, D., Thomas, D. Y., and Bergeron, J. J. M. (1991) SSRa and associated calnexin are major calcium binding proteins of the endoplasmic reticulum membrane. J. Biol. Chem. **266**, 19599–19610.

Wada, I., Ou, W. J., Liu, M. C., and Scheele, G. (1994) Chaperone function of calnexin for the folding intermediate of gp80, the major secretory protein in MDCK cells. Regulation by redox state and ATP. J. Biol. Chem. **269**, 7464–7472.

*Ware, F. E., Vassilakos, A., Peterson, P. A., Jackson, M. R., Lehrman, M. A., and Williams, D. B. (1995) The molecular chaperone calnexin binds Glc1Man9GlcNac2 oligosaccharide as an initial step in recognition unfolded glycoproteins. J. Biol. Chem. **270**, 4691–4704.

Watanabe, D., Yamada, K., Nishina, Y., Tajima, Y., Koshimizu, U., Nagata, A., and Nishimune, Y. (1994) Molecular cloning of a novel Ca(2+)-binding protein (calmegin) specifically expressed during male meiotic germ cell development. J. Biol. Chem. **26**, 7744–7749.

■ Ikuo Wada:
Department of Biochemistry,
Sapporo Medical University School of Medicine,
West-17, South-1, Sapporo 060, Japan
Tel.: 81 11 611 2111, ex. 2294
Fax: 81 11 612 5861
E-mail: wada@cc.sapmed.ac.jp

Calreticulin

Calreticulin is a ubiquitous and highly conserved Ca^{2+}-binding/storage protein associated with endo(sarco)plasmic reticulum membranes. Calreticulin is a multifunctional protein implicated to play a role in a variety of cellular functions ranging from Ca^{2+} homeostasis to the control of gene expression.

Rabbit calreticulin has a calculated molecular weight of 46, 567 (for recent reviews on the structure, function, amino acid sequence and localization of calreticulin see Michalak *et al.* 1992; Sontheimer *et al.* 1993; Burns *et al.* 1994; Nash *et al.* 1994 and references within). The protein migrates on SDS gels with an apparent molecular mass of 60 kDa (at pH 8.0) or of 55 kDa (at pH 7.0). The molecular weight of calreticulin estimated by sedimentation equilibrium is 55,000. The isoelectric point of the human protein is 4.65–4.67 and the protein stains blue with "Stains-All". Calreticulin contains potential glycosylation sites; however, only bovine and rat liver proteins are shown to be glycosylated. In CHO cells calreticulin undergoes a heat shock-induced glycosylation (Jethmalani *et al.* 1994). Bovine calreticulin has one disulfide bridge (Cys120–Cys146: Matsuoka *et al.* 1994).

■ Alternative names

The high-affinity calcium binding protein; calregulin (CAB-3); CRP55; Ro/SS-A; ERp60; calsequestrin-like protein; CaBP3; p425; *Aplysia* p407 "memory molecule"; P-SG67 (Jethmalani *et al.* 1994).

■ Identification/isolation

Calreticulin can be isolated from a variety of tissues and cultured cells by the ammonium sulfate precipitation method (Baksh *et al.* 1992). The protein precipitates in the presence of >85% ammonium sulfate and it is further purified by a series of chromatographic steps including MonoQ FPLC and hydroxylapatite. Recombinant calreticulin was also produced in *E. coli* (rabbit: Baksh *et al.* 1992).

■ Gene and sequences

cDNAs encoding calreticulin were isolated from rabbit (GenBank accession number: J05138), mouse (X14926), human (M32294, M84739), rat (X53363, S56918), bovine brain (L13462), *Aplysia* (S51239), *C. elegans* (X59589), *Xenopus* (X67597, X67598), *D. melanogaster* (Smith *et al.* 1992: X64461), *S. mansoni* (M93097), and barley (Chen *et al.* 1994: L27349, L27348). The amino acid sequence of different calreticulins is extremely similar. mRNA encoding calreticulin (approx. 1.9 kb) has been identified in a variety of different tissues. Larger, 3.75 kb in length,

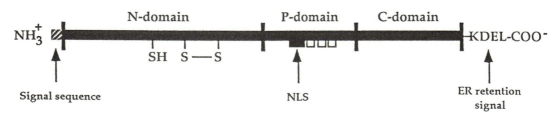

Figure 1. A schematic representation the various domains of calreticulin. Open boxes in the *P-domain* represent the PxxIxDPDAxKPEDWDE repeats. A putative nuclear localization signal (NLS) and disulfide bridge are shown.

mRNA can also be detected in some tissues. The human calreticulin gene exists in a single copy, occupies ~6 kd of genomic DNA and is localized to chromosome 19 (McCauliffe *et al.* 1992).

■ Protein

Calreticulin may be divided into distinct structural and functional domains (Fig. 1). The protein has an N-terminal signal sequence (Fig. 1). The *N-domain* (residues 7–180) is the most conserved domain among all calreticulins. This domain binds Zn^{2+} and interacts with the DNA-binding domain of the glucocorticoid receptor. Interestingly, the NH_2-terminal amino acid sequences of B50, mobilferrin, pvp2, and C1q receptor are similar to calreticulin. The *P-domain* (residues 180–280) is rich in proline and contains three sequence repeats of 17 amino acids (Fig. 1: open boxes). Two other ER membrane proteins contain similar amino acid repeats: calnexin (Bergeron *et al.* 1994) and calmegin (Watanabe *et al.* 1994). The *P-domain* contains the high affinity Ca^{2+} binding site (see below). This domain also contains a nuclear localization signal (NLS) (Fig. 1), which may be important in nuclear trafficking of the protein. The *C-domain* of calreticulin is very acidic and binds Ca^{2+}, Mg^{2+}, and Zn^{2+} with a relatively high capacity. This region may represent a Ca^{2+} storage site in the protein. The *C-domain* terminates with the KDEL ER retention signal and shares limited amino acid sequence similarities with calsequestrin and other ER resident protein of the KDEL family (PDI, BiP, endoplasmin). In the *O. vulvulus* calreticulin the *C-domain* is positively, rather than negatively, charged and does not terminate with the KDEL ER retention signal.

■ Antibodies

Anti-calreticulin antibodies are commercially available from Upstate Biotechnology, Inc.. This polyclonal antibody was raised in a goat and it recognizes rat, mouse, human, rabbit, *Aplysia*, and *Xenopus* calreticulin (Milner *et al.* 1991).

■ Localization

Calreticulin is found in every eukaryotic cell type (except for erythrocytes and yeast) so far examined, including plants. The protein is detected in high amounts in pancreas, liver, and testis, and in low amounts in muscle tissues. It is localized to endoplasmic reticulum (ER). By immunocytochemistry calreticulin is also found in the nuclear envelope, the nucleus, the acrosome of sperm cells, the cytotoxic granules in T cells, and neutrophil granules (Stendahl *et al.* 1994). Calreticulin can be isolated from human serum, suggesting that it may be secreted into the blood stream.

■ Biological activities

Purified calreticulin binds Ca^{2+} with high affinity and low capacity (K_d=~1 µM; B_{max}=1 mol of Ca^{2+}/mol protein: localized to the *P-domain*) and with low affinity and high capacity (K_d=~2 mM; B_{max} >25 moles of Ca^{2+}/mol of protein: localized to the *C-domain*). Calreticulin also binds Zn^{2+}, Fe^{3+}, and other metals. Recent reports indicate that the protein modulates steroid-sensitive gene expression (Burns *et al.* 1994) and affects adhesiveness of some cells (Leung-Hagesteijn *et al.* 1994). Calreticulin binds to blood clotting factors (factor IX, factor X, and prothrombin) and has antithrombotic activity. A chaperone function for the protein has also been suggested (Nauseef *et al.* 1995). Calreticulin has been proposed to be a human autoantigen associated with SLE and Sjögren's syndrome (Sontheimer *et al.* 1993). Antibodies against calreticulin are found in patients onchocerciasis (river blindness) caused by the filarial parasite *O. vulvalus* which expresses the RAL-1 antigen, a protein 64% homologous to calreticulin.

■ Biological regulation

The synthesis of calreticulin is induced in stimulated human and mouse T cells and the protein is localized to the lytic granules in cytolytic T lymphoctes, suggesting that it may play a role in the killing of target cells. Induction of expression of calreticulin (pvp2) was also observed in bovine papillomavirus type-I infected cells and in B16 melanoma cells. Amino acid starvation of the renal epithelial cell line NBL-1 leads to increased expression of calreticulin (Plakidou-Dymock and McGivan 1994). Cytomegalovirus-infected fibroblasts also express high levels of the protein (Zhu and Newkirk 1994). High levels of expression of calreticulin may be associated with actively proliferating cells.

■ Interactions

Many proteins have been shown to interact with calreticulin. The protein binds to the lung flavin-containing monooxygenase and interacts with the synthetic peptide KLGFFKR, which represents a highly conserved motif in the cytoplasmic domain of the α-subunit of the integrins. Calreticulin also interacts with the DNA-binding domain of glucocorticoid receptor. The protein binds to a set of low molecular weight proteins in the ER and the nucleus, via its *C-domain*. The identity of these membrane-associated proteins is not clear yet. Calreticulin interacts with perforin in the cytotoxic T-cell granules (Dupuis *et al.* 1993). Binding sites for Jaro spider toxin and anesthetic halothone have also been reported for calreticulin.

■ References

Baksh, S., Burns, K., Busaan, J., and Michalak, M. (1992) Expression and purification of recombinant and native calreticulin. Prot. Exp. Pur. **3**, 322–331.

Bergeron J.G.M., Brenner, M.B., Thomas,.D.Y., and Williams, D.B. (1994) Calnexin: a membrane-bound chaperone of the endoplasmic reticulum. TIBS **19**, 124–128.

*Burns, K., Atkinson, E.A., Bleackley, R.C., and Michalak, M. (1994) Calreticulin: from Ca²⁺ binding to control of gene expression. TICB **4**, 152–154.

Chen, F., Hayes, P.M., Mulrooney, D.M., and Pan, A. (1994) Identification and characterization of cDNA clones encoding plant calreticulin in Barley. Plant Cell, **6**, 835–843.

Dupuis, M., Schaerer, E., Krause, K.-H., and Tschopp, J. (1993) The calcium binding protein calreticulin is a major constituent of lytic granules in cytolytic T lymphocytes. J. Exp. Med. **177**, 1–7.

Jethmalani, S. M., Henle, K. J., and Kaushal, G. P. (1994) Heat shock-induced prompt glycosylation. Identification of P-SG67 as calreticulin. J. Biol. Chem. **269**, 23603–23609.

Leung-Hagesteijn, C. Y., Milankov, K., Michalak, M., Wilkins, J., and Dedhar, S. (1994) Integrin-mediated cell attachment to extracellular matrix substrates is inhibited upon downregulation of expression of calreticulin, an intracellular integrin α-subunit binding protein. J. Cell Sci. **107**, 589–600.

Matsuoka, K., Seta, K., Yamakawa, Y., Okuyama, T., Shinoda, T., and Isobe, T. (1994) Covalent structure of bovine brain calreticulin. Biochem. J. **298**, 435–442.

McCauliffe, D.P., Yang, Y.S., Wilson, J., Sontheimer, R.D., and Capra, J.D. (1992) The 5'-flanking region of the human calreticulin gene shares homology with the human GRP78, GRP94 and protein disulfide isomerase promoters. J. Biol. Chem. **267**, 2557–2562.

*Michalak, M., Milner, R.E., Burns, K., and Opas, M. (1992) Calreticulin. Biochem. J. **285**, 681–692.

Milner, R.E., Baksh, S., Shemanko, C., Vance, J.E., Carpenter, M., Smillie, L., Opas, M., and Michalak, M. (1991) Calreticulin, and not calsequestrin, is the major calcium binding protein of smooth muscle sarcoplasmic reticulum and liver endoplasmic reticulum. J. Biol. Chem. **266**, 7155–7156.

Nash, P.D., Opas, M., and Michalak, M. (1994) Calreticulin, not just another calcium binding protein. Mol. Cell. Biochem. **135**, 71–78.

Nauseef, W.M., McCormick, S.J., and Clark, R.A. (1995) Calreticulin functions as a molecular chaperone in the biosynthesis of myeloperoxidase. J. Biol. Chem. **270**, 4741–4747.

Plakidou-Dymock, S. and McGivan, J.D. (1994) Calreticulin—a stress protein induced in the renal epithelial cell line NBL-1 by amino acid deprivation. Cell Calcium **16**, 1–6.

Smith, M.J. (1992) Nucleotide sequence of a *Drosophila melanogaster* gene encoding a calreticulin homologue. DNA Seq. **3**, 247–250.

Sontheimer, R.D., Lieu, T.-S., and Capra, J. D. (1993) Calreticulin. The diverse functional repertoire of a new human autoantigen. Immunologist **1/5**, 155–160.

Stendahl, O., Krause, K.-H., Kirscher, J., Jerström, P., Theler, J.-M., Clark, R.A., Carpentier, J.-L., and Lew, D.P. (1994) Redistribution of intracellular Ca²⁺ stores during phagocytosis in human neutrophils. Science **265**, 1439–1441.

Watanabe, D., Yamada, K., Nishina, Y., Tajima, Y., Koshimizu, U., Nagata, A., and Nishimune, Y. (1994) Molecular cloning of a novel Ca²⁺-binding protein (calmegin) specifically expressed during male meiotic germ cell development. J. Biol. Chem. **269**, 7744–7749.

Zhu, J. and Newkirk, M. M. (1994) Viral induction of the human autoantigen calreticulin. Clin. Invest. Med. **17**, 196–205.

■ *Marek Michalak:*
MRC Group in Molecular Biology of Membranes,
Department of Biochemistry,
University of Alberta,
424 Heritage Medical Research Center,
Edmonton, Alberta,
Canada T6G 2S2
Tel.: 403 492 2256
Fax: 403 492 9753
E-mail: Marek.Michalak@ualberta.ca

Calsequestrin

Calsequestrin is the major Ca²⁺-binding protein in the sarcoplasmic reticulum (SR) of skeletal and cardiac muscle. It is concentrated in the terminal cisternae of the SR and suggested to function as a Ca²⁺-storage protein and to be involved in Ca²⁺ release by a mechanism not fully understood at present.

Calsequestrin (CS), a glycoprotein of the high mannose type, is expressed in isoforms specific to cardiac muscle (CSc) and fast-twitch skeletal muscle (CSs). CSc (dog heart) has a calculated molecular mass of 45,269 Da, migrates in SDS gels with an apparent molecular mass of 55 kDa at alkaline pH and 44 kDa at neutral pH, and has a calculated isoelectric point (pI) of 3.75 (Scott *et al.* 1988). CSs (rabbit) has a calculated molecular mass of 41,630 Da, migrates in SDS gels with an apparent molecular mass of 63 kDa at alkaline pH and 44 kDa at neutral pH, and has a calculated pI of 3.6 (Fliegel *et al.* 1987). CSs exhibits a Ca²⁺-dependent shift in SDS-PAGE. CS of either type becomes insoluble at Ca²⁺ > 0.4 mM, stains dark blue with Stains-all and red with Ruthenium red, stains with Schiff's reagent and binds concanavalin A. Ca²⁺-binding protects

CS against various proteinases. About 30% of the total amino acids of CSc and CSs are acidic residues, mainly concentrated within their carboxyl terminus. An even more acidic isoform has been cloned and sequenced from frog skeletal muscle with a calculated M_r of 45,941, 35% negatively charged residues and 77% amino acid sequence identity with rabbit CSs (Treves *et al.* 1992; X64324). The CSs transcript is the sole transcript in fast-twitch skeletal muscle and the major transcript in slow-twitch muscle, and is absent from cardiac muscle. The CSc transcript is the sole transcript in cardiac muscle and a minor transcript in slow-twitch muscle. It is absent from fast-twitch muscle. CS is also expressed in intestinal and vascular smooth muscle, chicken cerebellar neurons, and plant cells. In muscle, CS is localized within the terminal cisternae of the SR, close to the luminal site of the junctional membrane and in potential contact with the Ca^{2+}-release channels. It is suggested that it binds and stores rapidly exchangeable Ca^{2+} and contributes to the process of Ca^{2+} release by an as yet unknown mechanism.

Identification/isolation

Calsequestrin was identified and was originally purified from SR of rabbit fast-twitch skeletal muscle by MacLennan and Wong (1971). The original isolation procedure included extraction of isolated SR with sodium deoxycholate, fractionation of the extract with ammonium sulfate (CS precipitates only at ammonium sulfate saturation > 65%) followed by anionic exchange chromatography and gel-filtration. CS can be effectively extracted by various detergents and solutions that permeabilize SR vesicles. The most widely used are sodium deoxycholate and cholate, Triton X-100 or Na_2CO_3. Because it loses its hydrophobicity upon Ca^{2+}-binding, the protein can be precipitated from extracts with 4 mM $CaCl_2$ (Ikemoto et al. 1974) or purified by Ca^{2+}-dependent hydrophobic interaction chromatography on e.g. Phenyl-Sepharose (Cala and Jones 1983). The protein can also be isolated from total tissue homogenates by extraction with phosphate buffers and fractionation with ammonium sulfate (Slupsky et al. 1987). The cDNA encoding frog skeletal muscle CS has been expressed in COS-1 cells (Treves et al. 1992).

Gene and sequence

Two CS genes have been identified, one coding for cardiac CS and the other for fast-twitch muscle CS. The human CS genes have been assigned to chromosome 1 (CSc gene: bands 1p11–p13.3, CSs gene: band 1q21) (Fujii et al. 1990; Otsu et al. 1993). The existence of multiple cardiac CS-like sequences in the genome is suggested from analyses of canine genomic DNA (Scott et al. 1988). The sequence of dog cardiac CS (Scott et al. 1988; GenBank accession number: J 03766) and rabbit fast-twitch muscle CS (Fliegel et al. 1987) have 65% identity. CSc differs from CSs mainly by the following: its mRNA contains a second open reading frame that can code for a protein of 111 amino acids; it has an extended carboxyl terminus (residues 361–391) with 71% acidic residues containing a second glycosylation site (residues 376–378) and several consensus phosphorylation sites for casein kinase II (S378DEESN-DDSDDDDE-COOH) (Cala and Jones 1991). CSs is phosphorylated by casein kinase II at threonine 363. Conserved regions also detectable in frog skeletal muscle CS (Treves et al. 1992) are a glycosylation site at residues 316–318, five tryptophans within the carboxyl-terminal regions, and clusters of acidic residues throughout the sequence, but especially highly concentrated in the carboxy-terminal regions.

Protein

Sequence data do not support the presence of EF-hand domains or any related motifs that could provide defined Ca^{2+}-binding sites in CS isoforms. It has been proposed that the carboxy-terminal domain, containing the largest clusters of acidic residues, functions as a negatively charged surface that attracts Ca^{2+} electrostatically (e.g. Scott et al. 1988). Ca^{2+}-binding to CS causes the moving away of tryptophan residues from the solvent, and results in a large conformational change of the protein and in its loss of hydrophobicity (Ostwald and MacLennan 1974). The involved Ca^{2+}-regulated hydrophobic site has been assigned to residues 192–223 in CSc (e.g. Scott et al. 1988). Both rabbit skeletal muscle CS (Tanaka et al. 1986) and canine cardiac CS (Hayakawa et al. 1994) have been crystallized. The latter has been obtained in a monoclinic and a triagonal crystal form of X-ray quality, and initial analysis suggests the existence of a stable dimer. Secondary structure predictions on CS suggest a predominance of α-helix and β-sheet in the amino-terminal half of the molecule and a high potential for turn and coil conformations in the carboxy-terminal half (e.g. Scott et al. 1988). Hydropathy plot analysis suggests that there are no membrane-spanning domains.

Antibodies

Antibodies specific for cardiac muscle CS, which do not crossreact with fast-twitch skeletal muscle CS are commercially available through Swant.

Anatomical localization

CS is localized in the junctional SR of skeletal and cardiac muscle and concentrated at the cisternal site of the junctional membrane. An interaction between CS and junctional membrane elements (feet structures, Ca^{2+}-release channels) is suggested. CS seems to be also present in the corbular SR elements of cardiac muscle (Franzini-Armstrong and Jorgensen 1994, for recent review). CS isoforms have been detected in variable low concentrations in the endoplasmic reticulum of various smooth muscle tissues (Pozzan et al. 1994, for recent review). A chicken skeletal muscle isoform of CS is expressed in the endoplasmic reticulum of neurons of chicken cerebellum (Volpe et al. 1990). Until now this is the only certain evidence that CS is expressed in non-muscle tissue.

Biological activities

Purified canine cardiac and rabbit fast-twitch skeletal muscle CS were shown by equilibrium dialysis to have a comparable number of Ca^{2+}-binding sites (CSc, 35–40 mol/mol and CSs, 40–50 mol/mol) and similar binding affinities (K_d: 400–600 μM at 150 mM KCl and 100 μM at 20 mM KCl) (e.g. Mitchell et al. 1988). Sr^{2+} is bound with a comparable capacity at slightly higher affinity. CS of skeletal muscle has been shown to bind about 7 moles of Zn^{2+} per mole of protein with intermediate affinity (K_d: 15 μM) and 135 moles of Zn^{2+} per mole of protein with low affinity (K_d: 1.2 mM) (Ikemoto et al. 1974). The binding of Mg^{2+} and K^+ to CS has also been reported (e.g. Tanaka et al. 1986). The biological function of CS remains obscure. It has been suggested that the protein stores and concentrates Ca^{2+} near the junctional Ca^{2+}-release elements and participates in the regulation of Ca^{2+} release.

■ Biological regulation

The cardiac and skeletal muscle isoforms of CS are co-expressed in neonatal skeletal muscle and cultured myotubes. The synthesis of cardiac CS, which predominates, is turned off between two to four weeks post-natally. Cardiac muscle exclusively expresses cardiac CS at all stages of development. Gene expression in differentiating muscle seems to be under the control of the myogenic factor "myogenin" (Arai et al. 1992). CS is degraded with a half-life of about 23 h (Zubrzycka and MacLennan 1976). CS, a glycoprotein of the high mannose-type, was found to be a constituent of Golgi-derived clathrin-coated vesicles (CV). Secretion of CS has never been observed and selective CV-mediated transport of CS from the intermediate Golgi to the SR has been suggested (Thomas et al. 1989).

■ References

Arai, M., Otsu, K., MacLennan, D.H., and Periasamy, M. (1992) Regulation of sarcoplasmic reticulum gene expression during cardiac and skeletal muscle development. Amer. J. Physiol. **262**, C614–620.

*Cala, S.E. and Jones, L.R. (1983) Rapid purification of calsequestrin from cardiac and skeletal muscle sarcoplasmic reticulum vesicles by Ca^{2+}-dependent elution from Phenyl-Sepharose. J. Biol. Chem. **258**, 11932–11936.

Cala, S.E. and Jones, L.R. (1991) Phosphorylation of cardiac and skeletal muscle calsequestrin isoforms by casein kinase II. Demonstration of a cluster of unique rapidly phosphorylated sites in cardiac calsequestrin. J. Biol. Chem. **266**, 391–398.

Cala, S.E. and Miles, K. (1992) Phosphorylation of the cardiac isoform of calsequestrin in cultured rat myotubes and rat skeletal muscle. Biochim. Biophys. Acta **1118**, 277–287.

*Fliegel, L., Ohnisi, M., Carpenter, M.R., Khanna, V.K., Reithmeier, R.A.F., and MacLennan, D.H. (1987) Amino acid sequence of rabbit fast-twitch skeletal muscle calsequestrin deduced from cDNA and peptide sequencing. Proc. Natl. Acad. Sci. USA **84**, 1167–1171.

Franzini-Armstrong, C. and Jorgensen, A.O. (1994) Structure and development of E-C coupling units in skeletal muscle. Ann. Rev. Physiol. **56**, 509–534.

Fujii, J., Wilard, H.F., and MacLennan, D.H. (1990) Characterization and localization to human chromosome 1 of human fast-twitch skeletal muscle calsequestrin gene. Somat. Cell. Mol. Genet. **15**, 185–189.

Hayakawa, K., Swenson, L., Baksh, S., Wei, Y., Michalak, M., and Derewenda, Z.S. (1994) Crystallization of canine cardiac calsequestrin. J. Mol. Biol. **235**, 357–360.

Ikemoto, N., Nagy, B., Bhatnagar, G.M., and Gergely, J. (1974) Studies on a metal-binding protein of the sarcoplasmic reticulum. J. Biol. Chem. **249**, 2357–2365.

MacLennan, D.H. and Wong, P.T.S. (1971) Isolation of a calcium sequestering protein from sarcoplasmic reticulum. Proc. Natl. Acad. Sci. USA **68**, 1231–1235.

Mitchell, R.D., Simmermann, H.K.B., and Jones, L.R. (1988) Ca^{2+}binding effects on protein conformation and protein interactions of canine cardiac calsequestrin. J. Biol. Chem. **263**, 1376–1381.

Ostwald, T.J. and MacLennan, D.H. (1974) Effects of cation binding on the conformation of calsequestrin and the high affinity calcium-binding protein of sarcoplasmic reticulum. J. Biol. Chem. **249**, 5867–5871.

Otsu, K., Fujii, J., Periasamy, M., Difilippanto, M., Uppender, M., Ward, D.C., and MacLennan, D.H. (1993) Chromosome mapping of five human cardiac and skeletal muscle sarcoplasmic reticulum protein genes. Genomics **17**, 507–509.

Pozzan, T., Rizzuto, R., Volpe, P., and Meldolesi, J. (1994) Molecular and cellular physiology of intracellular calcium stores. Physiol. Rev. **74**, 595–636.

Sacchetto, R., Volpe, P., Damiani, E., and Margreth, A. (1993) Postnatal development of rabbit fast-twitch skeletal muscle: accumulation, isoform transition and fibre distribution of calsequestrin. J. Muscle Res. Cell Motil. **14**, 646–653.

* Scott, B.T., Simmerman, H.K.B., Collins, J.H., Nadal-Ginard, B., and Jones, L.R. (1988) Complete amino acid sequence of canine cardiac calsequestrin deduced by cDNA cloning. J. Biol. Chem. **263**, 8958–8964.

Slupsky, J.R., Ohnisi, M., Carpenter, M.R., and Reithmeier, R.A.F. (1987) Characterization of cardiac calsequestrin. Biochemistry **26**, 6539–6544.

Tanaka, M., Ozawa, T., Maurer, A., Cortese, J.D., and Fleischer, S. (1986) Apparent cooperativity of Ca^{2+}binding associated with crystallization of Ca^{2+}-binding protein from sarcoplasmic reticulum. Arch. Biochem. Biophys. **251**, 369–378.

Thomas, K., Navarro, J., Benson, R.J.J., Campbell, K.P., and Rotundo, R.L. (1989) Newly synthesized calsequestrin, destined for the sarcoplasmic reticulum, is contained in early/intermediate Golgi-derived clathrin-coated vesicles. J. Biol. Chem. **264**, 3140–3145.

Treves, S., Vilsen, B., Chiozzi, P., Andersen, J.P., and Zorzato, F. (1992) Molecular cloning, functional expression and tissue distribution of the cDNA encoding frog skeletal muscle calsequestrin. Biochem. J. **283**, 767–772.

Volpe, P., Alderson-Lang, B.H., Madeddu, L., Damiani, E., Collins, J.H., and Margreth, A. (1990) Calsequestrin, a component of the inositol 1,4,5-trisphosphate-sensitive Ca^{2+}-store of chicken cerebellum. Neuron **5**, 713–721.

Zubrzycka, E. and MacLennan, D.H. (1976) Assembly of the sarcoplasmic reticulum. Biosynthesis of calsequestrin in rat skeletal muscle cell cultures. J. Biol. Chem. **251**, 7733–7738.

■ *Claus Heilmann and Cornelia Spamer:*
Department of Gastroenterology,
University of Freiburg,
School of Medicine,
Hugstetter Str. 55,
D-79106 Freiburg,
Germany
Tel.: +49 761 270 3402
Fax: +49 761 270 3259

Crystallins

Crystallins are structural proteins that occur in high concentrations (up to 40% w/v) in the cytoplasm of eye lens cells. Four major groups of crystallins: α, β, and γ of the vertebrate lenses and δ-crystallin of all avian and reptilian lenses, have been distinguished based on size, charge, and immunological properties. The β- and δ-crystallins are Ca^{2+}-binding proteins (Sharma et al. 1989a; Balasubramanian and Sharma 1991). Since abnormal levels of Ca^{2+} (hypo- as well as hyper-) in the cytoplasm of lens cells have been implicated in cataractogenesis, Ca^{2+}-binding properties of these crystallins may have functional consequences in relation to lens transparency.

■ β-Crystallins

There are seven β-crystallins, each the product of a separate gene. Their molecular masses vary from 22 kDa to 32 kDa, and the N-terminus of all β-crystallins is blocked. They are classified into two groups, βA (acidic) and βB (basic), present in different multimeric forms and classified as βH (high molecular weight aggregate, about 200 kDa), βL1 (trimer) and βL2 (dimer).

■ Identification/isolation

β-Crystallins are purified from eye lens by gel filtration chromatography on Bio-Gel A-1.5m or Sephadex G-200 columns, as two different peaks (βH and βL). Further purification into the individual members is done using ion-exchange chromatography on FPLC with a Mono Q column (Slingsby and Bateman 1990).

■ Genes and sequences

In bovine β-crystallin, six or more chains are primary products, whereas some ten others arise by post-translational modifications. cDNAs have been sequenced for cow βA2 and βA4 (van Rens et al. 1991; EMBL accession no. M60329 and M60328), bovine βB1 (Quax-Jeuken et al. 1984; M11850), bovine βB2 (Hogg et al. 1987; M22466), human βB3 (Aarts et al. 1989; X15144), human βB2 (Aarts et al. 1989; X15144, X15146), human βA3/A1 (Hogg et al. 1986; M14301), human βB2 (Aarts et al. 1987; M18440, L10035), mouse βA3/A1 (Peterson and Piatigorsky 1986; M21472), mouse βB2 (Chambers and Russell, 1991; M60559), rat βB1 (den Dunnen et al. 1986; M13526), rat βB3 (den Dunnen et al. 1985; X05899), rat βA3/A1 (Aarts et al. 1989; X15143), chicken βA3/A1 (Peterson and Piatigorsky 1986; McDermott et al. 1992; M84460), chick βB1 (Hejtmancik et al. 1986; M11619), and for frog βA1 (Luchin et al. 1987; X06421).

■ Protein

β-Crystallin is a low affinity Ca^{2+}-binding protein which binds Ca^{2+} in the millimolar range. There is no EF-hand or helix–loop–helix motif in the amino acid sequence of any of its subunits (Sharma et al. 1989a). There is, however, one sequence rich in acidic amino acids which might act as a putative Ca^{2+}-binding site. βH-Crystallin was used in equilibrium dialysis experiments, and Ca^{2+}-binding sites and their affinities were measured. Ca^{2+}-ion binding can also be monitored by using lanthanide ions, such as terbium (Brittain et al. 1976); β-Crystallin binds terbium ions and, upon so doing, enhances the fluorescence quantum yield of the lanthanide. It also interacts with the Ca^{2+}-mimic carbocyanine dye "Stains-All", which changes colour upon binding to Ca^{2+} sites in the macromolecule. β-Crystallin binds Stains-all and generates the J band of the dye in the 610–620 nm region, just as the Ca^{2+}-binding protein parvalbumin does. The dye is released from the protein upon the addition of Ca^{2+} ions (Sharma et al. 1989b; Sharma and Balasubramanian 1991). Photolysis of β-crystallin, i.e. irradiation at 295 nm for extended periods, weakens its Ca^{2+}-binding ability (Sharma et al. 1993). It is not yet known whether any single subunit binds Ca^{2+} ions or whether the Ca^{2+}-binding site is located in the contacting interface of the supramolecular aggregate of β-crystallin.

The folding of the protein backbone (largely antiparallel β-sheet conformation) is highly symmetrical and forms four homologous motifs, organized into equivalent domains. Each motif is folded into a distinctive "Greek key" pattern (Bax et al. 1990). It has structural similarity with the *Myxococcous xanthus* spore coat protein S, a Ca^{2+}-binding protein, but the homology is not very strong in the region where protein S binds Ca^{2+} (Wistow et al. 1985; Bagby et al. 1994). Ca^{2+} binding does not appear to alter the conformation of β-crystallin markedly; however, Ca^{2+} binding induces a red shift in Trp fluorescence of the protein.

■ Anatomical localization

β-Crystallins are present intracellularly in the lens fibre cells.

δ-Crystallin

This protein is abundant in the lenses of almost all birds and reptiles, reaching levels of up to 70% of total protein in chicken and duck lenses. δ-Crystallin is highly homologous with argininosuccinate lyase (EC 4.3.2.1) (ASL), an enzyme of the urea cycle. δ-Crystallin is the product of two genes, δ1 and δ2. The gene product of δ2-crystallin is almost identical in its sequence to ASL, while δ1-crystallin shows significant variations; it neither binds the substrate nor displays ASL activity. The duck lens has considerable δ2-crystallin and has high ASL activity. In the chicken lens, however, the predominant protein is δ1-crystallin (less than 1% δ2), and ASL activity is negligible. Gene duplication thus may have allowed one copy of the δ genes, δ1, to code for a protein that has lost ASL activity, while maintaining its suitability as a lens structural protein (Piatigorsky et al. 1988; Bloemendal and de Jong 1990).

Identification/isolation

δ-Crystallin is purified from chicken lenses using a Sephacryl S-200 column in Tris buffer, pH 9.1 (Watanabe and Kawakami 1973; Narebor and Slingsby 1985), followed by DEAE-Sephadex chromatography. In SDS-PAGE, it shows two close bands of about 50 kDa molecular mass,

indicating the presence of δ1- and δ2-crystallins, the latter as a minor component.

Genes and sequences

The sequences of chicken δ1-crystallin gene (Ohno et al. 1985; EMBL accession no. X02222; Nickerson et al. 1985; M10806) and δ2-crystallin gene (Nickerson et al. 1986; M10806) have been determined and compared.

Protein

δ-Crystallin occurs as a tetrameric protein. Unlike α-, β-, and γ-crystallin, it is largely an α-helical protein. The crystal structure of δ-crystallin has recently been determined to a resolution of 2.5 Å (Simpson et al. 1994). Equilibrium dialysis studies have shown that each tetrameric molecule (the native form) has four Ca^{2+}-binding sites with K_d values of about 2 mM; each subunit has one site for Ca^{2+} binding. Whether Ca^{2+} binding affects the ASL activity of δ2-crystallin is not yet known. While the EF-hand or helix-loop-helix motif has been identified in the sequence of both δ1 and δ2 subunits, there is no Asp at the x coordinate of the loop region (Fig. 1). This protein also binds terbium ions, as well as

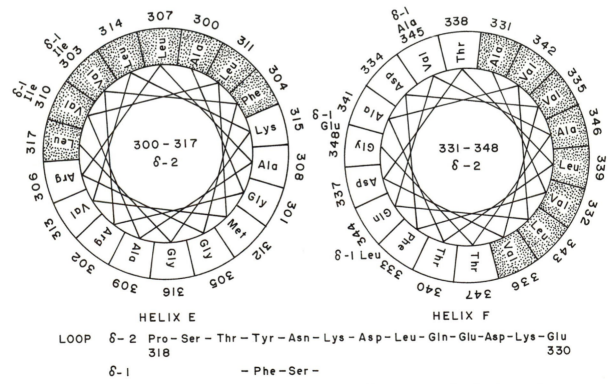

Figure 1. The helix wheel projection diagram of the δ1- and δ2-crystallin sequences, showing the putative amphiphilic helices E (residues 300–317) and F (331–348). The shaded region of the wheel is hydrophobic while the open region is largely polar. Other than the shown variations in the residues 303, 310, 321, 322, and 345, the two sequences are identical. The loop sequences are also shown. (Taken from Sharma et al. 1989a.)

Stains-All, and induces the g band of the dye near 500 nm, which is lost upon the addition of Ca^{2+} (Sharma et al. 1989b; Sharma and Balasubramanian 1991): Ca^{2+}-binding proteins with high helical conformation generate the g band of the dye, while those with the globular chain fold induce the J band.

■ Antibodies

Monoclonal antibodies specific to β-crystallins have been raised and have been useful in determining changes in crystallin profiles during development (Russell et al. 1985). Antibodies against pigeon lens δ-crystallin with low arginosuccinate lyase activity cross-react with enzymatically active δ-crystallins from duck lens (Chiou et al. 1992). No commercial preparations are available.

■ Anatomical localization

δ-Crystallin is abundantly present intracellularly in the fibre cells of the core region of eye lenses of avian and reptilian species.

■ Biological activities

δ2-Crystallin shows high level of argininosuccinate lyase activity while δ1-crystallin neither binds to the substrate nor displays activity. δ-Crystallin is an excellent example of heterologous recruitment of enzymes as structural proteins (Wistow and Piatigorsky 1987, 1988). Also, while δ-crystallin binds Ca^{2+} ions, this activity may or may not have any role in lenticular function.

■ References

Aarts, H.J., Den Dunnen, J.T., Lubsen, N.H., and Schoenmakers, J.G. (1987) Linkage between the βB2 and βB3 crystallin genes in man and rats: A remnant of an ancient β-crystallin gene cluster. Gene **59**, 127–135.

Aarts, H.J.M., Jacobs, E.H.M., Van Willingen, G., Lubsen, N.H., and Schoenmakers, J.G.G. (1989) Different evolution rates within the lens-specific β-crystallin gene family. J. Mol. Evol. **28**, 313–321.

Bagby, S., Harvey, T.S., Eagle, S.G., Inouye, S. and ikura, M. (1994) Structural similarity of developmentally regulated bacterial spore coat protein to β-crystallins of the vertebrate eye lens. Proc. Natl. Acad. Sci. **91**, 4308–4312.

* Balasubramanian, D. and Sharma, Y. (1991) Calcium binding crystallins. In *Novel calcium-binding proteins–fundamentals and clinical implications.* (ed. C.W. Heizmann), pp. 361–373. Springer-Verlag, Heidelberg.

Bax, B., Lapatto, R., Nalini, V., Driessen, H., Lindley, P.F., Mahadevan, D., Blundell, T.L., and Slingsby, C. (1990) X-ray analysis of β-crystallin and evolution of oligomeric lens proteins. Nature **347**, 776–780.

Bloemendal, H. and de Jong, W.W. (1990) Lens proteins and their genes. Prog. Nucleic Acids Res. Mol. Biol. **41**, 259–281.

Brittain, H.G., Richardson, F.S., and Martin, R.B. (1976) Terbium(III) emission as a probe of calcium(II) binding sites in proteins. J. Am. Chem. Soc. **98**, 8255–8260.

Chambers, C. and Russell, P. (1991) Deletion mutation in an eye lens β-crystallin. J. Biol. Chem. **266**, 6742–6746.

Chiou, S.H., Hung, C.C., and Lin, C.W. (1992) Biochemical characterization of crystallins from pigeon lenses: structural and sequence analysis of pigeon δ-crystallin. Biochem. Biophys. Acta **1160**, 317–324.

den Dunnen, J.T., Moormann, R.J., and Schoenmakers, J.G. (1985) Rat lens β-crystallins are internally duplicated and homologous to g-crystallins. Biochim. Biophys. Acta **824**, 295–303.

den Dunnen, J.T., Moormann, R.J., Lubsen, N.H., and Schoenmakers, J.G. (1986) Intron insertions and deletions in the β/γ-crystallin gene family: the rat βB1 gene. Proc. Natl. Acad. Sci. USA, **83**, 2855–2859.

Hejtmancik, J.F., Thompson, M.A., Wistow, G., and Piatigorsky, J. (1986) cDNA and deduced protein sequence for the βB1-crystallin polypeptide of the chicken lens: Conservation of the PAPA sequence. J. Biol. Chem. **261**, 982–987.

Hogg, D., Tsui, L.C., Gorin, M.B., and Breitman, M.L. (1986) Characterization of the human β-crystallin gene Hu-beta-A3/A1 reveals ancestral relationships among the βγ-crystallin superfamily. J. Biol. Chem. **261**, 12420–12427.

Hogg, D., Gorin, M.B., Heizmann, C., Zollmann, S., Mohandas, T., Klisak, I., Sparkes, R.S., Breitman, M., Tsui, L.C., and Horwitz, J. (1987) Nucleotide sequence for the cDNA of the bovine βB2-crystallin and assignment of the orthologous human locus to chromosome 22. Curr. Eye Res. **6**, 1335–1342.

Luchin, S.V., Zinovieva, R.D., Tomarev, S.I., Dolgilevich, S.M., Gause, G.G., Bax, J.B., Driessen, H., and Blundell, T.L. (1987) Frog lens βA1 crystallin: the nucleotide sequence of the cloned cDNA and computer graphics modelling of the three-dimensional structure. Biochim. Biophys. Acta **916**, 163–171.

McDermott, J.B., Peterson, C.A., and Piatigorsky, J. (1992) Structure and lens expression of the gene encoding chicken beta A3/A1-crystallin. Gene **117**, 193–200.

Narebor, E.M. and Slingsby, C. (1985) Characterization and crystallization of δ-crystallin from adult quail and young chick. Exp. Eye Res. **40**, 273–283.

Nickerson, J.M., Wawrousek, E.F., Hawkins, J.W., Wakil, A.S., Wistow, G.J., Thomas, G., Norman, B.L., and Piatigorsky, J. (1985) The complete sequence of the chicken δ1 crystallin gene and its 5' flanking region. J. Biol. Chem. **260**, 9100–9105.

Nickerson, J.M., Wawrousek, E.F., Borras, T., Hawkins, J.W., Norman, B.L., Filpula, D.R., Nagle, J.W., Ally, A.H., and Piatigorsky, J. (1986) Sequence of the chicken δ2 crystallin gene and its intergenic spacer. J. Biol. Chem. **261**, 552–557.

Ohno, M., Sakamoto, H., Yasuda, K., Okada, T.S., and Shimura, Y. (1985) Nucleotide sequence of a chicken δ-crystallin gene. Nucleic Acids Res. **13**:1593–1606.

Peterson, C.A. and Piatigorsky, J. (1986) Preferential conservation of the globular domains of the beta A3/A1-crystallin polypeptide of the chicken eye lens. Gene **45**, 139–147.

Piatigorsky, J., O'Brien, W.E., Norman, B.L., Kalumuk, D., Wistow, G.J., Borras, T., Nickerson, J.M., and Waweousek, E.F. (1988) Gene sharing by δ-crystallin and argininosuccinate lyase. Proc. Natl. Acad. Sci. USA, **85**, 3479–3483.

Quax-Jeuken, Y.E.F.M., Janssen, C., Quax, W.J., van den Heuvel, R., and Bloemendal, H. (1984) Bovine β-crystallin complementary DNA clones. J. Mol. Biol. **180**, 457–472.

Russell, P., Carper, D.A., Chiogioji, A., and Reddy, V. (1985) The comparison of human lens crystallins using three monoclonal antibodies. Invest. Ophthal. Vis. Sci. **26**, 1028–1031.

Sharma, Y. and Balasubramanian, D. (1991) Stains-all is a dye that probes the conformational features of calcium binding proteins. In *Novel calcium-binding proteins–fundamentals and clinical implications* (ed. C.W. Heizmann), pp. 51–61. Springer-Verlag, Heidelberg.

Sharma, Y., Rao, C.M., Narasu, M.L., Rao, S.C., Somasundaram, T., Gopalakrishna, A., and Balasubramanian, D. (1989a) Calcium ion binding to δ- and to β-crystallins. The presence of "EF-hand" motif in δ-crystallin that aids in calcium ion binding. J. Biol. Chem. **264**, 12794–12799.

Sharma, Y., Rao, C.M., Rao, S.C., Somasundaram, T., Gopalakrishna, A., and Balasubramanian, D. (1989b) Binding site conformation dictates the color of the dye Stains-all. A study of the binding of this dye to the eye lens proteins crystallins. J. Biol. Chem. **264**, 20923–20927.

Sharma, Y., Gopalakrishna, A., and Balasubramanian, D. (1993) Alteration of dynamic quaternary structure and calcium binding ability of β-crystallin by light. Photochem. Photobiol. **57**, 739–743.

* Simpson, A., Bateman, O., Driessen, H., Lindley, P., Moss, D., Mylvaganam, S., Narebor, E., and Slingsby, C. (1994) The structure of avian eye lens δ-crystallin reveals a new fold for a superfamily of oligomeric enzymes. Nature Struct. Biol. **1**, 724–734.

Slingsby. C. and Bateman, O.A. (1990) Rapid separation of bovine b-crystallin subunits βB1, βB2, βB3, βA3 and βA4. Exp. Eye Res. **51**, 21–26.

van Rens, G.L., Driessen, H.P., Nalini, V., Slingsby, C., de Jong, W.W., and Bloemendal, H. (1991) Isolation and characterization of cDNAs encoding βA2 and βA4-crystallins: Heterologous interactions in the predicted βA4-βB2 heterodimer. Gene **102**, 179–188.

Watanabe, H. and Kawakami, I. (1973) Fractionation of the soluble proteins of chick lens on Sephadex column. Exp. Eye Res. **17**, 205–207.

Wistow, G.J. and Piatigorsky, J. (1987) Recruitment of enzymes as lens structural proteins. Science **236**, 1554–1556.

Wistow, G.J. and Piatigorsky, J. (1988) Lens crystallins: The evolution and expression of proteins for a highly specialized tissue. Ann. Rev. Biochem. **57**, 497–504.

* Wistow, G., Summers, L., and Blundell, T. (1985) Myxococcus xanthus spore coat protein S may have a similar structure to vertebrate lens βγ-crystallins. Nature **315,** 771–773.

■ *Yogendra Sharma and Dorairajan Balasubramanian:*
Centre for Cellular and Molecular Biology (CCMB),
Uppal Road,
Hyderabad-500 007, India
Tel.: 91 40 673487
Fax: 91 40 671195
E-mail: dbala@ccmb.uunet.in

ER calcistorin/Protein disulfide isomerase (ECaSt/PDI)

ER calcistorin/Protein disulfide isomerase (ECaSt/PDI), identified in the endoplasmic reticulum (ER) of the sea urchin egg, is a high capacity, low affinity Ca^{2+}-binding protein which also has PDI activity. The molecule apparently has a dual function of Ca^{2+} storage and PDI activity in the ER of the sea urchin egg.

A 58 kDa calsequestrin-like protein was purified and partially characterized from microsomal fractions of sea urchin eggs (Oberdorf *et al.* 1988). Immunostaining of whole eggs demonstrated its diffuse distribution in the ER (Henson *et al.* 1989). Subsequent studies on Ca^{2+} binding, Ca^{2+}-induced conformational changes, and determination of its N-terminal sequence indicated its uniqueness (Lebeche and Kaminer 1992). From the cDNA sequence encoding this protein the deduced 496 amino acids contain a 17-residue NH2-terminal signal peptide and a KDEL COOH-terminal retention signal indicative of an ER-resident protein. Two thioredoxin-like domains, CGHC, are identical with those in mammalian PDI, and the sea urchin egg protein shares a 55% sequence identity with mammalian PDI. The enzyme activity of the protein purified from the eggs as described (Lucero *et al.* 1994) is 30% of that of the mammalian molecule.

■ Alternative names

58 kDa calsequestrin-like protein (Oberdorf *et al.* 1988; Henson *et al.* 1989; Lebeche and Kaminer 1992).

■ Isolation, purification, and cloning

Sea urchin species used *were Strongylocentrotus droebachiensis* and *Arbacia punctulata.* Dejellied eggs were washed in a buffered solution and homogenized, and a relatively pure microsomal fraction was obtained by differential centrifugation. Purification of the protein from isolated microsomes was attained by using DEAE (DE-52) and hydroxyapatite columns. The pure protein was identified on SDS gels stained with Stains-All (Oberdorf *et al.* 1988). The cDNA encoding this protein was cloned by immunoscreening from a cDNA expression library constructed from embryos obtained 4 h after fertilization and sequenced by conventional methods (Lucero *et al.* 1994).

Gene and sequence

The nucleotide sequence of the cDNA was submitted to GenBank (accession number UO6484). The cDNA transfected into Cos-7 cells was transcribed into the corresponding mRNA and detected by Northern blotting. A protein, immunoreactive with the antibody against the 58 kDa protein, was expressed in a crude membrane fraction of the transfected cells (Lucero et al. 1994).

Protein

The SDS electrophoretic mobility of the protein from the sea urchin egg is pH-dependent. Its molecular mass is 58 kDa under alkaline conditions (Laemmli) and 54 kDa at neutral pH (Weber-Osborn). The band on SDS gels stains blue with the carbocyanine dye Stains-All, as do calsequestrin and other Ca^{2+}-binding proteins. The 58 kDa molecule is a glycoprotein containing 8–9 glucose and 7–8 mannose residues per mol of protein (Lebeche and Kaminer 1992). It contains 25% acidic residues, and arginine and lysine constitute 10% of its amino acids, the composition of which, in general, resembles that of calsequestrin (Oberdorf et al. 1988). Ca^{2+} binding, however, induces UV difference spectra and intrinsic fluorescence changes in a direction opposite to those induced in calsequestrin. The N-terminal sequence is distinct from that in calsequestrin and is unique (Lebeche and Kaminer 1992).

Antibodies

A monospecific rabbit antiserum against the sea urchin protein has been produced (Oberdorf et al. 1988).

Localization

Immunostaining shows a diffuse distribution of the 58 kDa protein in the ER of the sea urchin egg (Henson et al. 1989). The corresponding mRNA, detected by Northern blotting, is found in oocytes, mature eggs, embryos, and differentiated tissues of the sea urchin in varying amounts (Lucero et al. 1994).

Biological activities

ECaSt/PDI has two putative functions, namely Ca^{2+} storage and PDI activity within the ER. The molecule binds 23 moles Ca^{2+} per mole of protein, as determined by equilibrium dialysis, with half-maximal binding values of 1.62 to 5.77 mM, depending on the ionic strength. Hill coefficients indicate mild binding cooperativity (Lebeche and Kaminer 1992). The number of paired carboxylic groups which are postulated to be the main Ca^{2+} low affinity binding sites, correspond approximately with the number of Ca^{2+} ions bound (Lucero et al. 1994). Similar Ca^{2+}-binding parameters were found in rabbit liver PDI: 19 moles Ca^{2+} bound per mole of protein with low affinity; half saturation values were 2.77 to 5.20 mM. Ca^{2+}-induced conformational changes were also similar (Lebeche et al. 1994).

The PDI activity of ECaSt/PDI was assayed by the reactivation of inactivated reduced RNase and scrambled RNase and also by measuring glutathione insulin transhydrogenase. The enzyme activities were about 30% of those of mammalian PDI (Lucero et al. 1994).

References

*Henson, J.H., Begg, D.A., Beaulieu, S.M., Fishkind, D.J., Bonder, E.M., Terasaki, M., Lebeche, D., and Kaminer, B. (1989) A calsequestrin-like protein in the endoplasmic reticulum of the sea urchin; localization and dynamics in the egg and first cell cycle embryo. J. Cell Biol. **109**, 149–161.

*Lebeche, D. and Kaminer, B. (1992) Characterization of a calsequestrin-like protein from sea urchin eggs. Biochem. J. **287**, 741–747.

Lebeche, D., Lucero, H.A., and Kaminer, B. (1994) Calcium binding properties of rabbit liver protein disulfide isomerase. Biochem. Biophys Res. Comm. **202**, 556–561.

Lucero, H.A., Lebeche, D., and Kaminer, B. (1994) ERcalcistorin/Protein disulfide isomerase (PDI): sequence determination and expression of a cDNA clone encoding a calcium storage protein with PDI activity from endoplasmic reticulum of the sea urchin egg. J. Biol. Chem. **269**, 23112–23119.

Oberdorf, J.A., Lebeche, D., Head, J., and Kaminer, B. (1988) Identification of a calsequestrin-like protein from sea urchin eggs. J. Biol. Chem. **263**, 6806-6809.

■ Hector Lucero, Djamel Lebeche, Benjamin Kaminer:
Department of Physiology,
Boston University School of Medicine,
80 E, Concord St., Boston, MA 02118 USA
Tel.: 617 638 4392
Fax: 617 638 4273
E-mail: bkaminer@acs.bu.edu

Appendix: List of companies selling antibodies

Name	Address	Tel. No.	Fax
Affinity Bioreagents Inc. email: affinity@bioreagents.com	14818 West 6th Ave. 13A Golden CO 80401	+1 303 278 4535	+1 303 278 2424
Alexis Corp.	P.O. Box 927190 San Diego CA 92192-7190	+1 619 658 0065	+1 619 658 9224
Biodesign International	105 York St. Kennebunk ME 04043 USA	+1 207 985 1944	+ 1 207 985 6322
Boehringer Mannheim Biochemicals	P.O. Box 50414 Indianapolis IN 46250-0414 USA	+1 800 262 1640	+1 317 576 2754
Biomedical Technologies	378 Page St. Stoughton MA 02072 USA	+1 617 344 9942 +1 800 854 3417	+1 617 341 1451
Calbiochem-Novabiochem Int.	P.O. Box 12087 La Jolla CA 92039-2087 USA	+1 619 450 9600	+1 800 776 0999
Chemicon International	28835 Single Oak Dr. Temecula CA 92590 USA	+1 909 676 8080 +1 800 437 7500	+1 909 676 9209
Dako A/S	Produktionvej 42 P.O. Box 1359 DK-2600 Glostrup Denmark	+45 44 920044	+45 42 841822
Dianova-Immunotech GmbH	Postfach 101705 Raboisen 5 D-2000 Hamburg 1 Germany	+49 40 32 30 74	+49 40 32 21 90
East-Acres Biologicals	Box 727 236 Blackmer Rd. Southbridge MA 01550 USA	+1 508 765 9580	+1 508 765 1288
ICN Immunologicals	3300 Hyland Ave. Costa Mesa CA 92626 USA	+1 714 545 0113 +1 800 854 0530	+1 714 557 4872 +1 800 334 6999
Santa Cruz Biotechnology Inc.	2161 Delaware Ave. Santa Cruz CA 95060 USA	+1 408 457 3800 +1 800 457 3801	+1 408 457 3801

Name	Address	Tel. No.	Fax
Serotec LTD.	22 Bankside Station field Indust. Est. Kidlington Oxford OX5 1JE England	+44 865 379 941	+44 865 373 899
Sigma Chemicals	P.O. Box 14508 St. Louis MO 63178 USA	+1 314 771 5765 +1 800 325 3010	+1 800 325 5052
Stressgen Biotechnologies email: info@stressgen.com	120-4243 Glanford Ave. Victoria BC V8Z 4B9 Canada	+1 604 744 2811	+1 604 744 2877
Swant http://www.swant.com email: info@swant.com	P.O. Box 2660 CH-6500 Bellinzona Switzerland	—	+41 91 825 76 08
Upstate Biotechnology Inc.	1601 Trapelo Rd. Waltham MA 02154 USA	+1 617 890 8845	+1 617 890 7738
Zymed Laboratories	458 Carlton Court South San Francisco CA 94080 USA	+1 415 871 4494 +1 800 874 4494	+1 415 871 4499

Index

18A2 132, 139, 141

29 kDa protein 26, 28
2A9 132, 143

32.5 calelectrin 192
35 α calcimedin 190
35 β calcimedin 192
35-g-calcimedin 194
35 kDa calelectrin 182, 194
36K phosphoprotein 187

42A 132, 139, 141
42C 132, 149, 150

5B10 132, 143
58 kDa calsequestrin-like protein 228

60B8Ag 132
67 kDa-calcimedin 198
67 kDa-calelectrin 198

73K 198

9 kDa calcium-binding protein 157
9 kDa cholecalcin 157

actin 16, 21–3, 48, 58–62, 71–2, 90–3, 134, 140, 149, 151, 154, 161, 172–5, 177, 183, 190, 199
  α 16, 21, 22, 58
  binding proteins 58, 88, 97, 107, 109, 154, 172–3, 177
  f 48, 172, 173, 187, 188
  filament 21, 22, 90–1, 189
adaptation 114–18, 135
adrenal medulla 181, 183, 199
aequorin 16–18, 58, 60–5
alkali LC 88
alpha-actinin 21, 22
αSp 172, 174
alternative splicing 26, 28, 29, 30, 31, 88, 200, 205, 213–15
Alzheimer's disease 19, 24, 154

amphioxus 2, 9, 10, 12, 59, 60–1, 63, 65, 66–7, 71–3, 78–80
anchorin CII 194
annexin 151, 181, 183–4, 186, 189, 191–2, 197, 199, 205
annexin I 144–5, 149–51, 156, 181–95, 198, 201
annexin II 151, 181, 183, 187–91
annexin III 190–1
annexin IV 192–3
annexin V 194–8
annexin VI 29, 181, 198–205
annexin VII 181, 183, 200–4
annexin XI 205–6
anticoagulant protein III 190
anticoagulant protein IV 187
anti-phospholipase A$_2$ 190–1, 193
antithrombotic activity 221
Aplysia p407 "memory molecule" 220
Arabidopsis 35, 41–3, 47–8, 74, 217, 219
astrocyte 170, 172, 174
autoimmune disease 96, 206
autoproteolysis 43
avian thymic hormone 16, 129, 130
axon 44, 68, 69, 84, 85, 108, 112, 114, 154, 172–5, 199, 200

BABP 172, 175
bacterial 34, 61, 80, 87, 108, 131, 148, 160, 209, 210, 211, 212, 227
basal bodies 49–51, 59, 87
bdr-1 111
biliary cirrhosis 144
bioluminescence 60, 62, 65
BM-40 169–71
brain 9, 17, 24–8, 30–2, 44, 52–3, 76, 79, 94, 98–102, 104–14, 120, 123, 135–6, 141, 143, 152, 154, 167, 169, 171–5, 193, 200–1
brain actin-binding protein 172
breast 41, 42, 134, 137
βSp 172–4

Ca[1] 149
Caenorhabditis elegans 41, 94, 96–7, 110–13, 117–18, 170
CaBP 1–10, 23, 27–8, 41–3, 58–60, 69, 70, 78, 84, 107, 132, 143
  CaBP3 220

CABP9k 10, 157–9
CaBP-22 41, 42, 43
CACY 1–2, 12, 136, 140–1, 143–5
cal-1 41
calbindin 8–9, 19, 23–5, 28, 125, 132, 157, 159, *see also* calretinin
  calbindin D-28k 16–19, 23–4, 26–7, 122, 130, 131
  calbindin-D9k 18, 157–9
calcineurin 18–20, 30–2, 39, 58, 87, 94, 105–6
calcitriol 157–9, *see also* Vitamin D3
calcium (Ca^{2+})
  ATPase 39, 212
  buffer 80
  channel 197–8, 200, 202, 209–11
  conformational change 10, 151, 228–9
  decalcification 1
  induced conformational changes 10, 228–9
  measurement 1
    equilibrium dialysis 99
    equilibrium gel filtration 5, 108
    flow-dialysis 155, 156
    protein kinase 46–8, 73–5
  pump 158
  regulator protein 34
  release 39, 167–8
  sensor 10, 34, 94, 97, 109–12, 114, 117–18, 120
  storage 85, 222, 228–9
  transport 211, 213, 215
  triggered synapses 113, 117
calcium vector protein 10, 61, 65, 80
calcyclin 132, 143–5, 161, 182, 205–6
calcyphosine 33–4
caldesmon 91, 93, 136, 144, 154
calerythrin 58, 60–1, 63–4, 77–9, 210
calgizzarin 132, 155–6
calgranulin 132, 147–8, 161
  calgranulin A 148
  calgranulin B 147
calmegin 215–18, 220–2
calmodulin 1, 2, 6–8, 10–12, 15–20, 22, 24, 30–44, 46–52, 54, 58, 60–1, 66–7, 73–7, 79–82, 84–5, 87–8, 91, 94, 98–9, 114, 116, 118–19, 126–8, 153, 156, 158, 165, 168, 172–6, 198, 209–15
  binding 8, 20, 30, 39, 44, 60–1, 66–7, 158, 172, 174–5, 210, 212–14